Basic Electrical Engineering

Basic Electrical Engineering

Pradip Kumar Sadhu PhD
Professor
Department of Electrical Engineering
Indian Institute of Technology (Indian School of Mines)
Dhanbad, India

Soumya Das PhD
Assistant Professor
Department of Electrical Engineering
University Institute of Technology
Burdwan University
West Bengal, India

Shiv Prakash Bihari ME
Associate Professor
Department of Electrical Engineering
Inderprastha Engineering College
Ghaziabad, Uttar Pradesh

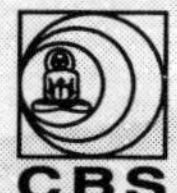

CBS Publishers & Distributors Pvt Ltd

New Delhi • Bengaluru • Chennai • Kochi • Kolkata • Mumbai
Bhopal • Bhubaneswar • Hyderabad • Jharkhand • Nagpur • Patna • Pune • Uttarakhand • Dhaka (Bangladesh)

Disclaimer

Science and technology are constantly changing fields. New research and experience broaden the scope of information and knowledge. The authors have tried their best in giving information available to them while preparing the material for this book. Although all efforts have been made to ensure optimum accuracy of the material, yet it is quite possible some errors might have been left uncorrected. The publisher, the printer and the authors will not be held responsible for any inadvertent errors or inaccuracies.

Basic Electrical Engineering

ISBN: 978-93-87964-31-0

First Edition: 2019

Published by Satish Kumar Jain and produced by Varun Jain for

CBS Publishers & Distributors Pvt Ltd

4819/XI Prahlad Street, 24 Ansari Road, Daryaganj, New Delhi 110 002, India.

Ph: 23289259, 23266861, 23266867 Fax: 011-23243014 Website: www.cbspd.com

e-mail: delhi@cbspd.com; cbspubs@airtelmail.in.

Corporate Office: 204 FIE, Industrial Area, Patparganj, Delhi 110 092

Ph: 4934 4934 Fax: 4934 4935 e-mail: publishing@cbspd.com; publicity@cbspd.com

Branches

- **Bengaluru:** Seema House 2975, 17th Cross, K.R. Road, Banasankari 2nd Stage, Bengaluru 560 070, Karnataka, India
  Ph: +91-80-26771678/79 Fax: +91-80-26771680 e-mail: bangalore@cbspd.com
- **Chennai:** 7, Subbaraya Street, Shenoy Nagar, Chennai 600 030, Tamil Nadu, India
  Ph: +91-44-26680620, 26681266 Fax: +91-44-42032115 e-mail: chennai@cbspd.com
- **Kochi:** 42/1325, 1326, Power House Road, Opposite KSEB Power House, Ernakulam 682 018, Kochi, Kerala, India
  Ph: +91-484-4059061-65 Fax: +91-484-4059065 e-mail: kochi@cbspd.com
- **Kolkata:** 6/B, Ground Floor, Rameswar Shaw Road, Kolkata 700 014, West Bengal, India
  Ph: +91-33-22891126, 22891127, 22891128 e-mail: kolkata@cbspd.com
- **Mumbai:** 83-C, Dr E Moses Road, Worli, Mumbai 400018, Maharashtra, India
  Ph: +91-22-24902340/41 Fax: +91-22-24902342 e-mail: mumbai@cbspd.com

Representatives

- **Bhopal** 0-8319310552 • **Bhubaneswar** 0-9911037372 • **Hyderabad** 0-9885175004 • **Jharkhand** 0-9811541605
- **Nagpur** 0-9421945513 • **Patna** 0-9334159340 • **Pune** 0-9623451994 • **Uttarakhand** 0-9716462459
- **Dhaka (Bangladesh)** 01912-003485

Printed at Glorious Printers, Daryaganj, Delhi, India

Preface

Basic Electrical Engineering has been designed as a textbook for electrical engineering as well as students pursuing their studies in civil, mechanical, mining, textile, chemical, industrial, environmental, aerospace, electronics and communication, computer science, information technology in BE/BTech, AMIE, diploma as well as for those preparing for other competitive examinations in India and overseas. It is equally helpful for aspiring engineers to understand the basic theoretical aspects. The book is easy to comprehend and inspiring in its direct approach.

The book provides an extensive range of topics under elementary concept of electrical engineering. It comprises fourteen chapters namely: Fundamentals of electrical engineering; electrical circuit analysis; AC fundamentals; steady state analysis of single phase AC circuits; DC network theorems; AC network theorems; three phase AC circuit; transients; measuring instruments; magnetic circuits; single phase transformer; DC machines; induction motors; three phase synchronous machines. Each chapter is fortified with elaborate illustrations, examples, solved university problems, problems for practice, short answer questions and multiple choice questions.

The presentation of the subject matter is very systematic and the language of the text is lucid and direct. We lay no claim to the original research in preparing the book. Liberal use of the materials available in the works of renowned authors has been made.

We welcome constructive criticism of the book and will be grateful for any appraisal by the readers.

Pradip Kumar Sadhu
Soumya Das
Shiv Prakash Bihari

Acknowledgements

We feel fortunate to receive many useful comments and suggestions from students, which have helped in improving the technical content and clarity of the book. We are grateful to them.

We are indebted to many readers in the academia and industry worldwide, for their valuable feedback and taking the trouble to draw our attention to the improvements required in the proposed manuscript.

We also thank the reviewers who took time from their busy schedules to send us suggestions.

Most importantly, we are extremely thankful and greatful to Mr Sathish Kumar Jain, (CMD) and Mr YN Arjuna (Senior Vice President Publishing, Editorial and Publicity), CBS Publishers & Distributors, New Delhi, for making this whole project a reality. We are grateful to the authorities of Indian Institute of Technology (Indian School of Mines), Dhanbad; University Institute of Technology, Burdwan University and Inderprastha Engineering College, Ghaziabad, for providing all the facilities while writing this book.

Finally, we are greatful to our families for their love, tolerance, patience and support throughout this very time consuming project. Readers of the book are welcome to send their comments and feedback.

Pradip Kumar Sadhu
Soumya Das
Shiv Prakash Bihari

Contents

Chapter

1

Fundamentals of Electrical Engineering Circuit Theory Concepts

1.1 INTRODUCTION

Electricity is modern society's most convenient, useful and popular form of energy. It has got numerous applications such as lighting, heating, cooling, transportation, entertainment and so on. Modern society is totally dependent on electricity and we cannot even think of life without it. In short, electricity has now become the universal medium of transmission and utilization of energy.

The subject of electrical engineering forms a basic course for AMIE, engineering graduates as it provides a foundation for all branches of engineering. In one way or the other, electricity, in turn, laws of electricity provides a base for all branches of engineering be it computer engineering or mechanical engineering, etc.

The beauty of electrical engineering lies in the fact that it is based on experimentally established laws only. To be precise, electrical engineering can be explained in terms of electric charge, voltage, and resistance and two fundamental laws–Ampere's law and Faraday's law of induction which govern electromechanical energy conversion. In this chapter, we shall discuss these five fundamentals which form the basics of this complete book. The reader has already some knowledge of these basic taught to him in physics in the chapter on electricity. Here, mathematical derivations and problems are deliberately avoided and only the application and physical significance part is explained in detail.

1.1.1 Electric Charge and Electric Current

All matters are made up of particles of electricity, viz. protons (positive charge) and electrons (negative charge). Whether a given body will exhibit electricity (i.e. charge) or not will depend upon the number of these charges.

When we are talking about electricity, the simplest pheomenon to prove its existence is the electricity produced when two bodies are rubbed with each other (e.g. silk cloth and glass rod). This is an example of frictional electricity. When a glass rod is rubbed with silk, the glass rod becomes positively charged while the silk becomes negatively charged. During the charge by friction, the body which loses electrons becomes positively charged while the other body which gains the electrons becomes negatively charged. The positive and negative charges which are produced simultaneously are equal in magnitude. It should be remembered that a neutral body has as many protons as electrons.

Now, think of a battery. It is also capable of producing electricity in a continuously flowing state in a wire. Initially, it was called current electricity to distinguish it from the frictional electricity. It has now been well established that the two are of the same kind. However, the difference is that static charges (charges at rest) produces only electric field while moving charges produce both electric and magnetic fields. The physical significance of moving charge is that energy is being transferred from one point to another. In other words, we can say that by controlling the rate, at which charge is put into motion, makes it possible to transmit information such as in communication devices.

Notes

1. When the number of protons is equal to the number ot electrons in a body, the resultant charge is zero. The body is electrically *neutral.*
2. When some electrons are removed from the body, there is deficiency of electrons in the body. The body attains a *positive charge.*
3. When a neutral body is supplied with electrons, there are excess electrons in it. The body attains a *negative charge.*

Electric current is defined as the time rate of change of charge passing through a specified area with respect to time.

$$i = \frac{dq}{dt}$$

where i is the instantaneous electric current, q is the net charge (may be positive or negative). Unit of charge is coulomb (C) and is defined as the charge transferred by a current of one ampere in one second. The SI unit of current is ampere. One ampere represents the passage of one coulomb of charge per second.

1.1.2 Direction of Current

We assume positive direction of current to be the direction in which the positive charge is moving (i.e. opposite to the direction of electron flow). A reference direction is usually assigned to the current by means of an arrow marked on the current path as shown in Fig. 1.1a. Here it is emphasized that the reference arrow does not show the direction of actual current flow. It is an indication of the direction with respect to other currents specified in a circuit. For the direction of current shown in Fig. 1.1a will prevail if the value of I comes out to be –2A, it signifies that current is flowing in the opposite direction of the assumed direction, i.e. current of 2A is flowing from B to A.

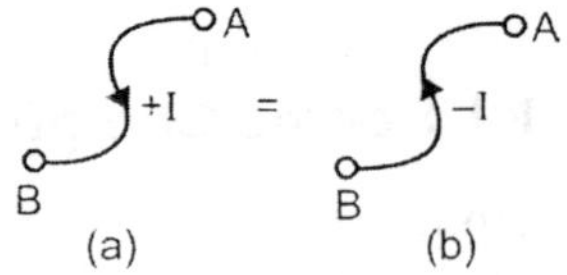

The two currents $+I$ and $-I$ in Figs 1.1a and 1.1b are equal. It is basically two methods of representing the same current. There are two types of electric current:

A
+I
=
B
(a)
A
–I
B
(b)

Fig. 1.1: Direction of current flow

i. ***Direct current* (*DC*):** If the polarity and direction of the potential difference never changes, i.e. the current always flows in one direction (unidirectional). It is called *direct current.* Unless otherwise specified, it is assumed to have a constant value with time as shown in Fig. 1.2a. As evident from the figure, the output of such sources (voltage or current) with respect to time is a straight line parallel to time axis.
ii. ***Alternating current*** **(*AC*):** If the electric current first flows in one direction and then reverses and flows in the other, such type of current is called *alternating current.* In more restricted sense, alternating current is a periodically varying

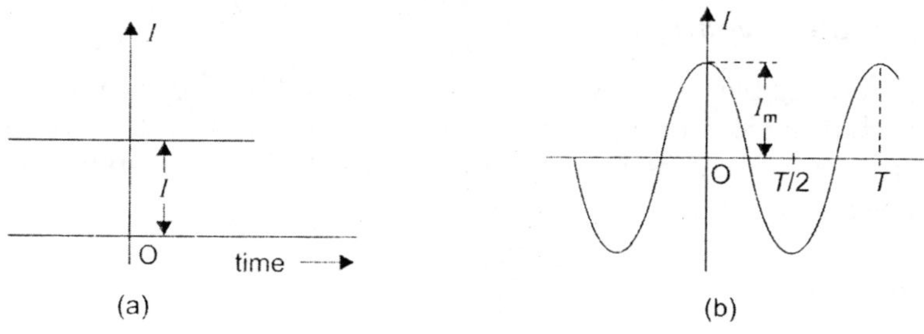

Fig. 1.2: (a) Direct current (b) Alternating current

current, the average value of which, over a period, is zero. Such a type of current is shown in Fig. 1.2b. The current wave shape shown in Fig. 1.2b is sinusoidal which is a common occurrence in electrical and electronic circuits. The power of a sinusoidal curve lies in the fact that its derivative and integral are also sinusoids of the same frequency.

1.1.3 Coulomb's Law

The force of attraction or repulsion (F) between two point charges q_1 and q_2 at a distance r is directly proportional to the product of the magnitude of the two charges and inversely proportional to the square of the distance between them. The force between the two charges always acts along a straight line joining the point charges. Thus

$$F \propto q_1 q_2 \text{ and } F \propto 1/r_2 \text{ or } F \propto q_1 q_2/r^2$$

$$\therefore \quad F = \frac{1}{4\pi\varepsilon_0} \times \frac{q_1 q_2}{r_2} \quad \text{(in vaccum)}$$

or

$$F = 9 \times 10^9 \times \frac{q_1 q_2}{r_2} \text{ N}$$

where q_1 and q_2 are in coulomb, r in metre; and $\varepsilon_0 = 8.854 \times 10^{-12}$ F/m is called the *permittivity of free space.*

$$\left[\frac{1}{4\pi\varepsilon_0} = 9 \times 10^9 \text{ Nm}^2/\text{C}^2\right]$$

For any other medium

$$F = \frac{1}{4\pi\varepsilon_0 K} \times \frac{q_1 q_2}{r^2}$$

where K is called the dielectric constant of the medium.

$$F = 9 \times 10^9 \times \frac{1}{K} \times \frac{q_1 q_2}{r^2} \text{ N}$$

The dielectric constant (K) or relative permittivity (ε_r) of the medium is given by

$$K = \frac{F_a}{F_m}$$

where F_a = Force between the two charges in air and F_m = Force between the same two chages in any other medium.

1.2 ELECTROMOTIVE FORCE AND POTENTIAL DIFFERENCE

The ability of the source to push charges to an external circuit is called *electromotive force* (emf). When a source of potential difference is in open circuit, i.e. no current is drawn from it, then the absolute potential difference between the two terminals of the source is called as electromotive force or emf of the source.

Potential Difference or Voltage

The potential difference between two points is measured by the amount of work done to transfer unit charge from one point to the other, or when a unit charge ($q = 1$) is passed between two points, then the amount of work done is equal to the potential difference between two points.

Mathematically, pd or voltage (V) = $\dfrac{W(\text{J})}{q(\text{C})}$

Hence, we can say that one volt is the potential difference between two points when one joule of work is done to transfer one coulomb of charge from one point to another.

If two points of an external circuit have a potential difference V then a charge q is passing between the two circuit points does an amount of work qV as it moves from the higher to the lower potential point, i.e. it gives up energy. Conversely, when a unit charge moves from a point of lower potential to one of higher potential, it will receive energy. This is the physical significance of potential difference or voltage.

The direction of current is always from higher potential to lower potential showing that either positive charges are moving from higher potential to lower potential or negative charges are moving from lower potential to higher potential.

Electromotive force, potential difference and voltage drop are all measured in units of voltage, i.e. volt (V). One volt is the voltage between two points when one joule (1 J) of energy is required to transfer 1 coulomb (1 C) of charge from one point to the other.

Reference Polarity

Reference polarity for voltage across an element is provided by marking a + sign on one end and a – sign on the other. In Fig. 1.3 end A is marked positive + implying A is at higher potential than B which is marked by a – sign. When we move from A to B we experience a voltage drop. Similarly when we move from B to A we experience a voltage rise.

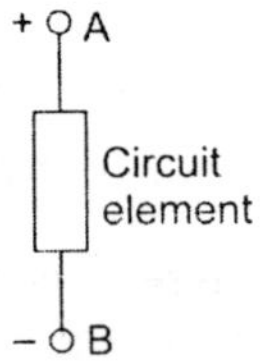

+ A

Circuit element

– B

Fig. 1.3: Polarity to voltage across an element

Difference between emf and Potential Difference

Emf is the energy imparted by the source to each coulomb of charge passing through it, whereas, potential difference between any two points in an electric circuit is the difference in their electrical state which causes the flow of electric current.

Electrical Power and Energy

The work done when a current i ampere flows for a time t second between two points having a potential difference V volt is

$$W = Vi\,t \text{ Joule (or W·s)} \tag{1.1}$$

Equation (1.1) gives the total energy absorbed or given out.

When t is one second, then $W = Vi =$ Power, thus work done in unit time is defined as *power*. It is measured in watt. However, the commercial unit of electrical energy is kilo-watt-hour or kWh. The energy consumed when a power of one kW is consumed or delivered in one hour is called kilowatt-hour. One kWh is often referred to as one unit of electrical energy.

1.3 OHM'S LAWS

The direct proportionality between the current in a metallic conductor and the potential difference between its terminals was first of all discovered by scientist Simon Ohm and is known as Ohm's law.

According to Ohm's law, if the physical conditions such as temperature remains constant, the current between two points in a conductor is proportional to the potential difference between these two points, i.e.

$$i \propto V \text{ or } V/i = R$$

where the constant of proportionality R is known as resistance of the conductor.

In SI units R is in ohm if i is in ampere and V is in volt. One ohm is the resistance of a conductor in which a current of one ampere exists when the potential difference between its ends is one volt.

Notes

1. The resistance of a conductor is the property which depends on its dimensions, material and temperature determines the current produced in it by a given potential difference across its ends.
2. The conductors which obey Ohm's law are called ohmic conductors. For ohmic conductors (metals and alloys), the graph between current and potential difference is a straight line passing through the origin.
3. For devices exhibiting a nonlinear V-I characteristics (e.g. incandescent lamp) Ohm's law is expressed in differential form, i.e.
$$dv = Rdi$$
where R is the slope of the nonlinear curve corresponding to a given point on the curve. If this point is changed, the value of resistance as applied to that point also changes.
4. Ohm's law can be expressed in three different ways, viz.
$$i = \frac{V}{R}, V = Ri \text{ and } R = \frac{V}{i}$$
Other relation derived from Ohm's law is
$$\text{Power } (W) = VI = \frac{V^2}{R} = I^2 R$$
5. **Limitations of Ohm's law:** Ohm's law is not applicable to nonlinear unilateral devices such as diode value, junction diodes, etc. as they exhibit discontinuity and different characteristics in either direction.
6. **Concept of open and short circuits:** By open circuit or simply open, we mean that current is zero regardless of the voltage. Figure 1.4a shows the representation of an open circuit implying that resistance is *infinite* between the two points A and B. From Ohm's law $R = V/I \because I = 0, R = \infty$.
By short circuit or simply short, we mean that voltage between the two points is zero regardless of the current through it. Fig. 1.4b shows the representation of a short circuit implying that resistance is zero between the two points A and B from Ohm's law $R = V/I \because V = 0, R = 0$.

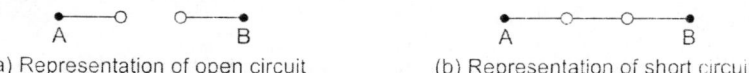

(a) Representation of open circuit (b) Representation of short circuit

Fig. 1.4: Representation of open and short circuits

1.4 BASIC PARAMETERS OF CIRCUIT (R–L–C)

Before discussing the three basic parameters of electric circuit theory, let us study some definitions of the terms which are used extensively in electrical engineering:

1. **Circuit:** An electric circuit is a closed path, composed of active and passive elements to which current flow is confined. Broadly speaking a circuit consists of a *source* of energy, a load which utilises the energy and two conductors connecting the source and the load to transfer the energy.
2. **Circuit parameters:** A parameter is a constant, the value of which characterizes the relationship between two variables. Hence, the various elements of an electric circuit are called its parameters like resistance, inductance and capacitance.
3. **Electric network:** A combination of various electric elements connected in any manner whatsoever is called an electric network.
4. **Excitation:** The input to a network is referred to as excitation, i.e. it represents energy supplied to the network from an external source.
5. **Response:** The output of a network is called response, i.e. it represents utilization of energy supplied by excitation. For electrical networks, the excitation and response functions are in terms of voltage and current, both being functions of time.
6. **Active elements:** Any source of energy (a voltage source or a current source) is said to be an active element. A battery or a generator is an example of a voltage source while an amplifier tube is an example of a current source.
7. **Passive elements:** An element which is not an energy source is a passive element. A passive element transforms or stores energy. Resistors, inductors and capacitor are examples of passive elements.
8. **Bilateral and unilateral elements:** Bilateral elements are those which transmit equally well in either direction. On the other hand, unilateral elements transmit equally in the two directions, for they have different laws relating to voltage and current for different directions of flow of current.
   Example of bilateral elements — High conductivity metals
   Example of unilateral elements — Vacuum tubes, metal rectifiers
9. **Linear and nonlinear elements:** There are elements where response is directly proportional to the excitation; for example, if the input is doubled, the output gets doubled. Such elements are called linear elements. Mathematically, an element which is governed by a linear differential equation for all values of applied input and expected output, is called linear element. If the element does not satisfy this condition, it is called as nonlinear element.
10. **Lumped and distributed elements:** Physically separate elements such as resistors, inductors and capacitors are known as lumped elements. Distributed elements on the other hand are those elements which are not separated for analytical purposes. An example of a circuit with distributed elements is a transmission line which has distributed resistance, inductance and capacitance along its entire length.
    There are three ideal circuit elements, viz. resistance, inductance and capacitance. By an ideal element we mean that their voltage and current are linearly related. Now we shall discuss the three elements one by one and observe that these elements are linear, bilateral, time invariant and lumped.

1.4.1 Resistance

Resistance is the property of a material by virtue of which it tends to oppose the flow of current through it. In opposing the flow of electric current energy loss takes place in the form of heat. Therefore, the resistance is a dissipative element which converts electric energy into heat, when the current flows through it in any direction. Figure 1.5 shows the schematic representation of resistance. As evident from Fig. 1.5, the element has two terminals A and B which are also called nodes. Current flows from a point of higher potential (node A) to another point of lower potential (node B). In the process voltage drop occurs across the element in the direction of current flow (i). The terminal at which the current enters, acquires a positive polarity with respect to the terminal at which the current exits. A practical element that possesses the property of resistance is called a resistor.

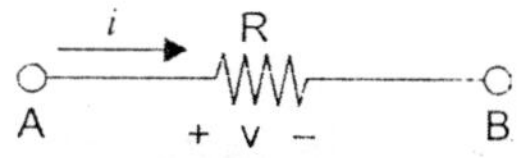

Fig. 1.5

Resistance comes into picture both in AC as well as DC circuits but the opposition offered by a resistor to the flow of AC is slightly more than that of DC (due to skin effect).

Mathematically, $$R = \rho \frac{l}{A}$$

where ρ is specific resistance. l and A are length and area respectively.

If $A = 1$, $l = 1$ then $R = \rho$,

i.e. specific resistance of the material of a conductor is defined as the resistance of the conductor of unit length and unit area of cross-section. Its unit is ohm-metre.

Electrical conductivity of a material is defined as the reciprocal of the resistivity, i.e.

electrical conductivity $\sigma = \frac{1}{\text{resistivity}}$; $\sigma = l/RA$ and its unit is (ohm-metre)$^{-1}$ or mho/metre.

Resistances in Series

Figure 1.6 shows three resistances R_1, R_2 and R_3 connected in series.

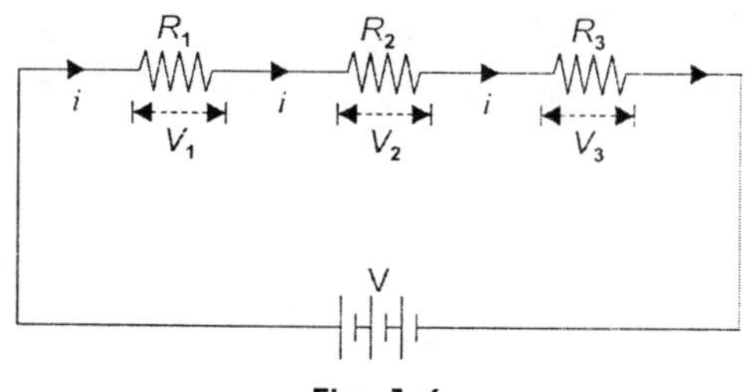

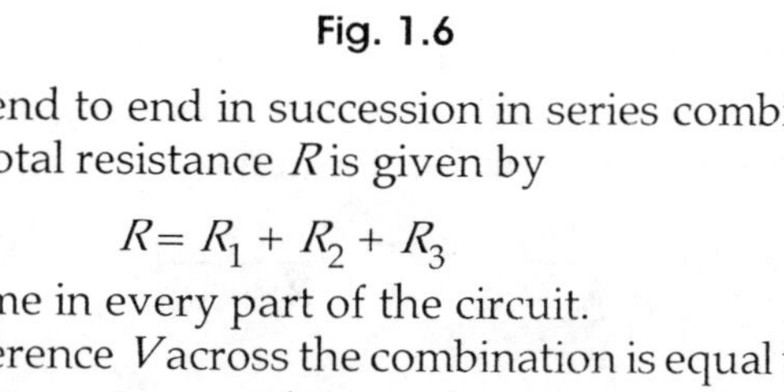

Fig. 1.6

They are connected end to end in succession in series combination.

i. The effective or total resistance R is given by

$$R = R_1 + R_2 + R_3$$

ii. The current is same in every part of the circuit.

iii. The potential difference V across the combination is equal to the sum of individual potential difference across a resistance, i.e.

$$V = V_1 + V_2 + V_3$$

or $$V_1 : V_2 : V_3 :: R_1 : R_2 : R_3$$

iv. If we want to determine V_1, V_2 and V_3 in terms of the total voltage V, then we can use the voltage-divider equations.

Current in the circuit, $i = \dfrac{V}{R_1 + R_2 + R_3} = \dfrac{V}{R}$

and $V_1 = R_1 i$

or $V_1 = R_1 \dfrac{V}{R}$

Similarly $V_2 = \dfrac{R_2}{R} V$ and $V_3 = \dfrac{R_3}{R} V$

Resistances in Parallel

Figure 1.7 shows three resistances R_1, R_2 and R_3 connected in parallel. Here one end of each of them is connected at one point and the other end of each of them is connected to other point.

In parallel combination:

i. The equivalent resistance R is given by

$$\frac{1}{R} = \frac{1}{R_1} + \frac{1}{R_2} + \frac{1}{R_3}$$

ii. The current is different in different resistances. The sum of the currents in different resistances is equal to the main current of the circuit, i.e.

$$i = i_1 + i_2 + i_3$$

iii. The potential difference across each resistance is the same.

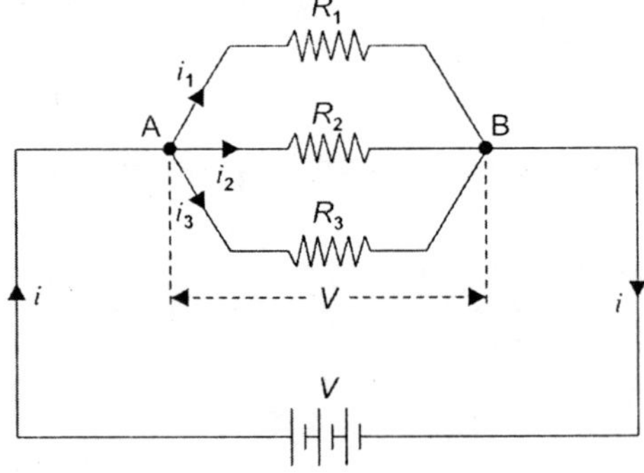

Fig. 1.7

iv. Consider the circuit shown in Fig. 1.8. Here R_1 and R_2 are two resistances connected in parallel having currents i_1 and i_2 flowing in them. The total current in the two branches is i. Then, current i_1 in the resistance R_1 is given as

$$i_1 = \frac{R_2}{R_1 + R_2} i \; ; \; i_2 = \frac{R_1}{R_1 + R_2} i ,$$

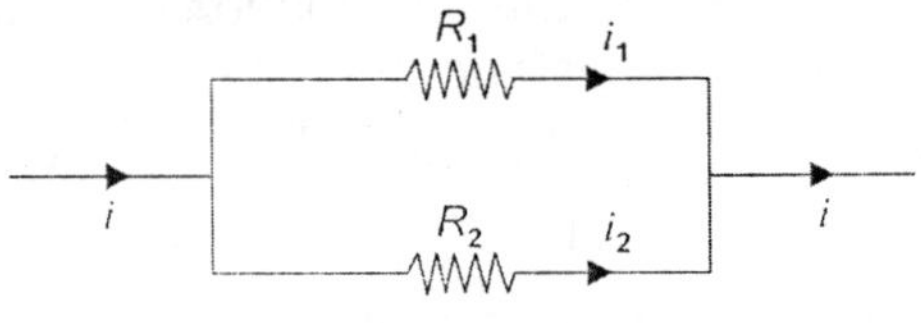

Fig. 1.8

i.e. currents are shared in the inverse ratio of the resistances. These equations are called *current-divider equations*. They show how the total current is divided in separate branches of parallel combination of resistors.

Concept of Resistance as a Circuit Parameter

Resistance is a proportionality factor in Ohm's law relating current to potential difference. By opposing the flow of electrons it converts electrical energy into heat energy.

$$V = R_i$$

Power loss or power absorbed by resistor $P = I_2 R$.

The corresponding amount of energy converted to heat in time interval $(t_2 - t_1)$ is

$$W = \int_{t_1}^{t_2} I^2 R\,dt \text{ J}$$

when I is a constant quantity

$$W = I^2 R\,t \text{ J}$$

where $t = t_2 - t_1$ second

Resistance is thus the electrical system characteristic which manifests itself in the expenditure of energy (in the form of heat) and is sometimes called 'sink' or energy dissipative element.

Effect of Temperature on Resistance

1. To increase the resistance of pure metals or we can say that metals have a positive temperature coefficient of resistance.
2. To increase the resistance of alloys. This increase is small and irregular.
3. To decrease the resistance of insulators and electrolytes or in other words they have a negative temperature coefficient of resistance.
   Mathematically, $R_t = R_0(1 + \alpha t)$ and $R_2 = R_1[1 + \alpha_1(t_2 - t_1)]$
   where R_t is resistance at temperatue t, R_0 is resistance at 0°C, R_2 and R_1 is are resistances at temperature t_2 and t_1 respectively and α is temperature coefficient of resistance. α is defined as the fractional increase in the resistance of the conductor per unit increase in its temperature.

1.4.2 Inductance

Inductance is that property of a circuit element by which energy is stored in a magnetic flux field. Inductance comes into picture only when there is time rate of change:

Mathematically, $$V_L = L\frac{di}{dt}$$

where V_L is the voltage across inductor.

Inductance is represented as shown in Fig. 1.9. Whenever a coil carries a current, a magnetic field (space flux) is created. If the current changes, the magnetic flux linked with the coil also changes. This change in flux induces an emf in the coil. This emf is known as statically induced emf because it is induced due to its own current. The direction of this emf is so as to oppose the change in current. That is, if the current increases, this self induced emf opposes the current. However, if the current decreases this emf acts in the same direction as the current.

Self induced emf is given by

$$V_L \propto di/dt$$

or

$$V_L = L\,di/dt$$

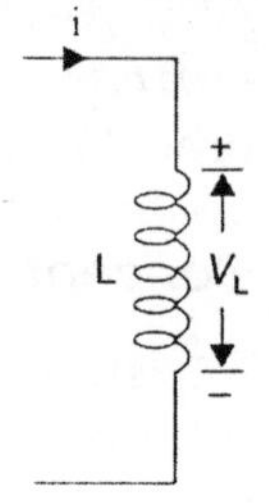

Fig. 1.9

where L is coefficient of self inductance or simply inductance. The SI unit of inductance is henry. A coil has an inductance of 1 H if a current changing at a rate 1.8 of 1 A/s causes an emf of 1 V to develop across it.

The inductance exists in AC circuits and DC transient circuits only. In AC circuits the current changes continuously and the effect of inductance can be observed. In case of DC transient circuits where emf is suddenly applied to or removed from a network-inductance as well as capacitance, also come into picture.

The important point to note is that inductance parameter stays constant for all values of current if current and flux remain proportional. Such inductances are known as linear inductances (Fig. 1.9). A practical inductance is called an inductor.

Inductances in Series

Figure 1.10 shows three inductances L_1, L_2 and L_3 connected in series. The current through all the inductances is *i*, and rate of change of current is *di*/*dt*.

i. The total inductance L is given by

$$L = L_1 + L_2 + L_3$$

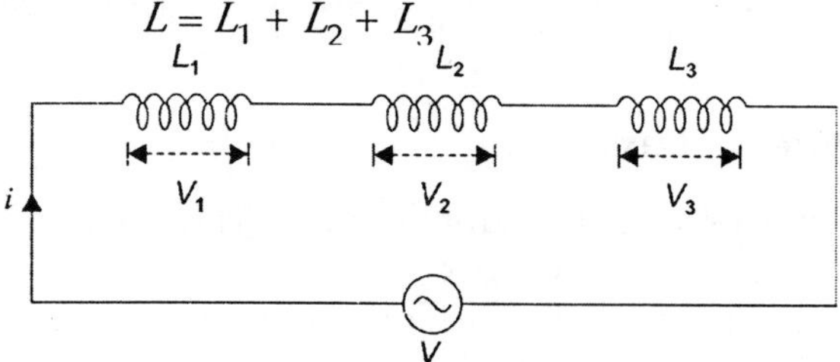

Fig. 1.10

ii. The total voltage across the series combination is the sum of voltages induced across the three inductances

$$V = V_1 + V_2 + V_3$$

$$= L_1 \frac{di}{dt} + L_2 \frac{di}{dt} + L_3 \frac{di}{dt}$$

Inductances in Parallel

Figure 1.11 shows three inductances L_1, L_2 and L_3 connected in parallel. The voltage induced across each inductance is V. It is also assumed that initially there is no current flowing in the circuit which is represented as $i(0) = 0$.

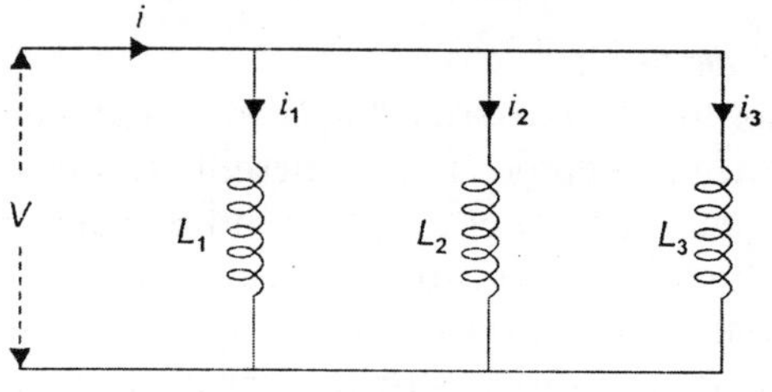

Fig. 1.11

i. The equivalent inductance L is given by

$$\frac{1}{L}=\frac{1}{L_1}+\frac{1}{L_2}+\frac{1}{L_3}$$

ii. The currents i_1, i_2 and i_3 are given by

$$i_1=\frac{1}{L_1}\int_0^t V\,dt,\; i_2=\frac{1}{L_2}\int_0^t V\,dt \text{ and } i_3=\frac{1}{L_3}\int_0^t V\,dt$$

iii. The total current i is given by

$$i=i_1+i_2+i_3=\left[\frac{1}{L_1}+\frac{1}{L_2}+\frac{1}{L_3}\right]\int_0^t V\,dt$$

Concept of Inductance as a Circuit Parameter

Inductance is the property of a circuit element which opposes the change of current. The current in an inductor cannot change abruptly in zero time since a finite change in current in zero time requires an infinite voltage to appear across the inductor. This is physically impossible.

If i is the current which is made to flow through a coil and V is the voltage across it and assuming zero initial current [$i(0) = 0$], the total energy received in the time interval from zero to t is given by

$$W=\int_0^t V i\,dt \text{ J}$$

Putting the value of $V = L\,di/dt$, we get

$$W=\int_0^t\left(L\frac{di}{dt}\right)i\,dt=\int_0^t L i\,di \text{ or } =\frac{1}{2}Li^2$$

This parameter can also be defined in terms of amount of energy stored in its magnetic field corresponding to its instantaneous current.

$$L=\frac{2W}{i^2}\text{ H}$$

It can also be shown that like resistance, inductance is dependent upon the geometry of physical dimensions and the magnetic property of the medium. In the case of a linear inductor with iron core inductance is given by

$$L=\frac{N^2\mu A_m}{l}$$

where N is the number of turns of coil, μ is permeability of the iron core A_m is the cross-sectional area of the core, l is the length of the iron-core.

Self Inductance

Inductance is the property of a circuit element in which a voltage is induced by changing the current in its own circuit, the property is called the self-inductance or simply *inductance.*

In other words, the flux will link the solenoid and the amount of flux connected with each turn be ϕ. So total flux linked with the solenoid is $N\phi$ (where N is the number of turns). $N\phi$ is known as the flux linkage of the solenoid. This flux linkage is directly proportioned to the current.

So,
$$N\phi \propto i$$
$$N\phi = Li \quad \text{...(1.1)}$$

The proportionality constant L is called self-inductance.

Taking derivatives both side of Eq. (1.1), we get

$$N\frac{d\phi}{dt} = L\frac{di}{dt}$$

and we know $e = N\frac{d\phi}{dt}$, where e = self induced voltage.

$$\therefore \quad e = L\frac{di}{dt} \text{ V}$$

The proportionally constant L is called the self inductance. The unit of self-inductance is henry (H).

If $\quad \frac{di}{dt} = 1 \text{ A/s, and e} = 1 \text{ V}$

then $\quad L = 1 \text{ H}$

Thus, henry is defined as a circuit element having a self inductance of 1 H when a voltage of 1 V is induced in it by a current in the element changing at the rate of 1 A/s. The direction of induced voltage is given by Lenz's law. Hence, the induced voltage is given by

$$e = -L\frac{di}{dt}$$

The negative sign is used to satify Lenz's law, since when the rate of current is positive the induced voltage is negative. Thus, it acts in a negative the circuit to oppose the change in current.

1.4.3 Capacitance

Capacitance is that property of a circuit element by which energy is capable of being stored in an electric field. It exists only when there is a changing voltage across the terminals of the element. Hence, whereas resistance dissipates electrical energy, inductance and capacitance store the same. Inductance stores the energy in a magnetic flux field and the capacitance stores the energy in an electric field.

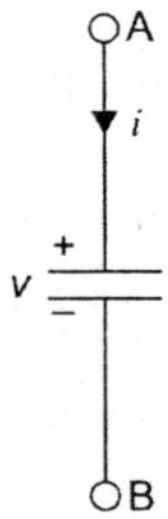

Fig. 1.12

Figure 1.12 shows the schematic representation of a capacitance. There is a voltage drop in the direction of current with the terminal (A) where the current flows in acquiring positive polarity with respect to the terminal (B) at which the current leaves the element. When a charge is given to an isolated conductor of any shape, its potential increases. The potential acquired by the isolated conductor is directly proportional to the charge given to it, i.e.

$$Q \propto V \text{or } Q = CV \text{or } C = Q/V$$

where C is the constant of proportionality and is known as capacity or capacitance of a conductor.

If $\quad V = 1$ then $C = Q$

Thus, the capacitance of a conductor is numerically equal to the quantity of charge required to raise the potential of that conductor by unity. The unit of capacitance is farad = coulomb/volt. A practical element possessing the property of capacitance is known as a *capacitor or condenser*. A condenser has a capacitance of one farad if the addition of one coulomb of charge to it raises its potential by one volt.

$$1\ \mu F = 10^{-6} \text{ farad}$$

and $$1 \text{ pF (pico farad)} = 10^{-12} \text{ farad}$$

An arrangement which is capable of changing the capacitance of a conductor is called condenser or capacitor. It consists of two plates placed close together and insulated from one another by air or some dielectric medium. In other words, a device or arrangement which can store considerable amount of charge is called a condenser or capacitor.

Capacitors in Series

When a number of capacitors having capacities C_1, C_2, C_3, etc. are connected in series, then the resultant capacitance C is given by

$$\frac{1}{C} = \frac{1}{C_1} + \frac{1}{C_2} + \frac{1}{C_3} + \ldots$$

Capacitors in Parallel

When a number of capacitors having capacities C_1, C_2, C_3 ... etc. are connected in parallel, then the resultant capacitance C is given by

$$C = C_1 + C_2 + C_3 + \ldots$$

Concept of Capacitance as a Circuit Parameter

We have already seen that

$$Q = CV$$

As $i = dQ/dt$, we may also write

$$i = C\frac{dV}{dt} \qquad \ldots(1.2)$$

From Eq. (1.2) it follows that capacitor is a circuit element which has the property of yielding a current directly proportional to the rate of change of voltage across its terminals. In case of two parallel plates separated by a distance d metre, the capacitance is equal to

$$C = \varepsilon\frac{A}{d}$$

where A is the area of plates in m^2, d is the distance of separation of plates, and E is the permittivity of the material (medium).

If the capacitor is given a charge q coulomb so that its potential is raised by V volt, then the energy W joule stored is given by

$$W = \frac{1}{2}qV = \frac{1}{2}CV^2 = \frac{1}{2}\frac{q^2}{C}$$

where C is in farad.

1.4.4 Capacitance in Series

In Fig. 1.13, three capacitors of capacitance C_1, C_2 and C_3 are connected in series across a DC supply of potential difference V through a switch K. On closing the switch, the capacitors got charges and at steady state the *pd* across C_1, C_2 and C_3 are V_1, V_2, V_3 respectively while the charge in each capacitor is Q (since, the capacitors are connected in series, same charging occurred would flow resulting in accumulation of charge Q in each capacitor.)

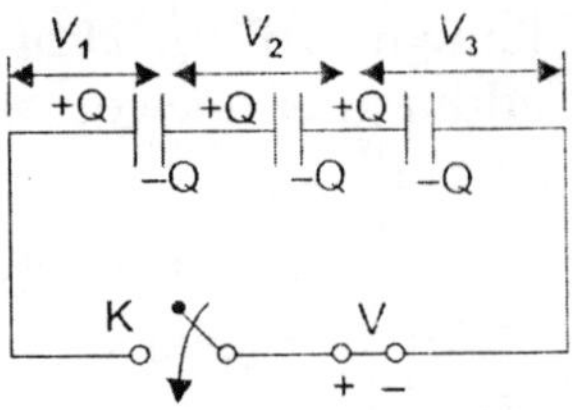

Fig. 1.13

$$V_1 = \frac{Q}{C_1},\ V_2 = \frac{Q}{C_2},\ V_3 = \frac{Q}{C_3}$$

$$V = V_1 + V_2 + V_3$$

$$\frac{Q}{C} = \frac{Q}{C_1} + \frac{Q}{C_2} + \frac{Q}{C_3} \text{ or } \frac{1}{C} = \frac{1}{C_1} + \frac{1}{C_2} + \frac{1}{C_3}$$

1.4.5 Capacitance in Parallel

On closing K, charge Q_1, Q_2, Q_3 would accumulate in capacitances C_1, C_2 and C_3 during steady state while the voltage will remain V across each capacitors in the parallel combination (Fig. 1.14a).

$$Q = Q_1 + Q_2 + Q_3$$

Where Q is the total charge obtained from the source.

$$CV = C_1V + C_2V + C_3V$$

$$C = C_1 + C_2 + C_3$$

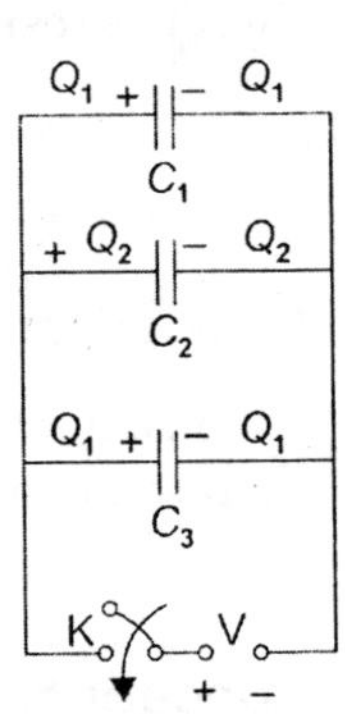

Fig. 1.14a

1.4.6 Capacitance of a Parallel Plate Capacitor

Let us consider two identical plates A and B are kept in close shown in Fig. 1.14. proximity and parallel to each other which are separated by dielectric medium of thickness (x) and relative permittivity (ε) (Fig. 1.14b).

Let us connect the parallel plates with a potential difference (V) volts and we assume Q coulombs of charge is accumulated by the parallel plate combination acting on a parallel plate capacitor. The electric flux is ψ is due to Q coulombs and the area of each plate is considered to be A square meters.

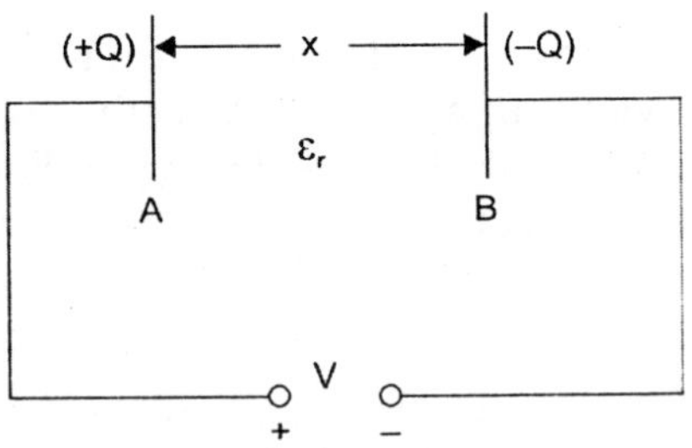

Fig. 1.14b

Since the charge Q is distributed uniformly over each plate, the electric field between the plates is nearly uniform. Let δ represent the electric flux density while E the intensity (or the potential gradient) and C the capacitance in farad for this parallel plate capacitor.

Here $$\delta = \frac{\psi}{A} = \frac{Q}{A} \text{ coulomb/square meter}$$

$$E = \frac{V}{x};\ V \text{ being the potential}$$

Total number of electric field lines is called *electric flux*. One coulomb of flux is defined as the flux originating at a positive charge of one coulomb and terminating at a negative charge of one coulomb.

$$\frac{\delta}{E} = \in$$

or $$\frac{Q/A}{V/x} = \in = \in_0 \in_r$$

or $$\frac{Q}{V} = C = \frac{\in_0 \in_r A}{x}$$

If the dielectric medium of the capacitance $\in_r$ is in vacuum, $\in_r = 1$ and hence

$$C = \frac{\in_0 A}{x}$$

$\in$ is the absolute permitivity, $\in_0$ is the permittivity of free space (8.854×10^{-12} F/m) and $\in_r$ is the relative permitivity of a dielectric medium.

1.4.7 Capacitance of Concentric Spheres

A pair of concentric sphere S_1 and S_2 of radius r_1 and r_2 metre, separated by a dielectric medium of permittivity $\in_r$ forms a spherical capacitance. We will consider two cases of this spherical capacitor.

Case A: S_2 (the outer sphere) is earthed: Let the inner sphere S_1 be charged by $+Q$ coulomb of charge. It will induce $-Q$ coulomb charge at the inner surface of S_2 and $+Q$ coulomb charge at the outer surface of S_2. But as the outer surface of S_2 is earthed, this charge at the outer surface of S_2 will escape (e_1) to the earth, shown in Fig. 1.15.

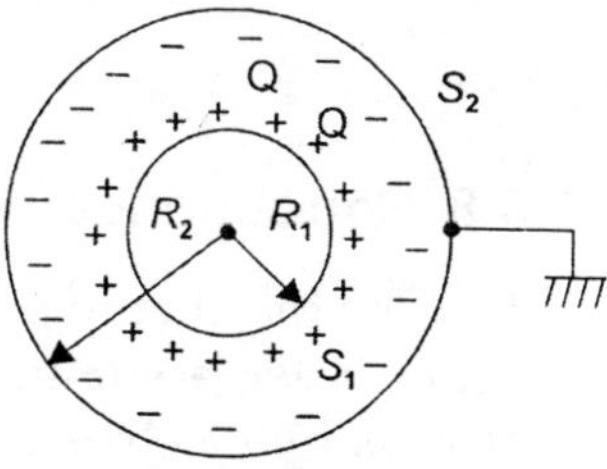

Fig. 1.15

Surface potential of S_1 is

$$V_{S_1} = \frac{+Q}{4\pi \in_0 \in_r R_1}$$

Surface potential of S_2 is

$$V_{S_2} = \frac{-Q}{4\pi \in_0 \in_r R_2}$$

Potential difference between S_1 and S_2 is

$$V = \frac{Q}{4\pi \in_0 \in_r}\left[\frac{1}{R_1} - \frac{1}{R_2}\right] = \frac{Q}{4\pi \in_0 \in_r} \times \frac{R_2 - R_1}{R_2 R_1}$$

$$\therefore \quad C = \frac{Q}{V} = \frac{Q}{\dfrac{Q}{4\pi \in_0 \in_r} \times \dfrac{R_2 - R_1}{R_2 R_1}} = \frac{4\pi \in_0 \in_r}{\left(\dfrac{R_2 - R_1}{R_2 R_1}\right)} \text{ farad}$$

Case B: S_i (the inner sphere) is earthed: This time the outer sphere S_2 is given a charge of $+Q$ coulomb. This charge is uniformly distributed in the outer and inner surface of S_2. We assume $+Q_2$ charge remain at the outer surface while $+Q_1$ at the inner surface of S_2 in Fig. 1.16.

The charge $+Q_1$ at the inner surface of S_2 would induce a charge of coulomb on the outer surface of S_1. $+Q_2$ charge induced in the inner surface of S_1 would pass to the earth as the inner surface of S_1 is earth.

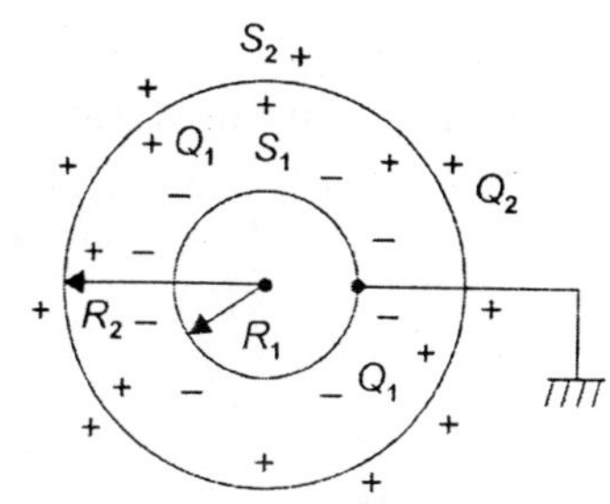

Fig. 1.16

The system is now composed of two subsystems of capacitors as described below:

i. Capacitor formed by inner surface of S_2 and outer surface of S_1 and is similar to the case we described in case A.
Its capacitance

$$C_1 = 4\pi \in_0 \in_r \left[\frac{1}{R_2} - \frac{1}{R_1}\right]^{-1} = \frac{4\pi \in_0 \in_r}{\left(\frac{R_1 - R_2}{R_2 R_1}\right)} \text{ farad.}$$

ii. Capacitor formed by the outer surface of outer sphere S_2 and earth with air as dielectric.

∴ Its capacitance $C_2 = 4\pi \in_0 \in_r R_2$
Since these two subsystems of capacitors are electrically parallel, we can find the total capacitance

$$C = C_1 + C_2$$

$$= 4\pi \in_0 \in_r \left[\frac{R_1 - R_2}{R_1 R_2}\right]^{-1} + 4\pi \in_0 \in_r R_2$$

$$= 4\pi \in_0 \in_r \left[\left(\frac{R_1 - R_2}{R_1 R_2}\right)^{-1} + R_2\right]$$

1.4.8 Capacitance of Two Coaxial Cylinders

Let $+Q$ be the charge per metre length at inside surface of the outer cylinder (assuming the outer surface of the outer cylinder earthed), by electrostatic induction, $-Q$ charge per meter is induced at the outer surface of inner cylinder.

Let us assume another imaginary coaxial cylinder having radius x and length one metre between the two given cylinders. Let $\in_r$ be the permitivity of medium in between the two cylinders of radius R_1 and R_2 as shown in Fig. 1.17.

Electric flux density δ on the surface of the imaginary cylinder is given by

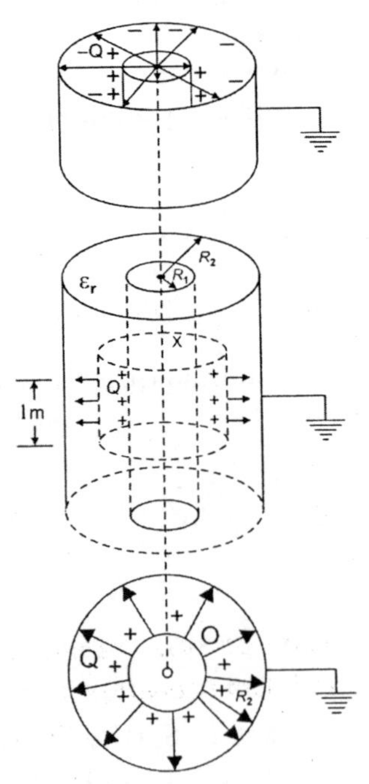

Fig. 1.17

$$\alpha = \frac{\psi}{A} = \frac{Q}{A} = \frac{Q}{2\pi x \times 1} \text{c/m}^2$$

[∵ curved surface area of a cylinder is $2\pi rL$ and here $r = x$, $L = 1$ ml]

∴ Electric field intensity is obtained as

$$E = \frac{\delta}{\varepsilon_0 \varepsilon_r} \text{V/m} = \frac{Q}{2\pi \in_0 \in_r x} \text{V/m}$$

Hence, we can write

$$\int_0^V dV = \int_{R_1}^{R_2} E\,dx$$

$$V = \int_{R_1}^{R_2} \frac{Q}{2\pi \in_0 \in_r^x} dx = \frac{Q}{2\pi \in_0 \in_r^x} \int_{R_1}^{R_2} \frac{1}{x} dx$$

$$= \frac{Q}{2\pi \in_0 \in_r} \left|\ln x\right|_{R_1}^{R_2} = \frac{Q}{2\pi \in_0 \in_r} en(Q_2 / Q_1)$$

Since capacitance $C = Q/V$ we have,

$$C = \frac{Q}{(Q/2\pi \epsilon_0 \epsilon_r)\pi(R_2/R_1)} = \frac{2\pi \epsilon_0 \epsilon_r}{\pi(R_2/R_1)} \text{F/m}$$

1.5 ELECTROMAGNETIC INDUCTION

Faraday in 1831, discovered that whenever magnetic flux associated with a coil changes, an emf is induced in it. If the circuit is closed, a current flows through it as long as the magnetic flux is changing. The current is called as *induced current.* The emf produced in the coil is called as *induced emf.* This phenomenon is called as *electromagnetic induction.* To show the phenomenon of electromagnetic induction, we describe the following two experiment:

Experiment 1: Figure 1.18 shows a copper coil whose ends are connected to a sensitive galvanometer. When the north pole of a powerful bar magnet is quickly pushed towards the coil, the galvanometer shows deflection while magnet is moving.

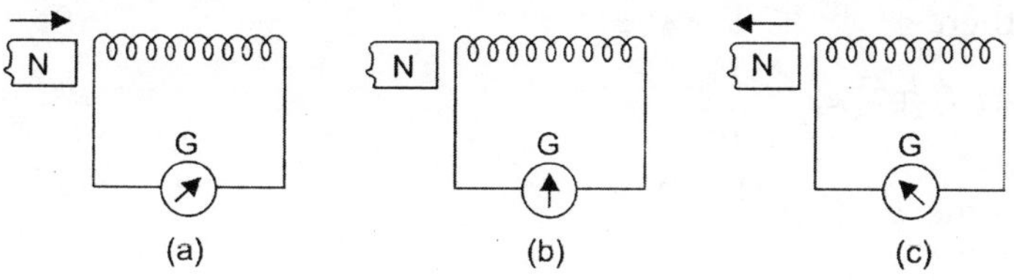

Fig. 1.18

If the magnet is held stationary (Fig. 1.18b), the galvanometer does not show any deflection. Again if the magnet is taken away from the coil (Fig. 1.18c) the galvanometer again shows deflection but in the opposite direction. Similarly, if the experiment is repeated by bringing the south pole of the magnet towards coil, the experiment works in the same way but the deflections are reversed.

Experiment 2: Figure 1.19 shows the experimental arrangement in which the primary coil is connected to battery and a key, while secondary is connected to a galvanometer. When a current is set up in the primary by closing K, the galvanometer shows a momentary deflection. A current is set up in secondary in opposite direction. When the key is opened, again there is momentary deflection in the galvanometer in the same direction of the current. So when the current is changing (increasing or decreasing) in the primary, an induced emf is developed in secondary.

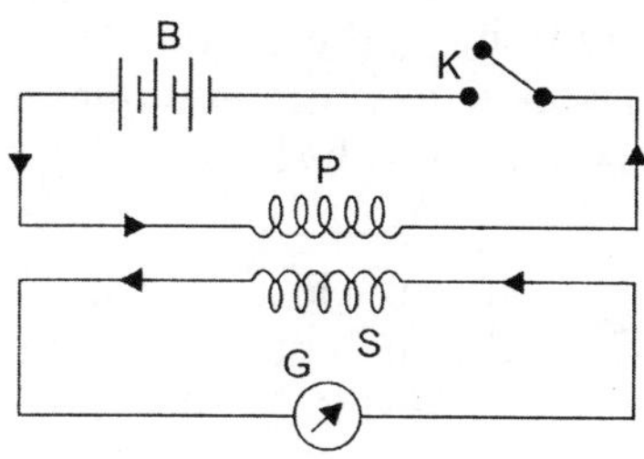

Fig. 1.19

1.6 LAWS OF ELECTROMAGNETIC INDUCTION

There are two laws governing the phenomenon of electromagnetic induction, known as Faraday's laws. These two laws are stated below.

i. Whenever there is a change in the magnetic flux linkage in a circuit an emf is induced in it.

ii. The magnitude of the induced emf is directly proportional to the rate of change of flux linkage.

If a flux of ϕ weber (Wb) links with a coil of N turns, the induced emf in the coil is given by

$$e \propto \frac{d(\phi N)}{dt} = k\frac{d(\phi N)}{dt}$$

In SI the proportionality constant $k = 1$ and

$$e = N\frac{d\phi}{dt} \quad ...(1.3)$$

Lenz's law: Faraday's law, that gives the magnitude of induced emf. The polarity of the induced emf is determined by Lenz's law. It states that the polarity of the induced emf is such as to opposes the change which produces it.

Remembering Lenz's law, Faraday's law is written as

$$e = -N\frac{d\phi}{dt} \quad ...(1.4)$$

If ϕ_1 be the magnitude of the flux linked with a circuit initially and ϕ_2 be the flux after t second, then

rate of change of flux = $\frac{\phi_1 - \phi_2}{t}$

The induced emf, $e = -N\frac{\phi_1 - \phi_2}{t}$

1.7 KIRCHHOFF'S LAWS

Ohm's law is unable to give current in complicated circuits. Kirchhoff in 1842, gave two general laws which are extremely useful in electrical circuits. These are:

i. The algebraic sum of the currents at any junction in a circuit is zero, i.e.

$$\Sigma i = 0$$

This means that there is no accumulation of electric charge at any point in the circuit. The currents which flow towards a point are taken as positive while those flowing away from the point are taken as negative. From Fig. 1.20, we have

$$i_1 - i_2 - i_3 + i_4 - i_5 + i_6 = 0$$

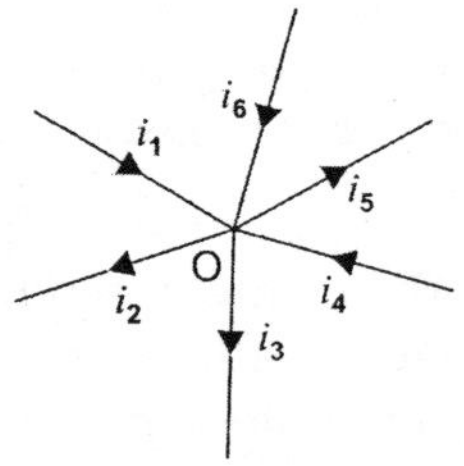

Fig. 1.20

ii. In any closed circuit, the algebraic sum of the products of the current and resistance of each part of the circuit is equal to the total emf in the circuit, i.e.

$$\Sigma iR = \Sigma E$$

The product of current and resistance is taken as positive when we traverse in the direction of current. The emf is taken positive when we traverse from negative to positive electrode through electrolyte.

Before discussing Kirchhoff's law, we shall now define certain basic terms associated with electrical circuits.

i. *Node* is a junction where two or more elemental points meet.
ii. *Path* is the route through elements from one node to another without going through the same node twice.
iii. *Branch* is a path between two adjoining nodes.
iv. *Loop* is a closed path where the route ends upon the starting node.
v. *Mesh* is a loop that does not contain any other loop within it.

Let us now apply Kirchhoff's second law to Fig. 1.21

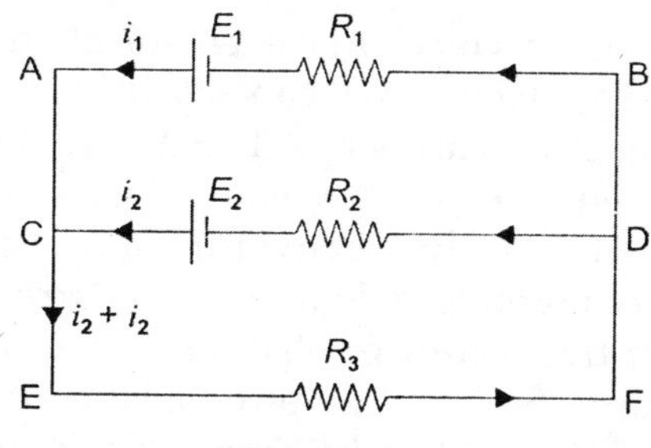

Fig. 1.21

For the mesh ACDBA,

$$i_1R_1 - i_2R_2 = E_1 - E_2 \qquad ...(1.3)$$

For the mesh EFDCE,

$$i_2R_2 + (i_1 + i_2)R_3 = E_2 \qquad ...(1.4)$$

For the mesh EFBAE,

$$i_1R_1 + (i_1 + i_2)R_3 = E_1 \qquad ...(1.5)$$

Method for Solving Problems Applying KVL

In applying KVL to a mesh of network, the proper sign must be assigned to the potential difference across a branch and to the source present in that mesh. For this, minus sign can be given to a fall in potential, positive sign to a rise in potential. It is important that once a particular direction has been assumed, the same should be used throughout the solution for that problem. If the assumed direction of current is not the actual direction, then while solving the problem, the current will be found to have a minus sign. If the answer is positive, then the assumed direction is the same as the actual direction. This shall be clear from the solved examples based on Kirchhoff's laws.

1.8 AMPERE'S LAW

Ampere's law states that the line integral of magnetic induction around any closed path is numerically equal to the product of permeability and current enclosed by the path, i.e. the strength of a magnetic field due to current depends on permeability of the medium μ.

$$\oint B d_1 = \mu i$$

It is defined as the characteristic of the material which indicates the ease with which magnetic flux can be set up in the material. The permeability of free space is denoted by μ_0 and equals $4\pi \times 10^{-7}$ H/m. For all other materials permeability is defined as the product of μ_0 and relative permeability μ_r. Thus

$$\mu = \mu_0\mu_r$$

Hence μ_r indicates the extent to which the given material is a better conductor of magnetic flux than air (or free space).

Ampere's law is helpful for camputing magnetic field induction.

1.9 SOURCES

A source is a device which converts mechanical, chemical, thermal or some other form of energy into electrical energy. Hence, we can say that source is an active network element meant for generating electrical energy. The different types of sources available are voltage sources and current sources. A voltage source has the forcing function of emf whereas the current source has the forcing function of current. Examples of voltage sources are batteries and alternators. Examples of current sources are photo-electric cells, collector current of transistors, etc. These sources are further categorised as ideal source or practical source. Sources can also be categorised as dependent source or independent source. This classification has been shown in Fig. 1.22.

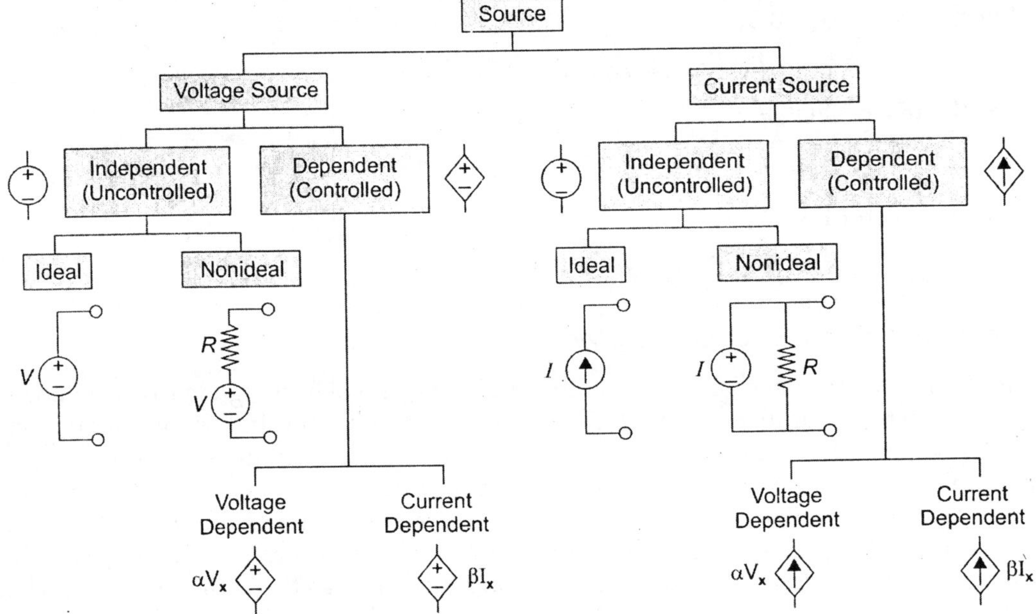

Fig. 1.22

An ideal source is one whose magnitude (voltage or current) does not change and remains constant. Hence, an ideal curent source supplies a given number of coulombs per second regardless of the energy which is required. In simple words, an ideal current source produces a fixed current no matter what voltage is across it. It should be kept in mind that when this source is turned off [i.e., $i(t) = 0$], the source is equivalent to an open circuit. Figure 1.23a shows the symbol and characteristics of an ideal current source.

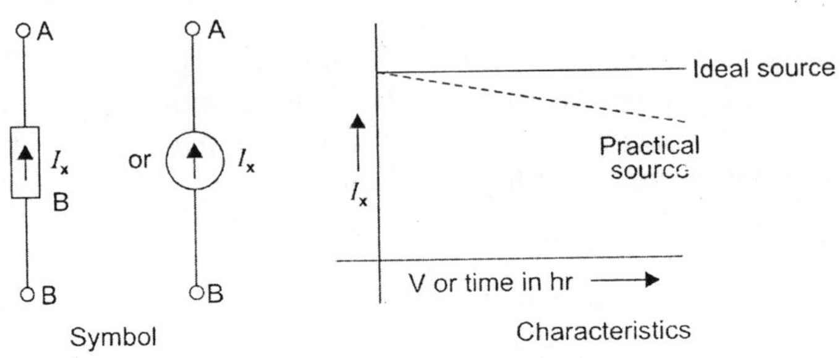

Fig. 1.23a

On the other hand an ideal voltage source supplies an arbitrary number of coulombs each possessing a fixed amount of energy. In this case the voltage across the terminal is constant and is independent of the current drawn from it. When this source is turned off [$v(t) = 0$], the source is equivalent to a short circuit. Figure 1.23b shows the symbol and characteristics of an ideal voltage source.

A practical source like battery has the characteristics of drooping, i.e. decay down and has some internal resistance as shown in Fig. 1.24. The two types of sources

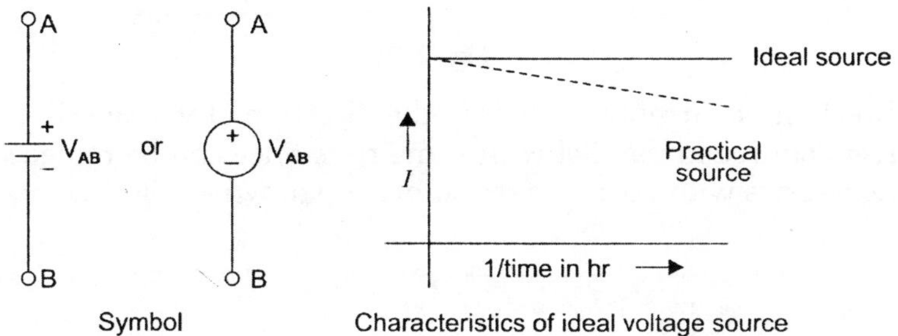

Fig. 1.23b

described above come under the category of independent sources, i.e. their magnitude does not depend on the circuit condition. The current or voltage is fixed and is not adjustable. They are represented by a circle as shown in Fig. 1.24. In a dependent or controlled source, the source output is not fixed but is dependent on a voltage or current at some other location in the network. As their magnitude depends upon the circuit conditions their equivalent circuit of short circuit or open circuit (two ports) is not possible. A different approach is taken for these sources for finding the equivalent circuit which is in the form of four port equivalent circuit. They are represented by a diamond shaped box as shown in Fig. 1.24.

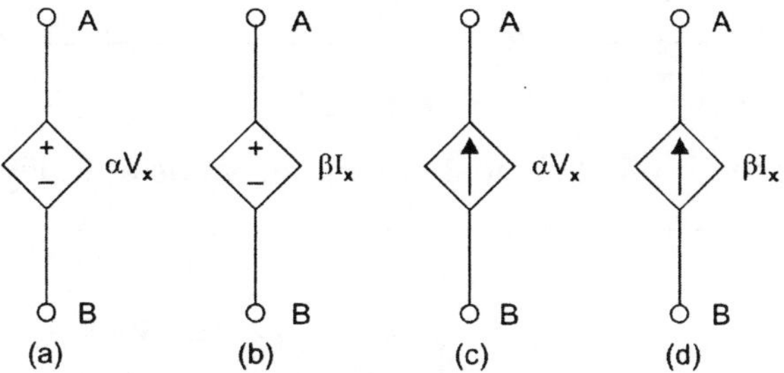

Fig. 1.24

The dependent sources can be categorised as:

1. Voltage dependent voltage source Fig. 1.24a
2. Current dependent voltage source Fig. 1.24b
3. Voltage dependent current source Fig. 1.24c
4. Current dependent current source Fig. 1.24d.

1.9.1 SOURCE TRANSFORMATION

It is the most important part of the circuit analysis. To simplify a circuit, certain rules have been framed which are given in the figures that follow.

a. A voltage source having some internal resistance can be replaced by the current source in parallel with the resistance as shown in Fig. 1.25.

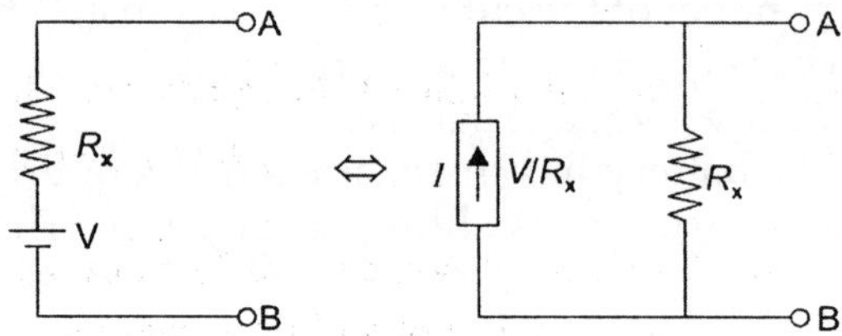

Fig. 1.25

The direction of current source is in the direction of voltage rise.

b. A current source in parallel with some resistance can be replaced by a voltage source in series with the same resistance as shown in Fig. 1.26

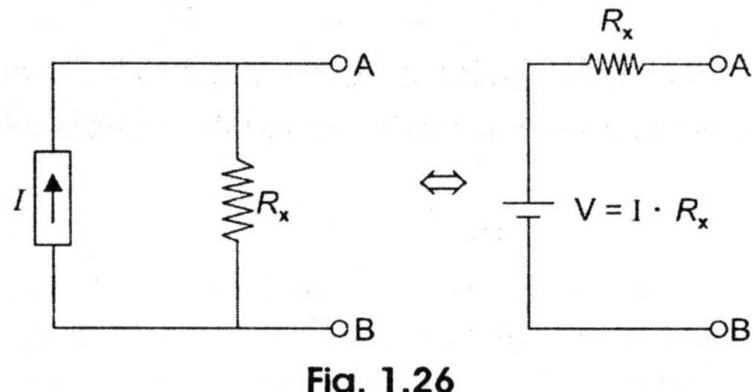

Fig. 1.26

c. Voltage sources in series are transformed, as in Fig. 1.27.

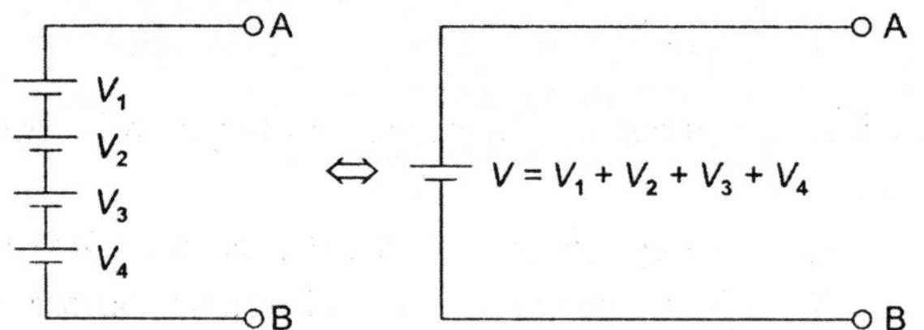

Fig. 1.27

d. Voltage sources in parallel must have same value as in Fig. 1.28.

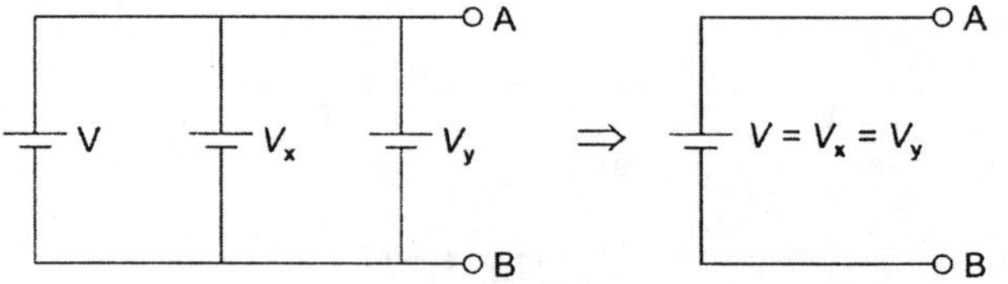

Fig. 1.28

e. Current sources in parallel are transformed as shown in Fig. 1.29.

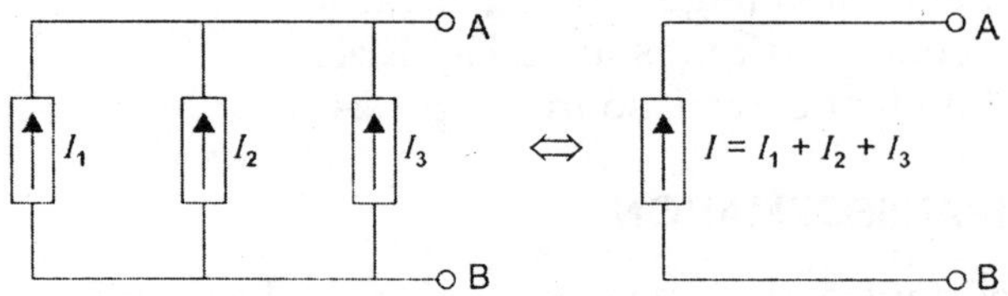

Fig. 1.29

f. Current sources in series must have same value.
g. Resistances in series and in parallel can be replaced by a single resistance of equivalent value.
h. Current shift property as shown in Fig. 1.30.

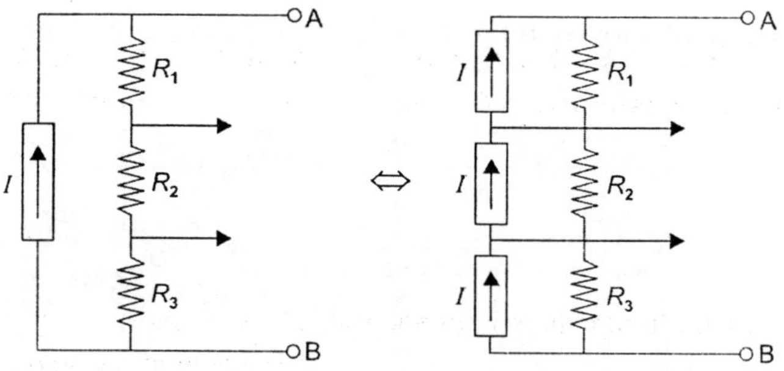

Fig. 1.30

i. Voltage shift property as shown in Fig. 1.31.

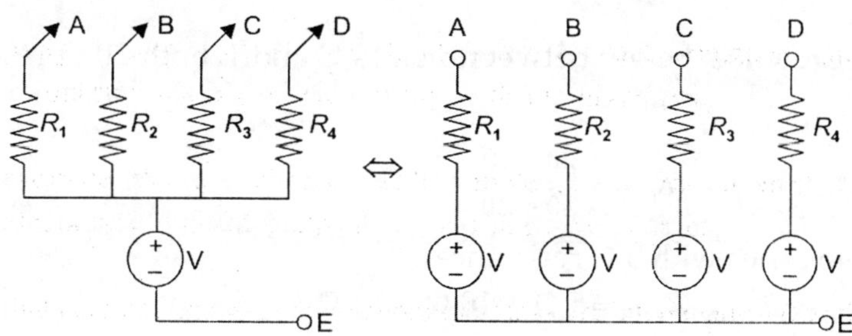

Fig. 1.31

The abovementioned rules are very helpful in circuit analysis for simplifying the circuit.

SOLVED EXAMPLES

Example 1: The resistance of two wires is 25 Ω when they are connected in series and 6 Ω when they are connected in parallel. Calculate the resistance of each wire.

Solution: Let R_1 and R_2 be the two resistances

then $$R_1 + R_2 = 25\ \Omega \text{ and } \frac{1}{R_1} + \frac{1}{R_2} = \frac{1}{6}$$

or $$\frac{R_1 + R_2}{R_1 R_2} = \frac{1}{6} \text{ or } R_1 R_2 = 6(R_1 + R_2) \text{ or } R_1 R_2 = 150$$

or $$R_1 = 150 / R_2$$

Putting this value of R_1, we get

$$150 / R_2 + R_2 = 25$$

$$150 + R_2^2 = 25 R_2 \text{ or } R_2^2 - 25 R_2 + 150 = 0$$

$$R_2 = \frac{+25 \pm \sqrt{625 - 4 \times 150}}{2} = \frac{+25 \pm 5}{2}$$

∴ Either $R_2 = 15\ \Omega$ or $10\ \Omega$ and $R_1 = 25 - R_2$.

Similarly, $R_1 = 10\ \Omega$ or $15\ \Omega$.

Example 2: In the circuit shown in figure below, find the equivalent resistance at points A and B.

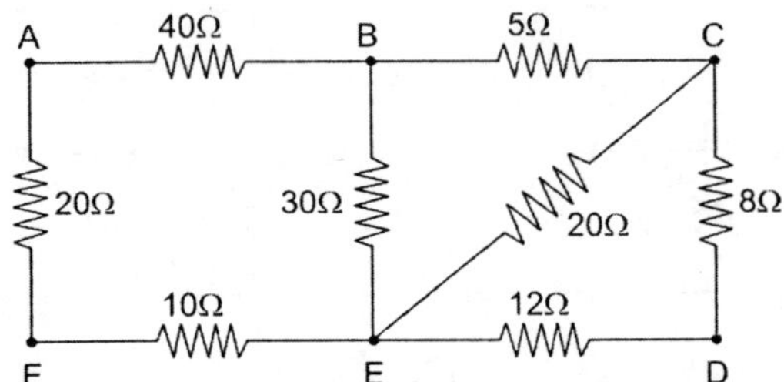

Solution: Observe the figure above carefully. We find that 20 Ω and 10 Ω resistances are in series (from point AFE). Similarly 12 Ω and 8 Ω resistances are in series (from point EDC).

Figure is redrawn as below between points C and E both 20 Ω resistances are in parallel.

$$\therefore \quad R_{CE} = \frac{20 \times 20}{20 + 20} = 10\ \Omega$$

This R_{CE} is in series with 5 Ω resistance

$$\therefore \quad R_{BCE} = 5\ \Omega + 10\ \Omega = 15\ \Omega$$

(a)

(b)

(c)

Now 30 Ω and 15 Ω are in parallel

$$R_{BCE} = \frac{30 \times 15}{30 + 15} = 10\ \Omega$$

30 Ω resistance and R_{BE} are in series, so figure (b) becomes figure (c) as

$$\therefore \quad R_{AB} = \frac{40 \times 40}{40 + 40} = 20\ \Omega$$

Example 3: A coil made of copper wire of 1 mm diameter and 1 km length is connected in parallel with another coil of Al wire of 1 mm diameter. The resistance of the combination is 9.738 Ω. If resistivity of copper is 1.72 × 10^{-8} Ω m while that of Al is 2.8 × 10^{-8} Ω m, what is the length of Al wire?

Solution:

$$D_{Al} = D_{Cu} = \frac{\pi d^2}{4} = \frac{\pi\left(1 \times 10^{-3}\right)^2}{4} = 7.853 \times 10^{-7}$$

$$R_{eq} = 9.738\ \Omega = R_{cu} \parallel R_{A1}$$

$$\rho_{Cu} = 1.72 \times 10^{-8}\ \Omega\text{ m and } \rho_{Al} = 2.8 \times 10^{-8}\ \Omega\text{ m}$$

$$\text{Resistance of copper } (R_{Cu}) = \rho_{Cu}\frac{l_{Cu}}{A_{Cu}} = 1.72 \times 10^{-8} \times \frac{1000}{7.853 \times 10^{-4}}$$

$$= 21.89 = 22\ \Omega$$

Now R_{Cu} and R_{Al} are in parallel as shown in figure below and R_{eq} is 9.738 Ω

$$R_{eq} = \frac{R_{Cu} R_{Al}}{R_{Cu} + R_{Al}}$$

$$9.378 = \frac{22 \times R_{Al}}{22 + R_{Al}}$$

$$22 + R_{Al} = 2.5\ R_{Al}$$

$$22 = 1.5\ R_{Al}$$

or

$$R_{Al} = \frac{22}{1.5} = 14.6\ \Omega$$

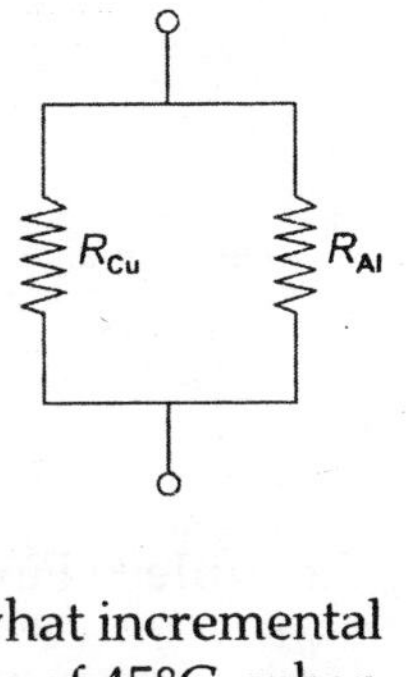

Since

$$R_{Al} = \rho_{Al}\frac{l_{Al}}{A_{Al}}$$

$$\therefore \quad 2.8 \times 10^{-8} \times \frac{l_{Al}}{7.853 \times 10^{-7}} = 14.6$$

Thus

$$l_{Al} = 411 \text{ metre}$$

R_{Cu} R_{Al}

Example 4: A field coil of motor has resistance of 250 Ω at 15°C. At what incremental value, will the resistance increase if motor attains average temperature of 45°C, when running. Assume temperature coefficient of resistance of Cu to be 0.00426°C at 0°C.

Solution:

$$R_1 = 250\ \Omega;\ t_1 = 15°\text{C}$$

$$R_2 = ?;\ t_2 = 45°\text{C}$$

$$\alpha_0 = 0.00426°\text{C}$$

We know

$$R_1 = R_0(1 + \alpha_0\ t_1)$$

$$250 = R_0(1 + 0.00426 \times 15) \quad ...(1)$$

$$R_2 = R_0 (1 + \alpha_0 t_2)$$

$$= R_0 (1 + 0.00426 \times 45) \quad ...(2)$$

Dividing Eq. (2) by Eq. (1)

$$\frac{R_2}{250} = \frac{1 + 0.00426 \times 45}{1 + 0.00426 \times 15}$$

$$R_2 = 280.03\ \Omega$$

Increase in resistance of field coil

$$= (R_2 - R_1) = 280.03 - 250 = 30.03\ \Omega$$

Example 5. If α_1 and α_2 are the temperature coefficients of resistance at t_1 and t_2 respectively, then show that: $\alpha_2 = \frac{\alpha_1}{1+\alpha_1(t_2 - t_1)}$

Solution: (*i*) We know that $R_t = R_0(1 + \alpha t)$

If we cool conductor from t°C to 0°C, then

$$R_0 = R_t[1 + (a_t(0-t)] = R_t(1 - \alpha_t t)$$

$$\alpha_1 = \frac{R_t - R_0}{R_t \times t} = \frac{R_0(1+\alpha_0 t) - R_0}{R_0(1+\alpha_0 t)\times t} = \frac{\alpha_0}{(1+\alpha_0 t)} \quad ...(1)$$

From above Eq. (1) we get

$$\alpha_1 = \frac{\alpha_0}{(1+\alpha_0 t_1)} \text{ and } \alpha_2 = \frac{\alpha_0}{(1+\alpha_0 t_2)}$$

or
$$1/a_1 = (1+\alpha_0 t_1)/\alpha_0 \quad ...(2)$$

and
$$1/a_2 = (1+\alpha_0 t_2)/\alpha_0 \quad ...(3)$$

Subtracting Eq. (3) from Eq. (2), we get

$$\frac{1}{\alpha_2} - \frac{1}{\alpha_1} = \frac{\alpha_1 - \alpha_2}{\alpha_1\alpha_2} = \frac{(1+\alpha_0 t_2)-(1+\alpha_0 t_1)}{\alpha_0} = (t_2 - t_1)$$

$$= \quad \text{Now } \frac{1}{\alpha_2} = \frac{1}{\alpha_1 + (t_2 - t_1)} = \left[\frac{1+\alpha_1(t_2 - t_1)}{\alpha_1}\right]$$

$$\therefore \quad \alpha_2 = \frac{\alpha_1}{1+\alpha_1(t_2 - t_1)}$$

Example 6: Find source current in given figure.

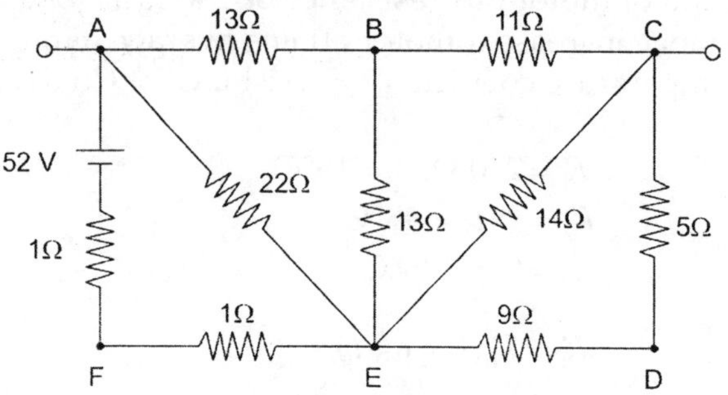

Solution: 5 Ω and 9 Ω resistances are in series

Thus $$R_{CDE} = 5 + 9 = 14\ \Omega$$

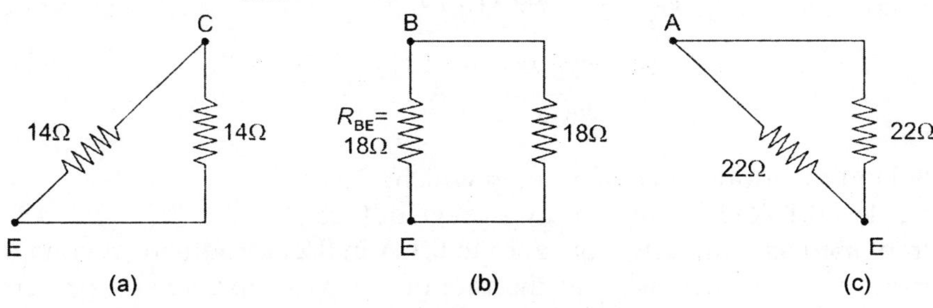

(a) (b) (c)

Now 14 Ω and 14 Ω are in parallel as shown in figure (a)

Thus, $$R_{EC} = \frac{14 \times 14}{14 + 14} = 7\ \Omega$$

Similarly, $$R_{BCE} = 11 + 7 = 18\ \Omega$$

Now R_{BE} is parallel to R_{BC} as shown in figure (b)

Thus, $$R_{eq} = \frac{18 \times 18}{18 + 18} = 9\ \Omega$$

Example 7: For the circuit shown in figure below, use the method of series-parallel combination and find V_1 and I_2 marked in the figure.

Solution: 10 Ω, 50 Ω, 20 Ω resistances are in

$$\therefore \quad \frac{1}{\text{eq.}} = \frac{1}{10} + \frac{1}{50} + \frac{1}{20} = \frac{8.5}{50}$$

or $$R_{eq} = \frac{50}{8.5}\ \Omega$$

Now R_{eq} and 25 Ω and 2.5 Ω resistances are in series

$$\therefore \quad R_{total} = 50/8.5 + 25 + 2.5 = 33.38\ \Omega$$

Now current flowing from the supply is

$$I = \frac{V}{R_{total}} = \frac{10}{33.38} = 0.299\ \text{A}$$

Voltage across 2.5 Ω resistor, $V_1 = R_1 = 2.5 \times 0.299 = 0.748$ V

Voltage across $R_{eq} = R_{eq}\ I = \dfrac{50}{8.5} \times 0.299 = 1.75$ V

$$\therefore \qquad I_2 = \frac{1.75\text{ V}}{50\ \Omega} = 0.35\text{ A}$$

Example 8: Find the inductance of a coil in which:

a. A current of 0.1 A yields an energy storage of 0.05 J.

b. A current increases linearly from zero to 0.1 A in 0.2 s producing a voltage of 5 V.

c. A current of 0.1 A increasing at the rate of 0.5 A/s represents a power flow of 0.5 W.

Solution: a. Given $I = 0.1$ A, $W = 0.05$ J

Now $$W = \frac{1}{2}LI^2 \text{ or } L = 2\,W/I^2$$

$$L = \frac{2 \times 0.05}{(0.1)^2} = 10\text{ H}$$

b. Given $$V_L = 5\text{ V and } di/dt = (0.1 - 0)/0.2 = 0.5\text{ A/s}$$

$$V_L = L\,di/dt \text{ or } L = V\,J(di/dt)$$

$$L = 5/0.5 = 10\text{ H}$$

c. Given $$i = 0.1\text{ A and } di/dt = 0.5\text{ A/s}$$

$$\text{power} = vi = L\frac{di}{dt}i$$

or $$L = \frac{0.5}{0.5 \times 0.1} = 10\text{ H}$$

Example 9: Find the capacitance of a circuit element in which:

a. A voltage of 100 V yields an energy storage in an electric field of 0.05 J.

b. A voltage increases linearly from zero to 100 V in 0.2 s causing a current of 5 mA to flow.

c. Two flat parallel plates are separated by a 0.1 mm layer of mica and have a total area of 0.113 m^2.
Assume mica to have a relative permittivity of 10. Find the capacitance.

Solution: a. Energy stored in a capacitor $= \dfrac{1}{2}CV^2$

or $$0.05 = \frac{1}{2} \times C \times (100)^2 \text{ or } C = 10\ \mu\text{F}$$

b. $$\frac{dV}{dt} = \frac{dV}{dt} = \frac{(100 - 0)}{0.2} = 500\text{ V/s}$$

$$i = CdV/\,dt \text{ or } C = 5 \times 10^{-3}/500\ \mu\text{F}$$

c. We know that $C = \varepsilon\, A/d = \varepsilon_0\, \varepsilon_r\, A/d$

$$C = 8.854 \times 10^{-12} \times 10 \times \frac{0.113}{0.1 \times 10^{-3}} = 0.1\ \mu\text{F}$$

Example 10: A DC circuit comprises of two resistors; resistor A of value 25 Ω resistor B of unknown value connected in parallel. A third resistor C of value 5 Ω is now connected in series with the parallel branch. Find the voltage to be applied across the whole circuit and the value of resistor B if the potential difference across C is 90 V and the total power consumed is 4320 W.

Solution: The circuit diagram is drawn as shown in the figure.

$$\text{Current through 5 } \Omega \text{ resistor} = \frac{V}{R} = \frac{90}{5} = 18\text{ A}$$

$$\text{Power consumed} = VI$$

or

$$V = \frac{\text{Power consumed}}{\text{Current through circuit}} = \frac{4320}{18} = 240\text{ V}$$

Voltage drop across parallel combination = Total voltage – Voltage drop across 5 Ω
= 240 – 90 = 150 V

$$\text{Current through 25 } \Omega \text{ resistor} = \frac{V}{R} = \frac{150}{25} = 6\text{ A}$$

∴ Current through resistor B = Total current – Current through 25 resistor
= 18 – 6 = 12 A

$$\therefore \quad \text{Value of resistor } B,\ R = \frac{V}{I} = \frac{150}{12} = 12.5\ \Omega$$

Example 11: In the circuit shown in figure, find values and directions of I_1, I_2 and I_3.

Solution: Let $I_1 = X$, $I_2 = Y$, $I_3 = x + y$

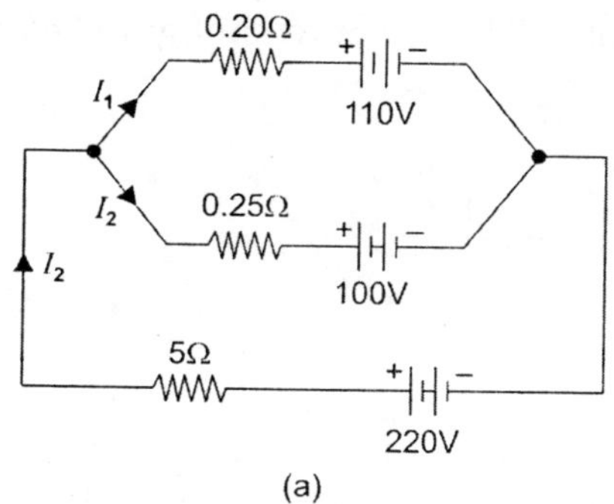

(a)

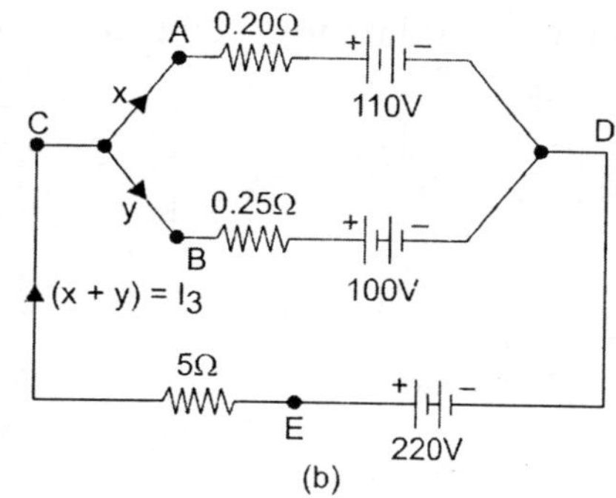

(b)

Assume direction of current as shown in figure, applying Kirchoff's law to the two loops.

loop $CADEC \rightarrow$ $0.2x + 110 - 220 + 5(x + y) = 0$

$$5.2x + 5y = 110 \qquad ...(1)$$

loop $CBDEC \rightarrow$ $0.25y + 100 - 220 + 5(x + y) = 0$

$$5x + 5.25y = 120 \qquad ...(2)$$

Solving (1) and (2), we get

$$x = 11.7\text{ A and } y = 32.17\text{ A}$$

$I_1 = -11.7$ A (opposite direction), $I_2 = 32.17$ A and $I_a = 20.47$

A check loop CADBC = $0.2 \times 110 - 100 - 0.25y = 0$

Example 12: Two batteries A and B are connected in parallel and a load of 10 Ω is connected across their terminals. A has an emf of 12 V with an internal resistance of

2 Ω and B has an emf of 8 V with an internal resistance of 1 Ω. Using appropriate method determine the magnitude of current and also the directions in each of the batteries. Also determine the potential difference across the external resistance.

Solution: The circuit is drawn as shown in the figure below.

Applying Kirchoff's second law (or KVL) for mesh ACDBA

$$2(I_1) - 1(I_2) = 12 - 8 \quad ...(1)$$

For mesh EFDCE $1(I_2) + (I_1 + I_2)10 = 8$ ...(2)

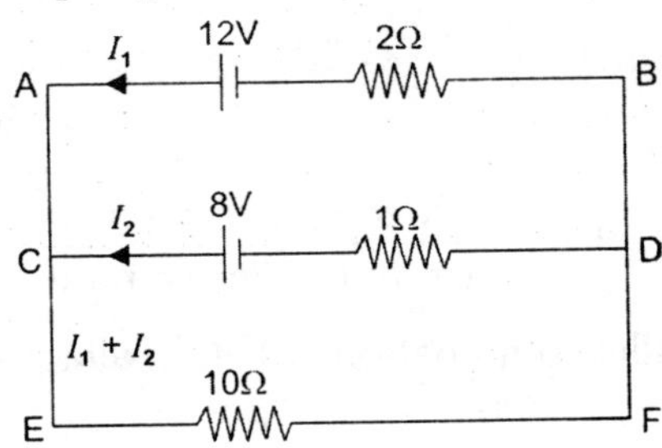

Solving Eqs (1) and (2) we get

$$I_1 = 1.625 \text{ A and } I_2 = -0.75 \text{ A}$$

Negative sign of I_2 indicates that the current is actually flowing opposite to the assumed direction of current flow.

Potential difference across external resistance, i.e. 10 Ω is given by

$$R_1 = 10\ (11 + 12) = 8.75 \text{ V}$$

Example 13: Three batteries consisting of 50, 55 and 60 cells in series respectively supply in parallel, a common load of 100 amp. Each cell has an emf of 2 V and and internal resistance of 0.005 Ω, determine the current supplied by each battery and the load voltage.

Solution: According to given problem circuit will be as shown in figure below.

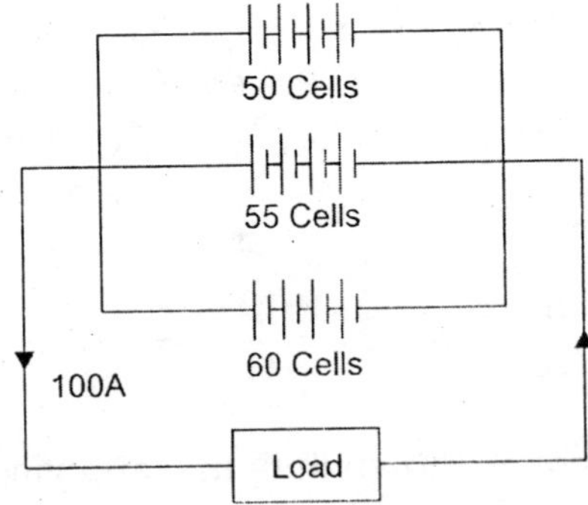

i. Consider first battery

No. of cell = 50

voltage = 50 × 2 = 100 V

Resistance = 50 × 0.005 Ω = 0.250 Ω

ii. Consider second battery

Voltage = 55 × 2 = 110

Resistance = 55 × 0.005 = 0.2750

iii. Consider third battery

Voltage = 60 × 2 = 120 V

Resistance = 60 × 0.005 = 0.300 Ω

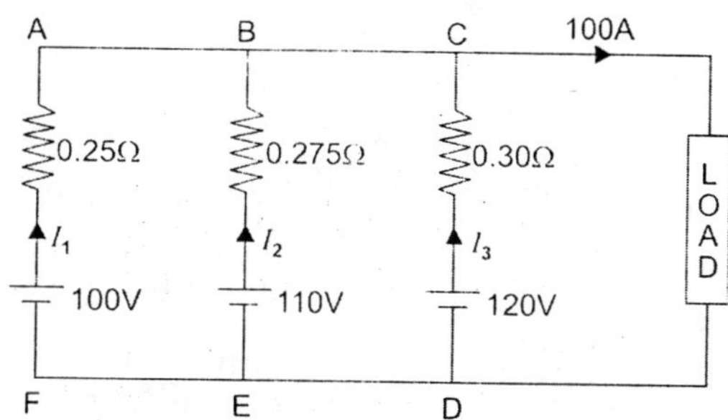

The equivalent circuit will be as shown in figure.

$$I_1 + I_2 + I_3 = 100$$

$$I_3 = 100 - (I_1 + I_2)$$

KVL in ABEFA

$$0.25I_1 + 0.275I_2 - 110 + 100 = 0$$

$$0.25I_1 + 0.275I_2 = 10 \qquad ...(1)$$

KVL in BCDEB

$$-0.275I_2 + 0.3I_3 - 120 + 110 = 0$$

$$-0.275I_2 + 0.3(100 - I_1 - I_2) = 10$$

$$0.275I_2 + 30 - 0.31I_1 - 0.3I_2 = 10$$

$$0.575\ I_2 - 0.3\ I_1 = -20$$

$$0.3\ I_1 + 0.575\ I_2 = 20 \qquad ...(2)$$

Multiplying Eq. (1) by 0.3

$$0.075\ I_1 + 0.0825\ I_2 = 3 \qquad ...(3)$$

Multiplying Eq. (2) by 0.25

$$0.075\ I_1 + 0.14375\ I_2 = 5 \qquad ...(4)$$

Adding Eq. (3) and Eq. (4), we have

$$0.22625\ I_2 = 8 \qquad \therefore\ I_2 = 35.359\text{ A}$$

From Eq. (1)

$$-0.25\ I_1 + 0.275 \times 35.359 = 10$$

Now

$$I_3 = 100 - (I_1 + I_2) = 65.746\text{ A}$$

∴ Current supplied by batteries are

$$\text{First } (I_1) = 1.105\text{ A}$$

$$\text{Second } (I_2) = 35.359\text{ A}$$

$$\text{Third } (I_3) = 65.746\text{ A}$$

$$\text{Potential across load} = 120 - (0.3 \times 13)$$

$$= 120 - (0.3 \times 65.7461)$$

$$= 100.27617\text{ volt}$$

Example 14: Using Kirchoff's law find the currents in all branches of the network shown in the figure given.

Solution: Let current in branch EF be IA. By using KCL at junctions A, B, C, D, E and F, the currents in all six branches are marked in terms of I on the figure. Applying KVL on the loop ABCDEFA, we get

$$0.02(I+50) + 0.01(I-10) + 0.03(I+50) + 0.01(I-70)$$

$$+0.01(I) + 0.02(I-30) = 0$$

$$I = -11\text{ A}$$

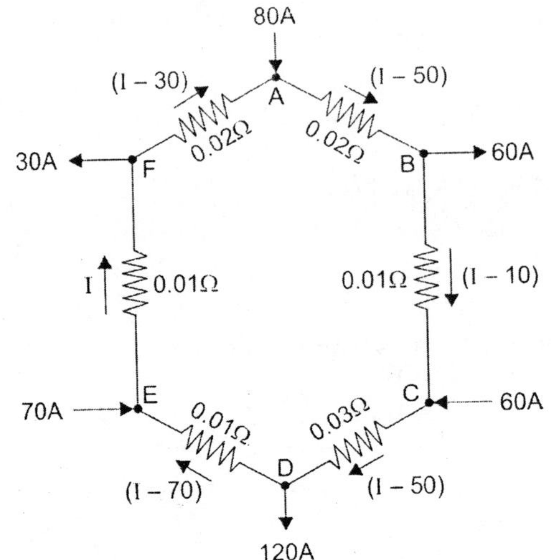

Negative sign signifies that the current is flowing in the reverse direction of the assumed direction of flow of current.

Current in different branches are:

$$AB = I + 50 = (-11 + 50)\text{ A} = 39\text{ A}$$
$$CB = I - 10 = (-11 - 10)\text{ A} = -21\text{ A}$$
$$CD = I + 50 = (-11 + 50)\text{ A} = 39\text{ A}$$
$$DE = I - 70 = (-11 - 70)\text{ A} = -81\text{ A}$$
$$EF = I = -11\text{ A}$$
$$FA = I - 30 = (-11 - 30)\text{ A} = -41\text{ A}$$

Example 15: Convert the voltage source as shown in the following figure into an equivalent current source.

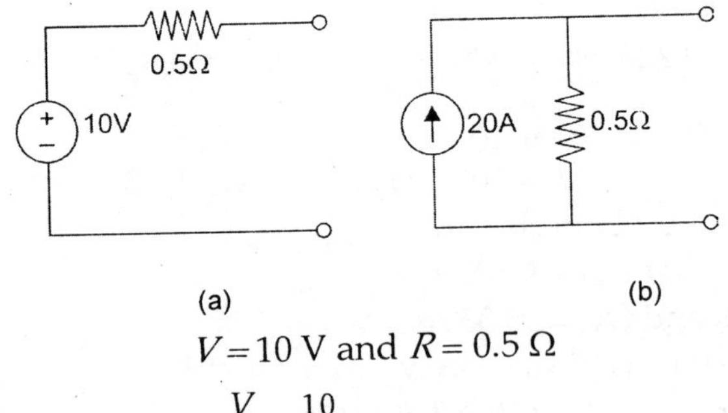

Solution: $V = 10\text{ V}$ and $R = 0.5\ \Omega$

$$\therefore \quad I = \frac{V}{R} = \frac{10}{0.5} = 20\text{ A}$$

Hence current source is drawn as shown in figure.

Example 16: Determine power consumed by 10 ohm resistor in the circuit shown in figure below.

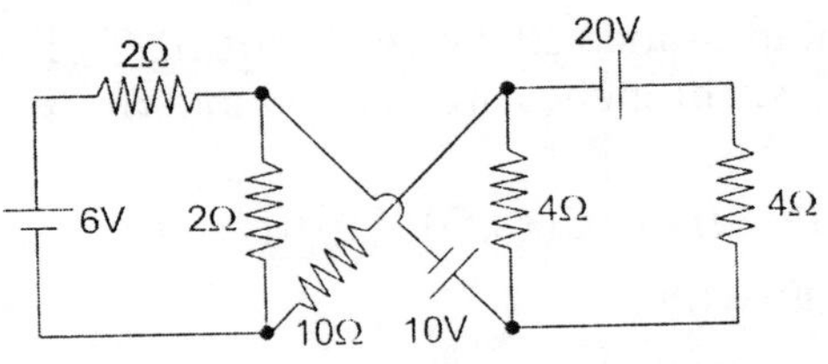

Solution: The circuit is redrawn as shown in figure (a).

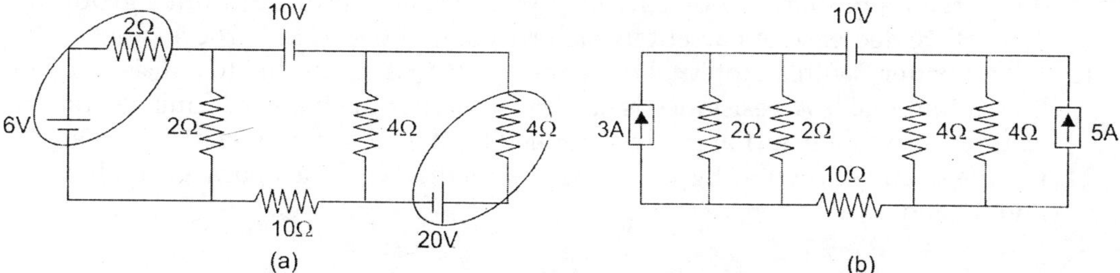

(a) (b)

Now the voltage source with resistance in series are converted into equivalent current source with resistance in parallel and circuit is obtained as shown in Fig. (b).

Again source transformation is applied and we obtain a simple circuit as shown in figure.

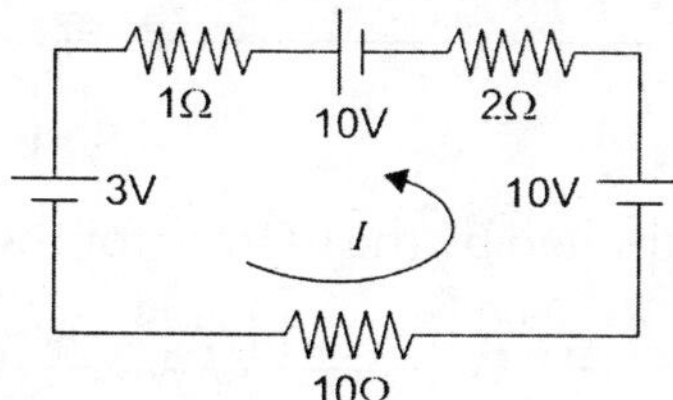

Current through 10 Ω resistance is

$$I = \frac{V}{R} = \frac{10 + 10 - 3}{2 + 1 + 10} = \frac{17}{13} = 1.307 \text{ A}$$

Power consumed by 10 Ω resistor,

$$P_{10\Omega} = I^2R = (1.307)^2 \times 10 = 17.1 \text{ watt.}$$

EXERCISES

1. What is the difference between field produced by static charges and moving charges?
2. What is the difference betwen direct current and alternating current?
3. Explain Coulomb's law with its limitations.
4. Distinguish among emf, potential difference, voltage, voltage drop and voltage rise.
5. Describe Ohm's law. What are its limitations.
6. Distinguish between the terms:
   a. Resistance and resistor
   b. Inductance and inductor
   c. Capacitance and capacitor
7. If heat is constantly being added to a current-carrying resistor, why does the resistor temperature not rise indefinitely?
8. Explain why it is that current flowing through an inductor is not allowed to change instantaneously.
9. How can one determine that in an electric circuit containing a single element, the element is capacitor.
10. Define and explain Kirchoff's current and voltage laws.
11. Three resistors are connected in series across a 12 V battery. The first resistor has the value of 1 ohm, second has a voltage drop of 4 V and third has a power dissipation of 12 W. Calculate the value of each resistance and circuit current.

    [**Hint**: Circuit current 6 A or 2 A, R_2 or 2 A, $\frac{2}{3}$ Ω]
12. A constant voltage E is applied to N groups of rheostats in series, where each group

has M identical rheostats in parallel. If one rheostat burns out in one group, find the percentage increase of current in each rheostat of the faulty group and percentage decrease of current in each rheostat of the sound group.

13. A 20 V battery with an internal resistance of 45 Q is connected to a resistor of x Q. If an additional 6 W resistance is connected across the battery terminals, find the value of x so that external power supplied by the battery remains the same.
14. For the circuit shown in figure, using the method of series-parallel combination, find V_1 and V_2.

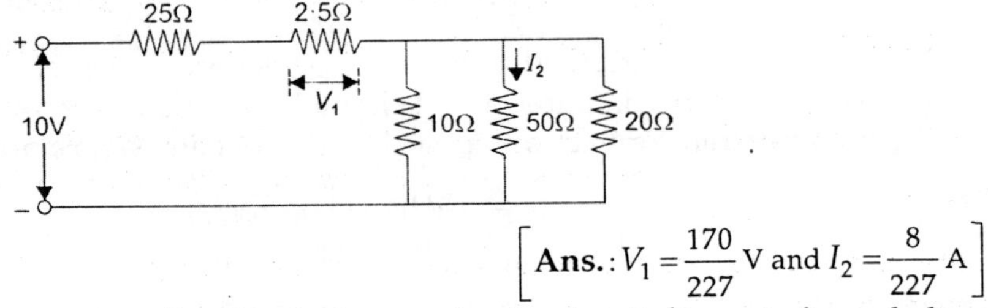

$$\left[\textbf{Ans.}: V_1 = \frac{170}{227}\text{ V and } I_2 = \frac{8}{227}\text{ A}\right]$$

15. Determine the current supplied by the battery for the circuit shown in figure below.

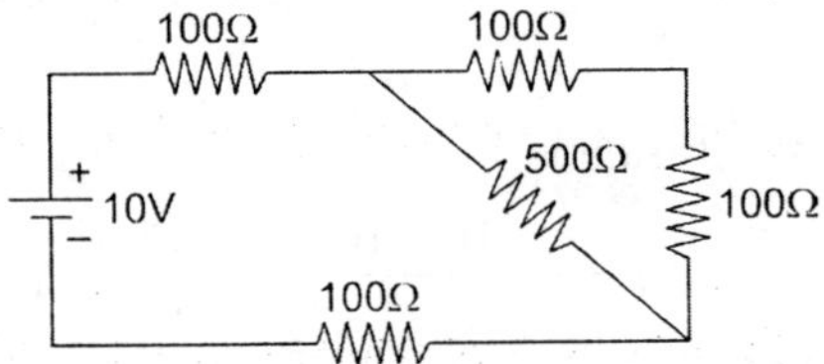

16. Find the value of resistance R and the current, I_R in figure below when the branch AD carries no current. **[Ans.** $R = 8\ \Omega$, $I_R = 0.25$ A**]**

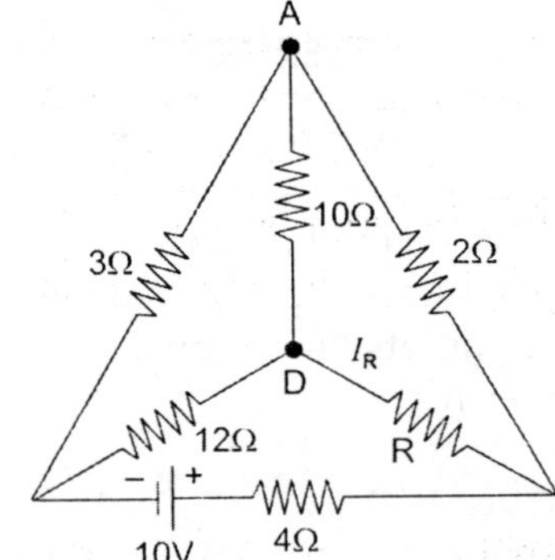

17. Calculate the current through the galvanometer in the bridge circuit shown in figure below.

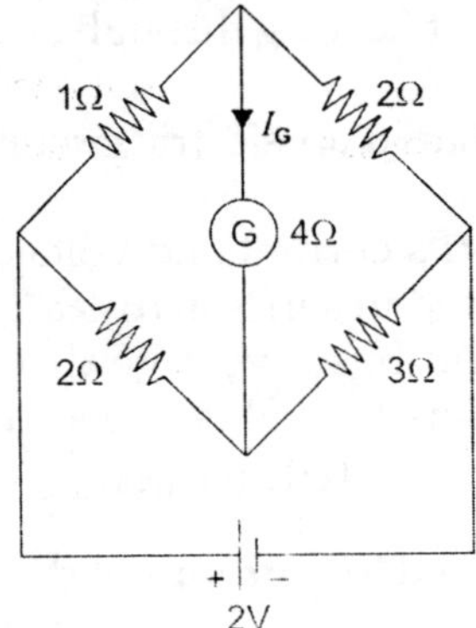

Chapter

2 Electrical Circuit Analysis

2.1 CIRCUIT CONCEPTS

Introduction: In this chapter, we are going to discuss different theorems and their use for the simplification of DC circuits. Before doing so, let us discuss some important definitions related with the networks.

2.1.1 Concept of Network/Circuit

Definition: It is an electrical configuration in which various components such as resistors, inductors, capacitors, etc. and voltage sources or current sources are electrically connected to each other (Fig. 2.1).

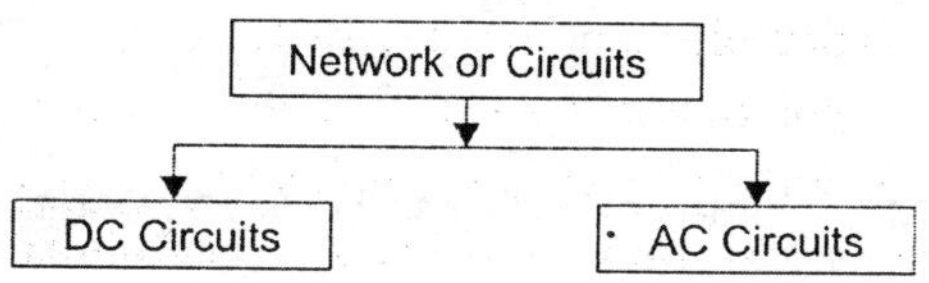

Fig. 2.1: Block diagram of a network

DC circuit: The DC circuit consist of only resistance and DC source of energy. *Example:* Battery

Symbol: + –

AC circuits: The AC circuit consist of resistor, inductor, capacitor and AC source of energy. *Example:* AC supply mains

Symbol: + –

2.2 NETWORK TERMINOLOGY

1. **Circuit element:** Any individual circuit elements with two terminals which can be connected to other circuit elements is called a circuit or network elements (Fig. 2.2).

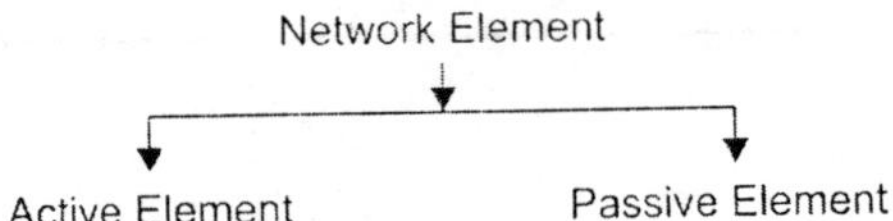

Fig. 2.2: Block diagram of network elements

a. **Active element:** Active elements are those elements which deliver energy (Fig. 2.3).

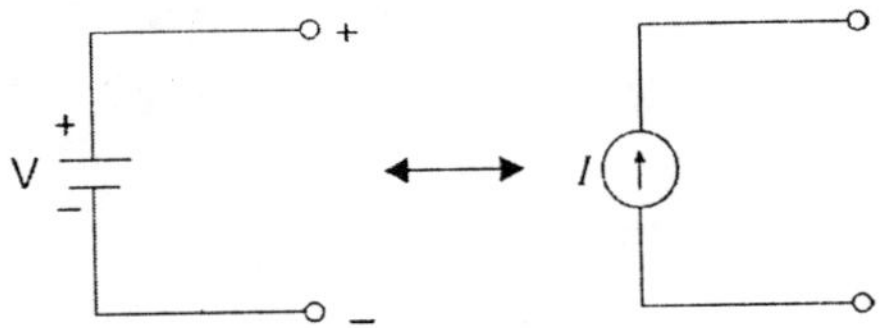

Fig. 2.3: Active element

Example: Voltage source and current source.

b. **Passive element:** The circuit elements which can not generate energy are known as the passive elements. These elements either dissipate or store energy. *Example:* Resistor, inductor and capacitor.

2. **Open circuit:** Two points in a circuit are said to be open circuited if there is no circuit element or connection present between them (Fig. 2.4).

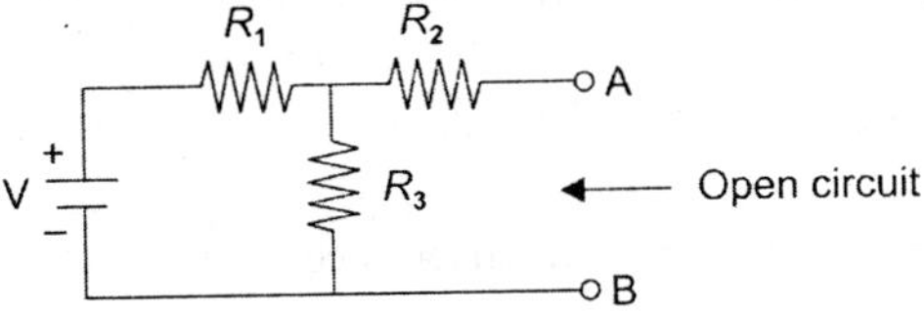

Fig. 2.4: An open circuit exists between points A and B

3. **Short circuit:** Two points in a circuit are said to be short circuited when they are connected with each other by a good conducting wire.

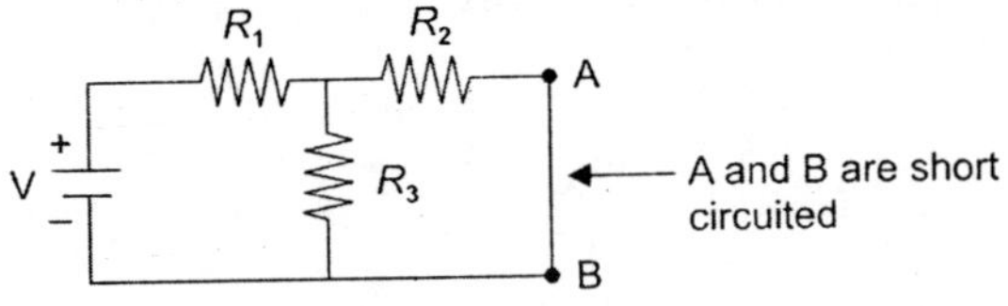

Fig. 2.5: Points A and B are short circuited

4. **Branch:** A branch of a network is defined as the group of elements connected in series or parallel and which has two terminals from connections. *Example:* The branches are: AB, BC, BDC, AE in Fig. 2.5.

5. **Loop:** Any closed path in a network is called loop. *Example:* A-B-C-E-A, closed path B-D-C-D, closed path A-B-D-C-E-A are the loops in Fig. 2.6.

6. **Mesh:** A mesh is the most elementary form of a loop and cannot be further divided into other loops. Thus a loop may contain mesh, but a mesh can not contain a loop. *Example:* ABCEA as BDCB are meshes.

7. **Node or junction:** It is a common point in a network at which two or more branches meet. *Example:* Points A, B, C and D are nodes in Fig. 2.6.

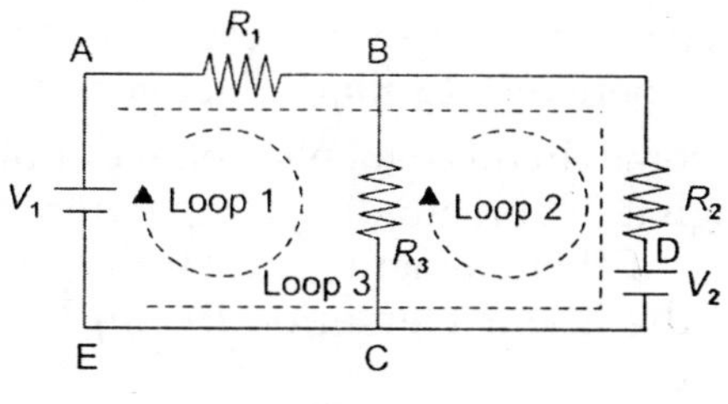

Fig. 2.6

2.3 CLASSIFICATION OF ELECTRICAL NETWORKS

The classification of a network depends on the characteristics and behaviour of its elements.

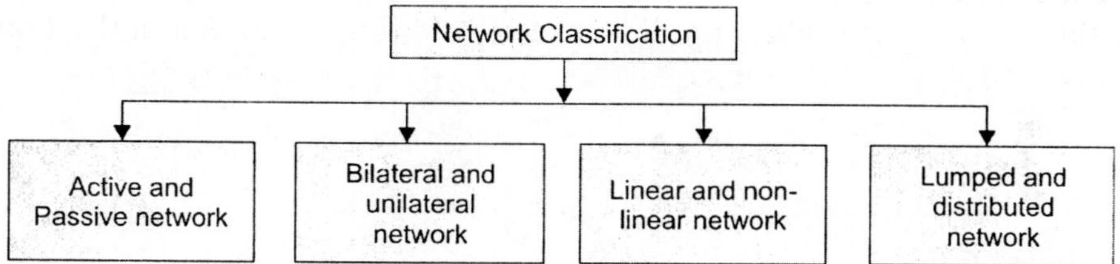

Fig. 2.7: Classification of electrical network

1. **Active network:** A network which contains at least one source of energy is called active network (Fig. 2.7a).

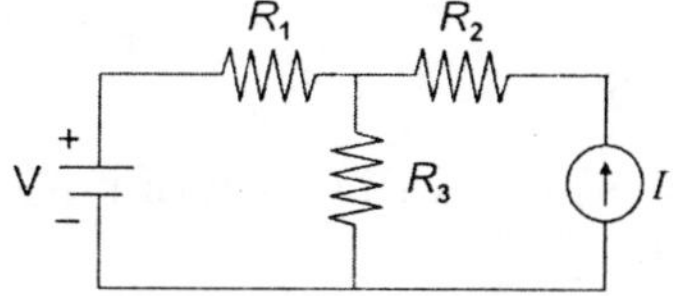

Fig. 2.8: Active network

2. **Passive network:** A network which does not contain any energy source is called passive network (Fig. 2.9).

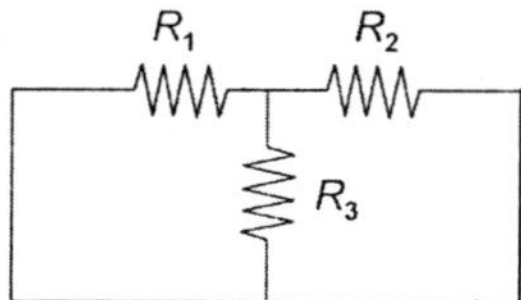

Fig. 2.9: Passive network

3. **Unilateral network:** A network whose working properties as well as behavior can be defined only in one direction. (Fig. 2.10). ***Example:*** Diode rectifier

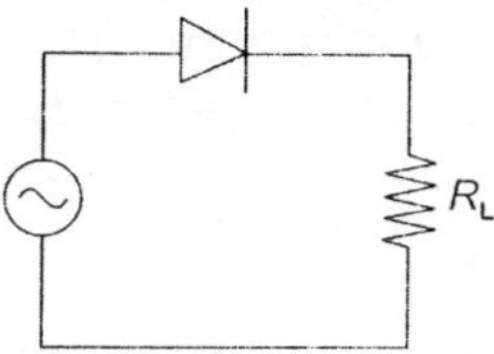

Fig. 2.10: Unilateral network

4. **Bilateral network:** A network whose properties does not depend on the direction of current is called bilateral network. ***Example:*** Network containing resistors only.

5. **Linear network:** For some circuit elements, voltage applied is directly proportional to the current flow through it (if surrounding temperature is constant). So the *V-I* characteristics of this elements is a straight line and this elements are known as the linear elements. ***Example***: Resistance, inductance, capacitance, etc.

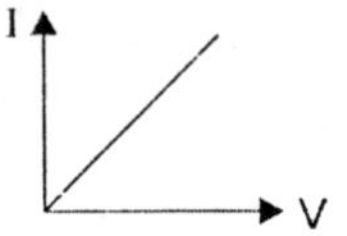

From ohm's law it is known that $V = IR$. So if R is assumed to be constant, V becomes directly proportional to I. $Y \propto X$, i.e. $Y = mX$ (Fig. 2.11). It is an equation of straight line passing through the origin. Therefore, resistance is a linear element.

I

V

Fig. 2.11

Ohm's law can be applied to linear network only.

6. **Nonlinear element:** Those circuit elements for which volt-ampere is not a straight line, rather a curve are called nonlinear elements (Fig. 2.12). ***Example:*** Transistor, diode, etc.

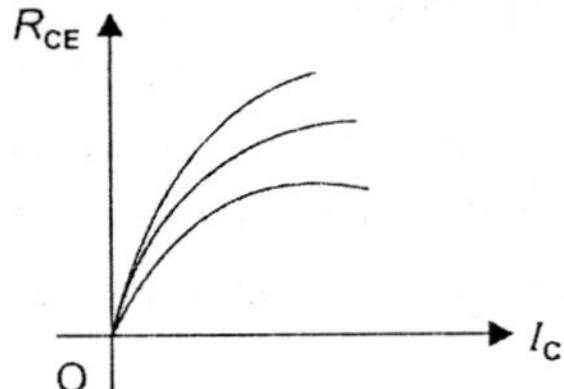

Fig. 2.12: *V–I* characteristics of nonlinear elements

2.4 BASIC CIRCUIT ELEMENTS

Figure 2.13 shows the illustrated block diagram of basic circuit elements.

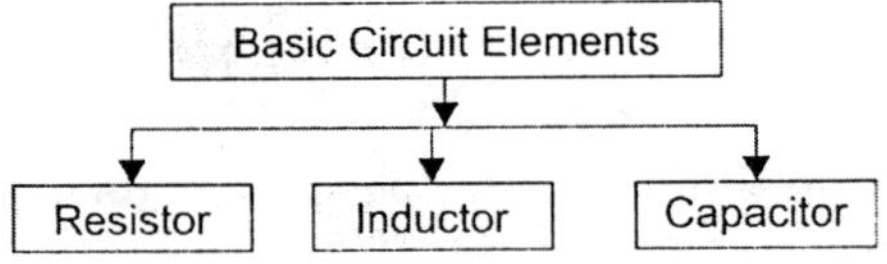

Fig. 2.13: Block diagram of basic circuit elements

1. **Resistor:** A circuit element which opposes the flow of current is called resistor (Fig. 2.14).

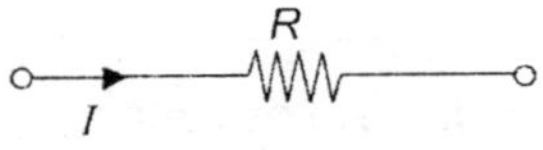

R

I

Fig. 2.14: A resistor

Resistance: It is the property of material by which it opposes the flow of current through it. It is denoted by R and unit is ohm (Ω).

Explanation: The resistance of a given material depends on the physical properties of that material.

$$\therefore \quad R = \rho \frac{l}{a}$$

where l = length in meter, a = cross-sectional in square metres, ρ = resistivity in ohm-metre, R = resistance in ohms

2. **Inductor:** A circuit element in which energy is stored in the form of electromagnetic field is known as inductor (Fig. 2.15).

Inductance: It is the property of our inductor by which it opposes the flow of current change in circuit. It is denoted by L and unit is henry.

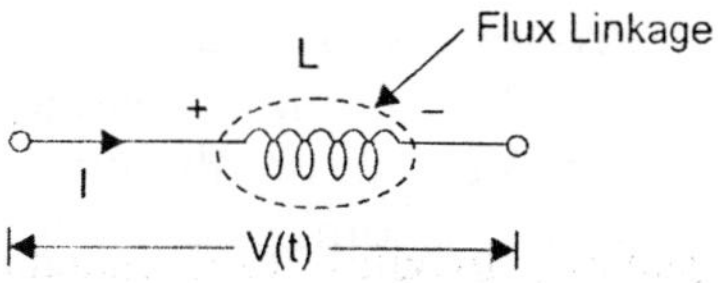

Fig. 2.15

$$L = \frac{N\phi}{I}$$

where N = no. of turns, ϕ = flux, I = current

3. **Capacitor:** A circuit element in which energy is stored in the form of an electrostatic field is known as capacitor. It is made up of two conducting plates separated by a dielectric material (Fig. 2.16).

Capacitance: It is the property of a capacitor by which it measures store charge in electric field. It is denoted by C and units is farad.

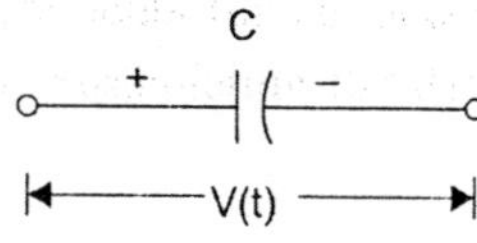

Fig. 2.16

$$C = \frac{q}{V}$$

where C = capacitance, q = charge, V = applied voltage

Note: When we supply the electrical energy to the circuit element, this electrical energy is either consumed or stored. If the electrical energy is completely consumed than the element will be a pure resistor. If the electrical energy is completely stored in a magnetic field the circuit element is an inductor, if it is stored in an electric field it is a capacitor.

2.5 ENERGY SOURCES

Figure 2.17 shows the block diagram of energy sources.

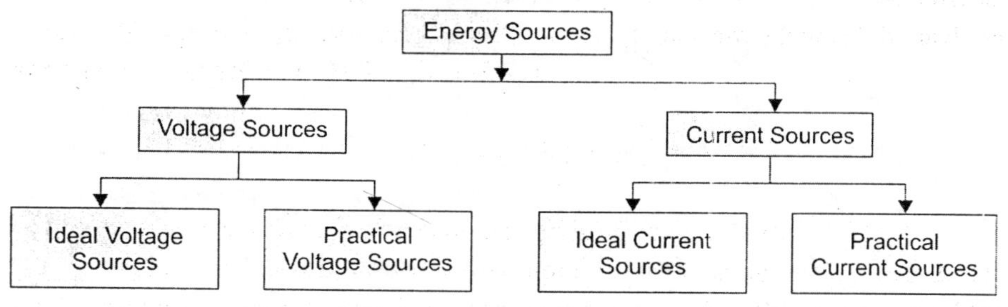

Fig. 2.17: Block diagram of energy sources

1. **Ideal voltage source:** It is defined as the energy source which gives constant voltage across its terminals irrespective of load current. The ideal voltage source is having zero internal resistance (Fig. 2.18).

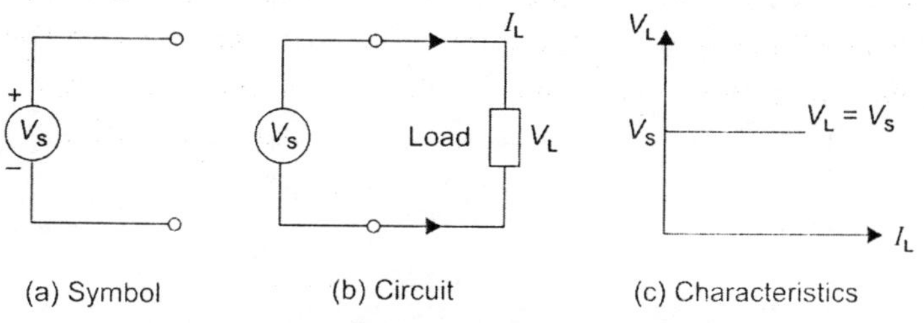

Fig. 2.18: Ideal voltage source

Properties of ideal voltage source

(i) The terminal voltage remains constant irrespective of the load current.

(ii) Voltage regulation is zero.

(iii) The source resistance is zero.

(iv) The power loss taking place in the source is zero.

2. **Practical voltage source:** In practice, an ideal voltage source does not exist. Practically every voltage source has small internal resistance R_{se} connected in series with voltage source as shown in Fig. 2.19.

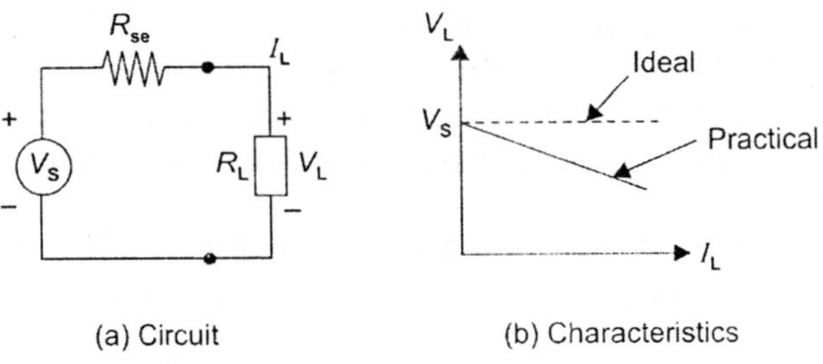

(a) Circuit (b) Characteristics

Fig. 2.19: Practical voltage source

Properties of practical voltage sources

(i) Voltage regulation should be as low as possible.

(ii) Terminal voltage decreases with increase in load current for a nonideal voltage source.

(iii) The source resistance should be as small as possible.

3. **Ideal current source:** Ideal current source is the source which give constant current to the circuit. An ideal current source is having infinite internal resistance (Fig. 2.20).

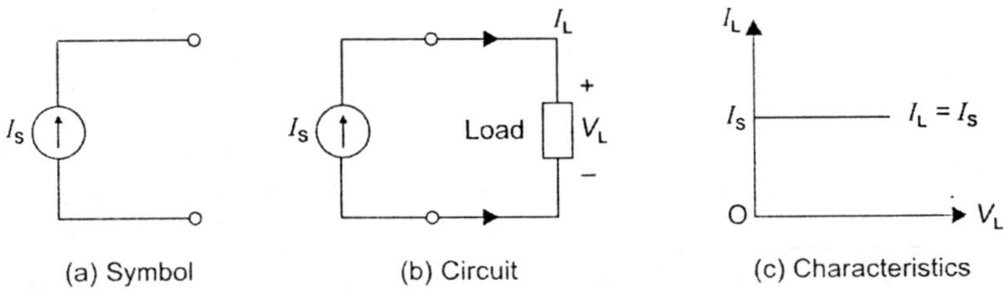

(a) Symbol (b) Circuit (c) Characteristics

Fig. 2.20: Ideal current source

4. **Practical current source:** In practice, an ideal current source does not exist. Practically every current source have high internal resistance connected in parallel with current source (Fig. 2.21).

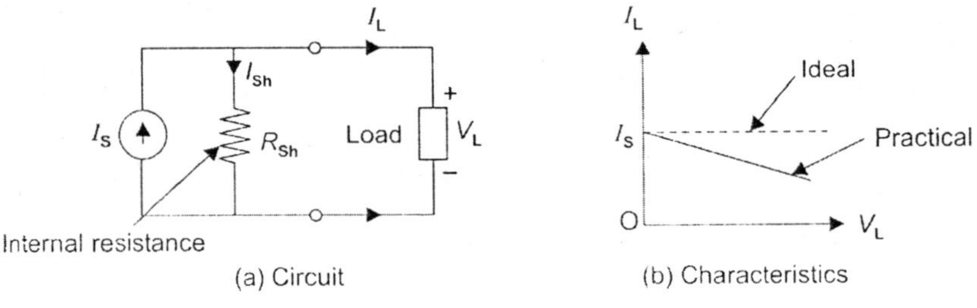

(a) Circuit (b) Characteristics

Fig. 2.21: Practical current source

2.6 CURRENT DIVISION RULE

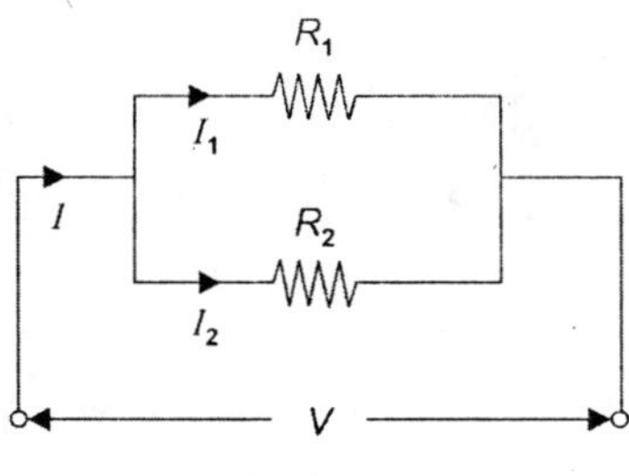

Fig. 2.22

$$I_1 = I \times \left(\frac{R_2}{R_1 + R_2} \right)$$

$$I_2 = I \times \left(\frac{R_1}{R_1 + R_2} \right)$$

2.7 VOLTAGE DIVISION RULE

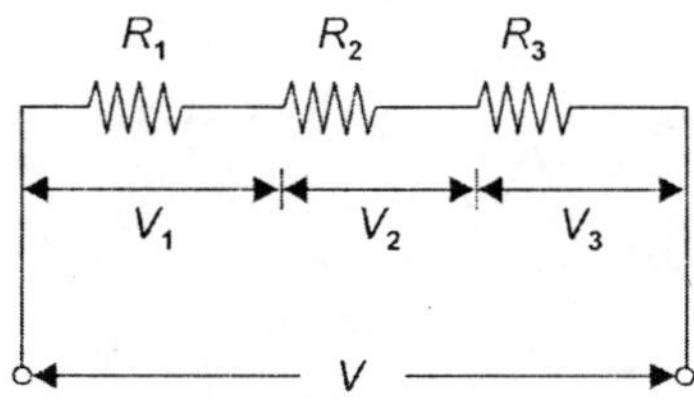

Fig. 2.23

$$V_1 = \frac{V R_1}{R_1 + R_2 + R_3}$$

$$V_2 = \frac{V R_2}{R_1 + R_2 + R_3}$$

$$V_3 = \frac{V R_3}{R_1 + R_2 + R_3}$$

2.8 SOURCE TRANSFORMATION

For the simplification of complex networks the transformation of voltage source to an equivalent current source or vice-versa is often necessary.

Definition of equivalent sources

Two sources are said to be equivalent if they supply the same load current for the same load connected across their terminals.

2.8.1 Transformation of Voltage Source to Current Source

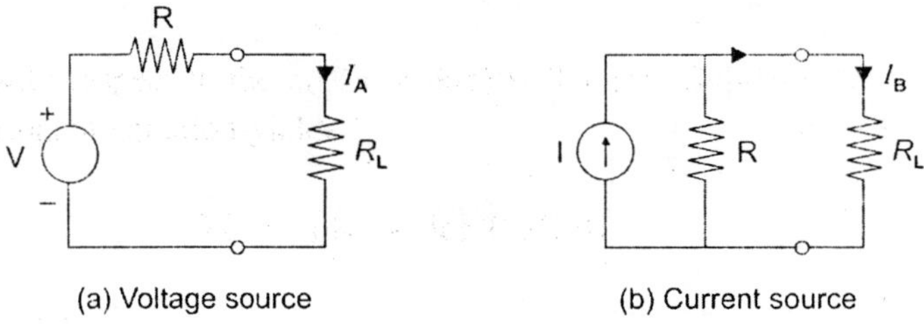

(a) Voltage source (b) Current source

Fig. 2.24

A voltage source in series with resistance R can be represented as current source in parallel with same resistance.

$$\therefore \qquad I = \frac{V}{R}$$

Explanation: The value of current I_A and I_B must be equal for Fig. 2.24.
For Fig. 2.25

$$I_A = \frac{V}{R + R_L}$$

For Fig. 2.25

$$I_B = I\frac{R}{R + R_L} \quad \text{(by current division rule)}$$

$$\therefore \qquad I_A = I_B$$

$$\therefore \qquad V = IR \text{ or } \frac{V}{R + R_L} = I\frac{R}{R + R_L}$$

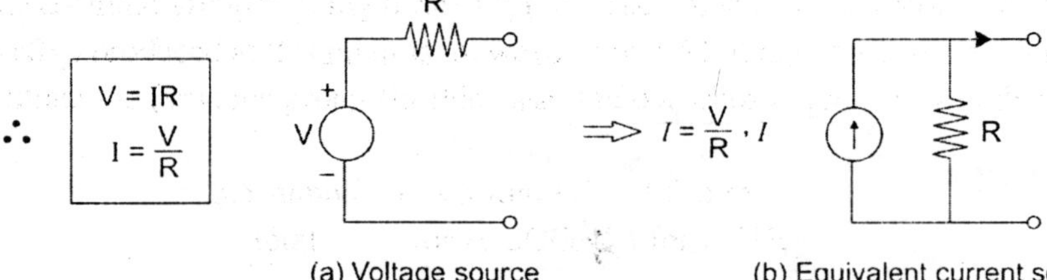

(a) Voltage source (b) Equivalent current source

Fig. 2.25

2.8.2 Transformation of Current Source to Voltage Source

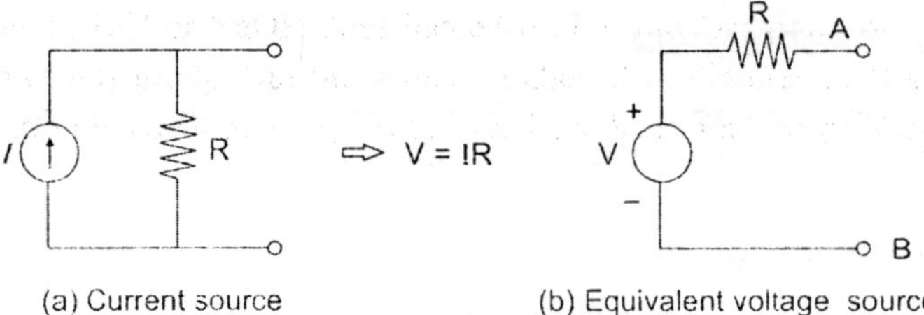

(a) Current source (b) Equivalent voltage source

Fig. 2.26

Example 2.1: Determine the flow of current in 28 Ω resistance by source transformation.

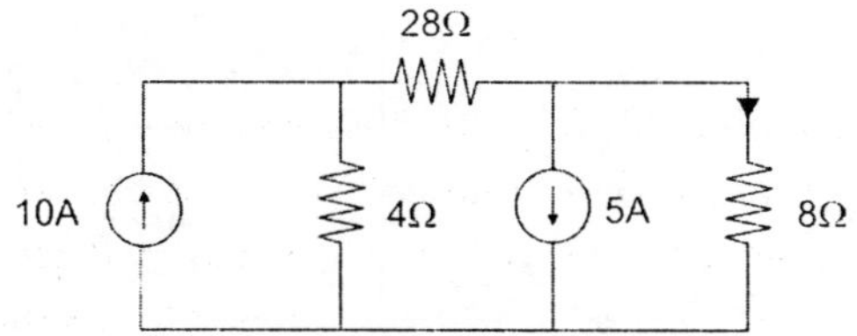

Solution: Step I: We convert 10 A current source to voltage source.

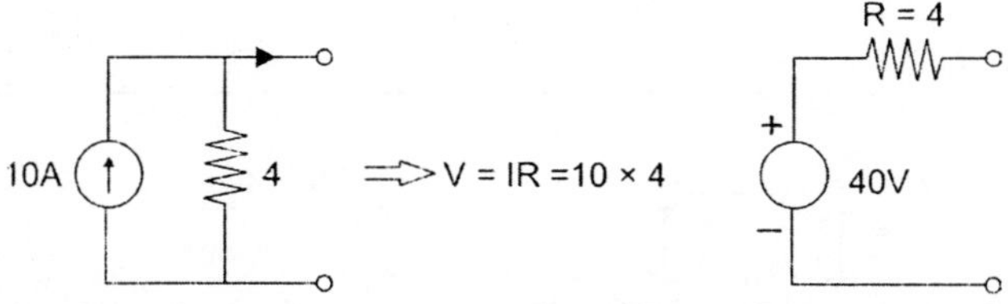

Step II: Convert 5 A current source to voltage source.

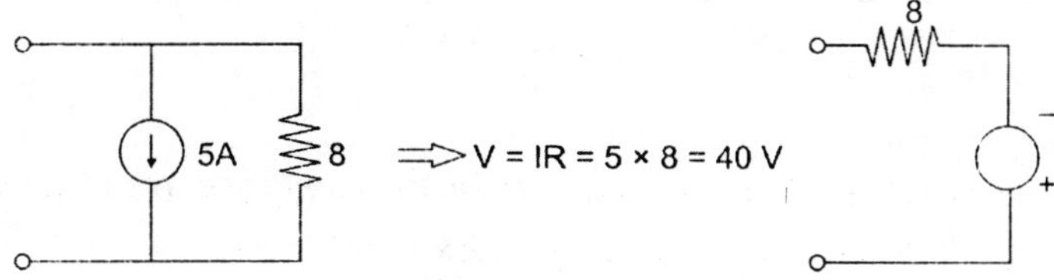

Step III: Joined step I and step II with above figure.

$$\therefore \quad \text{Current through } 28\ \Omega = \frac{40+40}{4+28+8} = \frac{80}{40} = 2\text{ A} \qquad \textbf{Ans.}$$

Example 2.2: Convert the following network into a circuit with one voltage source and one resistance.

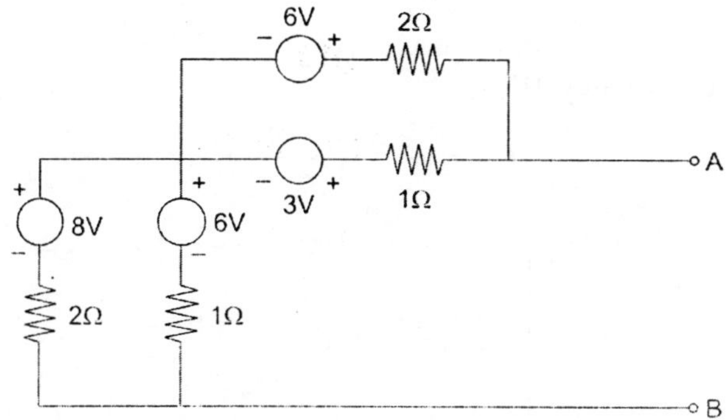

Solution: Step I: For the given figure convert all the voltage source to current source.

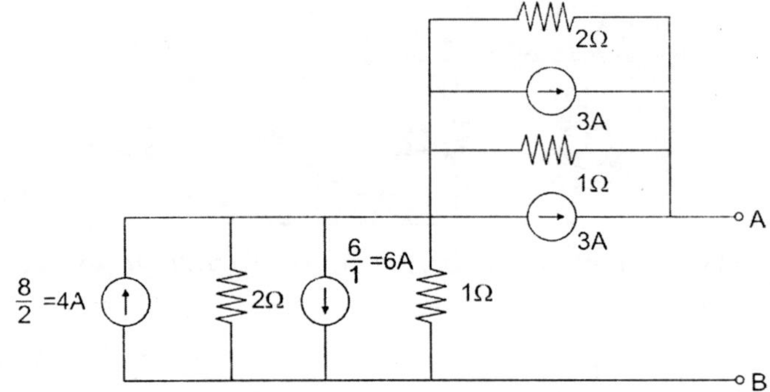

Step II:

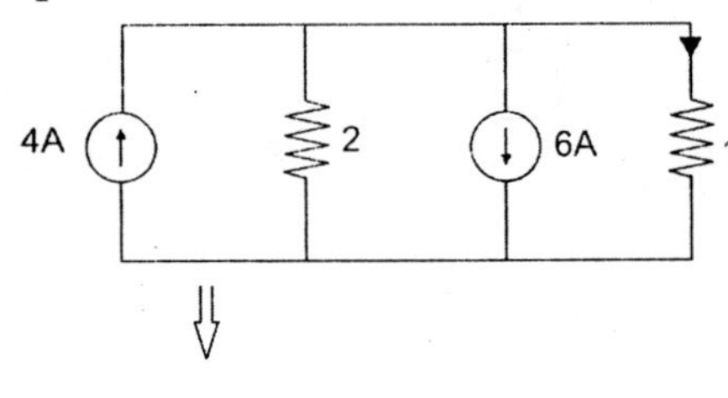

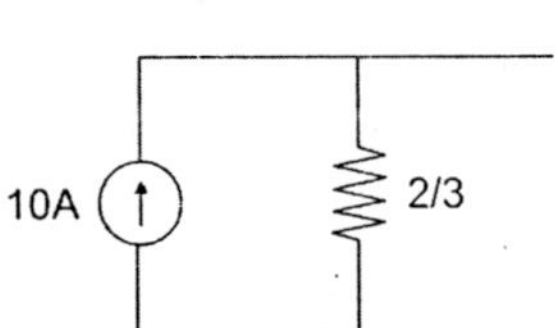

⇒ Both current are in parallal

$\therefore$ 4 + 6 = 10 A

⇒ Both resistance are in parallel

$$\therefore \frac{2 \times 1}{2+1} = \frac{2}{3}$$

Step III: Similarly

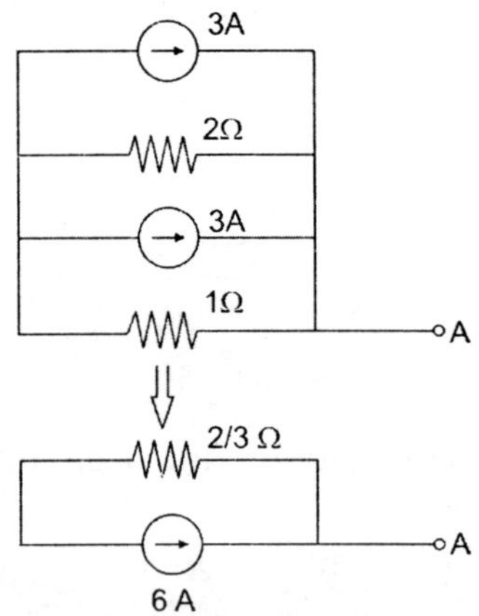

Step IV: From step II and step III

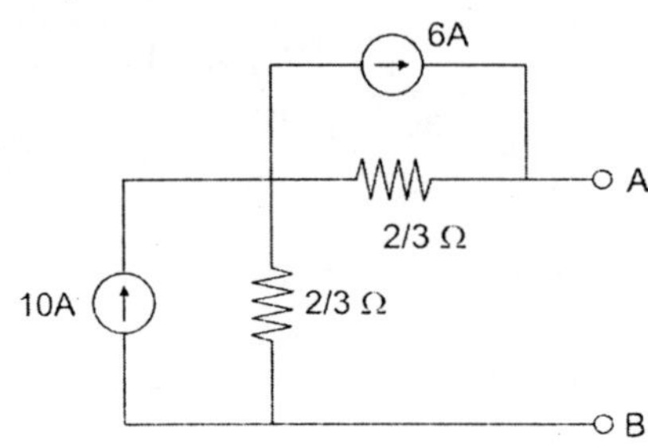

Convert both current source into voltage source.

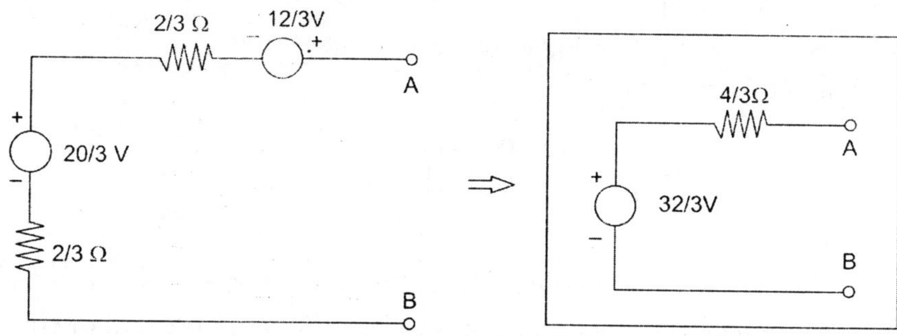

Ans.

Solution of Simultaneous Equation

By Cramer's rule

$$a_1x + b_1y = P \quad ...(2.1)$$

$$a_2x + b_2y = Q \quad ...(2.2)$$

Here x and y are unknown quantities, a_1, a_2, b_1, b_2 are the coefficient of unknown quantities, P and Q are constant.

⇒ In matrix form, this equation may be written as:

$$\begin{vmatrix} a_1 & b_1 \\ a_2 & b_2 \end{vmatrix} \begin{bmatrix} x \\ y \end{bmatrix} = \begin{bmatrix} P \\ Q \end{bmatrix}$$

$$\Delta = \begin{vmatrix} a_1 & b_1 \\ a_2 & b_2 \end{vmatrix} = a_1b_2 - a_2b_1$$

For finding unknown x, replace coefficients of x by constants of equation.

i.e.
$$\Delta_1 = \begin{vmatrix} P & b_1 \\ Q & b_2 \end{vmatrix} = Pb_2 - Qb_1$$

For finding unknown y, replace coefficients of y by constants of equation.

$$\Delta_2 = \begin{vmatrix} a_1 & P \\ a_2 & Q \end{vmatrix} = a_1Q - a_2P$$

∴ Using Cramer's rule

$$x = \frac{\Delta_1}{\Delta} = \frac{Pb_2 - b_1Q}{a_1b_2 - b_1a_2}$$

and
$$y = \frac{\Delta_2}{\Delta} = \frac{a_1Q - Pa_2}{a_1b_2 - b_1a_2}$$

⇒ Let us consider case of three simultaneous equation

$$a_1x + b_1y + c_1z = P \quad ...(2.3)$$

$$a_2x + b_2y + c_2z = Q \quad ...(2.4)$$

$$a_3x + b_3y + c_3z = R \quad ...(2.5)$$

In matrix form, we have

$$\begin{bmatrix} a_1 & b_1 & c_1 \\ a_2 & b_2 & c_2 \\ a_3 & b_3 & c_3 \end{bmatrix} \begin{pmatrix} x \\ y \\ z \end{pmatrix} = \begin{pmatrix} P \\ Q \\ R \end{pmatrix}$$

$$\Delta = \begin{vmatrix} a_1 & b_1 & c_1 \\ a_2 & b_2 & c_2 \\ a_3 & b_3 & c_3 \end{vmatrix}$$

$$\Rightarrow a_1(b_2c_3 - b_3c_2) - a_2(b_1c_3 - c_1b_3) + a_3(b_1c_2 - b_2c_1)$$

Unknown 'x' can be found by replacing coefficient of x by constant of equation

$$\Delta_1 = \begin{vmatrix} P & b_1 & c_1 \\ Q & b_2 & c_2 \\ R & b_3 & c_3 \end{vmatrix}$$

$$\Rightarrow P(b_2c_3 - c_2b_3) - Q(b_1c_3 - c_1b_3) + R(b_1c_2 - c_1b_2)$$

$$\therefore \quad x = \frac{\Delta_1}{\Delta}$$

Similarly for y

$$\Delta_2 = \begin{vmatrix} a_1 & P & c_1 \\ a_2 & Q & c_2 \\ a_3 & R & c_3 \end{vmatrix}$$

$$\Rightarrow a_1(Qc_3 - Rc_2) - a_2(Pc_3 - Rc_1) + a_3(Pc_2 - Qc_1)$$

$$\therefore \quad y = \frac{\Delta_2}{\Delta}$$

and for z

$$\Delta_3 = \begin{vmatrix} a_1 & b_1 & P \\ a_2 & b_2 & Q \\ a_3 & b_3 & R \end{vmatrix}$$

$$\Rightarrow a_1(b_2R - Qb_3) - a_2(b_1R - b_3P) + a_3(b_1Q - b_2P)$$

$$\therefore \quad z = \frac{\Delta_3}{\Delta}$$

2.9 KIRCHHOFF'S LAW'S

In 1847, Kirchhoff gave two fundamental laws which are very useful in electric circuits. These laws are more comprehensive than ohm's law and used for solving electrical network problems which may not be easily solved by the Ohm's law.

2.9.1 Kirchhoff's Current Law (KCL) or First Law

The algebraic sum of all the currents meeting at a junction is zero (Fig. 2.27)

$$\therefore \quad \sum_{i=0}^{n} I_i = 0$$

The current entering in a junction are assigned positive sign and current leaving the junction is assigned a negative sign. Apply KCL at the junction O (Fig. 2.27).

$$I_1 - I_2 + I_3 - I_4 - I_5 = 0$$

$$I_1 + I_3 = I_2 + I_4 + I_5$$

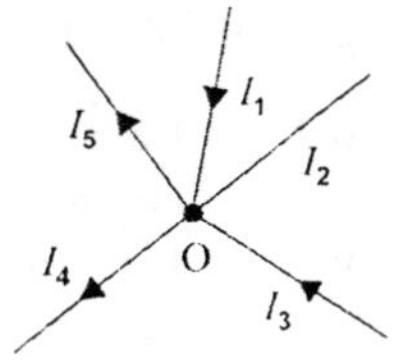

In other words sum of incoming current towards the junction is equal to the sum of outgoing current away from the junction.

Fig. 2.27

$$\therefore \quad I_1 + I_3 = I_2 + I_4 + I_5$$

2.9.2 Kirchhoffs Voltage Law (KVL) or Second Law

Second law is also known as Mesh law. The algebraic sum of voltage (or voltage drops) in any closed path of network that is traversed in a single direction is zero.

$$\therefore \quad \Sigma IR + \Sigma emf = 0$$

Sign conventions: While applying KVL, it is very important to assign a proper sign to emf and voltage drop in the closed circuit.

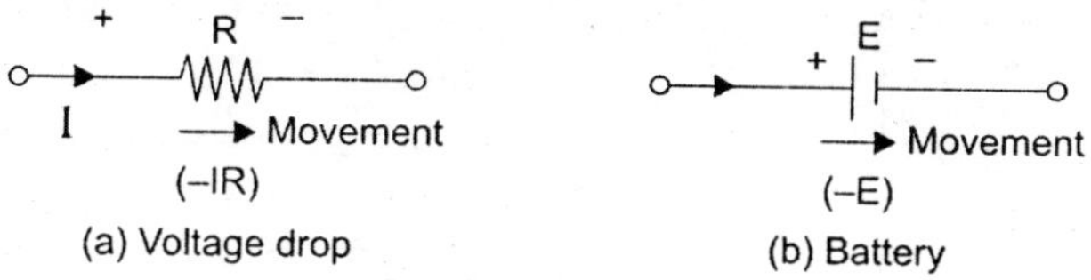

(–IR)

(a) Voltage drop

(–E)

(b) Battery

Fig. 2.28

If we move from positive terminal to negative terminal to resistor than voltage drop should assigned negative sign and vice-versa (Fig. 2.28a), and if we move from positive terminal to negative terminal of battery, the emf should be assigned negative sign and vice-versa (Fig. 2.28b).

Example 2.3: Write the equation of voltage by KVL.

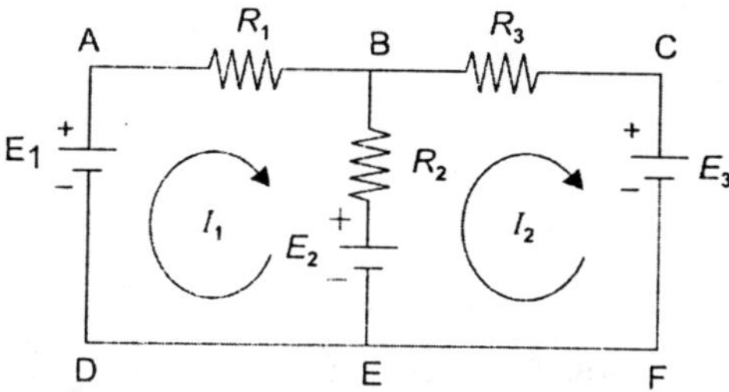

Apply KVL in closed path A – B – E – D – A.

$$E_1 - I_1 R_1 - R_2(I_1 - I_2) - E_2 = 0$$

Apply KVL in closed path B – C – F – E – B.

$$E_2 - R_2(I_2 - I_1) - R_3 I_2 - E_3 = 0$$

2.10 LOOP ANALYSIS OR MESH ANALYSIS

The loop or mesh analysis is based on Kirchhoff's voltage law. It is used to find out unknown currents in the mesh. In this method, each mesh is assigned a separate mesh current and KVL is applied to write mesh equation. The number of mesh equations are equal to the number of meshes in the circuit.

Steps for Solving Problems on Loop Analysis

Step I: Each mesh is assigned a separate mesh current in clockwise direction (usually clockwise direction is convenient).

Step II: Look for any current source, if current source is available, then convert it into voltage source.

Step III: Write KVL equation for each mesh.

Step IV: Solve the equation to find current in each element.

Example 2.4: Find the current in 10 Ω resistance by using mesh analysis.

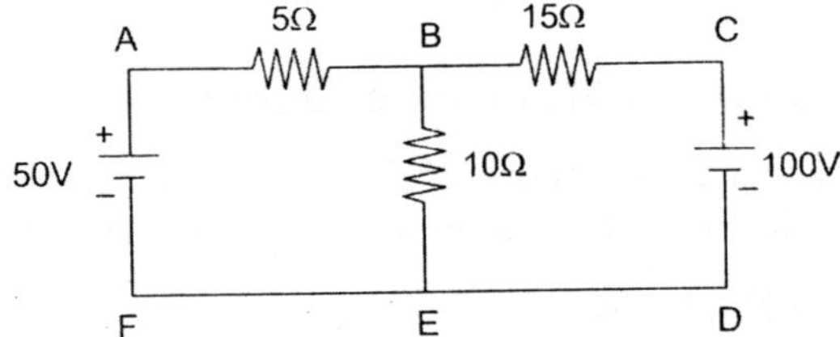

Solution: Step I: In Figure below, there are two meshes in the circuit and current I_1 and I_2 are flowing in clockwise direction.

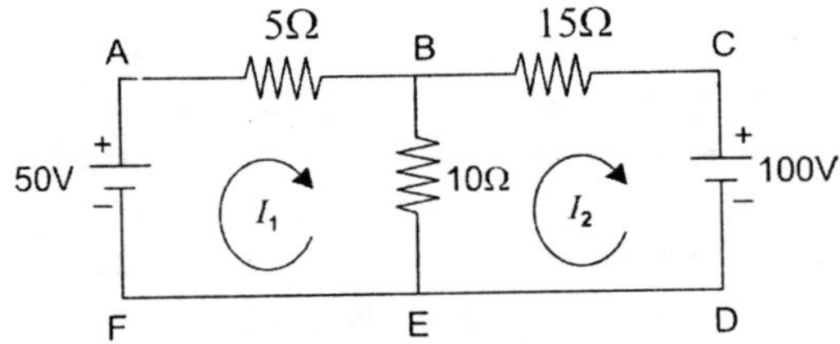

Step II: There is no current source exists in the circuit.

Step III: Apply KVL in mesh ABEFA

$$50 - 5I_1 - 10(I_1 - I_2) = 0$$

$$50 - 5I_1 - 10I_1 + 10I_2 = 0$$

$$15I_1 - 10I_2 = 50 \quad \text{...(2.6)}$$

Apply KVL in mesh BCDEB

$$-10(I_2 - I_1) - 15I_2 - 100 = 0$$

$$-25I_2 + 10I_1 = 100$$

$$10I_1 - 25I_2 = 100 \quad \text{...(2.7)}$$

Step IV: Solving Eqs (2.6) and (2.7), we get,

$$15I_1 - 10I_2 = 50$$

$$10I_1 - 25I_2 = 100$$

$$I_1 = \frac{10}{11} \text{ and } I_2 = -\frac{40}{11}$$

Current in 10 Ω is $I_1 - I_2$

$$I_1 - I_2 = \frac{10}{11} - \left(-\frac{40}{11}\right) = \frac{50}{11} = 4.54 \text{ A}$$

∴ Current in 10 Ω is 4.544 **Ans.**

2.11 NODAL ANALYSIS

The nodal analysis is based on Kirchhoff's current law. In this method, we define the voltage at each node as an independent variable. One of the node is taken as a reference node. Whose potential is assumed to be zero. It is also called as *zero potential node* or *datum node*. At other nodes the different voltages are measured with respect to the reference node. The reference node should be given a number zero and then the equation are to be written for all other nodes by applying KCL. The advantage of this method lies in the fact that we get $(n - 1)$ equation to solve if there are 'n' nodes.

Example 2.5: Find the branch current of the network in the given figure.

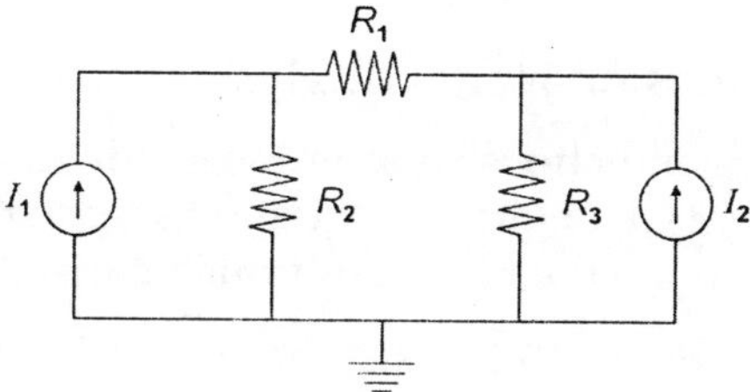

Solution:

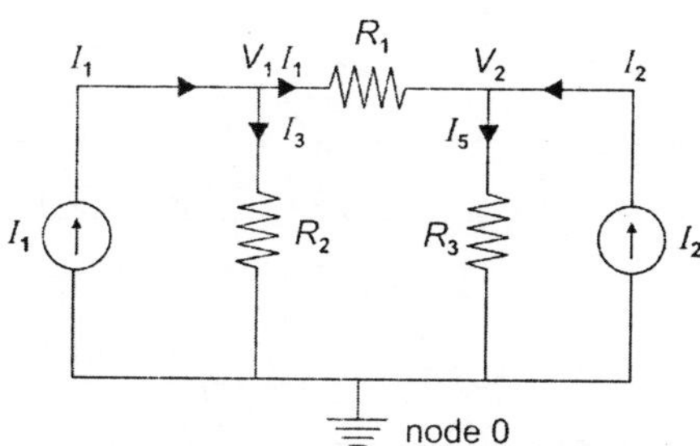

Let voltages at nodes 1 and 2 be V_1 and V_2 respectively.
Mark various branch current as shown in the above figure.
Now applying KCL at **node 1**

$$I_1 = I_3 + I_4 = \frac{V_1}{R_2} + \frac{V_1 - V_2}{R_1}$$

Applying KCL at node 2

$$I_2 + I_4 = I_5$$

$$I_2 + \frac{V_1 - V_2}{R_1} = \frac{V_2}{R_3}$$

As I_1 and I_2 are known, we get two equations with the two unknown V_1 and V_2 solving these equation simultaneously, the node voltage V_1 and V_2 can be determined.

Once V_1 and V_2 are known, current through any branch of the network can be determined.

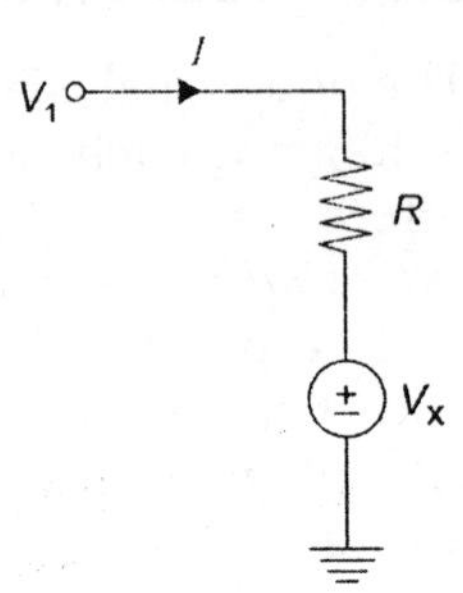

Note: If there exist a voltage source in any of the branches as shown in figure. Then that must be considered while writing the equation for current through the branch.

Now V_1 is at higher potential with respect to V_x, because current always flows from higher potential to lower potential.

So in such a case, equation of current becomes $I = \frac{V_1 - V_x}{R}$.

If the direction of current I is assumed entering the node then it is assumed that V_x is higher potential than V_1 and hence equation for current becomes

$$I = \frac{V_x - V_1}{R}$$

Steps for Solving Problems on Nodal Analysis

Identity the various nodes and choose a reference node (usually, the common node is the reference node). Using KCL determine equation at each node. Solve these equations to get node voltage. Determine the required branch current.

Example 2.6: Find the current in 10 Ω resistance by nodal analysis method.

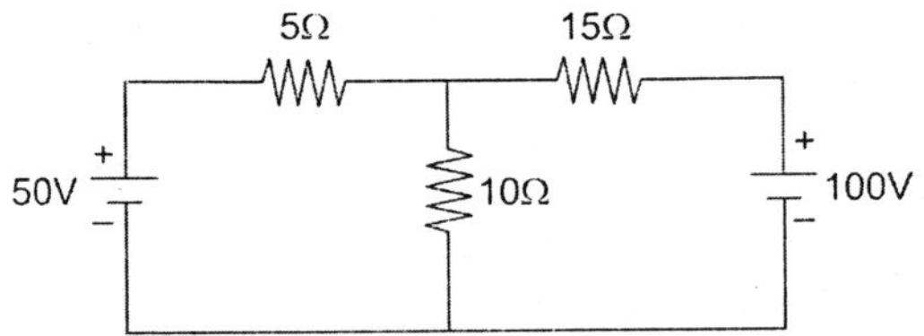

Solution:

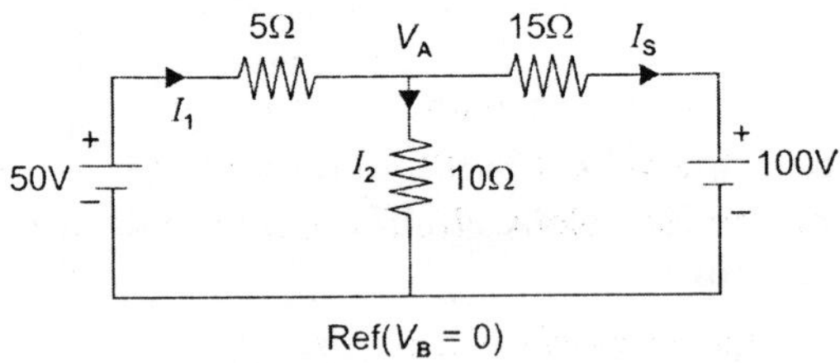

Step I: There are two nodes (A and B), V_A and V_B are corresponding voltage at node A and B we can choose node B as reference node because $V_B = 0$ as it is grounded.

Step II: By using KCL at node A

$$I_1 = I_2 + I_3$$

$$\frac{50 - V_A}{5} = \frac{V_A}{10} + \frac{V_A - 100}{15}$$

$$50 - V_A = \frac{V_A}{2} + \frac{V_A - 100}{3}$$

$$300 - 6\,V_A = 3V_A + 2V_A - 200$$

$$500 - 11\,V_A = 0$$

Step III: Now the node voltage is given by

$$500 = 11\, V_A$$

$$\therefore \qquad V_A = \frac{500}{11} \text{ volts}$$

Step IV: The current in 10 Ω is, $I_2 = \frac{V_A}{10}$

$$\therefore \qquad I_2 = \frac{500}{11 \times 10} = \frac{50}{11}$$

∴ Current in 10Ω is 4.53 A.

2.12 STAR-DELTA TRANSFORMATION

There are some network in which resistors are neither connected in series nor in parallel such as star-delta network. In such situation, it is not possible to simplify the network by series and parallel circuit rules. However, such network can be simplified by using star-delta and delta-star transformation techniques.

Star connection (Y): If the three resistors are connected in such a manner that one end of each is connected together to form a junction point called star point, the resistors are said to be connected in star as shown in Fig. 2.29.

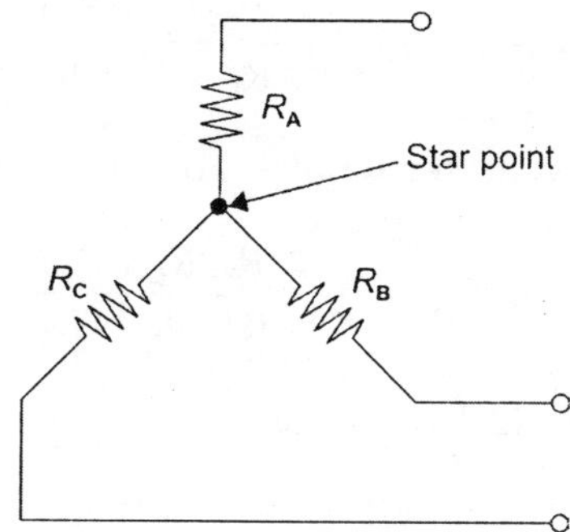

Fig. 2.29: Star-connection

Delta connection (Δ): If the three resistor are connected in such a manner that starting end of one is connected to terminating end of other to form a closed-loop is called delta connection as shown in Fig. 2.30.

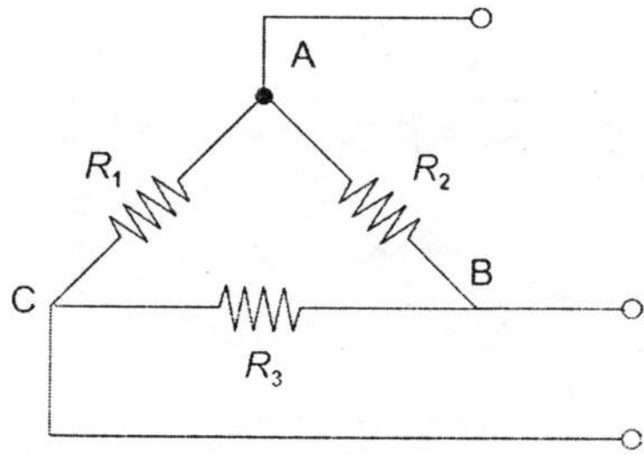

Fig. 2.30: Delta-connection

2.12.1 Network Reduction by Delta-Star and Star-Delta Transformation

For Delta to Star

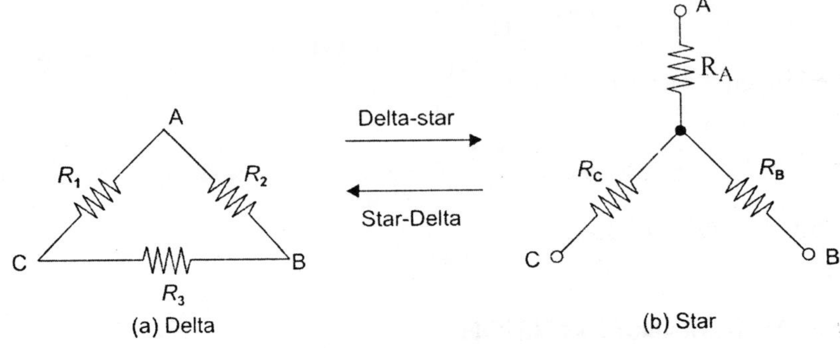

(a) Delta (b) Star

Fig. 2.31

Equate the resistance between terminal B and C

$$R_{BC} = R_B + R_C = \frac{R_3(R_1 + R_2)}{R_1 + R_2 + R_3} \quad ...(2.8)$$

Equate the resistance between terminal C and A

$$R_{CA} = R_C + R_A = \frac{R_1(R_2 + R_3)}{R_1 + R_2 + R_3} \quad ...(2.9)$$

Equate the resistance between terminal A and B

$$R_{AB} = R_A + R_B = \frac{R_2(R_1 + R_3)}{R_1 + R_2 + R_3} \quad ...(2.10)$$

Adding Eqs (2.8), (2.9) and (2.10), we get

$$2(R_A + R_B + R_C) = \frac{2(R_1R_2 + R_2R_3 + R_3R_1)}{(R_1 + R_2 + R_3)}$$

$$\therefore \quad R_A + R_B + R_C = \frac{R_1R_2 + R_2R_3 + R_3R_1}{R_1 + R_2 + R_3} \quad ...(2.11)$$

Substracting Eqs (2.8), (2.9), and (2.10) from Eq. (2.11), we get

$$\therefore \quad R_A = \frac{R_1R_2}{R_1 + R_2 + R_3} \quad ...(2.12)$$

$$R_B = \frac{R_2R_3}{R_1 + R_2 + R_3} \quad ...(2.13)$$

$$R_C = \frac{R_3R_1}{R_1 + R_2 + R_3} \quad ...(2.14)$$

For Star to Delta

Multiplying Eqs (2.12) and (2.13), (2.13) and (2.14) and (2.14) and (2.12) and then adding them, we get,

$$\therefore \quad R_A R_B + R_B R_C + R_C R_A = \frac{R_1 R_2^2 R_3 + R_1 R_3^2 R_2 + R_1^2 R_2 R_3}{(R_1 + R_2 + R_3)^2}$$

$$R_A R_B + R_B R_C + R_C R_A = \frac{R_1 R_2 R_3 (R_1 + R_2 + R_3)}{(R_1 + R_2 + R_3)^2}$$

$$\therefore \quad R_A R_B + R_B R_C + R_C R_A = \frac{R_1 R_2 R_3}{R_1 + R_2 + R_3} \qquad \text{...(2.15)}$$

Dividing Eq. (2.15) by Eqs (2.12), (2.13), and (2.14), separately, we get

$$R_3 = \frac{R_A R_B + R_B R_C + R_C R_A}{R_A} = R_B + R_C + \frac{R_B R_C}{R_A} \qquad \text{...(2.16)}$$

$$R_1 = \frac{R_A R_B + R_B R_C + R_C R_A}{R_B} = R_A + R_C + \frac{R_A R_C}{R_B} \qquad \text{...(2.17)}$$

$$R_2 = \frac{R_A R_B + R_B R_C + R_C R_A}{R_C} = R_A + R_B + \frac{R_A R_B}{R_C} \qquad \text{...(2.18)}$$

Converting Delta to Star

$$R_A = \frac{R_1 R_2}{R_1 + R_2 + R_3};$$

$$R_B = \frac{R_2 R_3}{R_1 + R_2 + R_3};$$

$$R_C = \frac{R_3 R_1}{R_1 + R_2 + R_3}$$

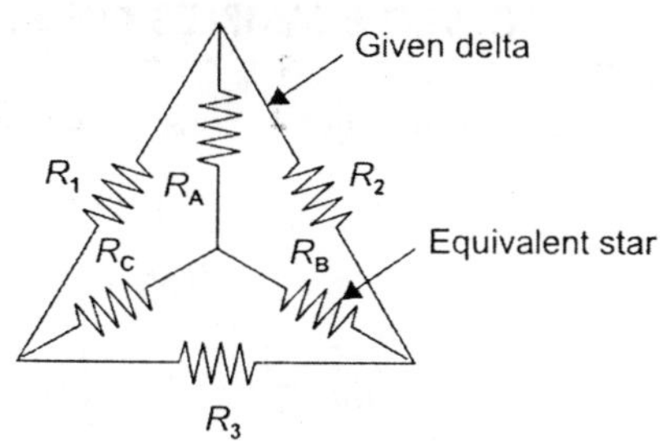

Fig. 2.32

Example 2.7: If all resistance in a delta connection have same magnitude say *R*, then its equivalent star will contain. What will be the magnitude of its equivalent star connection, if all resistances in a delta connection have the same magnitude *R*.

Solution: (i) $R_A = R_B = R_C = \dfrac{R \times R}{R_1 + R_2 + R_3} = \dfrac{R}{3}$

It means equivalent star contains three equal resistance, each of magnitude one third the magnitude of the resistance connected in delta.

(ii) Star to delta

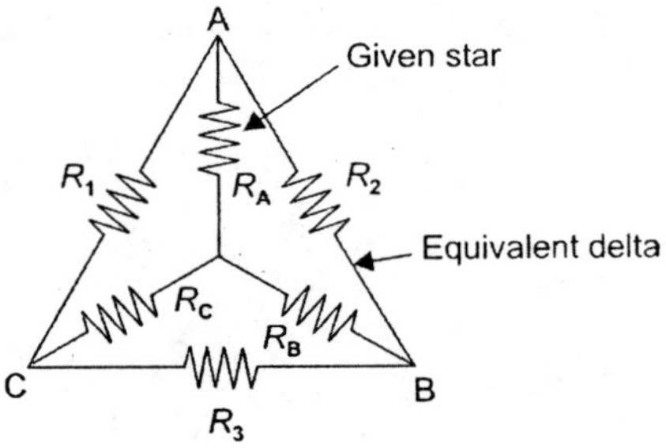

$$R_1 = \frac{R_A R_B + R_B R_C + R_C R_A}{R_B}$$

$$R_2 = \frac{R_A R_B + R_B R_C + R_C R_A}{R_C}$$

$$R_3 = \frac{R_A R_B + R_B R_C + R_C R_A}{R_A}$$

Example 2.8: If all the three resistances in a star connection are of same magnitude say R, then what will be the magnitude of its equivalent delta connection, if all three resistances in a star connection are *d* same magnitude *Q*.

Solution:

$$\therefore \quad R_1 = R_2 = R_3 = \frac{R \times R + R \times R + R \times R}{R} = 3R$$

It means equivalent delta contains three resistance each of magnitude thrice the magnitude of resistance connected in star.

SOLVED EXAMPLES ON SOURCE TRANSFORMATION

Example 1: Find the voltage across 4 Ω resistance by source transformation shown in figure.

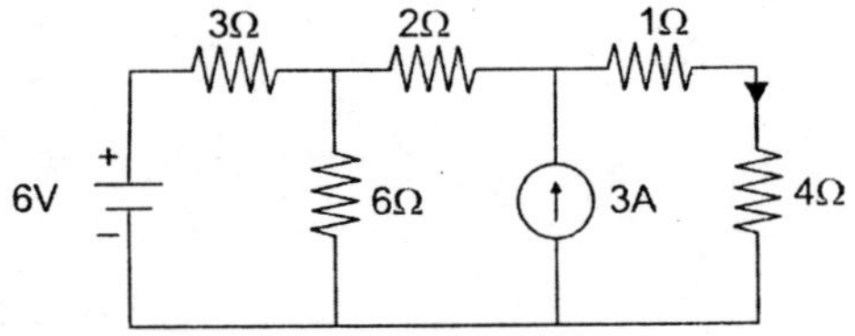

Solution: Step I: Convert the 6 V source into current source and draw the circuit.

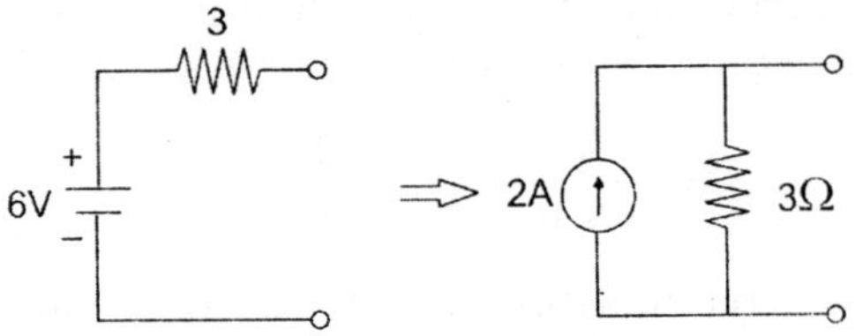

Conversion

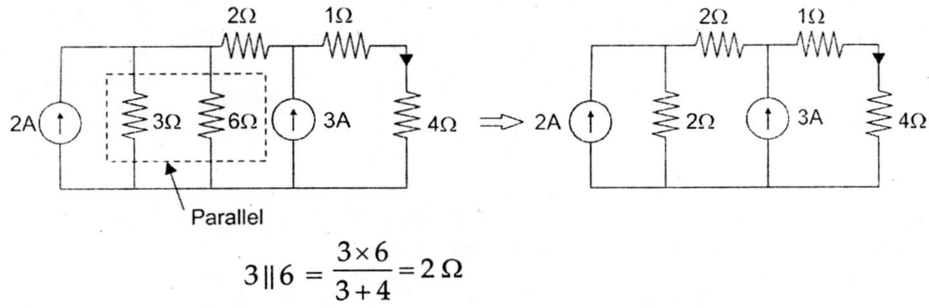

$$3 \| 6 = \frac{3\times 6}{3+4} = 2\ \Omega$$

Step II: Convert 2 A source to voltage source.

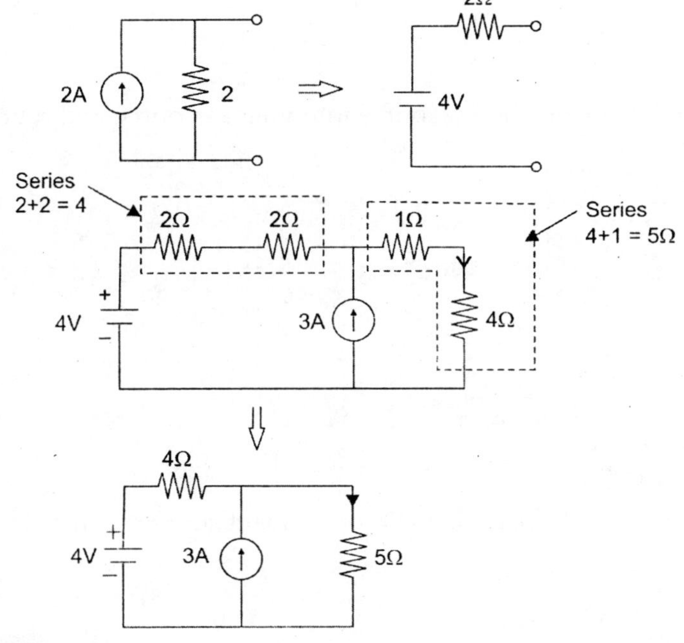

Step III: Convert the 4 V source to current source.

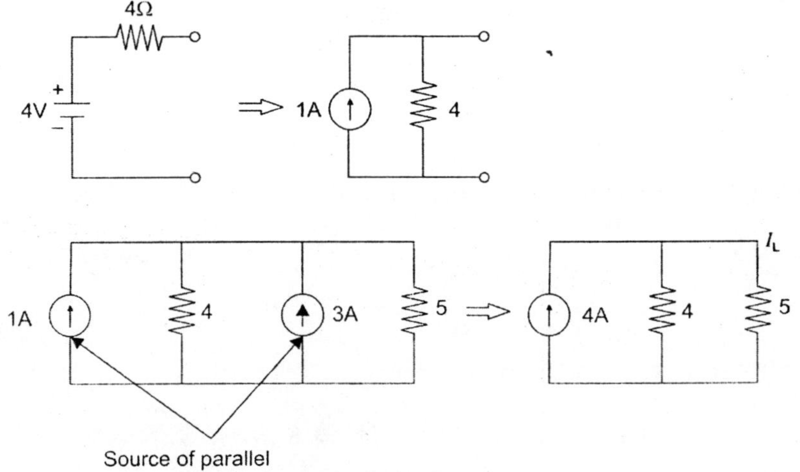

$\therefore \quad 1 + 3 = 4$ A

$$I_L = \frac{4 \times 4}{5 + 4} = \frac{16}{9}$$

$$\therefore \quad V_L = 4 \times I_L = 4 \times \frac{16}{9} = \frac{64}{9} \text{ volts}$$

Example 2: Reduce the circuit shown in figure into a single voltage source in series with single resistance using source transformation.

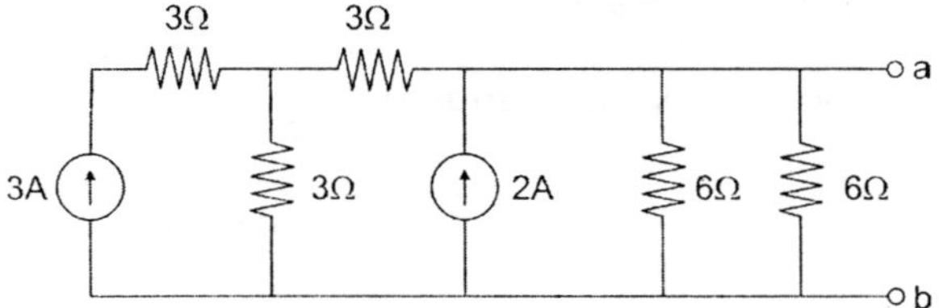

Solution: Step I: Convert the 3A source into voltage source and redraw the circuit.

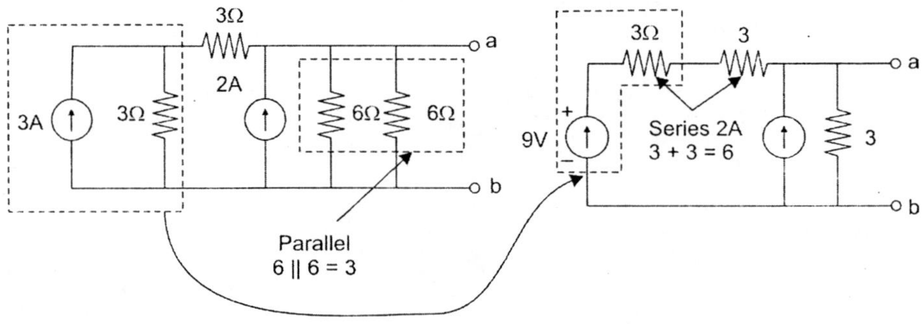

Step II: Now convert the 9 V source into a current sources and redraw.

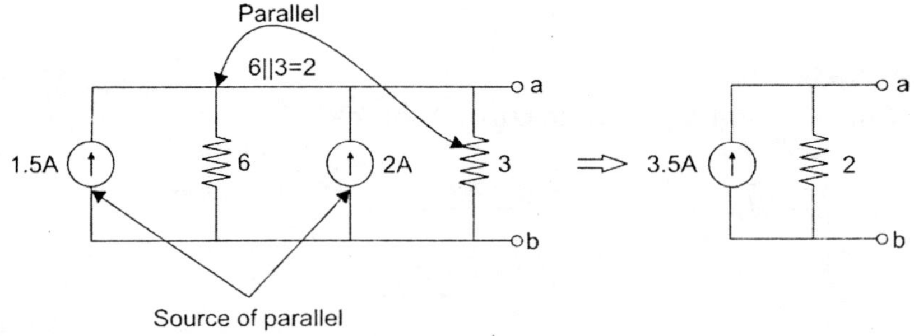

Step III: Finally convert the 3.5 A current source into a voltage source.

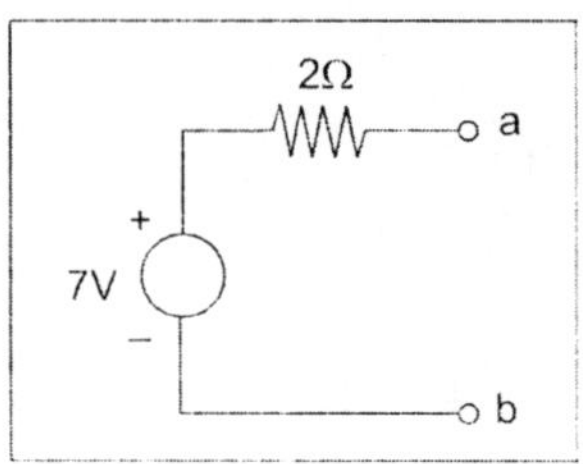

Example 3: Using source a transformation, convert the given circuit into a single source circuit at terminal ab.

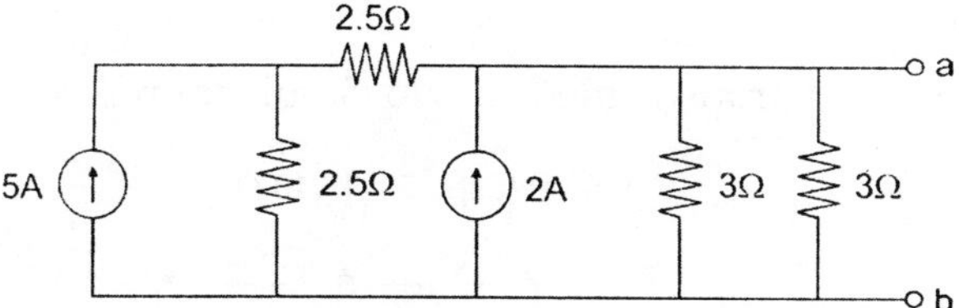

Solution: Step I: As shown in the figure below, two source transformations need to be applied along with network reduction of 3||3.

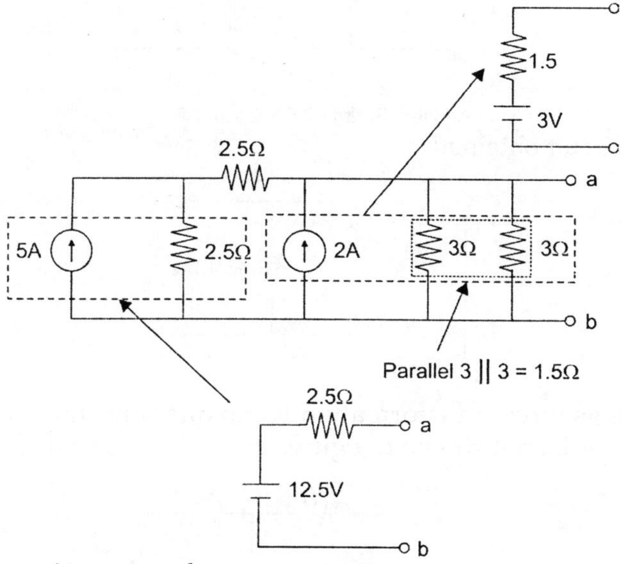

Step II: After transformation the circuit obtained as

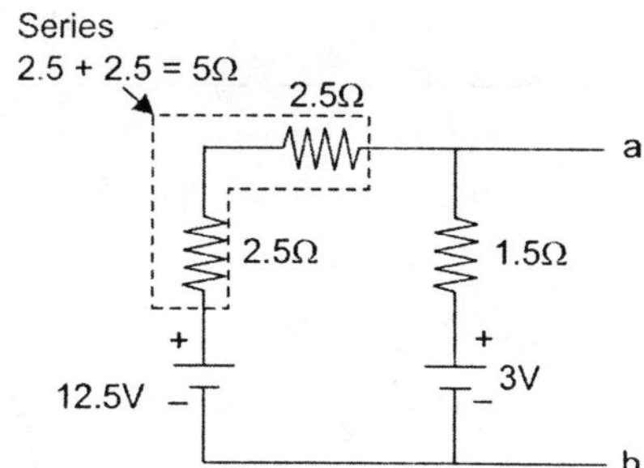

Step III: Combine 2.5 Ω and 2.5 Ω as series resistance to give $(2.5+2.5)\Omega = 5\,\Omega$ in series with 12.5 V source.

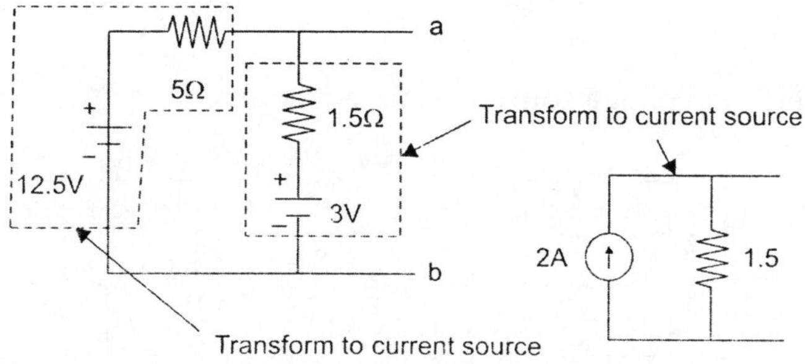

Step IV: 2.5A 5

Two voltage source are transformed to two circuit source.

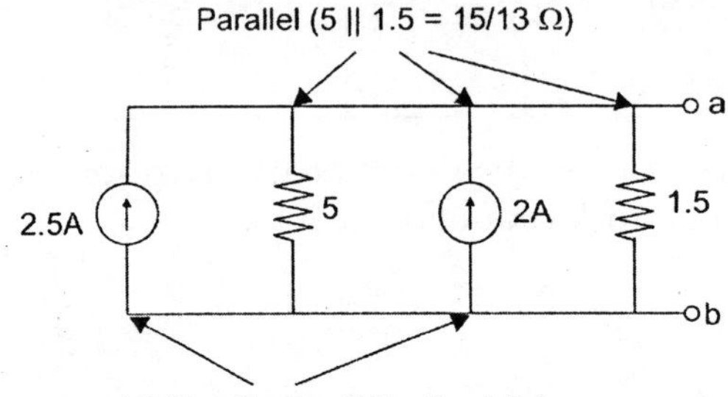

Step V: Final circuit obtained

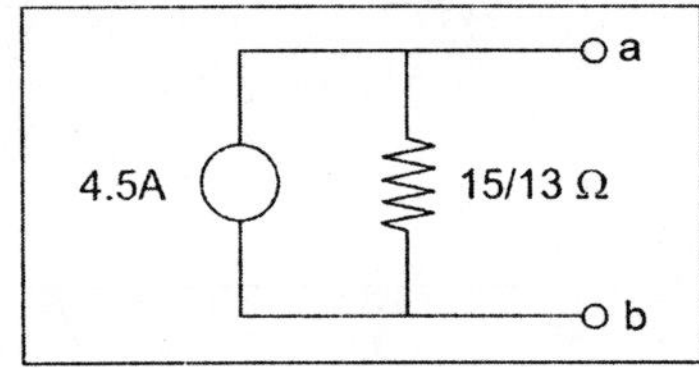

Example 4: Using source transformation technique, find the current through load resistance R_L of the circuit shown in figure.

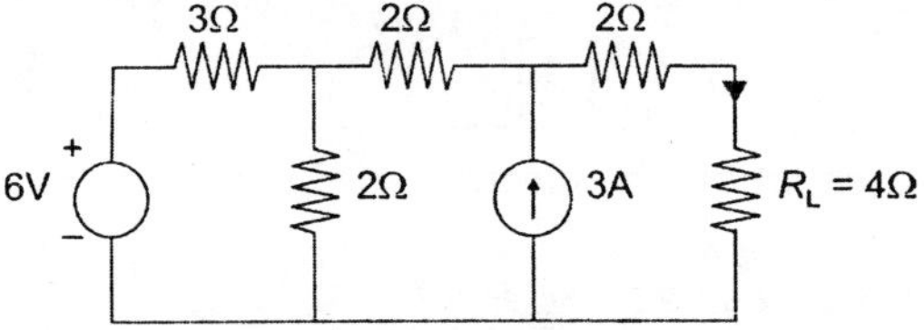

Solution:

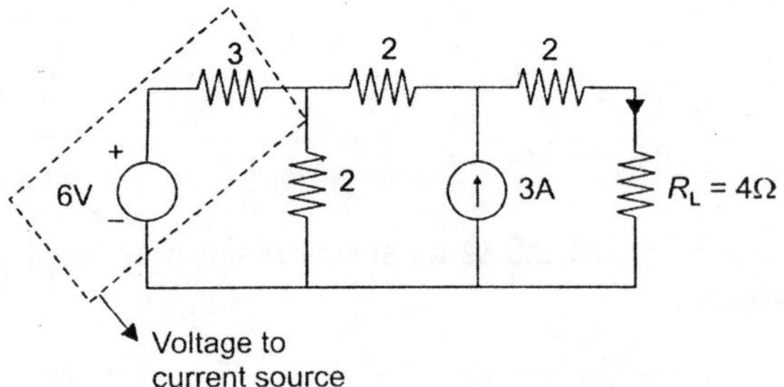

Step I: Convert the voltage source to current source.

$$I = \frac{V}{R} = \frac{6}{3} = 2A$$

Redraw the above circuit figure.

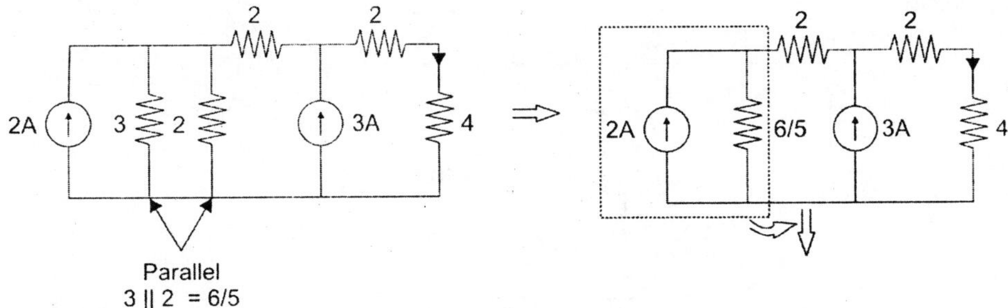

Convert the current source to voltage sources.

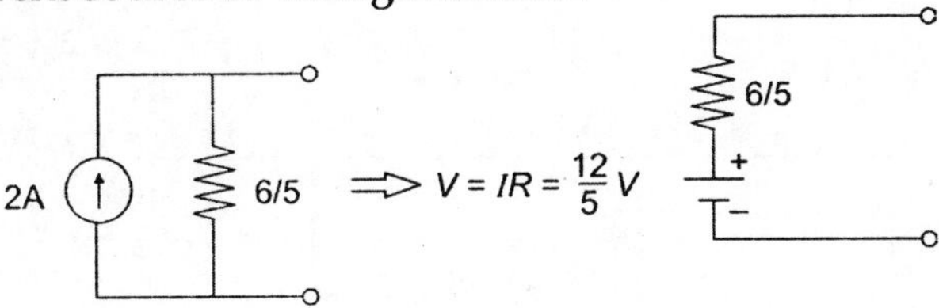

Above figure becomes

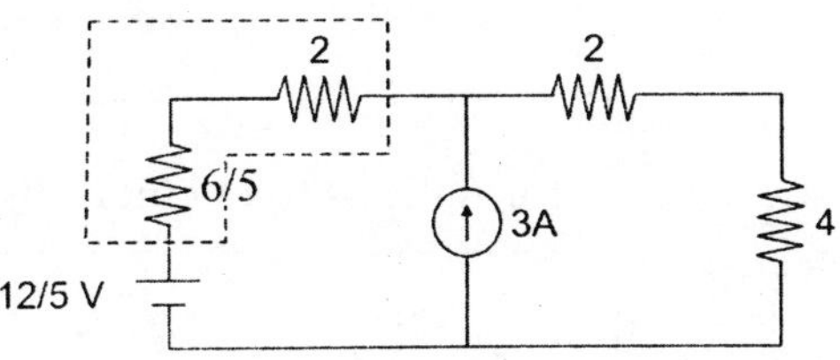

Again convert voltage source to current source.

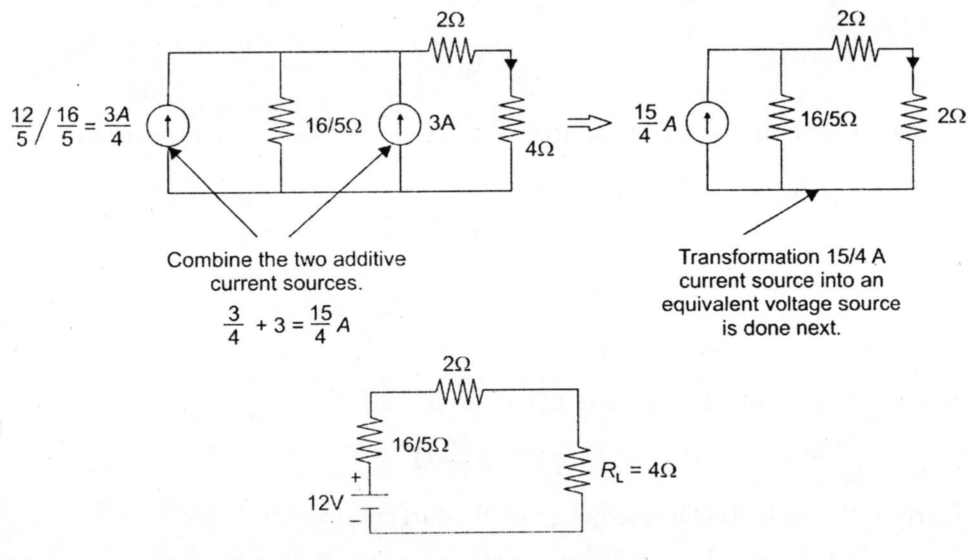

Current through 4 Ω is $I = \dfrac{12}{\dfrac{16}{5} + 2 + 4} = 1.303 \text{ A}$ **Ans.**

Example 5: Using the source transformation, find the voltage *V* in the circuit shown in figure below.

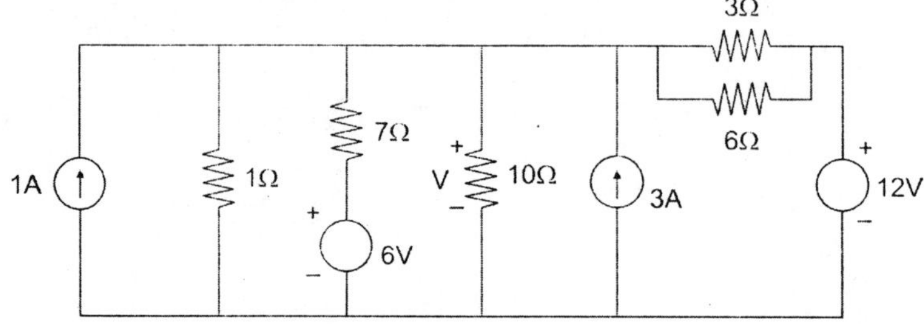

Solution: Step I: Apply circuit reduction in by combining parallel resistance of 3 Ω and 6 Ω as shown in figure.

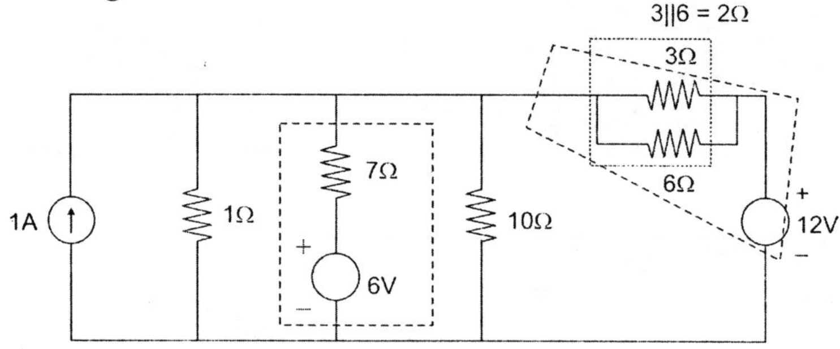

Step II: Apply two source transformations to circuit of figure.

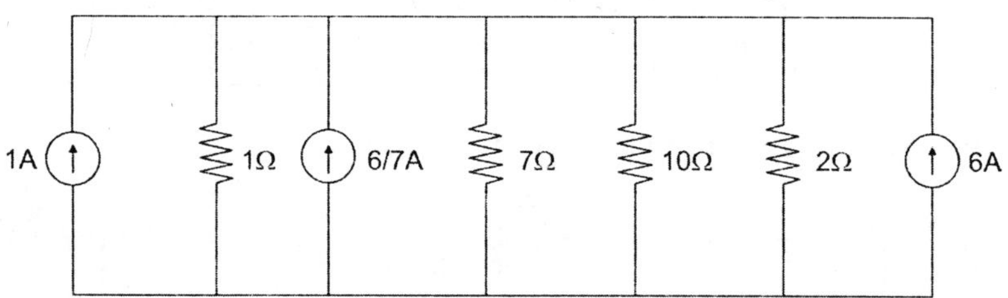

Step III: Combine the current source 1A, $\frac{6}{7}$A, 6A into a single current source of value $= 1 + \frac{6}{7} + 6 = \frac{55}{7}$A.

I_2
I
$\frac{55}{7}$ A
Req = $\frac{14}{23}$ Ω
+ V –
10Ω

Also, resistance of 1 Ω, 7 Ω and 2 Ω are in parallel.

i.e.,
$$R_{eq} = 1 \,||\, 7 \,||\, 2 = \frac{14}{23}\,\Omega.$$

Current through 10 Ω branch is given by current division rules.

∴ Here
$$I_2 = \frac{55}{7}\left(\frac{\frac{14}{23}}{\frac{14}{23} + 10}\right)$$

i.e. $I_2 = 0.4508$ Amperes.

Thus, voltage

$$V = 10I_2 = 10 \times 0.4508 = 4.508 \text{ volts}$$

SOLVED EXAMPLES ON KVL AND KCL (LOOP, MESH AND NODAL)

Example 1: Write and solve the node voltage equation for the circuit shown in figure. Find the current through 5 Ω resistance.

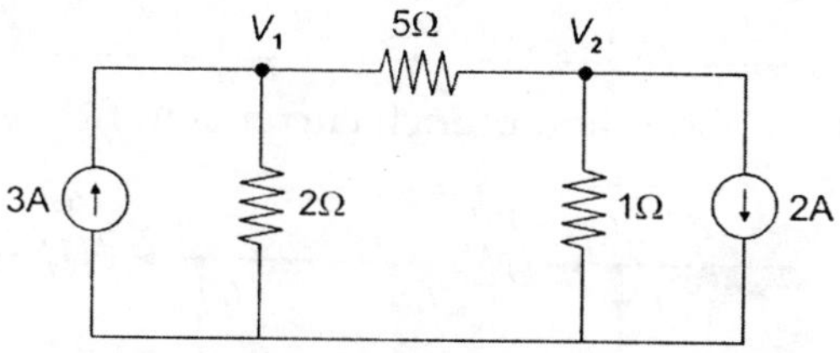

Solution: Step I: Redraw the circuit mark current in each branch.

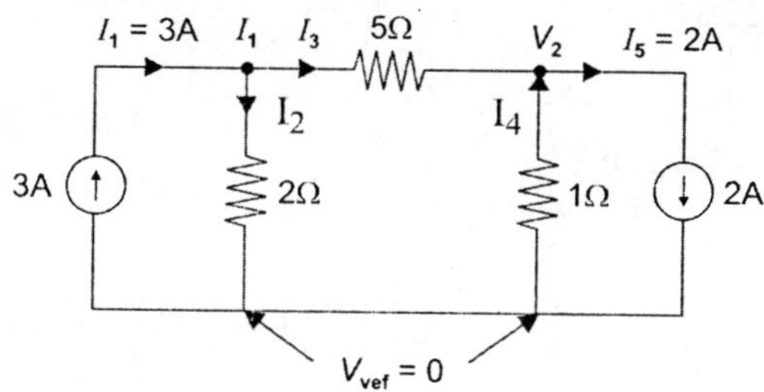

Step II: Apply KCL at node 1

$$I_1 = I_2 + I_3$$

$$3 = \frac{V_1}{2} + \frac{V_1 - V_2}{5} = \frac{5V_1 + 2(V_1 - V_2)}{10}$$

$\therefore$ $$30 = 7V_1 - 2V_2 \;\therefore 7V_1 - 2V_2 = 30 \quad \text{...(1)}$$

Step III: Apply KCL at node 2

$$I_3 = I_4 + I_5$$

$$\frac{V_1 - V_2}{5} = \frac{V_2}{1} + 2$$

$\therefore$ $$V_1 - V_2 = 5(V_2 + 2)$$

$\therefore$ $$V_1 - 6V_2 = 10$$

$\therefore$ $$V_1 = (10 + 6V_2) \quad \text{...(2)}$$

Solving Eqs (1) and (2), we get

$$V_1 = 4 \text{ and } V_2 = 1$$

$\therefore$ Current through 5 Ω resistance is

$$I_2 = \frac{V_1 - V_2}{5} = \frac{4-(-1)}{5} = 1 \text{ A}$$ **Ans.**

Example 2: Find current through 2 Ω and 3 Ω resistance using nodal analysis in the circuit shown in figure. **[UPTU 2006-07]**

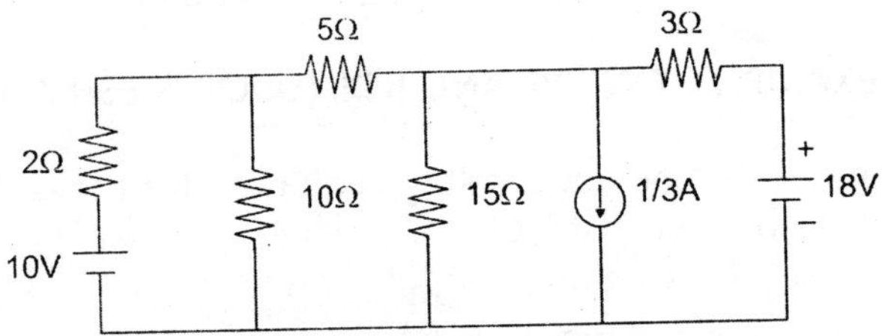

Solution: Step I: Mark nodes and branch currents in figure below.

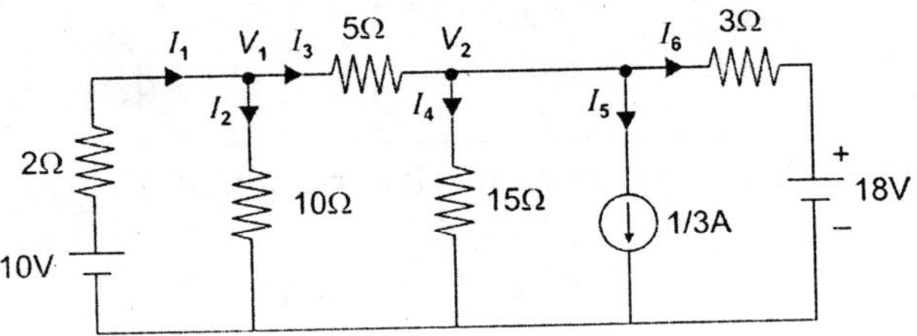

Step II: Apply KCL at node 1.

$$I_1 = I_2 + I_3$$

$$\therefore \quad \frac{10-V_1}{2} = \frac{V_1}{10} + \frac{V_1 - V_2}{5}, \quad 5(10-V_1) = V_1 + 2(V_1 - V_2)$$

$$8V_1 - 2V_2 = 50$$

$$\therefore \quad 4V_1 - V_2 = 25 \qquad \text{...(1)}$$

Step III: Apply KCL at node 2.

$$I_3 = I_4 + I_5 + I_6$$

$$\therefore \quad \frac{V_1 - V_2}{5} = \frac{V_2}{15} + \frac{1}{3} + \frac{V_2 - 18}{3}$$

$$\therefore \quad 3V_1 - 9V_2 = -85 \qquad \text{...(2)}$$

Step IV: Solving Eqs (1) and (2),we get

$$V_1 = 9.394V \text{ and } V_2 = 12.58 \text{ volt}$$

Current through 2 Ω is

$$I_1 = \frac{10 - V_1}{2} = \frac{10 - 9.394}{2} = \mathbf{0.303\ A}$$ **Ans.**

Current through 3 Ω is

$$I_6 = \frac{V_2 - 18}{3} = \frac{12.58 - 18}{3} = -1.807 \text{ A}$$

$$\therefore \quad I_6 = \mathbf{-1.807\ A}$$ **Ans.**

Example 3: Two batteries A and B are connected in parallel to a load of 10 Ω Battery A has an emf of 12 V and an internal resistance of 2 Ω and battery B has an emf of 10 V and internal resistance of 1 Ω. Using nodal analysis, determine the current supplied by each battery and load current. **[UPTU 2003-04, 06]**

Solution: Step 1: Draw circuit diagram according to given data.

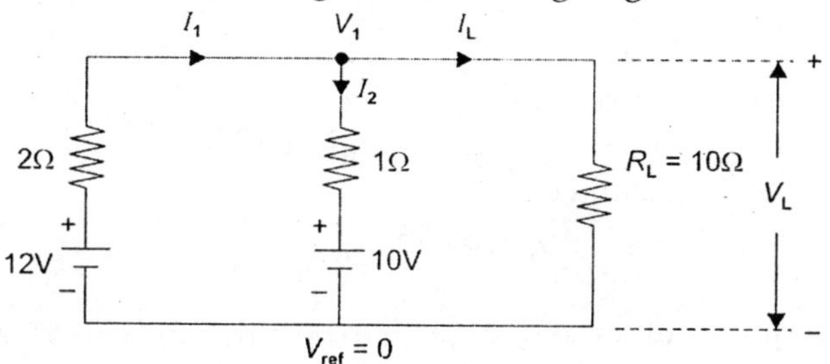

Step II: Find current I_1, I_2 and I_L.
Apply KCL at node 1

$$I_1 = I_2 + I_L$$

$$\therefore \quad \frac{12 - V_1}{2} = \frac{V_1 - 10}{1} + \frac{V_1}{10}$$

$$32 - 3V_1 = 0.2V_1 \quad \text{...(1)}$$

Solving Eq. (1), we get

$$\therefore \quad V_1 = 10\,V$$

$$I_1 = \frac{12 - V_1}{2} = \frac{12 - 10}{2} = 1\text{ A} \quad \textbf{Ans.}$$

$$I_2 = \frac{V_1 - 10}{1} = \frac{10 - 10}{1} = 0\text{ A} \quad \textbf{Ans.}$$

$$I_L = \frac{V_1}{10} = \frac{10}{10} = 1\text{ A} \quad \textbf{Ans.}$$

Example 4: For the circuit shown in figure, find voltage of node A and B and determine current in 8 Ω resistor. **[Sem-II, 03-04-05]**

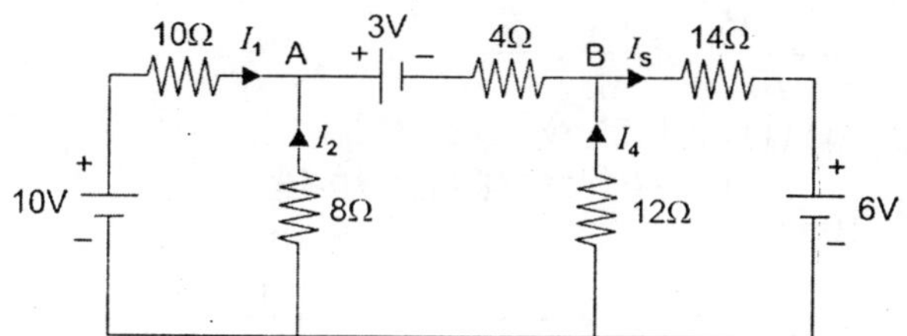

Solution: Step I: Apply KCL at node A.

$$I_1 = I_2 + I_3$$

$$\therefore \quad \frac{10 - V_A}{10} = \frac{V_A}{8} + \frac{V_A - 3 - V_B}{4}$$

$$\therefore \quad 8(10 - V_A) = 10V_A + 10 \times 2(V_A - 3 - V_B)$$

$$\therefore \quad 80 - 8V_A = 10V_A + 20V_A - 60 - 20V_B$$

$$\therefore \quad 19V_A - 10V_B = 70 \quad \text{...(1)}$$

Step II: Apply KCL at node B

$$I_3 = I_4 + I_5$$

$$\therefore \quad \frac{V_A - 3 - V_B}{4} = \frac{V_B}{12} + \frac{V_B - 6}{14}$$

$$\therefore \quad \frac{84(V_A - 3 - V_B)}{4} = 7V_B + 6(V_B - 6)$$

$\therefore \quad 21 V_A - 63 - 21 V_B = 7 V_B + 6 V_B - 36$

$\therefore \quad 21 V_A - 34 V_B = 27 \quad ...(2)$

Step III: Solving Eqs (1) and (2), we get

$\therefore \quad V_A = 3.096\, V \text{ and } V_B = 1.12 \text{ V}$

Current through 8 Ω resistance

$$I_2 = \frac{V_A}{8} = \frac{3.096}{8} = 0.387 \text{ A}$$

Example 5: Using the nodal analysis, find current through 10 Ω resistor as shown in figure. **[MTU 2009-10]**

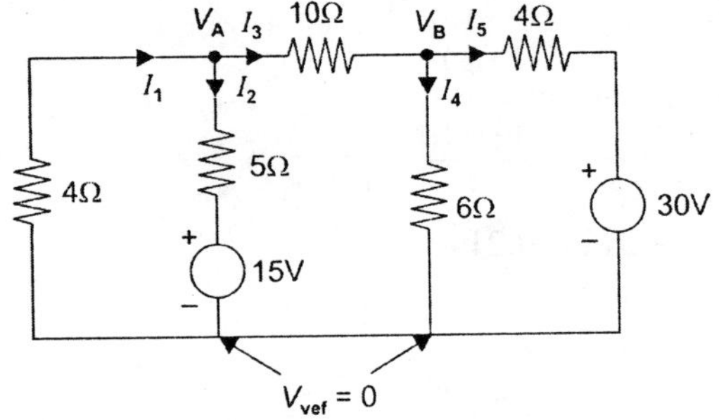

Solution: Step I: Apply KCL at node A.

$$I_1 = I_2 + I_3$$

$$-\frac{V_A}{4} = \frac{V_A - 15}{5} + \frac{V_A - V_B}{10} \quad ...(1)$$

Step II: Apply KCL at node B.

$$I_3 = I_4 + I_5$$

$$\frac{V_A - V_B}{10} = \frac{V_B}{6} + \frac{V_B - 30}{4} \quad ...(2)$$

Step III: Solving Eqs (1) and (2), we get

$$V_A = 8.39 \text{ and } V_B = 16.14$$

Current through 10 Ω

$$I_3 = \frac{V_A - V_B}{10} = \frac{8.39 - 16.14}{10} = -0.775 \text{ A} \quad \textbf{Ans.}$$

Therefore I_3 is flowing from B to A.

Example 6: Use nodal analysis to find the currents in varios resistors of the circuit shown in figure below. **[MTU Sem II, 05-06, 07-08]**

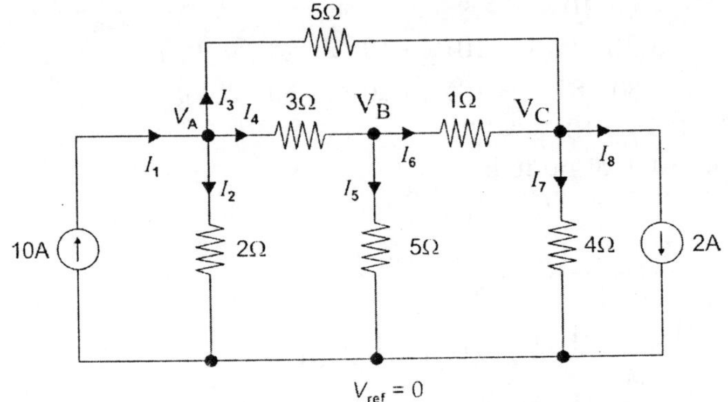

Solution: Step I: Apply KCL at node A

$$I_1 = I_2 + I_3 + I_4$$

$$\therefore \quad 10 = \frac{V_A}{2} + \frac{V_A - V_C}{5} + \frac{V_A - V_B}{3}$$

$$\therefore \quad 10 = \frac{15V_A + 6(V_A - V_C) + 10(V_A - V_B)}{30}$$

$$\therefore \quad 300 = 31V_A - 10V_B - 6V_C \qquad \text{...(1)}$$

Step II: Apply KCL at node B.

$$I_4 = I_5 + I_6$$

$$\therefore \quad \frac{V_A - V_B}{3} = \frac{V_B}{5} + \frac{V_B - V_C}{1}$$

$$\Rightarrow \quad 5(V_A - V_B) = 3V_B + 15(V_B - V_C)$$

$$\therefore \quad 5V_A - 23V_B + 15V_C = 0 \qquad \text{...(2)}$$

Step III: Apply KCL at node C.

$$I_3 + I_6 = I_7 + I_8$$

$$\therefore \quad \frac{V_A - V_C}{5} + \frac{V_B - V_C}{1} = \frac{V_C}{4} + 2$$

$$\therefore \quad 4(V_A - V_C + 5V_B - 5V_C) = 5V_C + 40$$

$$\therefore \quad 4V_A + 20V_B - 29V_C = 40 \qquad \text{...(3)}$$

Step IV: Solving Eq (1) (2) and (3), we get
By Cramer's rule:

$$\Delta = \begin{bmatrix} 31 & -10 & -6 \\ 5 & -23 & 5 \\ 4 & 20 & -29 \end{bmatrix} = 11377 - 2050 - 1152 = 8175$$

$$\Delta_1 = \begin{bmatrix} 300 & -10 & -6 \\ 0 & -23 & 15 \\ 40 & 20 & -29 \end{bmatrix} = 110100 - 6000 - 5520 = 98580$$

$$\Delta_2 = \begin{bmatrix} 31 & 300 & -6 \\ 5 & 0 & 15 \\ 4 & 40 & -29 \end{bmatrix} = -18600 + 61500 - 1200 = 41700$$

$$\Delta_3 = \begin{bmatrix} 31 & -10 & 300 \\ 5 & -23 & 0 \\ 4 & 20 & 40 \end{bmatrix} = -28520 + 2000 + 57600 = 31080$$

$$\therefore \quad V_A = \frac{\Delta_1}{\Delta} = \frac{98580}{8175} = 12.06\text{ V}\ ;\ V_B = \frac{\Delta_2}{\Delta} = \frac{41700}{8175} = 5.10\text{ V}\ ;\ V_C = \frac{\Delta_3}{\Delta} = \frac{31080}{8175} = 3.80\text{ V}$$

Step V: To find all the branch currents.

$$I_1 = 10\text{A (given)}$$

$$I_2 = \frac{V_A}{2} = \frac{12.06}{2} = 6.03\text{ A}$$

$$I_3 = \frac{V_A - V_C}{5} = \frac{12.06 - 3.80}{5} = 1.652 \text{ A}$$

$$I_4 = \frac{V_A - V_B}{3} = \frac{12.06 - 5.10}{3} = 2.32 \text{ A}$$

$$I_5 = \frac{V_B}{5} = \frac{5.10}{5} = 1.02 \text{ A}$$

$$I_6 = \frac{V_B - V_C}{1} = \frac{5.10 - 3.80}{1} = 1.30 \text{ A}$$

$$I_7 = \frac{V_C}{4} = \frac{3.80}{4} = 0.95 \text{ A}$$

$$I_8 = 2\text{A (given)}$$

Example 7: Use the nodal analysis to find the voltage across the 12 Ω resistance in the circuit shown in figure below.

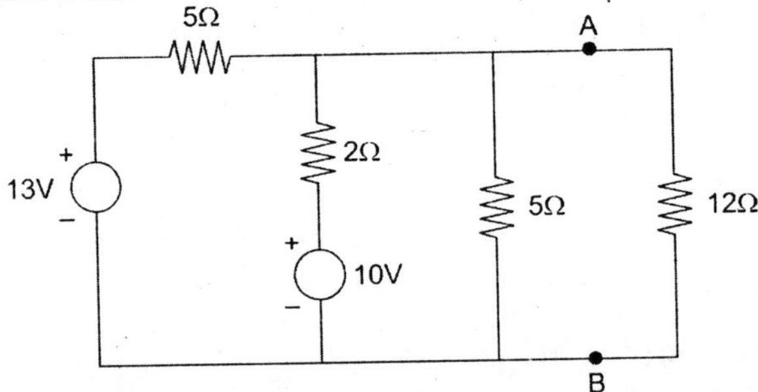

Solution: Step I: Convert the voltage sources to current sources.

$$I_1 = \frac{13V}{5} = 2.6 \text{ A} \; ; \; I_2 = \frac{10V}{2} = 5 \text{ A}$$

Redraw the above circuit

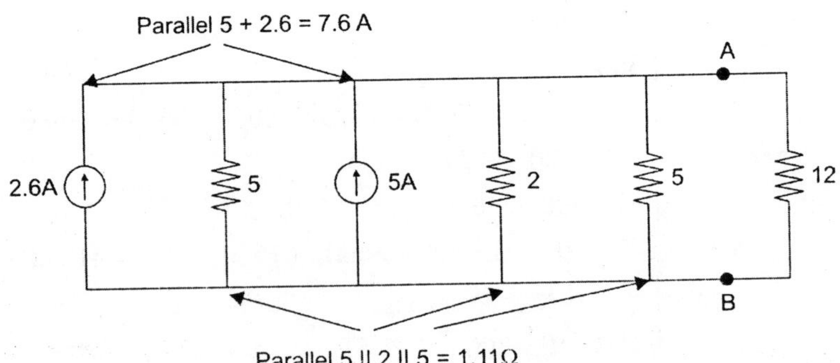

Step III: Apply KCL in figure below and find current in 12 Ω.

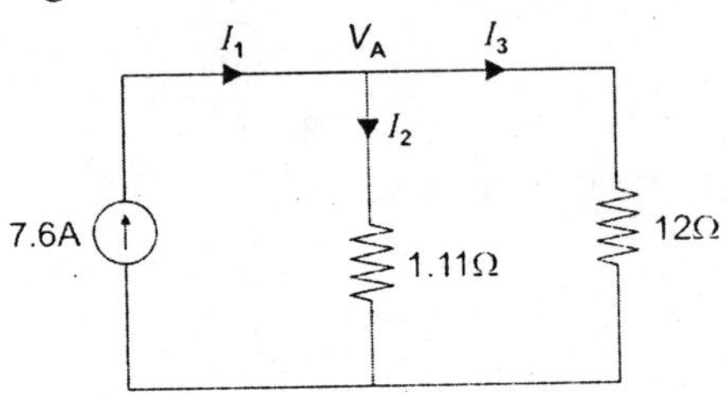

Apply KCL at node A.

$$I_1 = I_2 + I_3$$

$$7.6 = \frac{V_A}{1.11} + \frac{V_A}{12}$$

$\therefore$ Solving above expression, we get

$$V_A = 7.73 \text{ volts}$$

Current in 12 Ω is $I_3 = \frac{V_A}{12}$.

$$= \frac{7.73}{12} = 0.64 \text{ A}$$ **Ans.**

Example 8: Determine current in 30 Ω resistance for the current shown in figure.

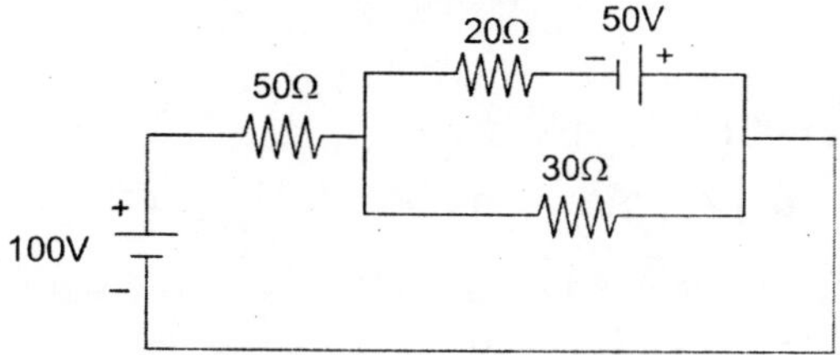

Solution: Step I: Mark currents and identify loops.

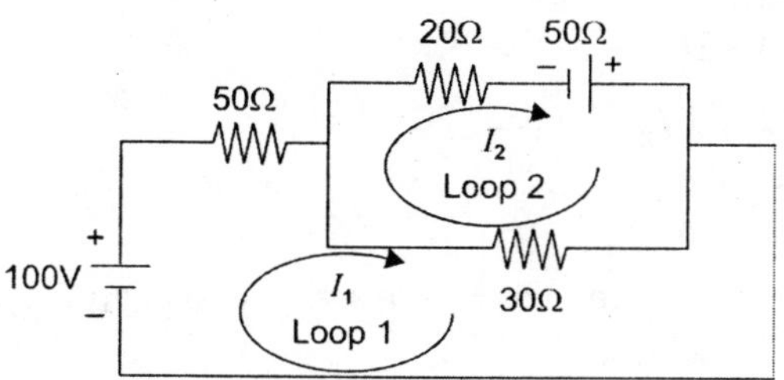

Step II: Apply KVL in loop 1

$$100 - 50I_1 - 30(I_1 - I_2) = 0$$

$$-8I_1 + 3I_2 = -10 \quad \text{...(1)}$$

Step II: Apply KVL in loop 2.

$$50 - 30(I_2 - I_1) - 20I_2 = 0$$

$$3I_1 - 5I_2 = -5 \quad \text{...(2)}$$

Step III: Solving Eqs (1) and (2)

$$I_1 = \frac{65}{31}\text{A}, I_1 = \frac{70}{31}\text{A}$$

Current through 30 Ω resistance is $I_1 - I_2 = -\frac{5}{31} = -0.1613$ A **Ans.**

Example 9: Using Kirchhoff's laws, find the current through 4 Ω resistor for circuit shown in figure.

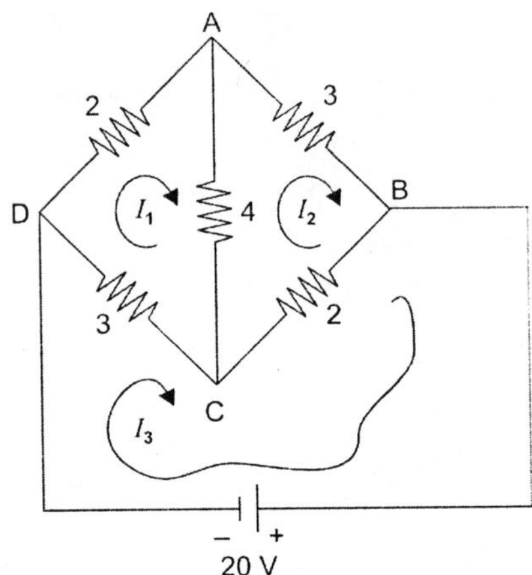

Solution: Step I: Mark the current and the three loops are identified as shown in figure.

Apply KVL in loop 1

$$\therefore \quad -2I_1-4(I_1-I_2)-3(I_1-I_3) = 0$$

$$\therefore \quad -9I_1+4I_2+3I_3 = 0 \qquad ...(1)$$

Apply KVL in loop 2

$$\therefore \quad -3I_2-2(I_2-I_3)-4(I_2-I_1) = 0$$

$$\therefore \quad 4I_1-9I_2+2I_3 = 0 \qquad ...(2)$$

Apply KVL in loop 3

$$\therefore \quad -20-3(I_3-I_1)-2(I_3-I_2) = 0$$

$$\therefore \quad 3I_1+2I_2-5I_3 = 20 \qquad ...(3)$$

Step II: By Cramer's rule:

$$\Delta = \begin{bmatrix} -9 & 4 & 3 \\ 4 & -9 & 2 \\ 3 & 2 & -5 \end{bmatrix} = -9(45-4)-4(-20-6)+3(8+27)$$

$$= -369+104+105 = -160$$

$$\Delta_1 = \begin{bmatrix} 0 & 4 & 3 \\ 0 & -9 & 2 \\ 20 & 2 & -5 \end{bmatrix} = -4(-40)+3(180) = 160+540 = 700$$

$$\Delta_2 = \begin{bmatrix} -9 & 0 & 3 \\ 4 & 0 & 2 \\ 3 & 20 & -5 \end{bmatrix} = -9(-40)+3(80) = 360+240 = 600$$

$$I_1 = \frac{\Delta_1}{\Delta} = \frac{700}{-160}, \quad I_1 = -4.375 \text{ A}$$

$$I_2 = \frac{\Delta_2}{\Delta} = \frac{600}{-160} = -3.75, \quad I_2 = -3.75 \text{ A}$$

Current through 4 Ω is $I_1 - I_2$

$$\Rightarrow \quad -4.375-(-3.75) = -0.625 \text{ A}$$ **Ans.**

Example 10: Determine the current and power consumed in the 3 Ω resistance of the circuit shown in figure below.

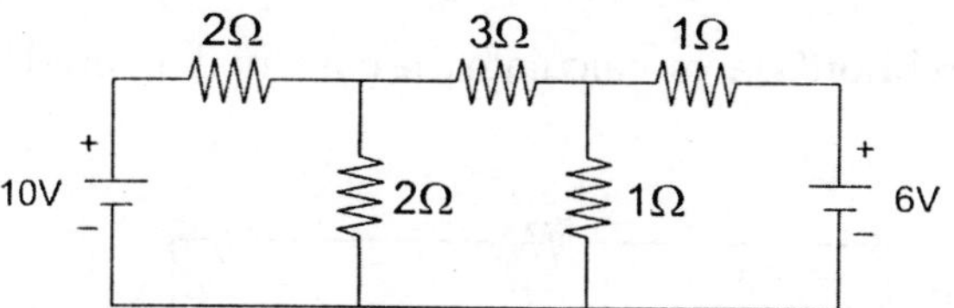

Solution: Step I: Mark the loop current and identify the loops shown in figure below.

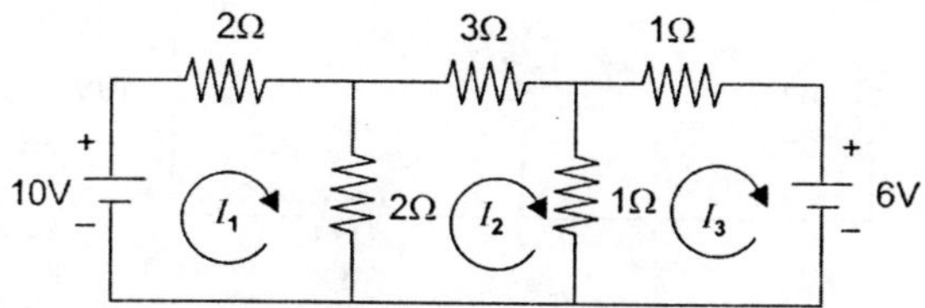

Step II: Using KVL write down the loop equations:

Apply KVL in loop 1.

$$\therefore \quad 10-2I_1-2(I_1-I_2)=0$$

$$\therefore \quad -4I_1+2I_2=-10$$

$$\therefore \quad 2I_1-I_2=5 \quad \text{...(1)}$$

Apply KVL in loop 2.

$$\therefore -2(I_2-I_1)-3I_2-1(I_2-I_3)=0$$

$$\therefore \quad -6I_2+2I_1+I_3=0$$

$$\therefore \quad 2I_1-6I_2+I_3=0 \quad \text{...(2)}$$

Apply KVL in loop 3.

$$\therefore \quad -1(I_3-I_2)-1(I_3)-6=0$$

$$\therefore \quad I_2-2I_3=6 \quad \text{...(3)}$$

The three loop equation are as follows:

$$2I_1-I_2=5$$

$$2I_1-6I_2+I_3=0$$

$$I_2+2I_3=6 \quad \text{...(4)}$$

Step III: By Cramer's rule

$$\Delta = \begin{bmatrix} 2 & -1 & 0 \\ 2 & -6 & 1 \\ 0 & 1 & -2 \end{bmatrix} = 18$$

$$\Delta_2 = \begin{bmatrix} 2 & 5 & 0 \\ 2 & 0 & 1 \\ 0 & 6 & -2 \end{bmatrix} = 8$$

Current through 3 Ω resistance is I_2

$$\therefore \quad I_2 = \frac{\Delta_2}{\Delta} = \frac{8}{18} = 0.444 \text{ A} \qquad \textbf{Ans.}$$

Power consumed in 3 Ω resistance

$$P = I_2^2 R = (0.444)^2 \times 3 = 0.5914 \text{ W}$$ **Ans.**

Example 11: Using Kirchhoff's laws, calculate the current delivered by the battery shown in figure below. **[UPTU 2003-04]**

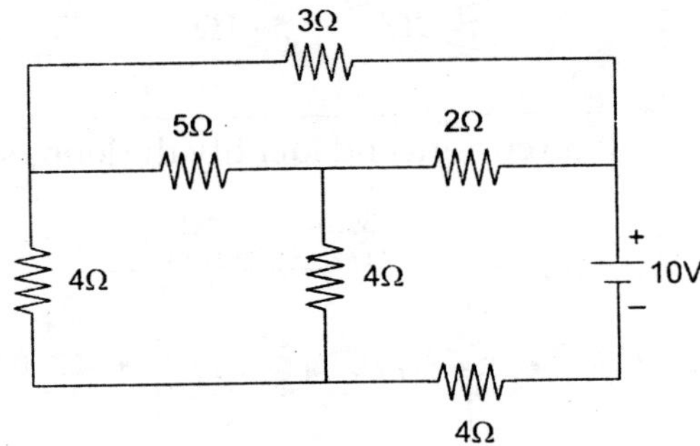

Solution: Step I: Identify the loops and loop current shown below.

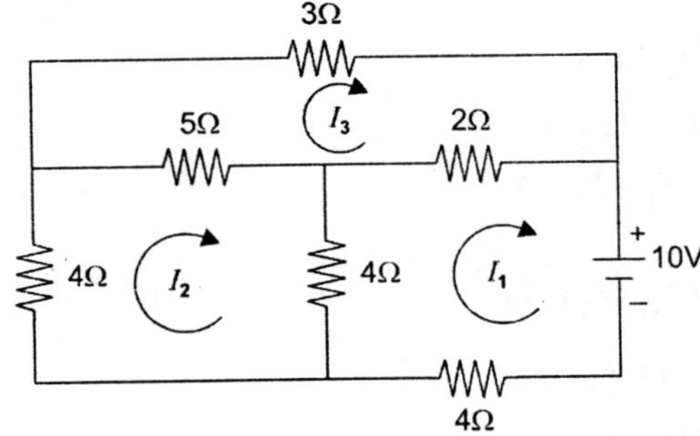

Step II: Write the loop equation.

Apply KVL in loop 1.

$$\therefore \quad -10 - 4I_1 - 4(I_1 - I_2) - 2(I_1 - I_3) = 0$$

$$\therefore \quad -4I_1 - 4(I_1 - I_2) - 2(I_1 - I_3) = 10$$

$$\therefore \quad -5I_1 + 2I_2 + I_3 = 5 \quad \text{...(1)}$$

Apply KVL in loop 2.

$$\therefore \quad -4I_2 - 5(I_2 - I_3) - 4(I_2 - I_1) = 0$$

$$\therefore \quad 4I_1 - 13I_2 + 5I_3 = 0 \quad \text{...(2)}$$

Apply KVL in loop 3.

$$\therefore \quad -3I_3 - 2(I_3 - I_1) - 5(I_3 - I_2) = 0$$

$$\therefore \quad 2I_1 + 5I_2 - 10I_3 = 0 \quad \text{...(3)}$$

Step III: From the loop equations are

By Cramer's rule

$$\Delta = \begin{bmatrix} -5 & 2 & 1 \\ 4 & -13 & 5 \\ 2 & 5 & -10 \end{bmatrix}$$

$$= -5(130 - 25) - 2(-40 - 10) + 1(20 + 26)$$

$$\Delta = -5(105) + 100 + 46 = -379$$

$$\Delta_1 = \begin{bmatrix} 5 & 2 & 1 \\ 0 & -13 & 5 \\ 0 & 5 & -10 \end{bmatrix}$$

$$= 5(130-25)-2(0)+1(0)=525$$

$$I_1 = \frac{\Delta_1}{\Delta} = \frac{525}{-379} = -1.385$$

Current through battery is 1.385 ampere in the direction opposite to I_1. **Ans.**

Example 12: Using the mesh current method, determine current I_x in the circuit shown in figure. **[Sem-I 05-06]**

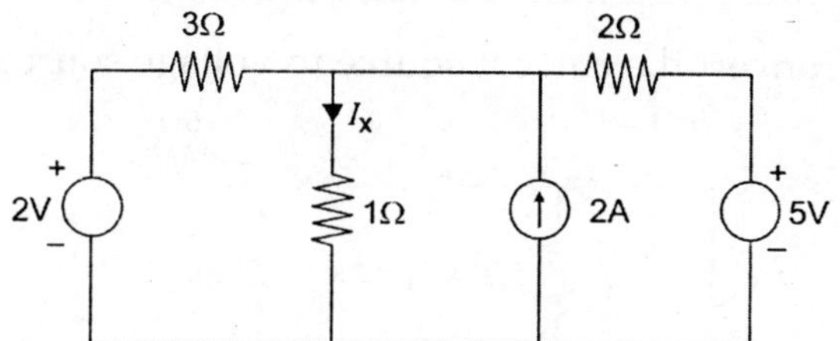

Solution: Step I: Convert the current source to voltage source.

$\therefore$ $$V = 2 \times 1 = 2\text{ V}$$

Step II: Identify the meshes and mesh current.

Apply KVL in mesh (A – B – C – D – A)

$\therefore$ $$2-3I_1-1(I_1-I_2)-2 = 0$$

$\therefore$ $$-4I_1+I_2 = 0$$

$$I_2 = 4I_1 \quad \text{...(1)}$$

Apply KVL in mesh 2 (B – E – F – C – B)

$\therefore$ $$-2I_2-5+2-1(I_2-I_1) = 0$$

$\therefore$ $$-3I_2+I_1-3 = 0 \quad \text{...(2)}$$

$\therefore$ From Eq. (1) $I_2 = 4I_1$ putting the value in Eq. (2), we get

$\therefore$ $$-3(4I_1)+I_1-3 = 0$$

$\therefore$ $$-11I_1-3 = 0$$

$\Rightarrow$ $$I_1 = -\frac{3}{11}$$

$\therefore$ $$I_1 = -0.273\ A$$

$\therefore$ $$I_2 = 4I_1 = 4\times 0.273 = -1.092\text{ A}$$

Current $I_x = I_1 - I_2$

$I_x = -0.273 - (-1.092) = 0.819$ A **Ans.**

Example 13: Using mesh equation method, find the current in resistance R_1 of network shown in figure. **[Sem-II, 04-05]**

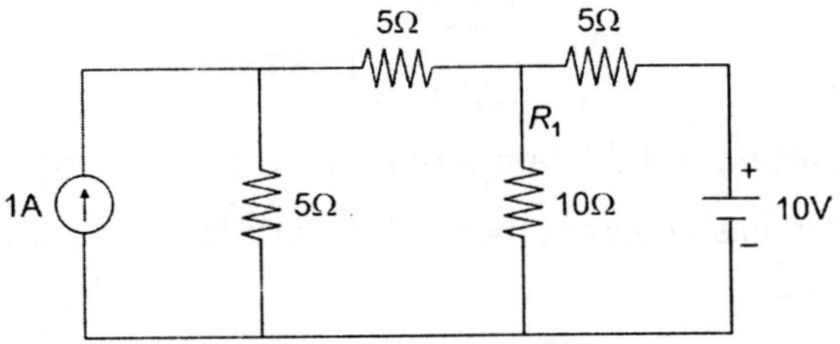

Solution: Step I: Convert the current source to voltage source.

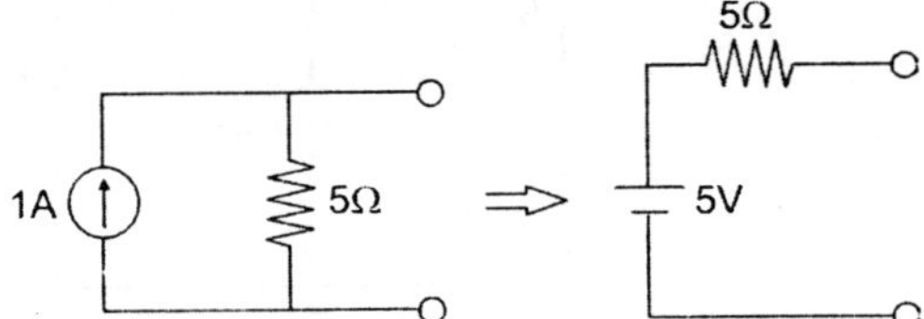

Redraw the figure.

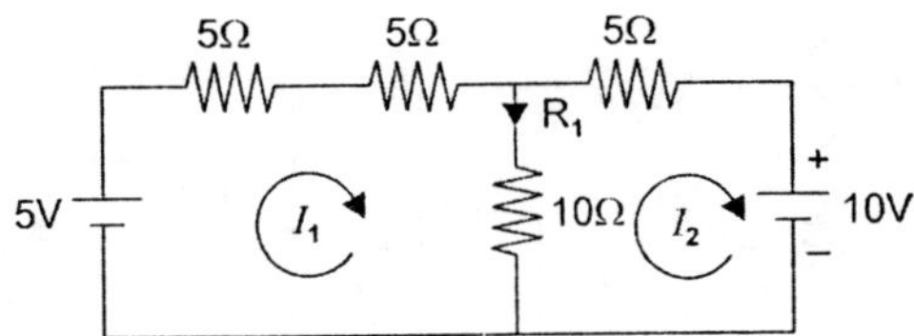

Step II: Identify the loops and loop current.
Apply KVL in loop 1.

$\therefore\ 5 - 5I_1 - 5I_1 - 10(I_1 - I_2) = 0$

$\therefore\ -20I_1 + 10I_2 = -5$

$\therefore\ 4I_1 - 2I_2 = 1$ ...(1)

Apply KVL in loop 2

$\therefore\ -10(I_2 - I_1) - 5I_2 - 10 = 0$

$\therefore\ 10I_1 - 15I_2 = 10$

$\therefore\ 2I_1 - 3I_2 = 2$ ...(2)

Step III: Solving Eqs (1) and (2), we get

$$I_2 = -\frac{6}{8} = -0.75 \text{ A}$$

From Eq. (1)

$4I_1 - 2 \times 0.75 = 1$

$I_1 = -0.125$ A

Current in resistance R_1 is

$I_1 - I_2 = -0.125 - (0.75) = 0.625$ A **Ans.**

Example 14: Calculate the current through the galvanometer of the bridge shown in figure.

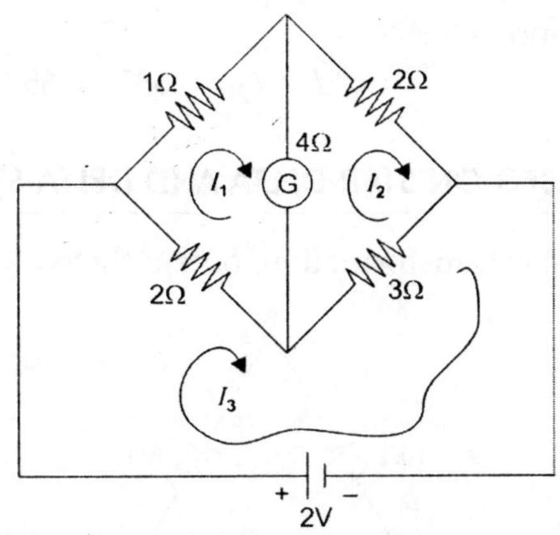

Solution: Step I: Identify the loop and loop current.

Apply KVL in loop 1.

$$\therefore \quad -1I_1 - 4(I_1 - I_2) - 2(I_1 - I_3) = 0$$

$$\therefore \quad -7I_1 + 4I_2 + 2I_3 = 0 \quad \text{...(1)}$$

Apply KVL in loop 2.

$$\therefore \quad -2I_2 - 3(I_2 - I_3) - 4(I_2 - I_1) = 0$$

$$\therefore \quad 4I_1 - 9I_2 + 3I_3 = 0 \quad \text{...(2)}$$

Apply KVL in loop 3.

$$\therefore \quad 2 - 2(I_3 - I_1) - 3(I_3 - I_2) = 0$$

$$\therefore \quad 2 + 2I_1 + 3I_2 - 5I_3 = 0$$

$$\therefore \quad 2I_1 + 3I_2 - 5I_3 = -2 \quad \text{...(3)}$$

Step II: Solving Eqs (1), (2) and (3), we get

By Cramer's rule

$$\Delta = \begin{vmatrix} -7 & 4 & 2 \\ 4 & -9 & 3 \\ 2 & 3 & -5 \end{vmatrix} = -88$$

$$\Delta_1 = \begin{vmatrix} 0 & 4 & 2 \\ 0 & -9 & 3 \\ -2 & 3 & -5 \end{vmatrix} = -60$$

$$\Delta_2 = \begin{vmatrix} -7 & 0 & 2 \\ 4 & 0 & 3 \\ 2 & -2 & -5 \end{vmatrix} = -58$$

$$I_1 = \frac{\Delta_1}{\Delta} = \frac{-60}{-88} = 0.682 \text{ A}$$

$$I_2 = \frac{\Delta_2}{\Delta} = \frac{-58}{-88} = 0.659 \text{ A}$$

Current through galvanometer

$$= I_1 - I_2 = 0.682 - 0.659 = 0.023 \text{ A} \qquad \textbf{Ans.}$$

SOLVED EXAMPLES BASED ON STAR-DELTA AND DELTA-STAR TRANSFORMATION

Example 1: Using delta-star transformation, obtain the equivalent star circuit.

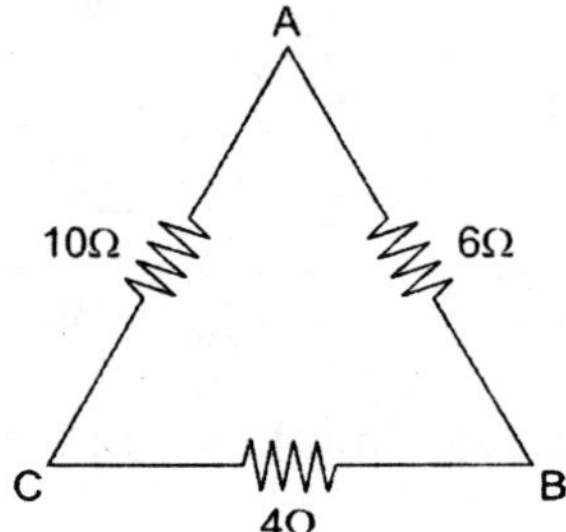

Solution: Step I: Draw dotted star resistances inside the Δ network as shown in figure.

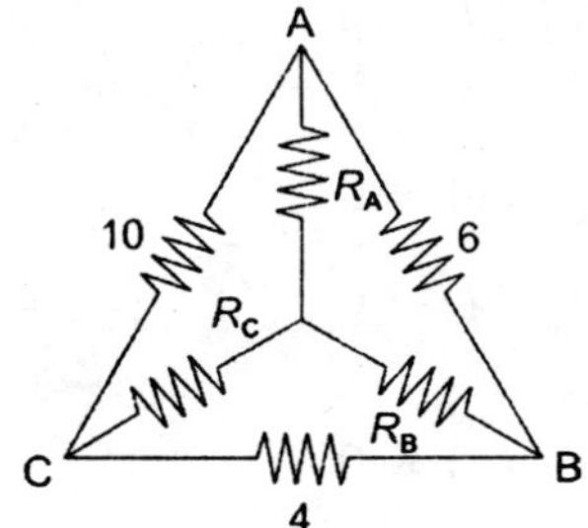

Step II: Calculate R_A, R_B and R_C using formulas.

$$R_A = \frac{10 \times 6}{10 + 6 + 4} = \frac{60}{20} = 3\ \Omega$$

$$R_B = \frac{6 \times 4}{10 + 6 + 4} = \frac{24}{20} = 1.2\ \Omega$$

$$R_C = \frac{4 \times 10}{10 + 6 + 4} = \frac{40}{20} = 2\ \Omega$$

A

$R_A = 3\Omega$

$R_C = 2\Omega$ $R_B = 1.2\Omega$

C B

Y-connected network

Example 2: Obtain an equivalent delta network for the circuit shown.

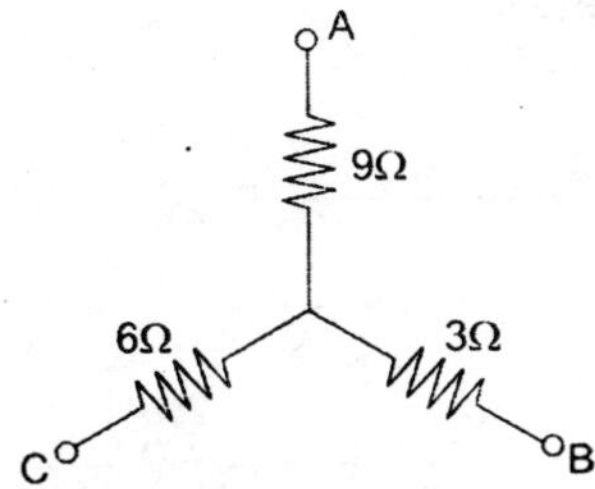

Solution: Step I: Draw a dotted Δ- connected network as the equivalent network between terminals A, B and C as shown in figure.

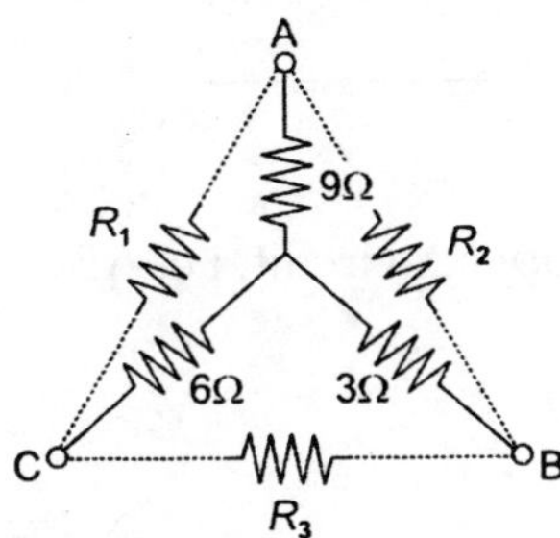

Step II: To find R_1, R_2 and R_3

$$R_1 = \frac{R_A R_B + R_B R_C + R_C R_A}{R_B}$$

$$R_1 = \frac{9 \times 3 + 3 \times 6 + 6 \times 9}{3} = 33\ \Omega$$

Similarly
$$R_2 = \frac{R_A R_B + R_B R_C + R_C R_A}{R_C}$$

$$R_2 = \frac{9 \times 3 + 3 \times 6 + 6 \times 9}{6} = 16.5\ \Omega$$

and
$$R_3 = \frac{R_A R_B + R_B R_C + R_C R_A}{R_A}$$

$$= \frac{9 \times 3 + 3 \times 6 + 6 \times 9}{9} = 11\ \Omega$$

Step III: Thus the equivalent Δ- connected network shown.

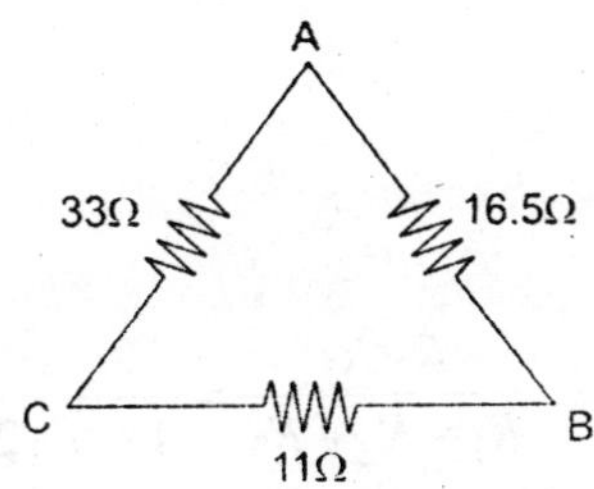

Example 3: Find the resistance between terminals XY of the bridge circuit shown in figure by using delta-star transformation.

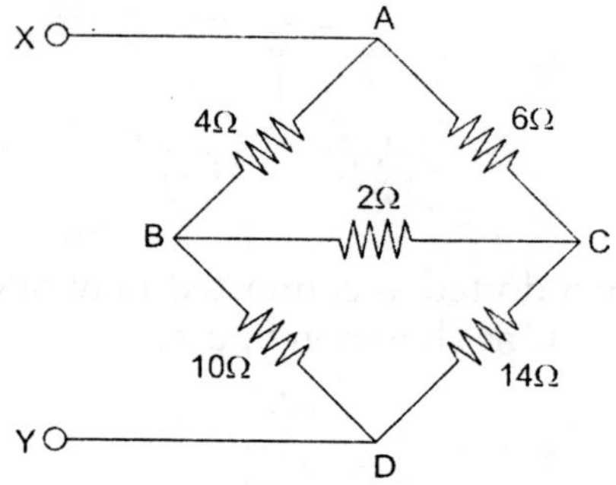

Solution: Step I: Choose upper Δ-circuit, i.e. ABC and obtain the equivalent star for it.

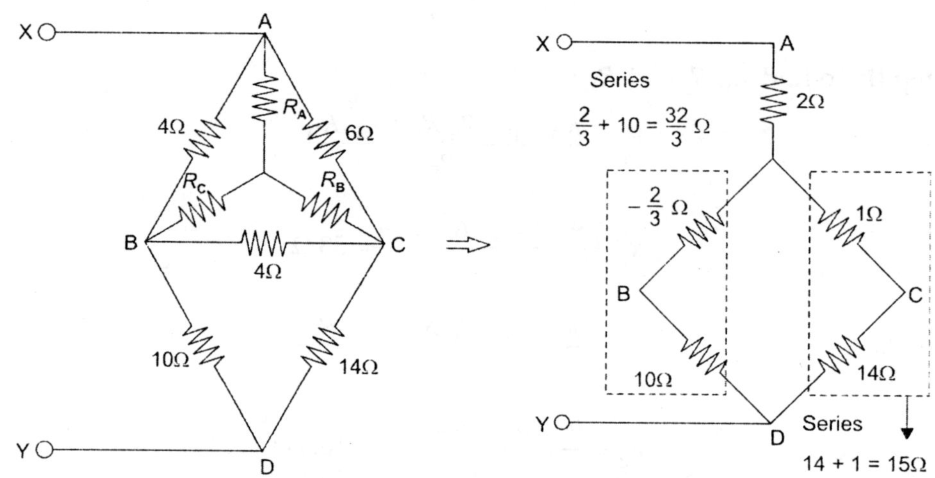

$$\Rightarrow \qquad R_A = \frac{R_1 R_2}{R_1 + R_2 + R_3} = \frac{4 \times 6}{4 + 6 + 2} = 2\ \Omega$$

$$\Rightarrow \qquad R_B = \frac{R_2 R_3}{R_1 + R_2 + R_3} = \frac{6 \times 2}{4 + 6 + 2} = 1\ \Omega$$

Similarly

$$\Rightarrow \qquad R_C = \frac{R_3 R_1}{R_1 + R_2 + R_3} = \frac{2 \times 4}{4 + 6 + 2} = \frac{2}{3}$$

Step II: After obtaining the series combination redraw the figure.

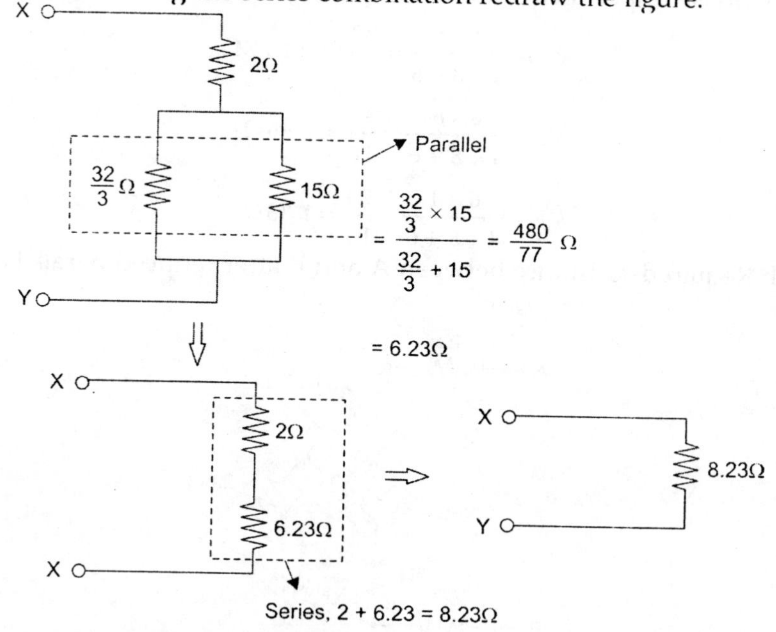

Resistance between terminal X and Y.

$$\therefore \qquad R_{XY} = 8.23\ \Omega$$

Ans.

Example 4: Find the input resistance between terminals A and B of the figure below.

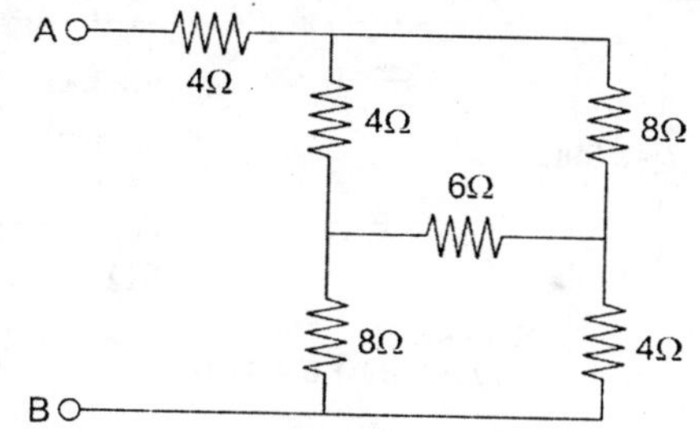

Solution: **Step I:** Redraw the given figure

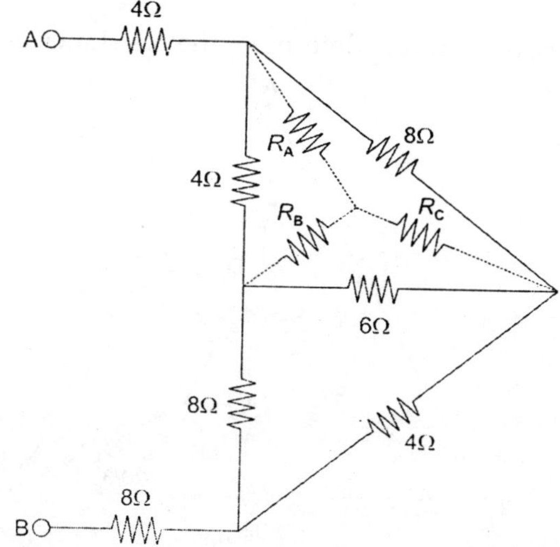

Step II: Choose upper Δ-circuit into Y-equivalent circuit.

$$R_A = \frac{4 \times 8}{4+8+6} = \frac{32}{18}\Omega = 1.77\,\Omega$$

$$R_B = \frac{8 \times 6}{4+8+6} = \frac{48}{18} = 2.66\,\Omega$$

$$R_C = \frac{6 \times 4}{4+8+6} = \frac{24}{18} = 1.33\,\Omega$$

Step III: Required resistance between A and B after reduced parallel combination.

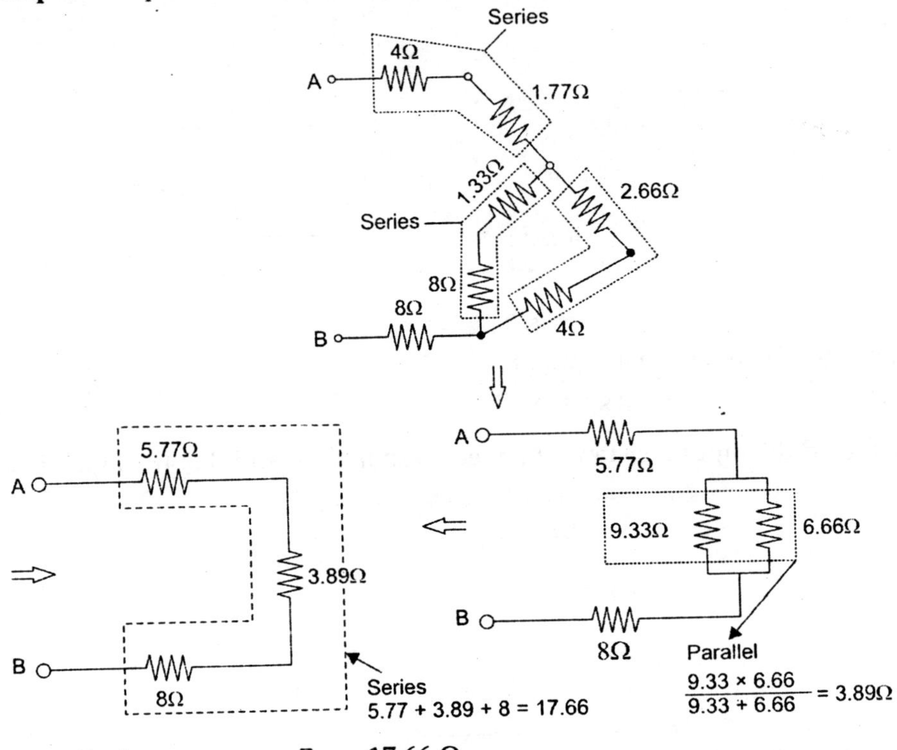

Required $R_{AB} = 17.66\ \Omega$ **Ans.**

Example 5: In the network shown, determine the resistance between A and B.

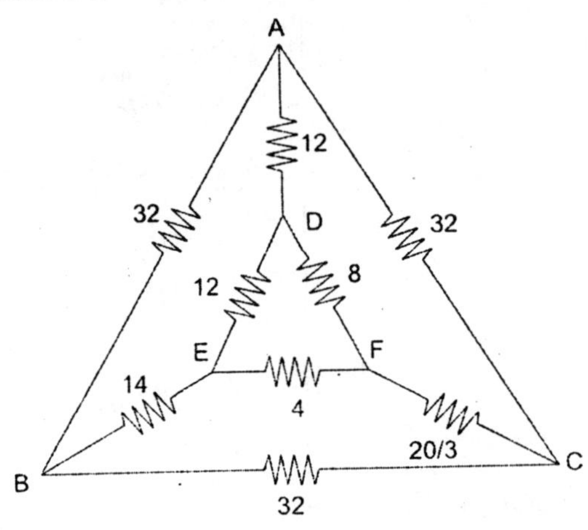

Solution: Step I: Consider the inner Δ-connected network DEF into *Y*-network.

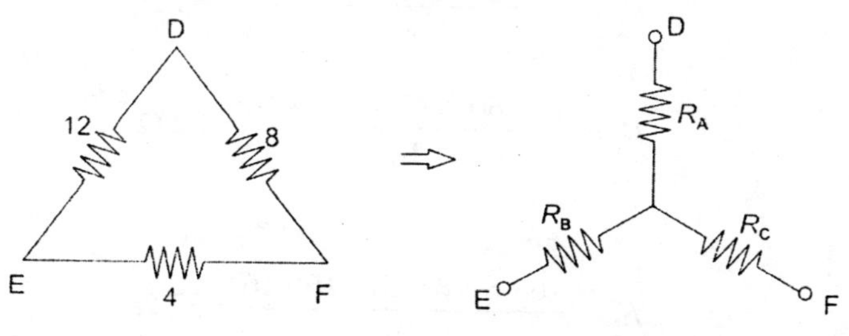

$$\Rightarrow R_A = \frac{12\times 8}{12+8+4} = \frac{96}{24} = 4\,\Omega;\ R_B = \frac{12\times 4}{12+8+4} = \frac{48}{24} = 2\,\Omega;\ R_C = \frac{8\times 4}{12+8+4} = \frac{32}{24} = \frac{4}{3}\Omega$$

Step II: The original network is reduced to the shape shown.

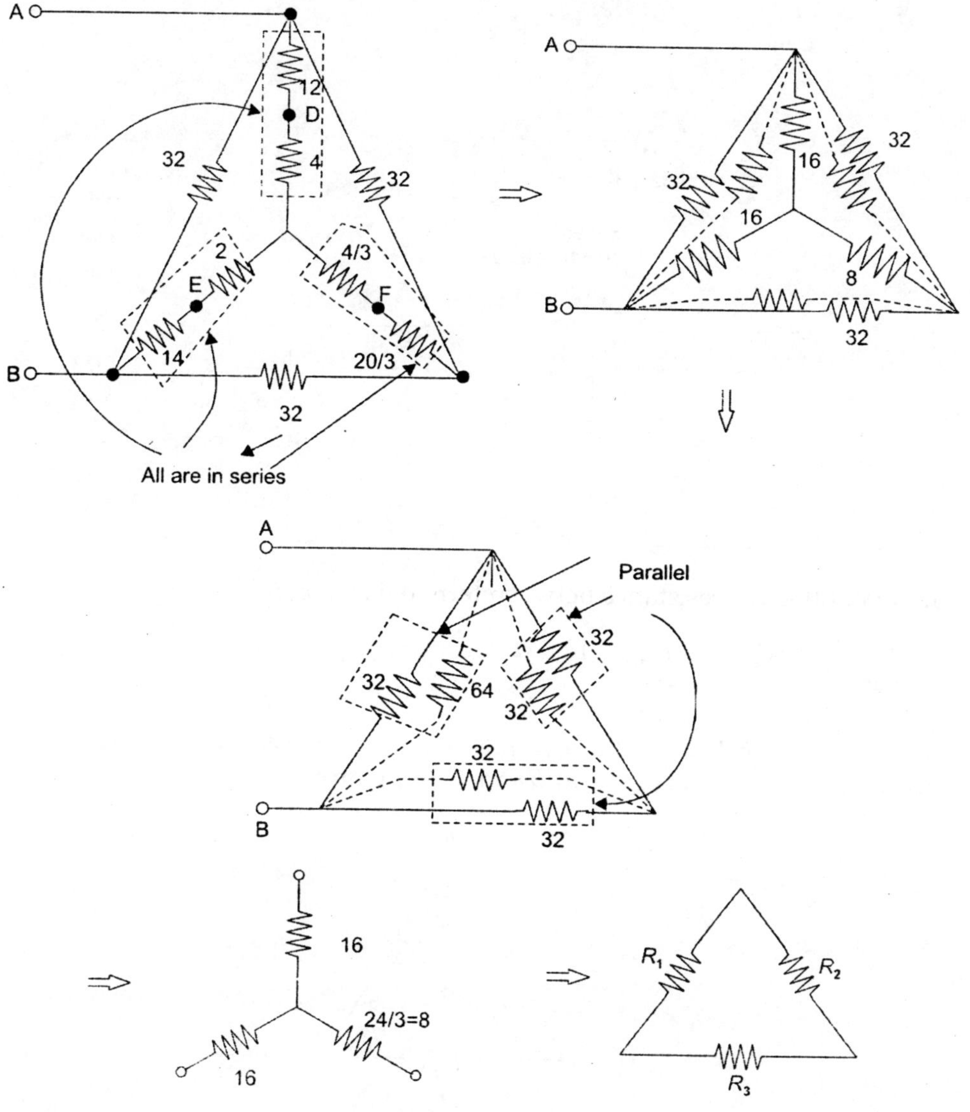

All are in series

Parallel

24/3=8

$$\Rightarrow \qquad R_1 = \frac{16\times 8 + 8\times 16 + 16\times 16}{8} = 64\ \Omega$$

$$\Rightarrow \qquad R_2 = \frac{16\times 8 + 8\times 16 + 16\times 16}{16} = 32\ \Omega$$

Similarly

$$\Rightarrow \qquad R_3 = \frac{16\times 8 + 8\times 16 + 16\times 16}{16} = 32\ \Omega$$

Step III: Redraw above after parallel combination.

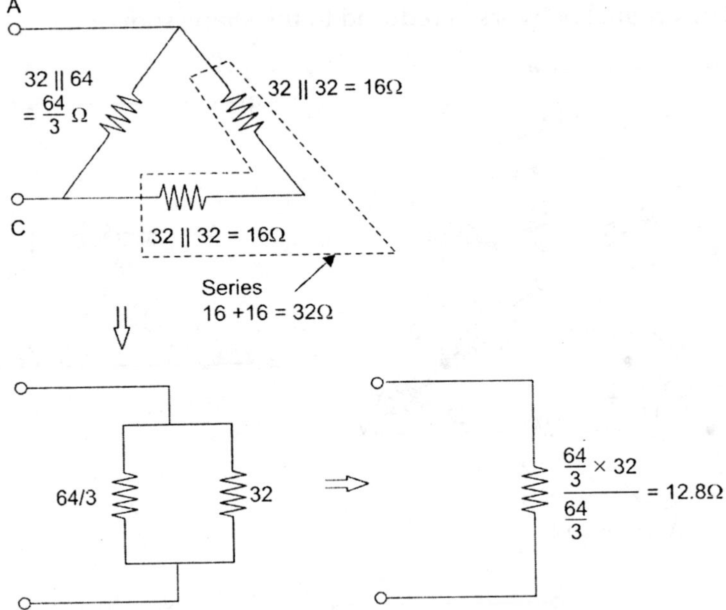

Step IV: Effective resistance between terminal A and B.

$$\therefore \qquad R_{AB} = 12.8\ \Omega$$

Example 6: A network of resistance is shown, compute the equivalent network resistance measured between (i) A and B, (ii) B and C, (iii) C and A.

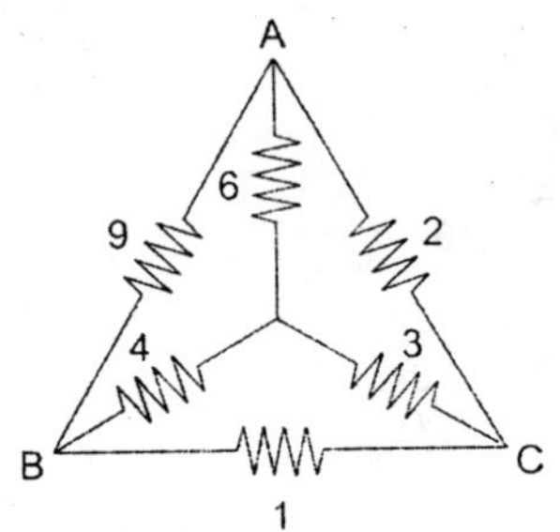

Solution: Step I: Convert the internal Y-network into Δ-network.

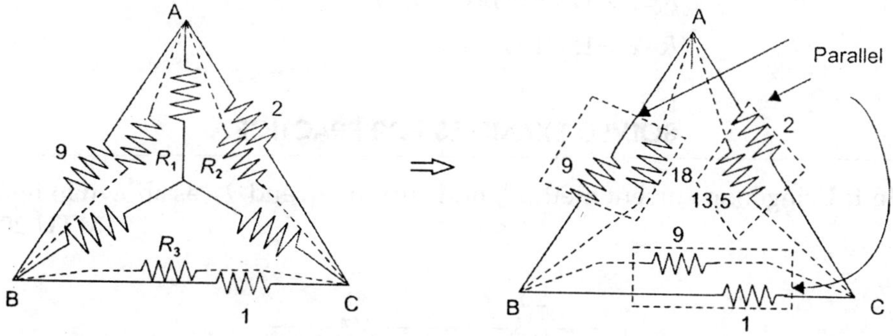

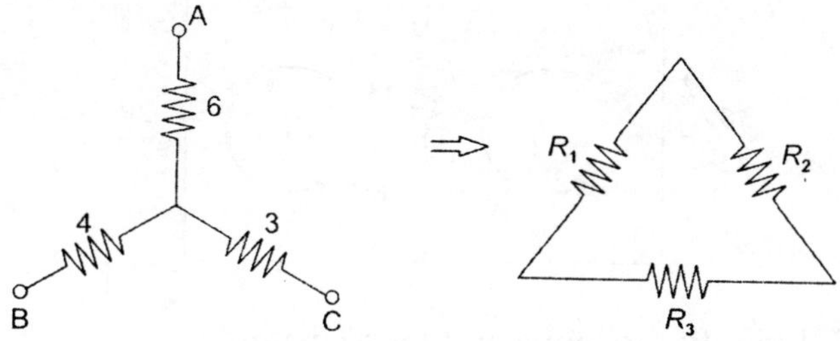

$$\Rightarrow \quad R_1 = \frac{4\times 3+6\times 3+4\times 6}{3} = 18\ \Omega$$

$$\Rightarrow \quad R_2 = \frac{4\times 3+6\times 3+4\times 6}{4} = 13.5\ \Omega$$

$$\Rightarrow \quad R_3 = \frac{4\times 3+6\times 3+4\times 6}{6}\ 9\ \Omega$$

$\Rightarrow$ Solved parallel (each branch)

$$9 \| 8 = 6\ \Omega$$

$$9 \| 1 = 0.9\ \Omega$$

$$2 \| 13.5 = 1.7419\ \Omega$$

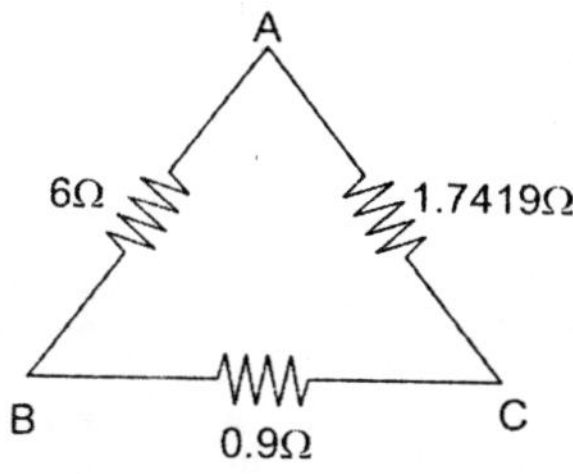

Resistance measured between A and B

$$R_{AB} = (6) \| (0.9+1.7419)$$

$$R_{AB} = 1.834\ \Omega$$ **Ans.**

Resistance measured between B and C

$$R_{BC} = (0.9) \| (6+1.7419)$$

$$R_{BC} = 0.806\ \Omega$$ **Ans.**

The resistance measured between C and A

$$R_{CA} = (1.7419) \| (6+0.9)$$

$$R_{CA} = 1.391\ \Omega$$ **Ans.**

SOLVED EXAMPLES FOR PRACTICE

Example 1: Using loop current method, find current I_1 and I_2 as shown in figure. **[MTU 2009-10]**

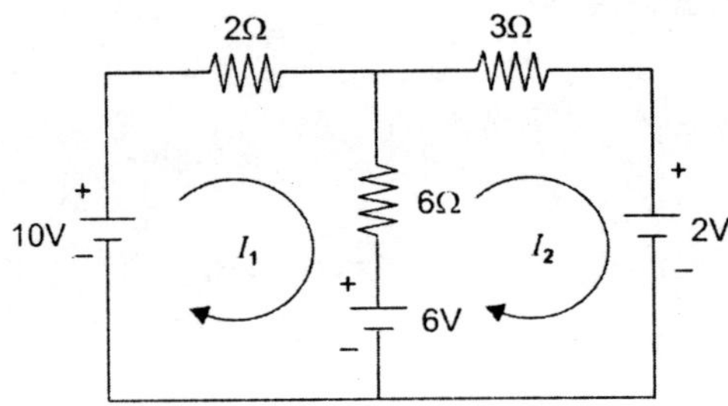

Solution: Step I: Identify the loops and loop current.

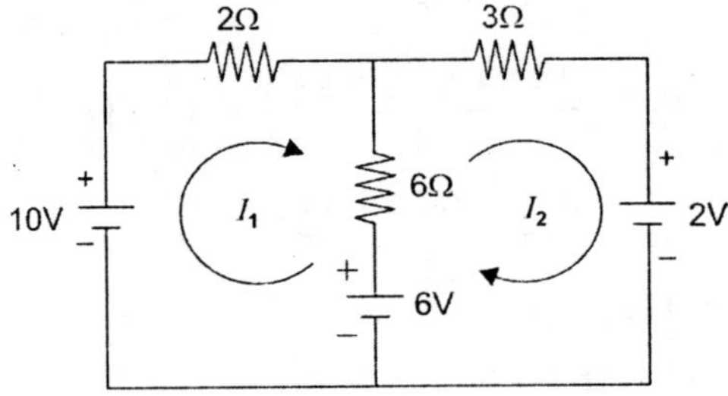

Step II: Apply KVL in loop 1 and loop 2.

Apply KVL in loop 1

$$\therefore \quad 10 - 2I_1 - (6I_1 - I_2) - 6 = 0$$

$$\therefore \quad 8I_1 - 6I_2 = 4$$

$$\therefore \quad 4I_1 - 3I_2 = 2 \qquad \text{...(1)}$$

Apply KVL in loop 2

$$\therefore \quad 6 - 6(I_2 - I_1) - 3I_2 - 2 = 0$$

$$\therefore \quad -6I_1 + 9I_2 = 4 \qquad \text{...(2)}$$

Step III: Solving the Eqs (1) and (2),we get

$$I_1 = 1.667\text{ A}$$

$$I_2 = 1.56\text{ A}$$

Example 2: Using Maxwell's loop current method, find I_1 and I_2.

[UPTU 2007-08, RTU 2006-07]

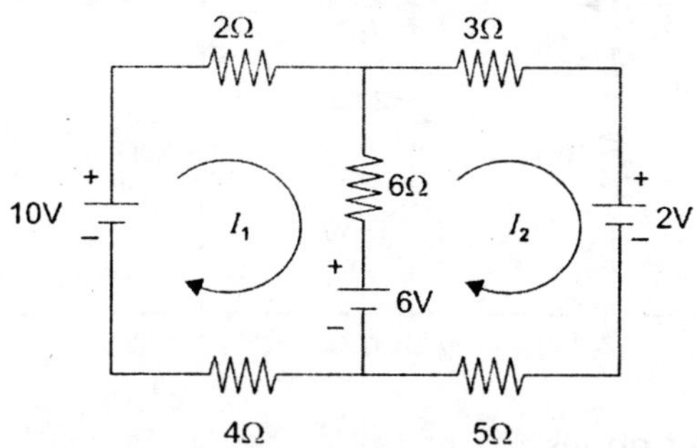

Solution: Step I: Identify the loops and loop current.

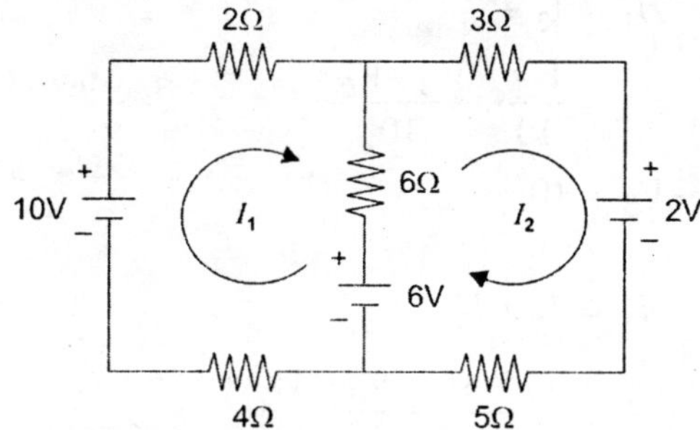

Step II: Apply KVL in loop 1 and loop 2.

Apply KVL in loop 1

$$\therefore \quad 10 - 2I_1 - 6(I_1 - I_2) - 6 - 4I_1 = 0$$

$$\therefore \quad 12I_1 - 6I_2 = 4$$

$$\therefore \quad 6I_1 - 3I_2 = 2 \quad \text{...(1)}$$

Apply KVL in loop 2

$$\therefore \quad -3I_2 - 2 - 5I_2 + 6 - 6(I_2 - I_1)$$

$$\therefore \quad -6I_1 + 14I_2 = 4 \quad \text{...(2)}$$

Step III: Solving the Eqs (1) and (2), we get

$$I_1 = 0.606 \text{ A}$$

$$I_2 = 0.545 \text{ A}$$

Example 3: Using nodal analysis method determine current in each branch.

(UPTU 2005-06)

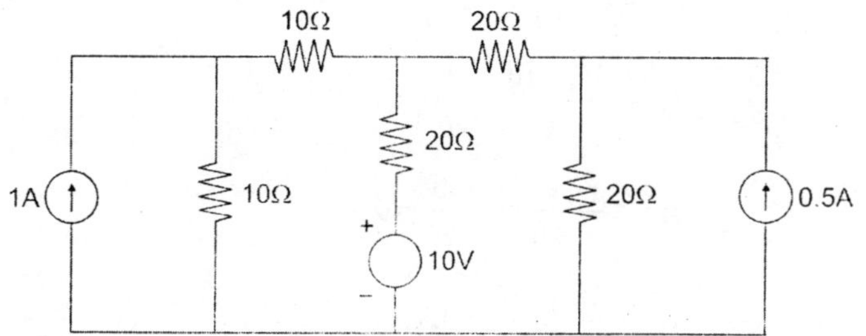

Solution: Step I: Identify the node and nodes voltages:

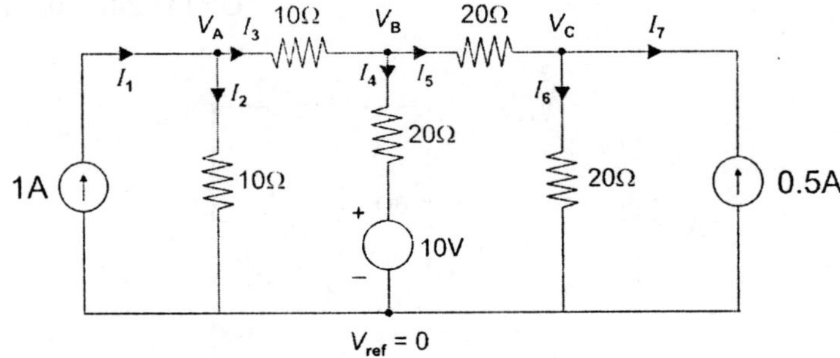

Step II:

Apply KCL at different nodes:

Apply KCL at node A

$$\therefore \quad I_1 = I_2 + I_3$$

$$1 = \frac{V_A}{10} + \frac{V_A - V_B}{10}$$

$$2V_A - V_B = 10 \quad \text{...(1)}$$

Apply KCL at node B

$$I_3 = I_4 + I_5$$

$$\therefore \quad \frac{V_A - V_B}{10} = \frac{V_B - 10}{20} + \frac{V_B - V_C}{20}$$

$$\therefore \quad 2V_A - 4V_B + V_C = -10 \quad \text{...(2)}$$

Now apply KCL at node C

$$I_5 = I_6 + I_7$$

$$\therefore \quad \frac{V_B - V_C}{20} = \frac{V_C}{20} - 0.5$$

$$\therefore \quad 2V_C - V_B = 10 \quad \text{...(3)}$$

Step III: Solving Eqs (1), (2) and (3), we get

$$V_A = 10\text{ V};\ V_B = 10\text{ V};\ V_C = 10\text{ V}$$

Step IV: Now the current in each branches given by

$$I_2 = \frac{V_A}{10} = \frac{10}{10} = 0.1\text{ A}$$

$$I_3 = \frac{V_A - V_B}{10} = \frac{0}{10} = 0\text{ A}$$

$$I_4 = \frac{V_B - 10}{20} = \frac{0}{20} = 0\text{ A}$$

$$I_5 = \frac{V_B - V_C}{20} = \frac{0}{20} = 0\text{ A}$$

$$I_6 = \frac{V_C}{20} = \frac{10}{20} = 0.5\text{ A}$$

EXERCISES

Short Answer Questions

1. Define the following terms:
   (i) Network.
   (ii) Source transformation
2. Give the difference between
   (i) Ideal voltage source and practical voltage source
   (ii) Ideal current source and practical current source
3. Explain current source to voltage source transformation.
4. Explain voltage source to current source conversion. Give an example with the help of a suitable diagram.
5. State and explain Kirchhoff's laws.
6. Derive expression for:
   (i) Star to delta transformation
   (ii) Delta to star transformation with example
   [UPTU 2004-05, 06-07, 09, 10-11, 12-13]
7. Distinguish the following terms with examples.
   [UPTU 2008-09, 09-10, 11-12, 12-13]
   (i) Active and passive elements.
   (ii) Linearity and nonlinearity.
   (iii) Unilateral and bilateral elements.

Descriptive Type Questions

1. Using the source transformation, find the voltage V in the circuit shown in figure below. **[Ans.** 4.508 V] [MTU 2008-09]

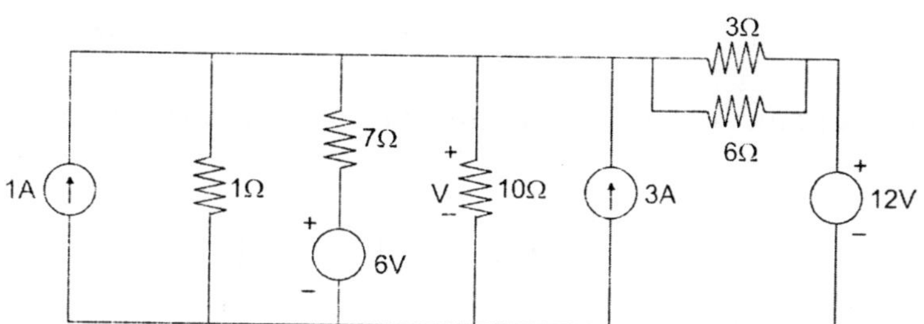

2. Using the source transformation techniques, find the current through 28 Ω branch of the circuit shown in figure below. **[Ans.** 2 A]

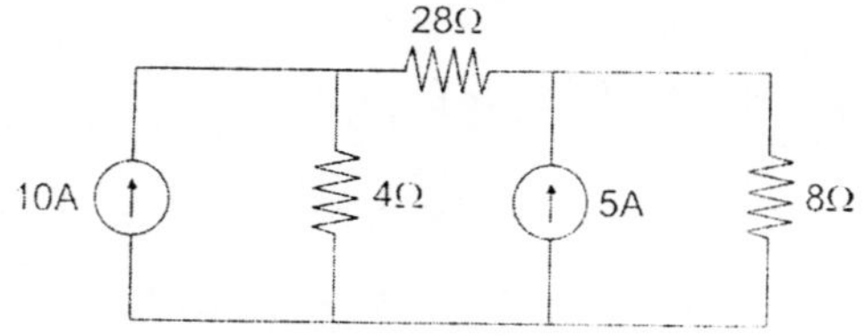

3. Using source conversion technique, find the current through load resistance R_L of the circuit shown in figure below. **[Ans.** 1.3043 A]

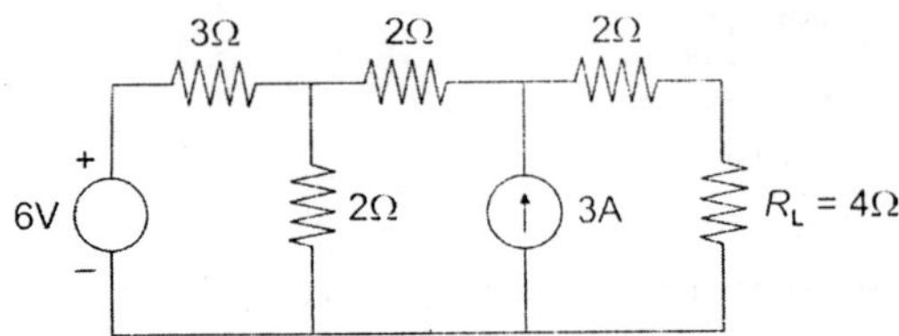

4. Find the branch currents in the circuit of figure shown by using
   (i) Nodal analysis
   (ii) Loop analysis

$$\left[\text{Ans. } \frac{7}{9}\text{A}, \frac{1}{3}\text{A}, -\frac{13}{12}\text{A}, \frac{4}{9}\text{A}, \frac{17}{12}\text{A}\right]$$

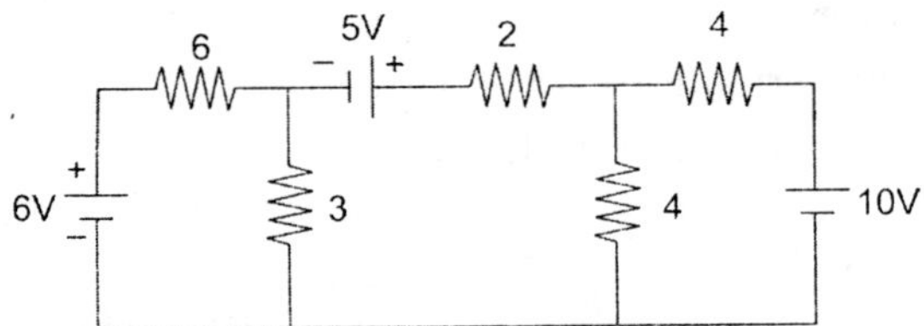

5. Apply loop current method to find loop current I_1, I_2 and I_3 in the circuit shown in figure below. **[Ans.** $I_1 = 3.75\text{A}, I_2 = 0\text{A}, I_3 = 1.25\text{A}$]

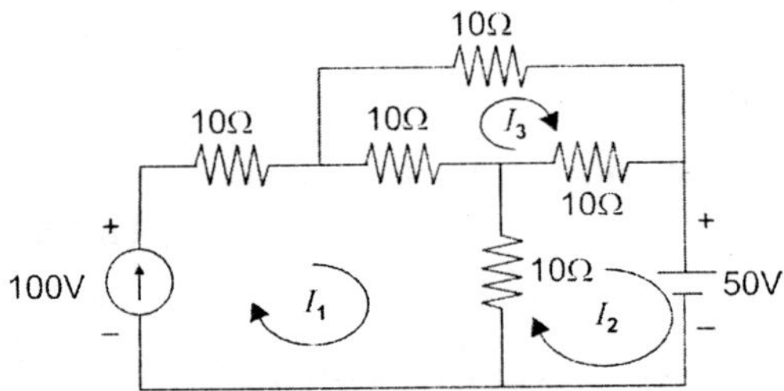

6. Using Mesh method, determine the current I_x in following circuit. **[Ans.** 1.92 A]

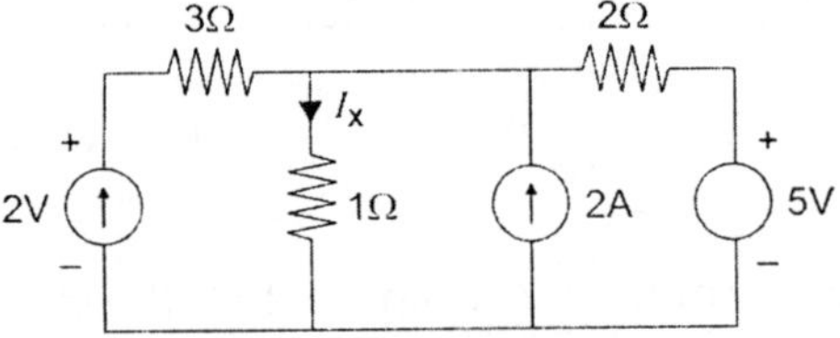

7. Calculate the node voltage V_B using nodal analysis. **[Ans.** V_B = 2.81 V]

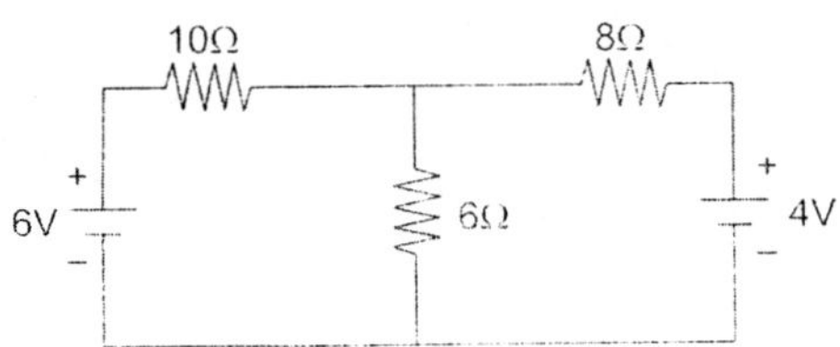

8. Determine the node voltage V_A and V_B by nodal analysis.

[**Ans.** $V_A = 8$ V, $V_B = 8$ V]

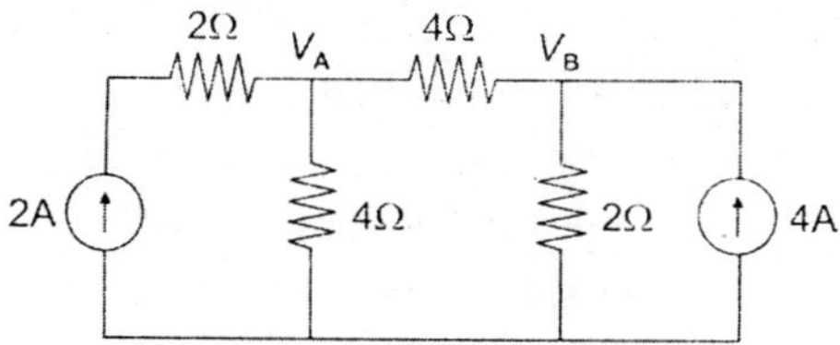

9. Determine the current through 5 Ω resistance using nodal analysis. [**Ans.** 3.105 A]

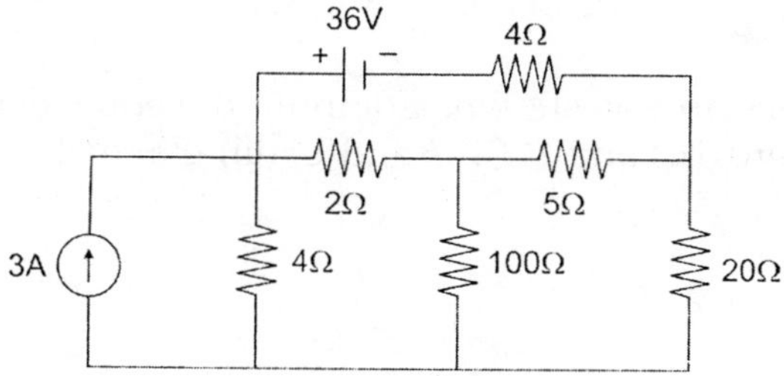

10. Find the input resistance between terminal *A* and *B* of the figure below.

[**Ans.** $R_{AB} = 11.667\ \Omega$]

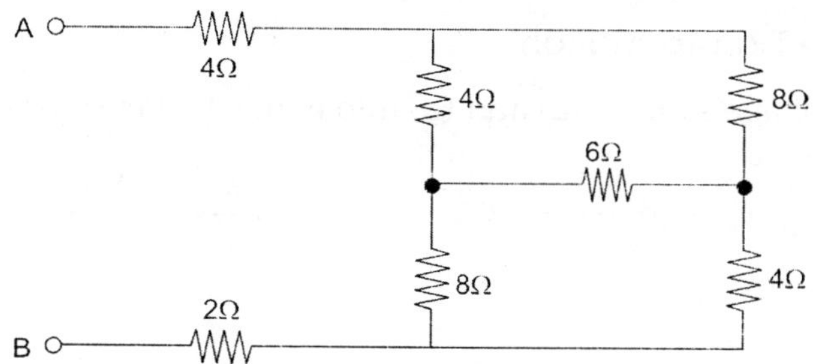

11. Using delta to star-transformation, determine the resistance between terminals *a-b* and the total power drawn from the supply in the circuit shown.

[**Ans.** P= 19.843 W]

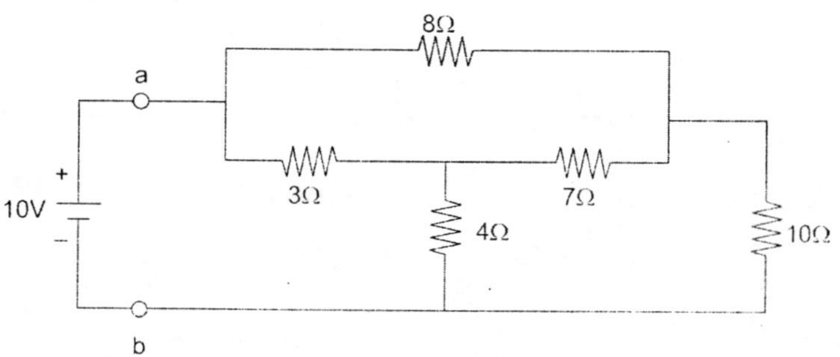

12. In the network shown determine the resistance between A and B.

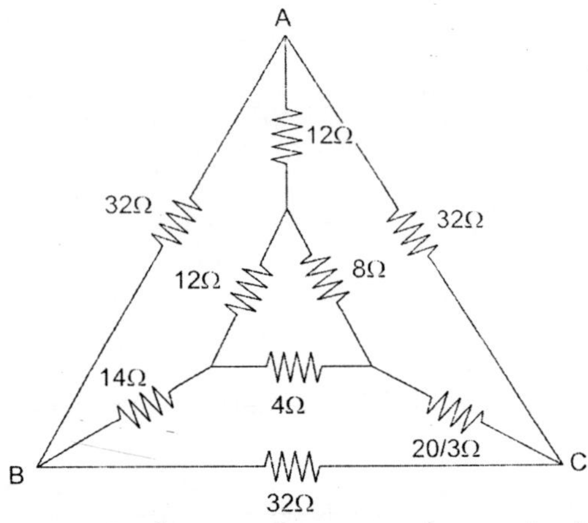

13. A network of resistance is shown. Compute the equivalent network resistance measured between. (i) A and B, (ii) B and C, (iii) C and A.

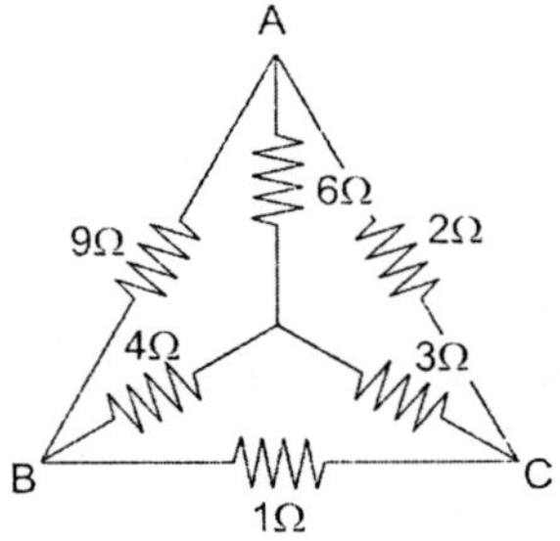

Based on Source Transformation

14. Transform voltage sources (a) and (b) into equivalent current sources.

[**Ans.** 10 A, 5 A]

2Ω A + 20V − B (a)

2Ω A + 10V − B (b)

15. Convert the arrangement into an equivalent single current source circuit.

$\left[\textbf{Ans. } 5\text{ A}, \frac{4}{3}\Omega\right]$

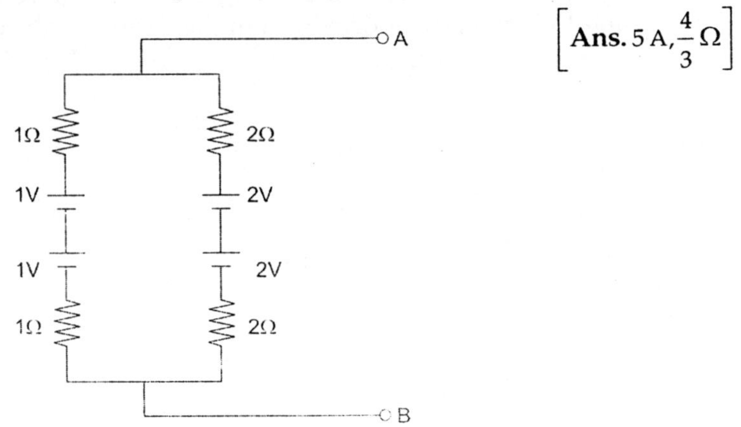

16. Using source transformation, find the voltage V in the circuit shown.

$$\left[\textbf{Ans. } 4.157\text{ V}, \ \frac{6}{171}\ \Omega\right]$$

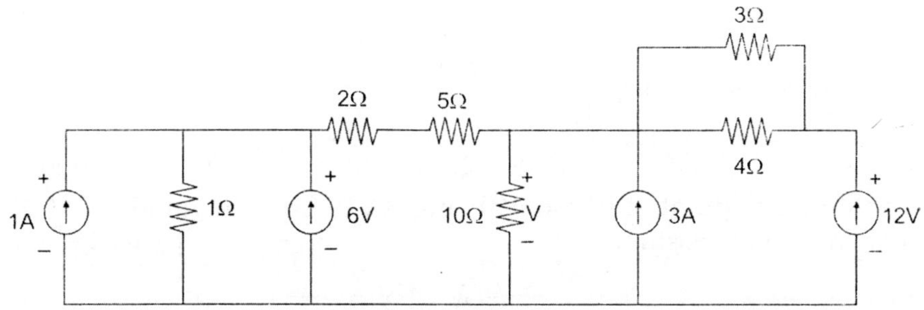

17. By using repeated source transformation, find the value of V. **[Ans.** 8 V]

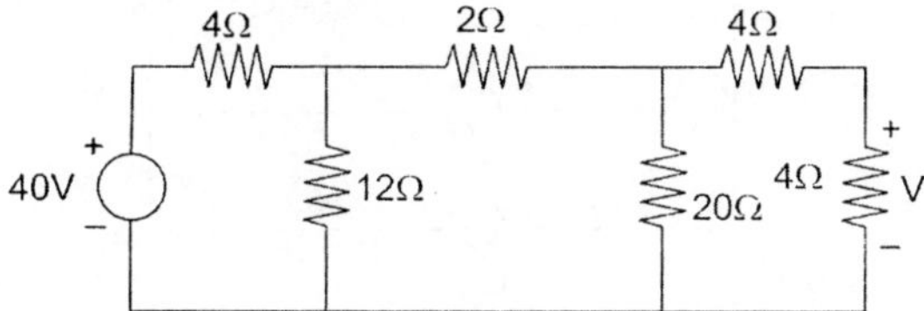

18. Find the current flowing through 2 Ω resistor using source transformation.

[Ans. 10 A]

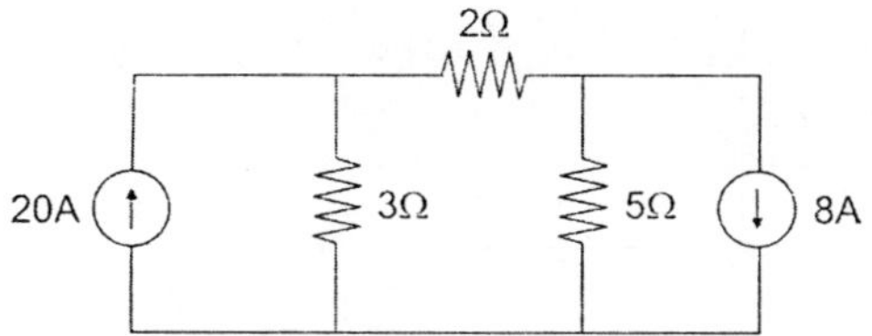

19. Use source conversion to find the load current I_L. **[Ans.** 2 A]

3Ω 2Ω 1Ω
6V 6Ω 3A 4 I_L R_L (3Ω)

Based on Kirchhoff's Laws

20. Use KVL, to find the values of V_1 and V_2 in the network shown. $\left[\text{Ans. } \begin{vmatrix} V_1 = 2\text{ V;} \\ V_2 = 5\text{ V} \end{vmatrix}\right]$

9V 18V
12V V_2 10V
V_1 3V

21. Use KVL, to find unknown current for circuit shown. [**Ans.** $I_1 = 2\,A, I_2 = 7\,A$]

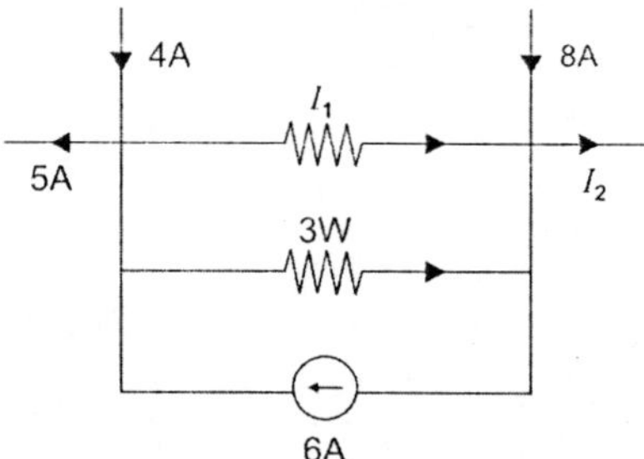

22. The potential of point *A* is –30 *V*, using KVL, find (*a*) value of '*V*' (*b*) power dissipated by 5 Ω resistance. [**Ans.** $V = 100$, 500 W]

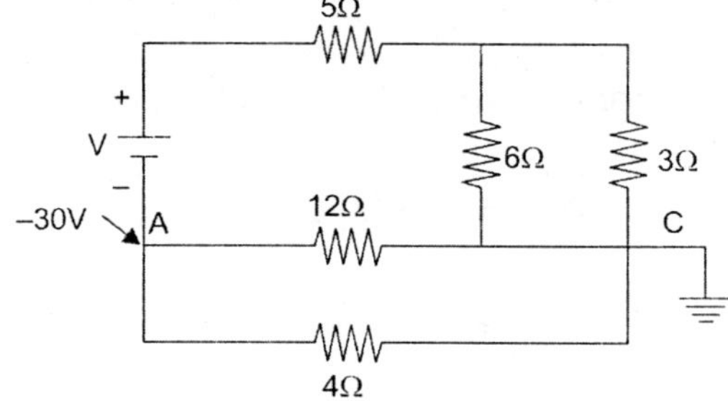

23. Using KCL and KVL, find the value of *V* and *I* for the circuits shown.

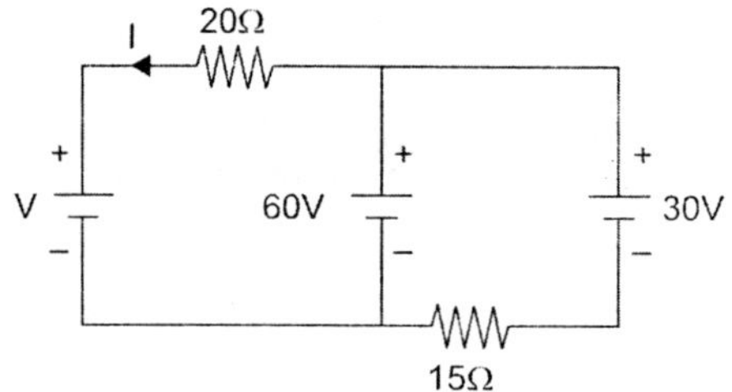

24. Find the current in 10 Ω branch using Kirchhoff's laws.

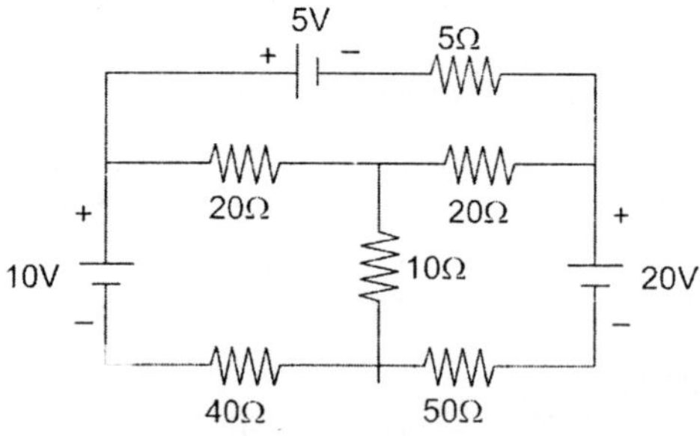

25. Calculate the current through 15 Ω branch using Kirchhoff's law and verify your answer using superposition theorem. [**Ans.** 2.281 A]

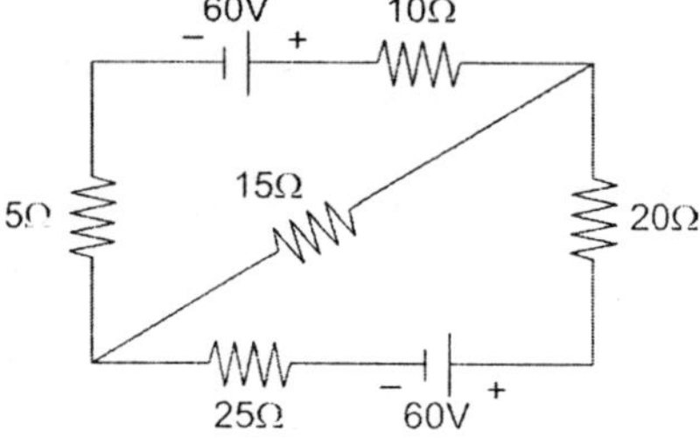

Based on Loop/Mesh Analysis

26. Find the ammeter current by using loop analysis. $\left[\textbf{Ans.} \frac{1}{7} \text{ A}\right]$

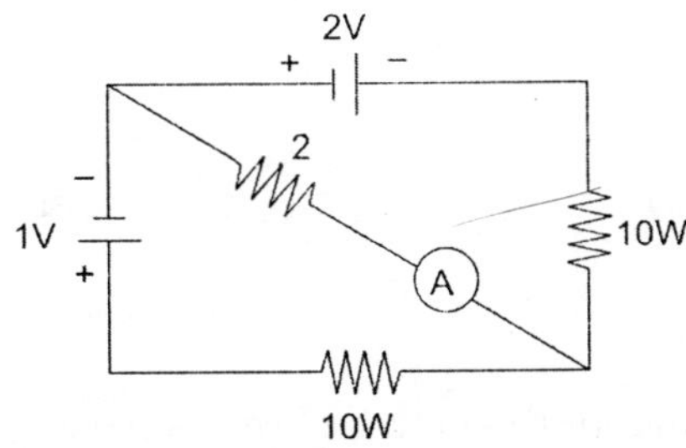

27. Using Mesh analysis, determine the voltage across 10 kΩ resistor at terminals *a, b* of the circuit shown. [**Ans.** 2.65 V]

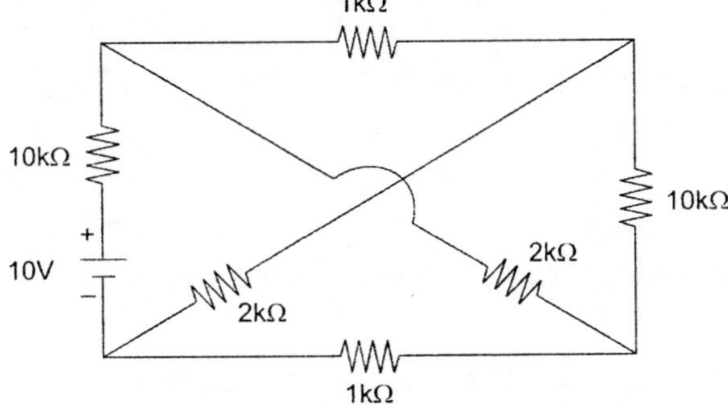

28. Apply loop current method to find loop currents I_1, I_2 and I_3 in the circuit. $\left[\textbf{Ans.}\ I_1 = 3.75 \text{ A}, I_2 = 0 \text{ A}, I_3 = 1.25 \text{ A}\right]$

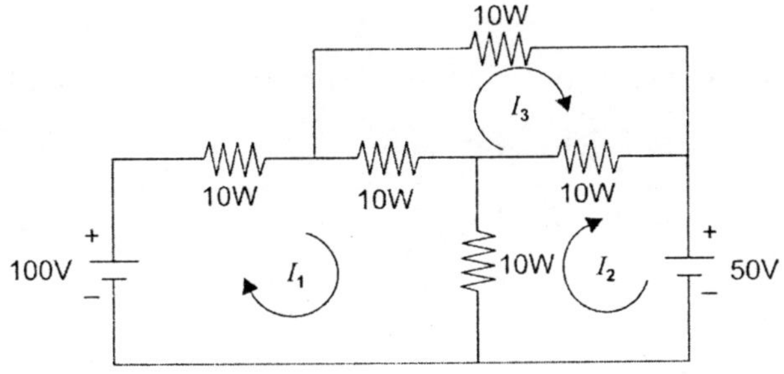

29. Using Mesh method, determines the current I_x in the following circuits. [**Ans.** –1.92 A]

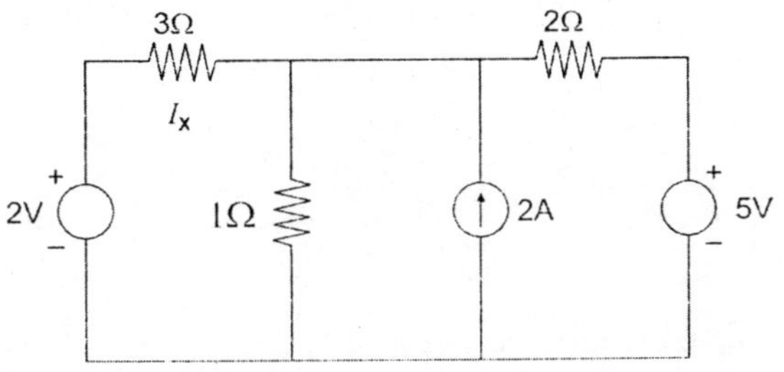

Based on Nodal Analysis

30. Calculate the node voltage V_B using nodal analysis. [**Ans.** 2.81 V]

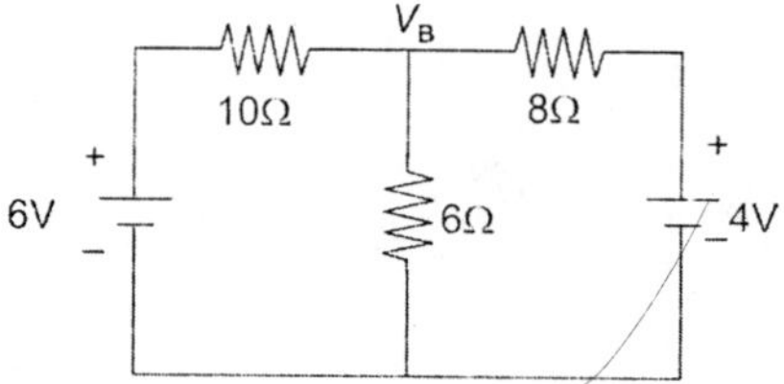

31. Solve for the branch current through 5 Ω resistor using nodal analysis. [**Ans.** 1 A]

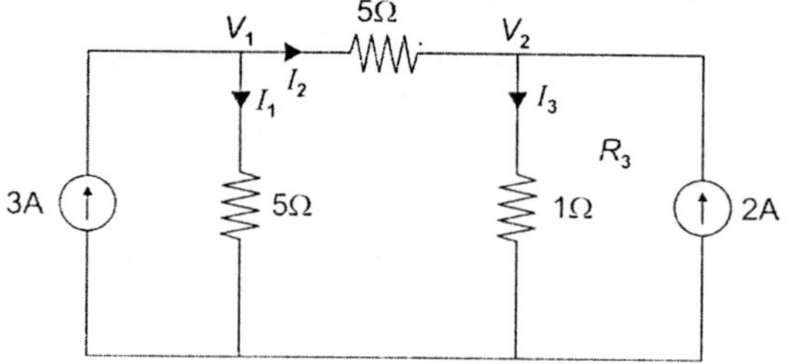

32. Find the current through 2 Ω and 3 Ω branch using nodal analysis.

[Ans. $I_{2\,\Omega} = 0.303$ A, $I_{3\,\Omega} = 1.807$ A]

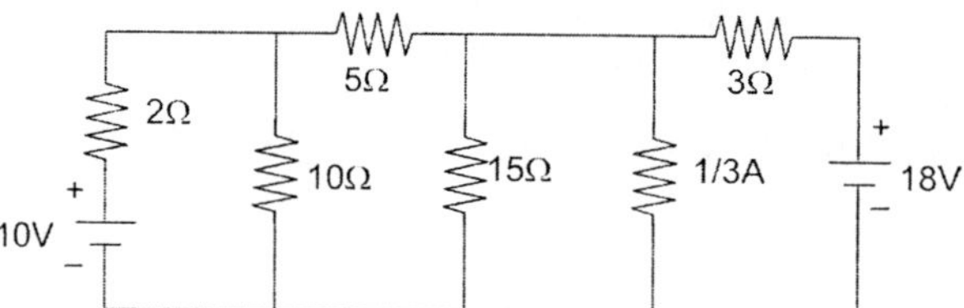

33. Determine the current through 5 Ω resistance using nodal analysis. [**Ans.** 3.105 A]

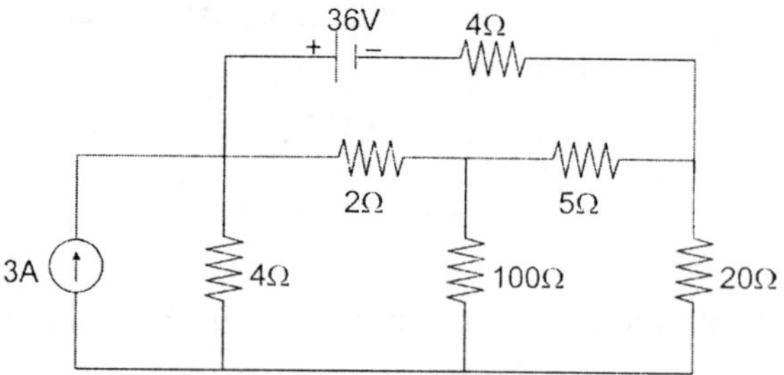

34. Using nodal voltagem method find the magnitude and direction of current I in the network.

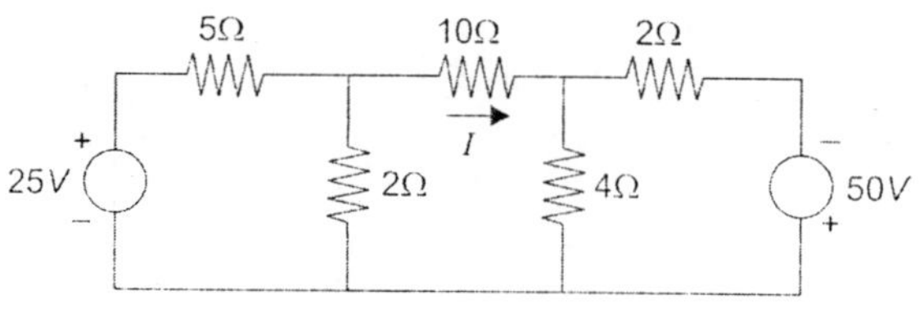

35. Calculate the power dissipated in the 9W resistor using nodal analysis method.
[**Ans.** 81 W]

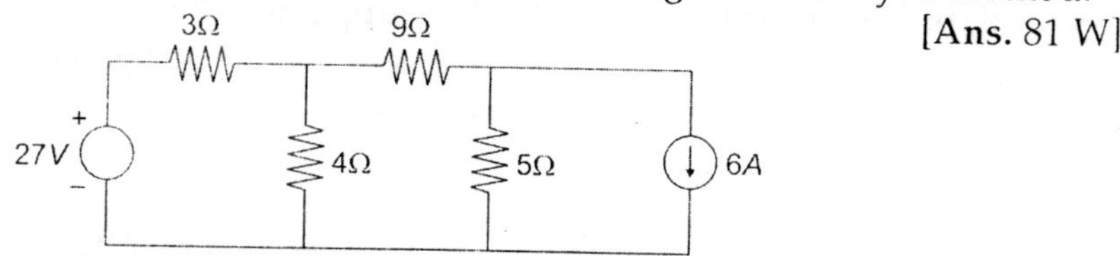

Based on Star/Delta Transformation

36. Find the current in the 17 Ω resistance in the network shown by using: Star-delta conversion.
$\left[\textbf{Ans.}\ \frac{10}{3}\ \text{A}\right]$

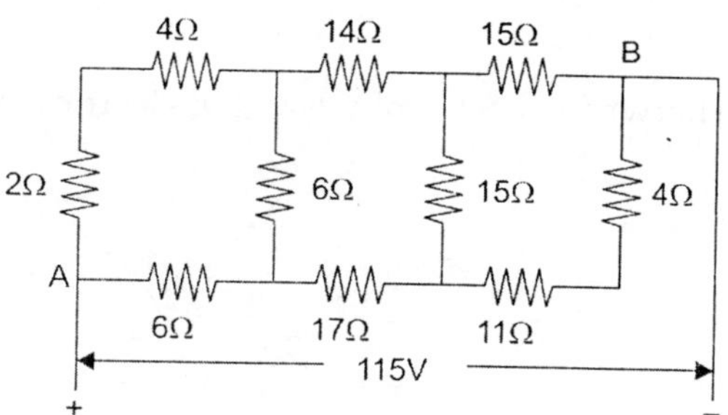

37. Determine the resistance between points A and B in the network shown. [**Ans.** 4.23 Ω]

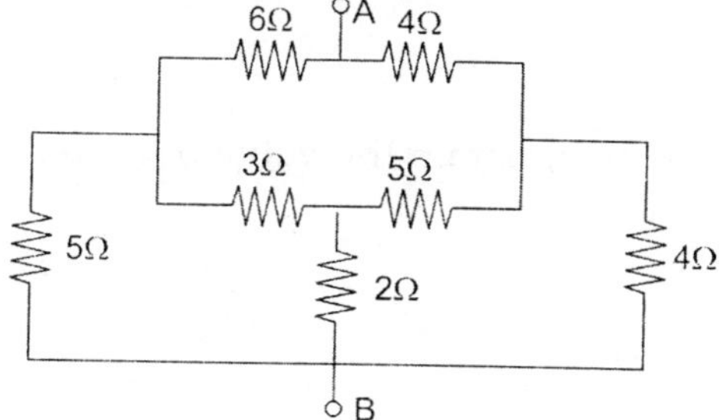

38. Using the delta-star transformation determine the current through the galvanometer in the wheat stone bridge.
[**Ans.** 0.025 A]

39. Obtain the circuit given on right side from the circuit given on left hand side using delta-star transformation.
[**Ans.** $R = 5.38\ \Omega$]

40. Using star-delta transformation, determine the resistance between terminals *a-b* and the total power drawn from the supply in the circuit shown.
[Ans. $R_{ab} = 5.04\,\Omega, p = 19.84$ W]

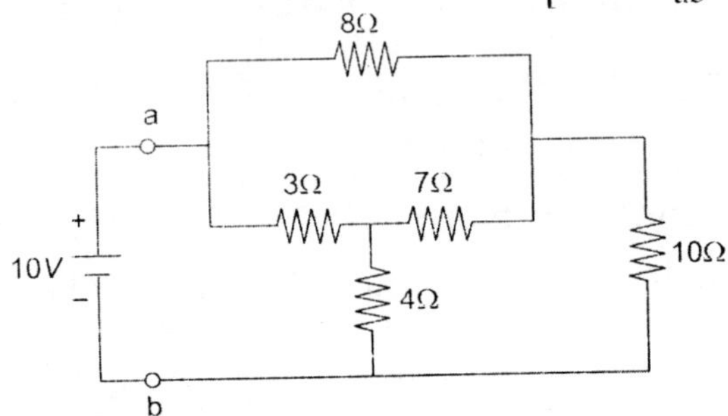

41. Find the resistance between A-B terminals in the electric circuit using $\Delta - Y$ transformation.
[Ans. 36 Ω]

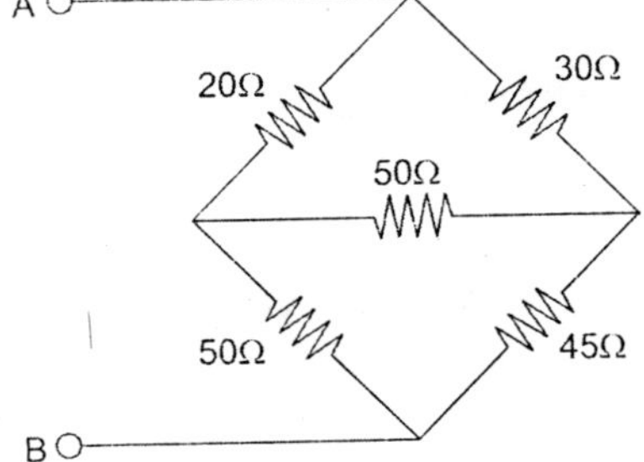

42. Using $Y - \Delta$ transformation, obtain the value of current supplied by the source shown in figure shown.
[Ans. 1 A]

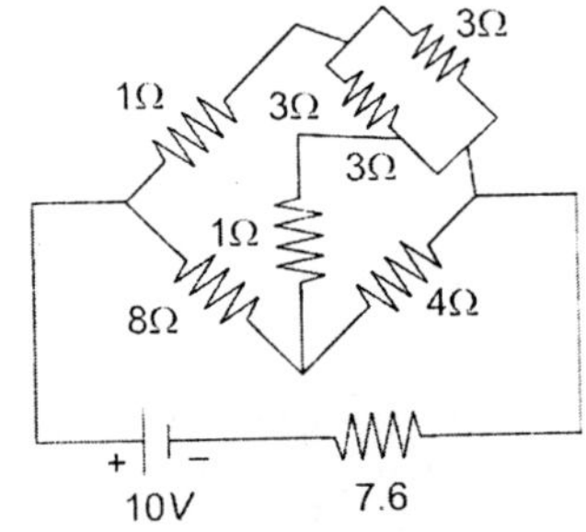

43. By using Δ / Y transformated on the mesh *ABC*, find the current by the source.
[Ans. 1 A]

40Ω A 20Ω

50Ω

D 10Ω C 30Ω B

30V 6Ω

Chapter

3 AC Fundamentals

3.1 INTRODUCTION

The acronym for alternative current is AC. In AC both the magnitude and direction changes. No such changes take place for the direct current (DC). An alternating current can be positive, negative or zero. It changes its polarity.

3.1.1 AC Quantity

Definition: An alternating (AC) quantity (voltage, current or power) is defined as the one which changes its magnitude as well as direction (polarity) with respect to time. Practically about 90% of the circuits use AC energy for their operation. The voltage supplied to us by the electricity board is also AC voltage. All appliances such as TV, refrigerator, washing machines, air conditioners, fans, etc. operate on the alternating voltage (AC voltage).

3.2 TYPES OF AC WAVEFORMS

Waveform: A waveform is a graphical representation of magnitude of any quantity with respect to time. We know that an alternating voltage is any voltage that varies both in magnitude and polarity with respect to time. Similarly, an alternating current is any current that varies in both magnitude and direction with respect to time. The schematic of types of AC waveforms are given in Fig. 3.1

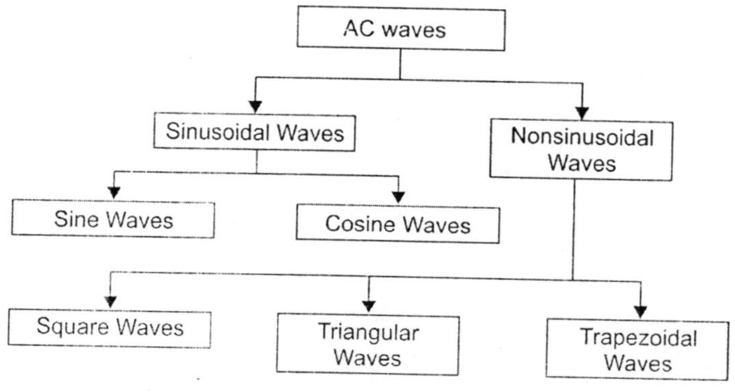

Fig. 3.1

Alternating quantity may be represented graphically. The shape of the curve obtained by plotting the value of voltage and current at different instants against time is called waveform or a waveshape (Fig. 3.2). Out of all these types of alternating waveforms, purely, sinusoidal waveform is preferred for AC system.

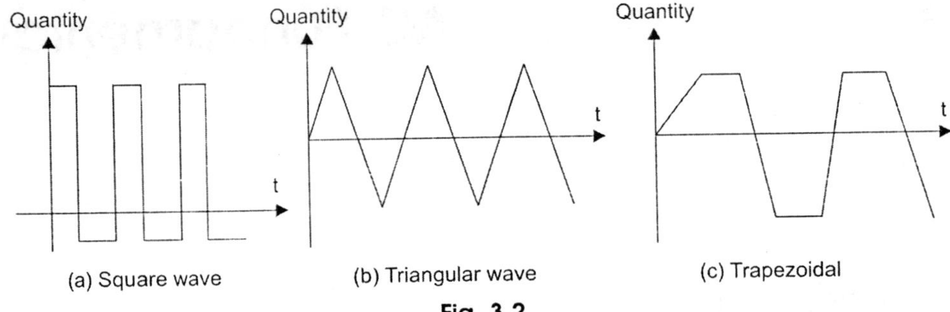

Fig. 3.2

3.3 ADVANTAGES OF SINUSOIDAL WAVEFORMS

The sinewave can be expressed in simple mathematical term or mathematically it is very easy to write the equation for purely sinusoidal waveform. Sinusoidal voltage and curent produce minimum disturbance in electrical circuit during operation. Sinusoidal voltage and current produce less interference (noise) on telephones lines. In AC machines, sinusoidal voltage and current produce less iron and less copper.

Note: It can be proved that any waveshape can be considered to be made up of various combination of sinewaves. Thus, sine wave is basic to all alternating voltages and currents. The quantities obeying sine laws are called sinusoidal quantities or sinusoids.

3.4 GENERATION OF ALTERNATING QUANTITY

According to Faraday's law of electromagnetic induction, when a coil is rotated in a magnetic field, an electromotive force (emf) is generated in it. This induced emf is directly proportional to the rate of change of flux. Figure 3.3a shows the basic principle of generation of alternating quantity.

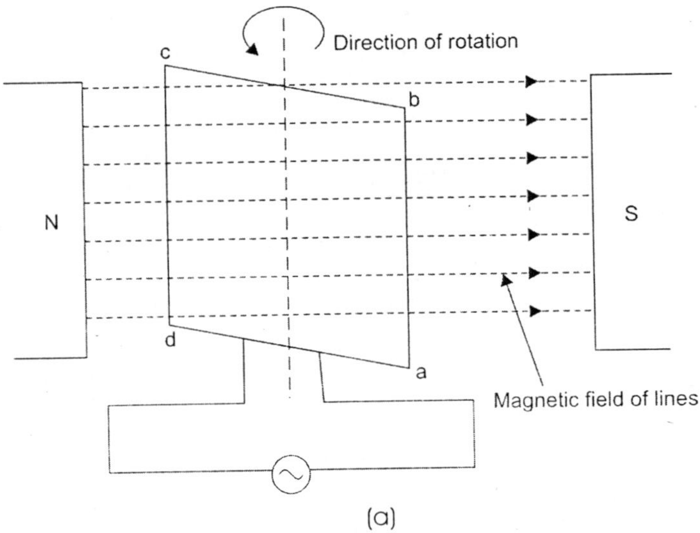

(a)

3.4.1 Equations of the Alternating Voltages and Currents

Consider a rectangular coil, having N turns and rotating in a uniform magnetic field with an angular velocity of ω radian/second, as shown in Fig. 3.3b. Let time be measured from the x-axis. Maximum flux ϕ_m is linked with the coil, when its plane coincides with the x-axis. In time t seconds, this coil rotates through an angle $\theta = \omega t$. In this deflected position, the component of the flux which is perpendicular to the plane of the coil is $\phi = \phi_m \cos \omega t$. Hence, flux linkages of the coil at any time are $N\phi = N\phi_m \cos \omega t$. According to Faraday's laws of electromagnetic induction, the emf induced in the coil is given by the rate of change of flux-linkages of the coil. Hence, the value of the induced emf at this instant (i.e. when $\theta = \omega t$) or the instantaneous value of the induced emf is

$$e = \frac{d}{dt}(N\phi)\,\text{volt} = -N\frac{d}{dt}(\phi_m \cos\omega t)\,\text{volt} = -N\phi_m\omega(-\sin\omega t)\,\text{volt}$$

$$= \omega N\phi_m \sin\omega t = \omega N\phi_m \sin\theta \qquad \text{...(3.1)}$$

When the coil has turned through 90°, then $\sin\theta = 1$, hence e has maximum value, say E_m,

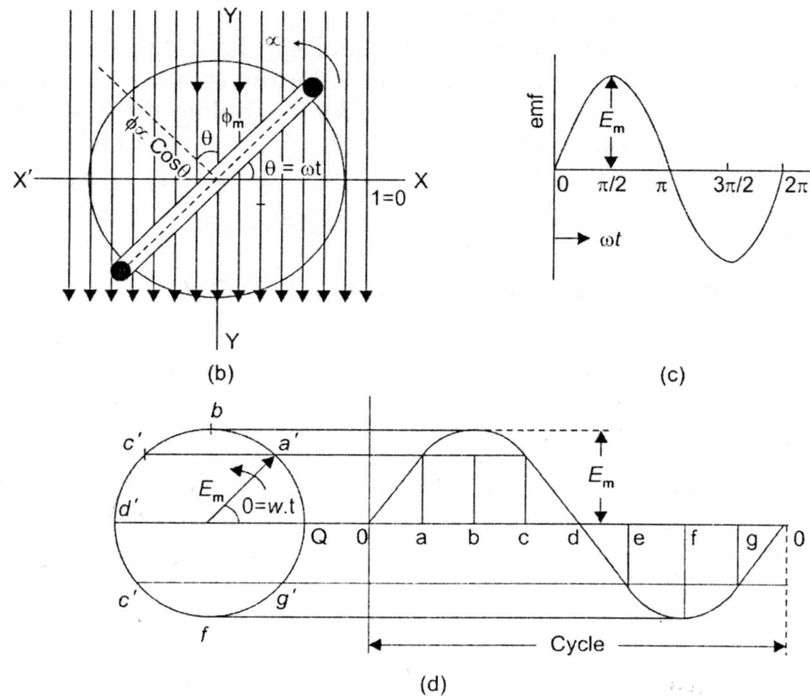

Fig. 3.3: Basic principle of generation of alternating quantities

Therefore, Eq. (3.1) we get

$$E_m = \omega N \phi_m = \omega N B_m A = 2\pi f N B_m A \qquad \text{...(3.2)}$$

B_m = maximum flux density Wb/m^2; A = area of the coil in m^2

f = frequency of rotation of the coil in rev/sec

Substituting this value of E_m in Eq. (3.1), we get

$$e = E_m \sin\theta = E_m \sin\omega t \qquad \text{...(3.3)}$$

Similarly, the equation of induced alternating current is

$$I = I_m \sin \omega t \quad ...(3.4)$$

provided the coil circuit has been closed through a resistive load.

Since $\omega = 2\pi f$, where f is the frequency of rotation of the coil, Eqs (3.3) and (3.4) of voltage and current can be written as $e = E_m \sin 2\pi ft = E_m \sin\left(\frac{2\pi}{T}\right)t$ and $i = I_m \sin 2\pi ft$ $= I_m \sin\left(\frac{2\pi}{T}\right)t$.

where T = time-period of the alternating voltage or current = $1/f$.

It is seen that the induced emf varies as sine function of the time angle wt and when emf is plotted against time, a curve similar to the one shown in Fig. 3.3c is obtained. This curve is known as sine curve and the emf which varies in this manner is known as sinusodial emf. Such a sine curve can be conveniently drawn as shown in Fig. 3.3d. A vector, equal in length to E_m is drawn. It rotates in the counter-clockwise direction with a velocity of ω radian/second, making one revolution while the generated emf maked two loops or one cycle. The projection of this vector on y-axis gives the instantaneous value e of the induced emf i.e. $E_m \sin \omega t$.

To construct the curve, lay off long x-axis equal angular distance *oa, ab, bc, cd,* etc. corresponding to suitable angular displacement of the rotating vector. Now, erect coordinates at the points *a, b, c* and *d* etc. (Fig. 3.3d) and then project the free ends of the vector E_m at the corresponding positions a', b', c', etc to meet these ordiates. Next draw a curve passing through these intersecting points. The curve so obtained is the graphic representation of Eq. (3.3) above.

63.5 IMPORTANT DEFINITIONS RELATED TO AC QUANTITY

(i) Instantaneous value (ii) Cycle (iii) Time period
(iv) Frequency (v) Amplitude (vi) Angular velocity

i. Instantaneous Value

Defintion: The instantaneous value of an AC quantity is defined as the value of that quantity at a particular instant of time. *Example:* $v_{(t_1)}$ is the instantaneous value of the AC voltage $v(t)$ at instant t_1 or $v(t_2)$ is its instantaneous value at instant t_2.

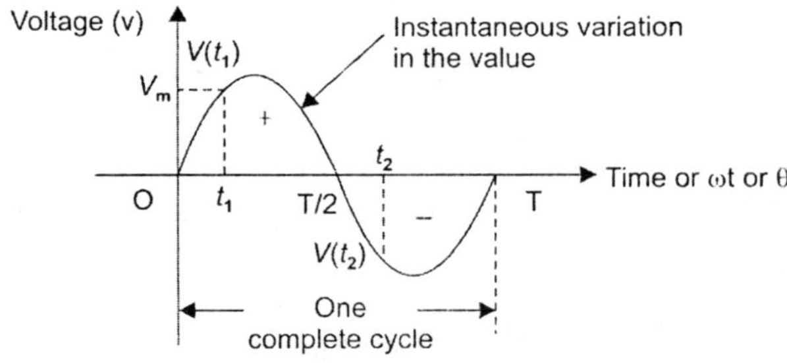

Fig. 3.4 Waveform of an AC voltage

$$v = V_m \sin \omega t$$

$$= V_m \sin \theta \text{ (instantaneous equation of voltage)}$$

V_m = peak value of voltage

Similarly for current

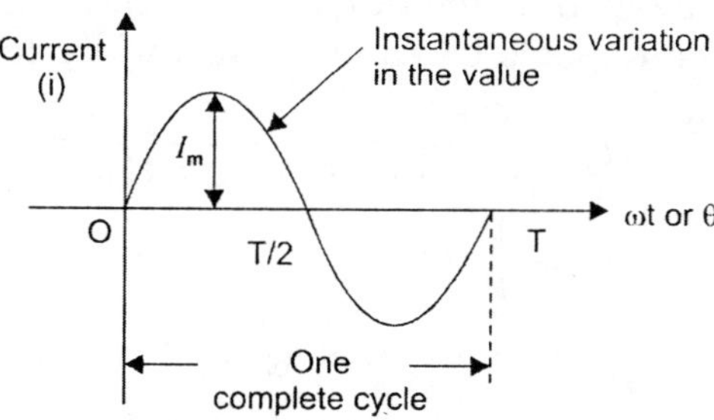

Fig. 3.5: Waveform of an AC current

$$i = I_m \sin \omega t$$

or $$i = I_m \sin \theta = \text{instantaneous equation of current}$$

where, I_m = peak value of current

ii. Cycle

Definition: In an AC waveform, each repetition consisting of one positive and one identical negative part is called as one cycle of the waveform (Fig. 3.6).

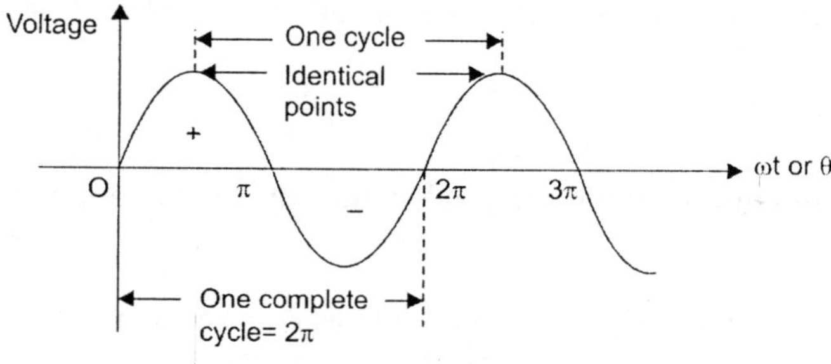

Fig. 3.6: Definition of a cycle

iii. Time Period or Periodic Time (*T*)

Definition: Time period (T) is defined as the time taken in seconds by the waveform of an AC quantity to complete one cycle.

After every T seconds, the cycle repeats itself as shown in Fig. 3.7.

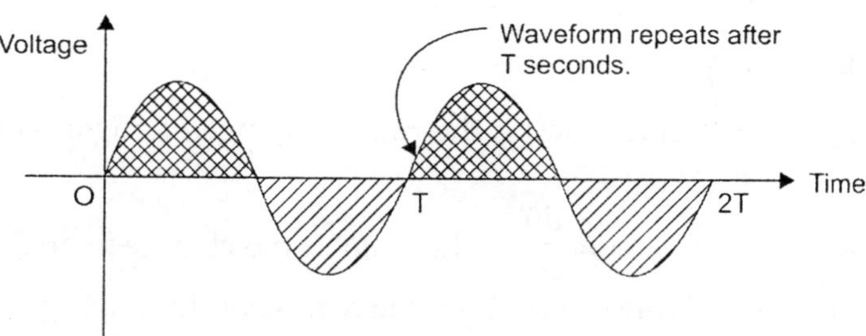

Fig. 3.7: Concept of time period (T)

∴ Time period T = time corresponding to one cycle

IV. Frequency

Defintion: Frequency is defined as the number of cycles completed by an altenating quantity in one second. It is denoted by f and its units are cycles/seconds or hertz (Hz).

$$\therefore \text{ Frequency } (f) = \frac{\text{Cycle}}{\text{Second}} = \frac{1}{\text{Second/Cycle}} = \frac{1}{T}$$

$$\therefore \quad f = \frac{1}{T} \text{Hz}$$

Voltage or current

O

T

Time

Time period T

(a) Low frequency

Voltage or current

O

T

Time

Time period reduced

(b) High frequency

Fig. 3.8: Effect of change in time period (T) on the value of frequency

v. Amplitude

Defintion: The maximum value or peak value of an AC quantity is called as its amplitude.

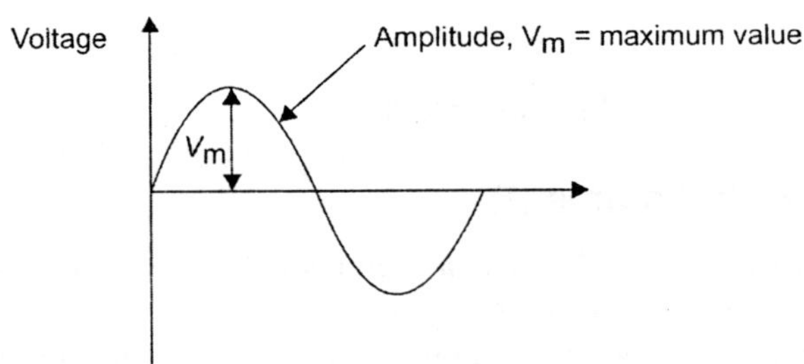

Fig. 3.9: Concept of amplitude

vi. Angular Velocity (ω)

Definition: The angular velocity (ω) is the rate of change of angle ω or θ with respect to time.

$$\therefore \quad \omega = \frac{d\theta}{dt}, \text{ where } d\theta \text{ is the change in angle in time } dt.$$

If $dt = T$, i.e. time period (one cycle), then the corresponding change in θ is 2π radians.

$$\therefore \quad d\theta = 2\pi$$

$$\therefore \quad \omega = \frac{2\pi}{T}.$$

But $\frac{1}{T} = f \therefore \omega = 2\pi f$

3.6 IMPORTANT VALUES OF ALTERNATING QUANTITIES

There are two types of values

(i) Effective value or RMS value.

(ii) Average value or mean value.

(i) **Effective value or RMS value:** The root mean square (RMS) value of an alternating current is equal to that value of direct current which will produce the same heat in the same time in the same resistor (Fig. 3.10).

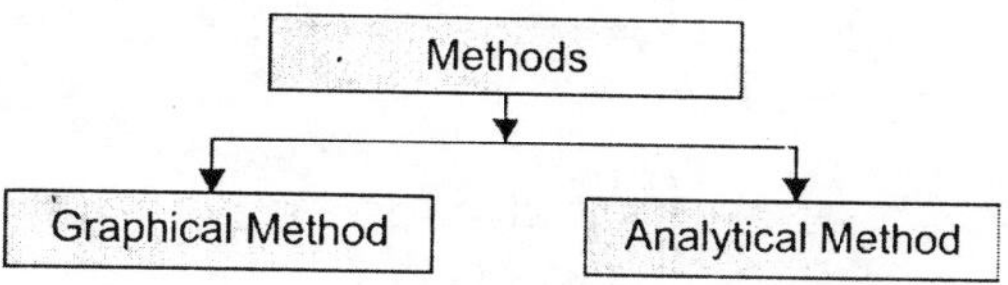

Fig. 3.10

Practical importance of RMS value: Worldwide, an alternating voltage or current is always specified in terms of RMS values. The domestic AC supply is 230 V, 50 Hz, it is the RMS value, it means that alternating voltage available has the same heating effect as 230 V DC. When we say that alternating current in a circuit is 5 A, we are specifiying the RMS value, it means that the alternating current flowing in the circuit has the same heating effect as 5 A DC. Ammeters and voltmeters record RMS value of alternating current and voltage, respectively.

(ii) **Average value or mean value:** The average value of an alternating quantity is defined as the value which is obtained by averaging all the instantaneous values over a period of half cycle (Fig. 3.11).

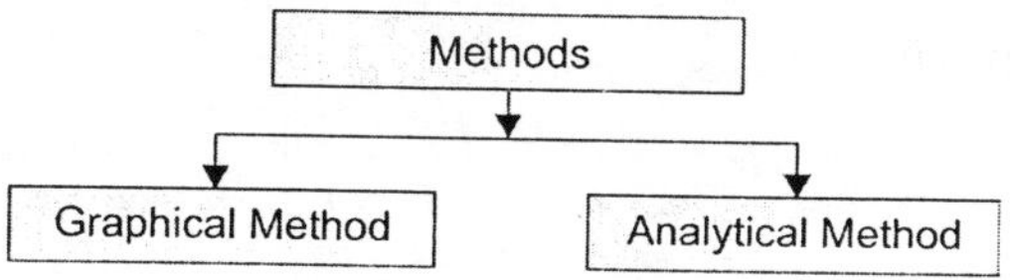

Fig. 3.11: Block diagram

Practical importance of average value: The average value is used for applications like battery charging and rectifier circuits, etc. The DC ammeters and voltmeters indicate the average values. The change transferred in capacitor circuit is measured using average value. The average value of purely sinusoidal waveform over a complete cycle is always zero.

3.7 ROOT MEAN SQUARE (RMS) OR EFFECTIVE VALUES, AVERAGE VALUE, FORM-FACTOR AND PEAK FACTOR OF ALTERNATING CURRENT AND ALTERNATING VOLTAGE FOR SINUSOIDAL WAVEFORM

(i) RMS Value (Root Mean Square Value)

RMS value of an AC is given by that steady current which when flowing through a circuit for a given time produces the same heat as produced by the AC when flowing through the same circuit for the same time.

Heat produced by an alternating current of instanteneous value i in resistor R in time dt is $i^2R\,dt$. Total heat produced in one cycle (i.e. in time T) is given by:

$$H_{ac} = \int_0^T i^2 R\,dt$$

Heat produced by the equivalent direct current I in resistor R in time T is given by

$$H_{DC} = I^2RT$$

$$H_{DC} = H_{AC}$$

$$I^2RT = \int_0^T i^2 R\,dt$$

$$I^2 = \frac{1}{T}\int_0^T i^2\,dt$$

$$= \frac{1}{2\pi}\int_0^{2\pi} i^2\,d\theta$$

$$= \frac{1}{2\pi}\int_0^{2\pi} I_m^2 \sin^2\theta\,d\theta$$

$$= \frac{I_m^2}{2\pi}\int_0^{2\pi}\frac{1}{2}(1-\cos 2\theta)\,d\theta$$

$$= \frac{I_m^2}{4\pi}\left[\theta - \frac{1}{2}\sin 2\theta\right]_0^{2\pi}$$

$$= \frac{I_m^2}{4\pi}[\theta]_0^{2\pi} - \frac{I_m^2}{8\pi}[\sin 2\theta]_0^{2\pi}$$

$$= \frac{I_m^2}{4\pi}(2\pi - 0) - \frac{I_m^2}{8\pi}(\sin 4\pi - \sin 0)$$

Now $\sin 4\pi = 0$, $\sin 0 = 0$

$$\therefore \quad I^2 = \frac{I_m^2}{4\pi}\times 2\pi \qquad \therefore I_{rms} = \frac{I_m}{\sqrt{2}} = 0.707\,I_m$$

Similarly $$V_{rms} = \frac{V_m}{\sqrt{2}} = 0.707\,V_m$$

(ii) Average Value

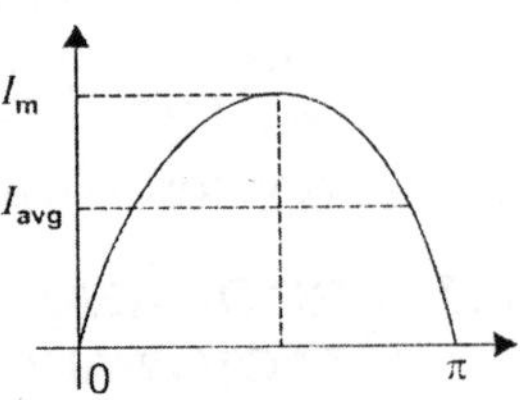

Fig. 3.12

The average value I_a of an alternating current is expressed by that steady current which transfer across any circuit the same change as transfered by that alternating current during the same time.

In the case of a symmetrical alternating current (i.e. one whose two half cycles are exactly similar, wheather sinusoidal or non-sinusoidal) the average value over a complete cycle is zero.

The standard equation of an alternating current $i = I_m \sin\theta$

$$I_{avg} = \int_0^{\pi}\frac{i\,d\theta}{(\pi - 0)} = \frac{I_m}{\pi}\int_0^{\pi}\sin\theta\,d\theta$$

$$= \frac{I_m}{\pi}[-\cos\theta]_0^{\pi} = \frac{I_m}{\pi}\left[+1-(-1)\right] = \frac{2I_m}{\pi} = \frac{I_m}{\pi/2}$$

$\therefore$ $I_{avg} = 0.637\ I_m$

Similary for voltage

$$V_{avg} = \frac{2V_m}{\pi} = 0.637\ V_m$$

(iii) Form Factor

The ratio of RMS value to the average value of an alternating quantity is called *form factor* and it is denoted by K_f

$$\therefore \qquad K_f = \frac{\text{RMS value}}{\text{Average value}}$$

For current, form factor is:

$$K_{fI} = \frac{I_{rms}}{I_{avg}} = \frac{0.707\ I_m}{0.637\ I_m} = 1.11$$

$$K_{fI} = \frac{\frac{I_m}{\sqrt{2}}}{\frac{2I_m}{\pi}} = \frac{\pi}{2\sqrt{2}} = 1.11$$

For voltage, form factor is

$$\therefore \qquad K_{fV} = \frac{V_{rms}}{V_{avg}} = \frac{\frac{V_m}{\sqrt{2}}}{\frac{2V_m}{\pi}} = \frac{\pi}{2\sqrt{2}} = 1.11$$

(iv) Peak Factor or Crest Factor

The ratio of maximum value to crest or amplitude factor value of an alternating quantity is known as peak factor. It is also known as crest or amplitude factor and it is denoted by K_a or K_p.

$$\therefore \qquad K_a \text{ or } K_p = \frac{\text{Maximum value}}{\text{RMS value}}$$

For current, peak factor

$$K_{pi} = \frac{I_m}{I_{rms}} = \frac{I_m}{\frac{I_m}{\sqrt{2}}} = 1.414$$

For voltage, peak factor

$$K_{pv} = \frac{V_m}{V_{rms}} = \frac{V_m}{\frac{V_m}{\sqrt{2}}} = \sqrt{2} = 1.414$$

SOLVED EXAMPLES FOR PRACTICE

Example: An alternating current of frequency 60 Hz has maximum value of 120 A. Write down the equation for instantaneous value of current. Find the time taken to reach 96 A for first time. **[UPTU 2006-07]**

Solution: Given data

$$I_m = 120 \text{ A}, f = 60 \text{ Hz}, i = 96 \text{ A}$$

We know that, instantaneous equation of current

$$i = I_m \sin \omega t, \quad \omega = 2\pi f$$

$$\therefore \quad i = 120 \sin 2\pi \times 60t = 120 \sin 120\pi t \text{ A.} \qquad \textbf{Ans.}$$

Time taken to reach 96 A

$$\therefore \quad 96 = 120 \sin (120\,\pi t)$$

$$t = \frac{1}{120\pi} \sin^{-1}\left(\frac{96}{120}\right)$$

$$= 0.00246 \text{ seconds} \qquad \textbf{Ans.}$$

Note: For any trigonometry (sin, cos, tan, cot, etc.) multiplication/ division 'π' is taken as 180°.

Example: The AC supply at a house is 230 V, 50 Hz, find maximum value, rms value, average value, form factor and peak factor of voltage.

Solution: The given data

$$V_{rms} = 230 \text{ V}, f = 50 \text{ Hz}$$

We know that $V_{rms} = \dfrac{V_m}{\sqrt{2}}$

RMS value of voltage $= 230$ V

$$\therefore \quad V_m = \sqrt{2} \times V_{rms}$$

$$= \sqrt{2} \times 230 = 325.27 \text{ V} \qquad \textbf{Ans.}$$

Average value of voltage

$$V_{avg} = \frac{2V_m}{\pi} = \frac{2 \times 325.27}{\pi} = 207.2 \text{ V} \qquad \textbf{Ans.}$$

Form factor of voltage

$$K_{fv} = \frac{V_{rms}}{V_{avg}} = \frac{\dfrac{V_m}{\sqrt{2}}}{\dfrac{2V_m}{\pi}} = \frac{\pi}{\sqrt{2}} = 1.11$$

Peak factor of voltage

$$K_{Pv} = \frac{V_m}{V_{rms}} = \frac{325.27}{230} = 1.414 \qquad \textbf{Ans.}$$

3.8 RMS VALUE OR EFFECTIVE VALUE, FORM FACTOR FOR HALF-WAVE VOLTAGE AND CURRENT

Waveform for half-wave rectifier (Fig. 3.13)

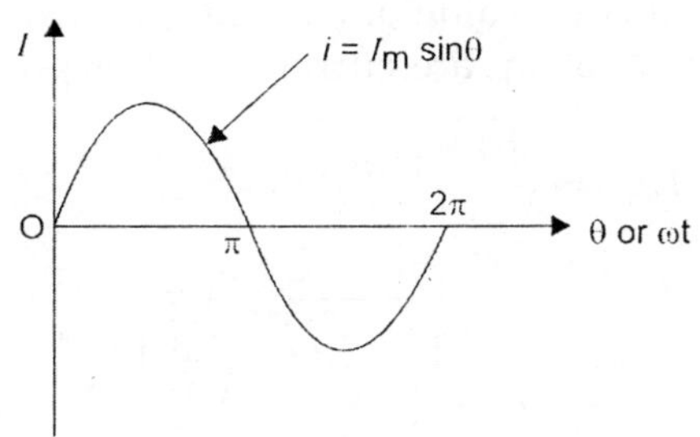

Fig. 3.13

$$\therefore \quad I_{\text{rms}} = \sqrt{\frac{1}{2\pi}\int_0^{\pi} i^2\, d\theta} = \sqrt{\frac{1}{2\pi}\int_0^{\pi} (I_m \sin\theta)^2\, d\theta}$$

$$= \sqrt{\frac{I_m^2}{2\pi}\int_0^{\pi} \sin^2\theta d\theta} = \sqrt{\frac{I_m^2}{2\pi}\int_0^{\pi} \frac{(1-\cos 2\theta)}{2} d\theta}$$

$$= \sqrt{\frac{I_m^2}{4\pi}\int_0^{\pi} (1-\cos 2\theta) d\theta} = \sqrt{\frac{I_m^2}{4\pi}\left[\theta - \frac{\sin 2\theta}{2}\right]_0^{\pi}}$$

$$= \sqrt{\frac{I_m^2}{4\pi}(\pi - 0)} = \frac{I_m}{2}$$

Similarly for voltage

$$V_{\text{rms}} = \frac{V_m}{2}$$

Form factor

For current

$$K_{\text{fI}} = \frac{I_{\text{rms}}}{I_{\text{avg}}} = \frac{I_m/2}{I_m/\pi} = \frac{\pi}{2} = 1.57$$

For voltage

$$K_{\text{fv}} = 1.57$$

Peak factor

For current $\quad K_{\text{PI}} = \dfrac{I_m}{I_{rms}} = \dfrac{I_m}{I_m/2} = 2$

Similary for voltage $\quad K_{\text{Pv}} = 2$

3.9 RMS VALUE, AVERAGE VALUE, FORM FACTOR AND PEAK FACTOR FOR SQUARE WAVE OF VOLTAGE AND CURRENT

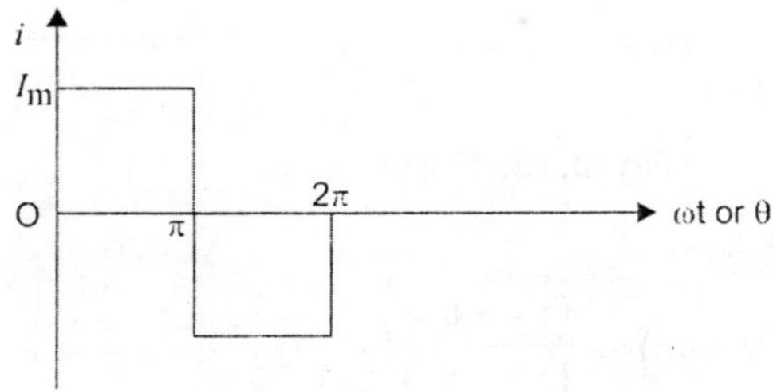

Fig. 3.14: Square wave

From waveform, instantaneous value of current given by, $I = I_m$ for $0 < \theta < \pi$.

RMS Value: The rms value of square current wave is given by

$$I_{rms} = \sqrt{\frac{1}{2\pi}\int_0^{2\pi} i^2 d\theta}$$

$$= \sqrt{\frac{1}{2\pi}\int_0^{\pi} I_m^{2\pi} d\theta} = \sqrt{\frac{I_m^2}{2\pi}[\theta]_0^{2\pi}} = \sqrt{\frac{I_m^2}{2\pi}2\pi} = I_m$$

$$\therefore \quad I_{rms} = I_m$$

Similarly for voltage

$$\therefore \quad V_{rms} = V_m$$

Average value: The average value of the square current wave is given by

$$I_{avg} = \frac{1}{\pi}\int_0^{\pi} I d\theta = \frac{1}{\pi}\int_0^{\pi} I_m d\theta$$

$$= \frac{I_m}{\pi}[\theta]_0^{\pi} = \frac{I_m}{\pi}\times\pi$$

$$\therefore \quad I_{avg} = I_m$$

Similarly for voltage

$$\therefore \quad V_{avg} = V_m$$

Form factor: The form factor of the square current wave is given by

$$K_{FI} = 1$$

Similary for voltage

$$K_{fV} = 1$$

Peak factor: The peak factor of the square current wave is given by

$$K_{PI} = 1$$

Similarly for voltage

$$K_{PV} = 1$$

3.10 RMS VALUE, AVERAGE VALUE, FORM FACTOR, PEAK FACTOR OF TRIANGULAR WAVE FOR CURRENT AND VOLTAGE

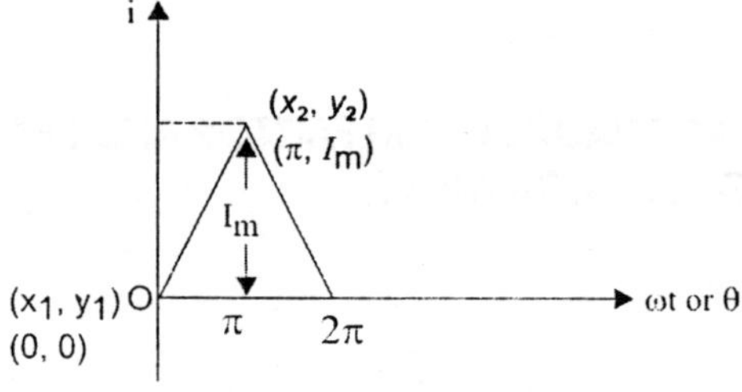

Fig. 3.15: Triangular-waveform

By using this formula

$$(y - y_1) = \frac{(y_2 - y_1)}{(x_2 - x_1)}(x - x_1)$$

$$(i-0) = \frac{(I_m - 0)}{(\pi - 0)}(\theta - 0)$$

$$\therefore \quad i = \frac{I_m}{\pi}\theta$$

So, the instantaneous value of current is given by

$$i = \frac{I_m}{\pi}\theta \text{ for } 0 < \theta < \pi$$

RMS value: The rms value of triangular current wave is given by

$$I_{rms} = \sqrt{\frac{1}{\pi}\int_0^{\pi} i^2 d\theta}$$

$$= \sqrt{\frac{1}{\pi}\int_0^{\pi}\left(\frac{I_m}{\pi}.\theta\right)^2 d\theta} = \sqrt{\frac{I_m^2}{\pi^3}\int_0^{\pi}\theta^2 d\theta}$$

$$= \sqrt{\frac{I_m^2}{\pi^3}\left(\frac{\theta^3}{3}\right)_0^{\pi}} = \sqrt{\frac{I_m^2}{\pi^3}\frac{\pi^3}{3}}$$

$$\therefore \quad I_{rms} = \frac{I_m}{\sqrt{3}} \text{ for } 0 < \theta < \pi$$

Similarly for voltage

$$\therefore \quad V_{rms} = \frac{V_m}{\sqrt{3}}$$

Average value: The average value of a triangular current wave is given by

$$I_{avg} = \frac{1}{\pi}\int_0^{\pi} i.\, d\theta$$

$$= \frac{1}{\pi}\int_0^{\pi}\frac{I_m}{\pi}\theta.\, d\theta = \frac{I_m}{\pi^2}\left(\frac{\theta^2}{2}\right)_0^{\pi} = \frac{I_m}{2}$$

Similarly for voltage

$$V_{avg} = \frac{V_m}{2}$$

Form factor: The form factor of triangular current wave is given by

$$\therefore \quad K_{PI} = \frac{I_{rms}}{I_{avg}} = \frac{\frac{I_m}{\sqrt{3}}}{\frac{I_m}{2}} = \frac{2}{\sqrt{3}}$$

Similarly for voltages $\quad K_{fV} = \frac{2}{\sqrt{3}}$

Peak factor: The peak factor of triangular current wave is given by

$$\therefore \quad K_{PI} = \frac{I_m}{I_{rms}} = \frac{I_m}{\frac{I_m}{\sqrt{3}}} = 1.732$$

Similarly for voltages $\quad K_{PV} = 1.732$

SOLVED EXAMPLES

Example 1: The equation of an alternating current $i = 42.42 \sin 628t$. Determine (i) its maximum value (ii) frequency (iii) rms value (iv) average value (v) form factor.

[Sem-I, 2004-05]

Solution: The given instantaneous value of alternating current $i = 42.42 \sin 628t$

$$I_m = 42.42 \text{ or } \omega = 628$$

(i) Its maximum value is

$$\therefore \quad I_m = 42.42 \text{ A} \qquad \textbf{Ans.}$$

(ii) $\omega = 628$ rad/sec

$$\therefore \quad \omega = 2\pi f = 628$$

$$f = \frac{628}{2\pi} = 100 \text{ Hz} \qquad \textbf{Ans.}$$

(iii) RMS value

$$\therefore \quad I_{rms} = \frac{I_m}{\sqrt{2}} = \frac{42.42}{\sqrt{2}} = 30 \text{ A} \qquad \textbf{Ans.}$$

(iv) Average value of current

$$\therefore \quad I_{avg} = \frac{2I_m}{\pi} = \frac{2 \times 42.42}{\pi} = 27 \text{ A} \qquad \textbf{Ans.}$$

(v) Its form factor $\quad K_{fI} = \dfrac{I_{rms}}{I_{avg}} = \dfrac{30}{27} = 1.11 \qquad$ **Ans.**

Example 2: Find RMS and average value for the waveform shown in figure below.

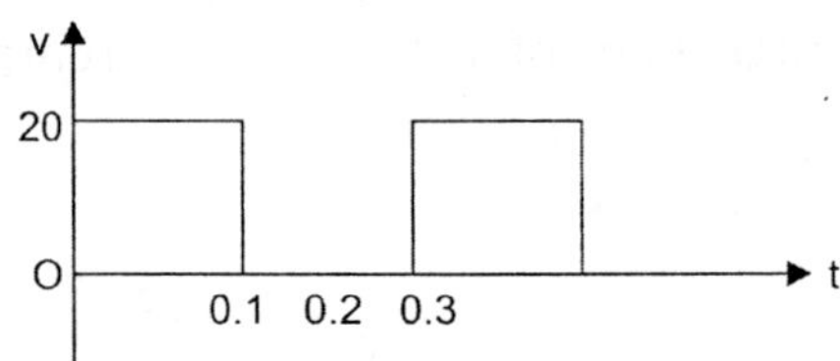

Solution: We know that the average value is given by

$$V_{avg} = \frac{1}{T}\int_0^T v\,dt = \frac{1}{0.3}\int_0^{0.1} 20dt = 6.67 \text{ volt} \qquad \textbf{Ans.}$$

The RMS value of given waveform

$$V_{rms} = \sqrt{\frac{1}{T}\int_0^T v^2\,dt} = \sqrt{\frac{1}{0.3}\int_0^{0.1}(20)^2\,dt} = 11.5 \text{ volt} \qquad \textbf{Ans.}$$

Example 3: Calculate from first principles, the rms value of a triangular voltgae wave in which the voltage rises from 0 to V_m and completes the cycle by falling instantly back to zero. Also, give the ratio of rms to mean value for the waveform (sawtooth wave).

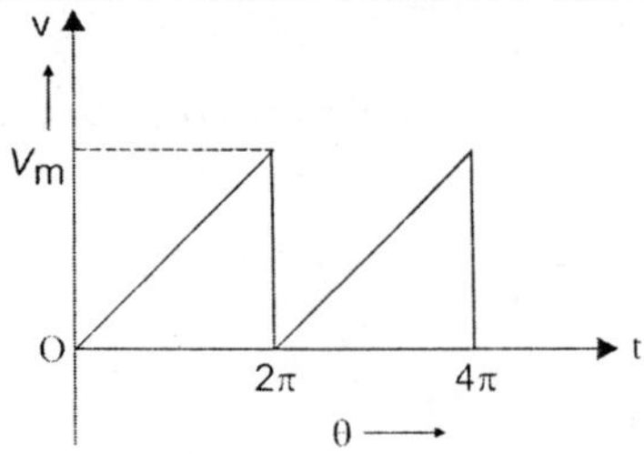

Solution: From above waveform, the instantaneous value of voltage can be expressed as follows.

∴ We know

$$v = K\theta$$

where K is the slope of the curve.

Let the maximum value of the voltage be V_m

⇒ Since $v = V_m$ when $\theta = 2\pi$

$$\therefore \qquad K = \frac{V_m}{2\pi}$$

The expression for the instantaneous voltage becomes

$$v = \frac{V_m}{2\pi}\theta$$

RMS value of the voltage wave

$$V_{rms} = \sqrt{\frac{1}{2\pi}\int_0^{2\pi} v^2\, d\theta} = \sqrt{\frac{1}{2\pi}\int_0^{2\pi}\left(\frac{V_m}{2\pi}\theta\right)^2 d\theta}$$

$$= \sqrt{\frac{V_m^2}{4\pi^3}\left(\frac{\theta^3}{3}\right)_0^{2\pi}} = \frac{V_m}{\sqrt{3}} \qquad \textbf{Ans.}$$

Mean value of the voltage wave

$$V_{avg} = \frac{1}{2\pi}\int_0^{2\pi} v\, d\theta = \frac{1}{2\pi}\int_0^{2\pi}\frac{V_m}{2\pi}\,\theta\, d\theta$$

$$= \frac{V_m}{4\pi}\times[\theta]_0^{2\pi} = \frac{V_m}{2} \qquad \textbf{Ans.}$$

Ratio of rms value to mean value for the given waveform

$$= \frac{V_{rms}}{V_{avg}} = \frac{\frac{V_m}{\sqrt{3}}}{\frac{V_m}{2}} = 1.155 \qquad \textbf{Ans.}$$

3.11 CONCEPT OF PHASOR

A sinusoidal quantity can be represented by a line of finite length rotating in counter clockwise direction with the same angular velocity as that of the sinusoidal quantity. Such rotating line is called phasor.

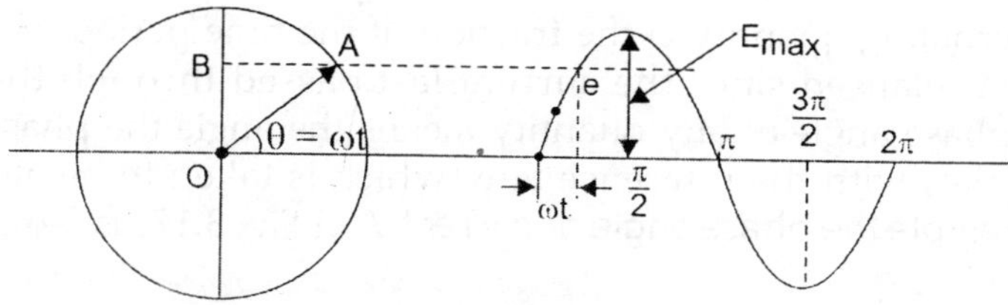

Fig. 3.16

In Fig. 3.16, line OA represented the maximum value of alternating quantity. $OB = OA \sin\theta = E_{max} \sin\omega t = e$ and phasor can be drawn on the basis of maximum/rms value.

Example: Phasor representation (unity pf load)

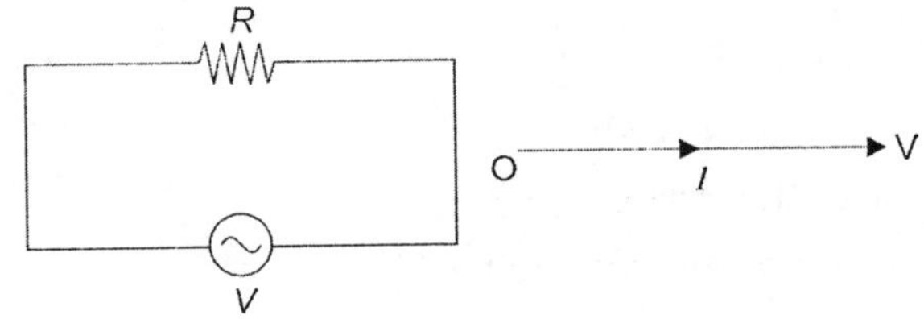

$$v = V_m \sin \omega t \,;\, i = I_m \sin \omega t$$

For lagging pf load:

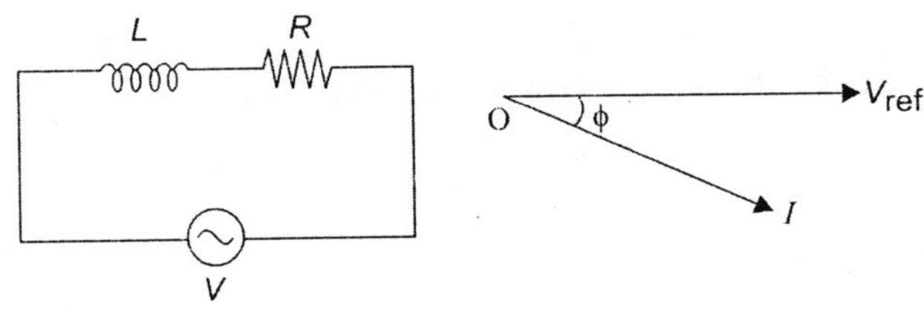

$$v = V_m \sin \omega t \,;\, i = I_m \sin (\omega t - \phi)$$

For leading pf load:

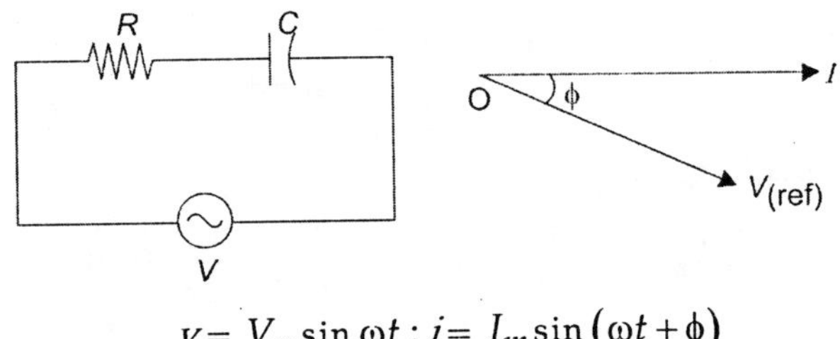

$$v = V_m \sin \omega t \,;\, i = I_m \sin (\omega t + \phi)$$

3.11.1 Phasor Diagram Using RMS Values

Since there is a definite relation between maximum value and rms value

$$\therefore \quad V_m = \sqrt{2}\, V_{rms}$$

The length of phasor OA can be taken equal to rms value if desired. But it should be noted that in such cases, the projection of rotating phasor on the vertical axis will not give the instantaneous value of that alternating quantity. The phasor diagram drawn in rms values of the alternating quantities helps in understanding the behaviour of the AC machines under different loading conditions.

3.11.2 Phase and Phase Angle

Phase of an alternating quantity is the fraction of the time period of that alternating quantity that has elapsed since the current last passed through the zero position reference. The phase angle of any quantity means the angle the phasor representing the quantity makes with the reference line (which is taken to be at zero degree or radians). For example the phase angle of current I_2 in Fig. 3.17c is $(-\phi)$.

3.11.3 Phase Difference

When two alternating quantites, say, two emf, or two currents or one voltage and one current are considered simultaneoulsy, the frequency being the same, they may not pass through a particular point at the same instant. One may pass through its maximum value at the instant when the other passes through the value other than its maximum one. These two quantities are said to have a phase difference.

The phase difference is measured by the angular distance between the points where the two curves cross the base or reference line in the same direction. The quantity ahead in phase is said to lead the other quantity while the second quantity is said to lag behind the first one.

In Fig. 3.16 current I_1 represented by phasor *OA* leads the current I_2 represented by phasor *OB* by θ or current I_2 lags behind the current I_1 by θ. The leading current I_1 goes through its zero and maximum value first and the current I_2 goes through its zero and maximum values after time angle θ.

The two waves representing these two currents are shown in Fig. 3.16. If I_1 is taken as reference phasor, the two currents can be expressed

$$i_1 = I_{m_1} \sin \omega t \text{ and } i_2 = I_{m_2} \sin(\omega t - \theta)$$

The two quantities are said to be in phase with each other if they pass through zero values at the same instant and rise in the same direction as shown in Fig. 3.17a. But the two quantities passing through zero values at the same instant but rising in opposite directions, as shown in Fig. 3.17c are said to be in phase opposition, i.e. phase difference is 180°. When the two alternating quantities have a phase difference of 90° or $\frac{\pi}{2}$ radians they are said to be in quadrature.

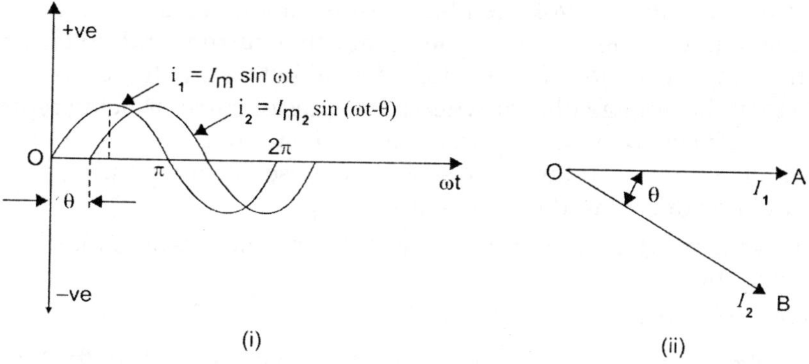

Fig. 3.17a

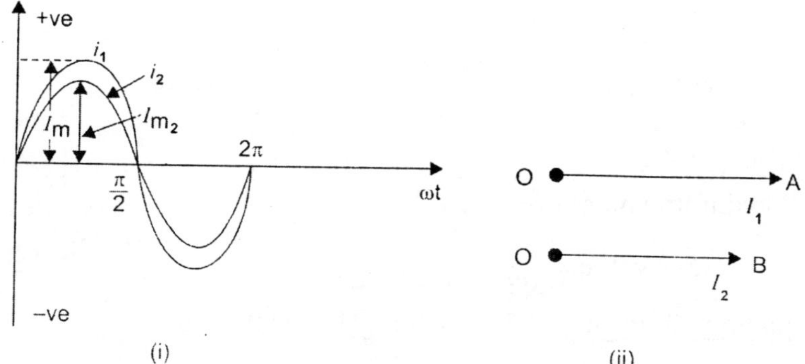

Fig. 3.17b

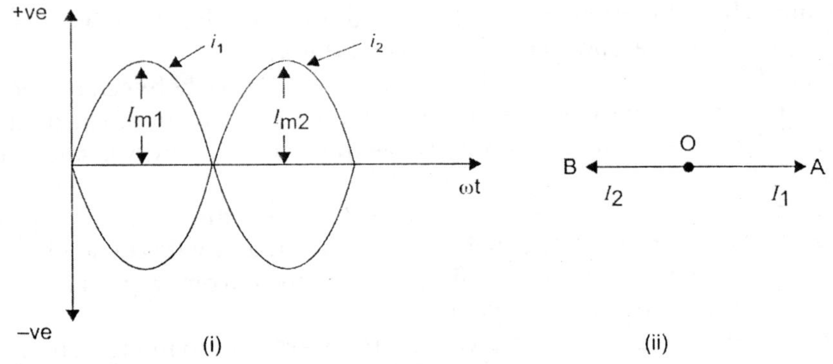

Fig. 3.17c

3.11.4 Conventions for Drawing Phasor Diagrams

Counterclockwise direction of rotation of phasors is usually taken as positive direction of rotation of phasor, i.e. a phasor rotated in a counter-clockwise direction from a given phasor is said to lead the given phasor while a phasor rotated in clockwise direction is said to lag in the given phasor.

For series circuit, in which the current is common to all parts of the circuit, the current phasor is usually taken as reference phasor for other phasors in the same diagram and drawn on horizontal line. In parallel circuits in which the voltage is common to all branches of the circuits, the voltage phasor is usually taken as reference phasor and drawn on the horizontal line. It is not necessary that current and voltage phasors are drawn to the same scale, in fact it is often desirable to draw the current phasor to a larger scale than the voltage phasor when the values of currents being represented are small. However, if several voltage phasors are to be used in the same phasor diagram, they should all be drawn to the same scale. Likewise all current phasors in the same diagram should be drawn to the same scale.

Example: Calculate (a) maximum value and (b) the root mean square values of the following quantities.

(i) 40 sin ωt (ii) *B*sin $B\sin(\omega t - \pi/2)$ and (iii) 10 sin ωt – 17.3 cos ωt

Draw the phasors showing the phase difference with respect to $A\sin(\omega t - \pi/6)$.

Solution:

(*i*) For the given, 40 sin ωt

(a) Maximum value = 40 **Ans.**

(b) $$\text{RMS value} = \frac{\text{Maximum value}}{\sqrt{2}} = \frac{40}{\sqrt{2}} = 28.28$$ **Ans.**

(*ii*) Given $B\sin(\omega t - \pi/2)$

(*a*) Maximum value = *B* **Ans.**

(*b*) $$\text{RMS value} = \frac{B}{\sqrt{2}}$$ **Ans.**

(*iii*) The equation 10 sin ωt – 17.3 cos ωt may be written as

$$20\left(\frac{1}{2}\sin\omega t - \frac{\sqrt{3}}{2}\cos\omega t\right)$$

or $$20\left(\cos\frac{\pi}{3}\sin\omega t - \sin\frac{\pi}{3}\cos\omega t\right)$$

or $$20\sin\left(\omega t - \frac{\pi}{3}\right) \quad \cos A.\sin B - \sin A \cos B = \sin(B - A)$$

(*a*) Maximum value = 20 **Ans.**

(*b*) RMS value $= \frac{20}{\sqrt{2}} = 14.14$ **Ans.**

Phasors showing the phase difference with respect to $A \sin\left(\omega t - \frac{\pi}{6}\right)$ are shown in figure below.

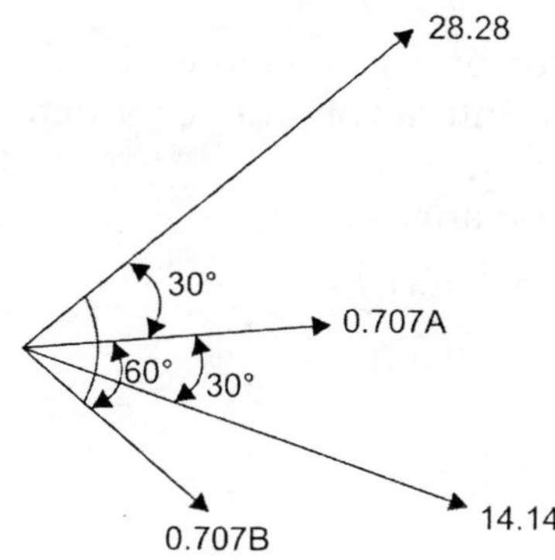

3.12 ADDITION AND SUBTRACTION OF ALTERNATING QUANTITIES

Let it is required to add two currents given by the equations.

$$i_1 = I_{m_1} \sin(\omega t + \phi_1)$$

$$i_2 = I_{m_2} \sin(\omega t + \phi_2)$$

Addition and subtraction of these equation by analytical method is given below.

Analytical Method

Resolving currents I_{m1} and I_{m2} along *x*-axis and *y*-axis, we have

Algebraic sum of *x*-components

$$= I_{m_1} \cos\phi_1 + I_{m_2} \cos\phi_2$$

Algebraic sum of *y*-components

$$= I_{m_1} \sin\phi_1 + I_{m_2} \sin\phi_1$$

Resultant of maximum value of current is

$$I_{mr} = \sqrt{(x \text{ component})^2 + (y \text{ component})^2}$$

Resultant phase difference is

$$\phi_R = \tan^{-1}\left(\frac{y \text{ component}}{x \text{ component}}\right)$$

Instantaneous equation of current is

$$i = I_{mr} \sin(\omega t \pm \phi_R)$$

Similarly, subtraction can be performed.

Algebraic difference of x-components

$$= I_{m_1} \cos\phi_1 - I_{m_2} \cos\phi_2$$

Algebraic difference of y-components

$$= I_{m_1} \sin\phi_1 - I_{m_2} \sin\phi_2$$

Resultant of maximum value of current is

$$I_{mr} = \sqrt{(x \text{ comp. difference})^2 + (y \text{ comp. difference})^2}$$

$$\theta_R = \tan^{-1}\left(\frac{y \text{ component difference}}{x \text{ component difference}}\right)$$

$$i = I_{mr} \sin(\omega t \pm \phi_R)$$

Example: Two alternating currents represented by the equation $i_1 = 7 \sin \omega t$ and $i_2 = 10 \sin(\omega t + \pi/3)$ are fed into a common conductor. Find the equation for the resultant current and its rms value. **[Sem-I, 06-07; UPTU, 09-10]**

Solution: The given equation are

$$i_1 = 7 \sin \omega t \qquad \therefore \quad \phi_1 = 0°$$

$$i_2 = 10 \sin\left(\omega t + \frac{\pi}{3}\right) \qquad \therefore \quad \phi_2 = \pi/3$$

The resultant current

$$I_r = I_1 + I_2$$

By Analytical method

Algebraic sum along x-axis

$$= 7\cos\theta° + 10\cos\frac{\pi}{3}$$

$$\therefore \quad x \text{comp} = 7 + 5 = 12$$

Algebraic sum along y-axis

$$\therefore \quad y \text{comp} = 7\sin 0° + 10 \sin\frac{\pi}{3} = 8.66$$

$$I_{mr} = \sqrt{(x \text{ component})^2 + (y \text{ component})^2}$$

$$= \sqrt{(12)^2 + (8.68)^2} = 14.8 \text{ A}$$

and phase difference of resultant is currrent is

$$\phi_R = \tan^{-1}\left(\frac{y \text{ comp}}{x \text{ comp}}\right) = \tan^{-1}\frac{8.60}{(12)} = 0.199\pi$$

$$I_r = I_{mr} \sin(\omega t \pm \theta_R) = 14.8 \sin(\omega t + 0.199\pi) \text{ A}$$ **Ans.**

$\therefore$ RMS value of current is

$$I_{rms} = \frac{I_{rms}}{\sqrt{2}} = \frac{14.8}{\sqrt{2}} \text{A}$$ **Ans.**

SOLVED EXAMPLES FOR PRACTICE

Example 1: An AC voltage of 50 Hz frequency has a peak value of 220 V, write down the expression for the instantaneous value of this voltage. **[UPTU 2007-08]**

Solution: The given data

$$f = 50 \text{ Hz}$$

$$V_m = 220 \text{ V}$$

∴ Expression for instantaneous value of AC voltage is

$$v = V_m \sin \omega t \qquad (\omega = 2\pi f)$$

$$v = 220 \sin 2\pi \times 50t = 220 \sin 314\, t$$ **Ans.**

Example 2: An alternating current of frequency 50 Hz has a maximum value of 100 A. Calculate (i) its value $\frac{1}{600}$ second, after the instant current, is zero and its value decreasing there afterwards. (ii) How many seconds after the instant, the current is zero (increasing there afterwards) and will the current attains the value of 86.6 A?

[UPTU 2005-06, AU 1991, NU 1999]

Solution: The given data,

$$f = 50 \text{ Hz}$$

$$I_m = 100 \text{ A}$$

From above waveform $I = 100 \sin 100\pi t$

(i) Since the current is measured from the instant the current is zero and is decreasing there afterwards (i.e. from point A in above figure)

∴ The equation for the alternating current with respect to the point A becomes

$$i = -100 \sin (100\pi t + \pi) = -100 \sin 100\pi t$$

For the given time $t = \frac{1}{600}$ sec

∴ $$I = -100 \sin 100\pi \times \frac{1}{600} = -100 \sin \frac{\pi}{6} = -50 \text{ A}$$ **Ans.**

(ii) Let the current attain the value of 86.6 A, t seconds after the zero value of the current.

∴ $$I = 86.6 \text{ A (given)}$$

$$86.6 \text{ A} = 100 \sin 100\pi t$$

∴ $$t = \frac{1}{100\pi} \sin^{-1}\left(\frac{86.6}{100}\right) = \frac{1}{300} \text{ sec}$$

Example 3: A sinusoidally varying alternating current of frequency 60 Hz has a maximum value of 15 A.

(i) Write down the equation for instantaneous value.

(ii) Find the value of current after $\frac{1}{200}$ sec.

(iii) Find the time taken to reach 10 A for the first time and

(iv) Find its average value. **[UPTU Sem-II, 2002-03]**

Solution: The given data

$$f = 60 \text{ Hz}$$

$$I_m = 15 \text{ A}$$

(i) The equation for instantaneous value of current.

$$i/= I_m \sin \omega t$$
$$= 15\sin 2\pi \times ft = 15\sin 2\pi \times 60t$$
$$i= 15\sin 120\pi t$$

(ii) For given $t= \frac{1}{200}$ second

Current becomes $i = 15\sin 120\pi \times t$

$$= 15\sin 120\pi \times \frac{1}{200} = 14.266 \text{ A}$$ **Ans.**

(iii) Let the instantaneous value of current be 10 A (given), then time becomes

$\therefore$
$$i= 15\sin 120\pi t$$
$$10 = 15\sin 120\pi t$$

$\therefore$
$$t= \frac{1}{120\pi}\sin^{-1}\left(\frac{10}{15}\right) = 0.001936 \text{ seconds}$$ **Ans.**

(*iv*) The average value of current is

$$I_{avg} = \frac{2I_m}{\pi} = \frac{2\times 15}{\pi} = 9.55 \text{ A}$$ **Ans.**

Example 4: An alternating current when passed through a resistance immersed in water for 5 minutes, just raised the temperature of water to boiling point. When a direct current of 4 amperes was passed through the same resistance under identical conditions it took 8 minutes to boil the water. Find the rms value of the alternating current.

Solution: Heat produced when an alternating current of I_{rms} amperes is passed through a resistance R immersed in water for 5 minutes.

$$= (I_{rms})^2 \times R\times 5\times 60 = 300 I_{rms}.R \text{ Joule}$$

Heat produced when a direct current of 4 A is passed through the same resistance R immersed in the water for 8 minutes.

$$= 4^2 \times R\times 8\times 60 = 7680R \text{ Joule}$$

Since heat produced in both the case is same,

$\therefore$ Equating equation (1) and (2) we get

$$300\ I_{rms}{}^2.R = 7680 \text{ R}$$

or
$$I_{rms} = \sqrt{\frac{7680}{300}} = 5.06 \text{ A}$$ **Ans.**

Example 5: An alternating current is given by $i= 20\sin 600t$ ampers. Find (i) frequency (ii) peak value of current and (iii) time taken from $t = 0$ for the current to reach a value of 10 A. **[UPTU 2004-05]**

Solution: The given instantaneous equation of current $i= 20\sin 600t$

$\therefore$
$$I_m = 20 \text{ A}$$
$$\omega = 600$$

(i) Frequency, $f= \frac{600}{2\pi} = 99.5$ Hz **Ans.**

(ii) Peak value of current.

$\therefore$
$$I_m = 20 \text{ A}$$ **Ans.**

(iii) Time taken from $t = 0$ for the current to reach a value of 10 A.

$$\therefore \quad t = \frac{1}{600}\sin^{-1}\left(\frac{10}{20}\right) = 0.872 \text{ m sec} \quad \textbf{Ans.}$$

Example 6: An alternating current varying sinusoidally with a frequency of 50 Hz has an rms value of 20 A. Write down the equation for the instantaneous value and find the value at (i) 0.0025 seconds (ii) 0.0125 seconds, after passing through a positive maximum value. At what time, measured from a positive maximum value, will the instantaneous current be 14.14 A? **[AU 1992]**

Solution: The given data

$$f = 50 \text{ Hz}$$
$$I_{rms} = 20 \text{ A}$$

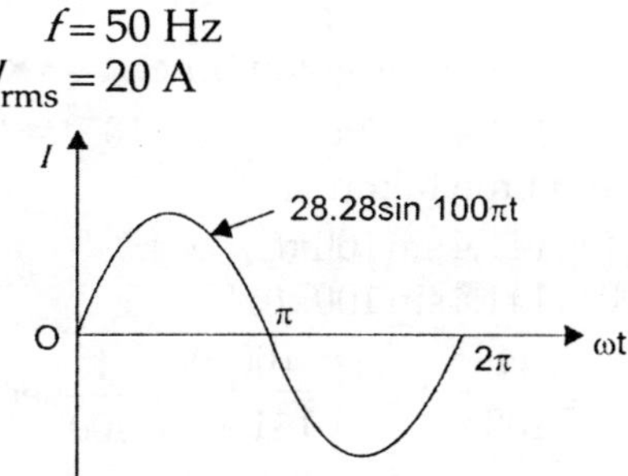

The peak value of current is

$$\therefore \quad I_m = \sqrt{2} \times I_{rms} = \sqrt{2} \times 20 = 28.28 \text{ A}$$

The equation of alternating current with respect to origin O is

$$i = I_m \sin 2\pi f t$$
$$= 28.28\sin 2\pi \times 50 t = 28.28\sin 100\pi t \quad \textbf{Ans.}$$

The above expression is valid when time is measured from the instant the current is zero and increasing in positive direction. After passing through a positive maximum value equation becomes:

$$\therefore \quad i = 28.28\sin\left(100\pi t + \frac{\pi}{2}\right) = 28.28\cos 100\pi t \quad \textbf{Ans.}$$

(i) When $t = 0.0025$ sec, the instantaneous value of current

$$i_1 = 28.28\cos 100\pi \times 0.0025 = 28.28\cos\frac{\pi}{4}\ 20 \text{ A} \quad \textbf{Ans.}$$

(ii) When $t = 0.0125$ sec, the instantaneous value of current,

$$i_2 = 28.28\cos 100\pi \times 0.0125 = -20 \text{ A} \quad \textbf{Ans.}$$

(iii) If $i = 14.14$ A (given), then, t we get

$$\therefore \quad 14.14 = 28.28\cos 100\pi t$$

$$t = \frac{1}{100\pi}\cos^{-1}\left(\frac{14.14}{28.28}\right) = \frac{1}{300}\text{sec} \quad \textbf{Ans.}$$

Example 7: An alternating voltage is given by $v = 141.4 \sin 314\, t$. Find (i) frequency (ii) rms value (iii) average value (iv) the instantaneous value of voltage when t is 3 ms (v) the time taken for the voltage to reach 100 V for the first time after passing through zero value. **[UPTU Sem-I, 2006-07]**

Solution: The instantaneous value of alternating voltage is given by expression

$$v = 141.4 \sin 314 t$$

$$\therefore \quad V_m = 141.4 \text{ V}$$

$$\omega = 314 \text{ rad/sec}$$

(i) The frequency is given by

$$\omega = 2\pi f$$

$$\therefore \quad f = \frac{\omega}{2\pi} = \frac{314}{2\pi} = 50 \text{ Hz}$$ **Ans.**

(ii) RMS value of given alternating voltage is

$$V_{rms} = \frac{V_m}{\sqrt{2}} = \frac{141.4}{\sqrt{2}} = 100 \text{ V}$$ **Ans.**

(iii) Average value of alternating voltage

$$V_{avg} = \frac{2V_m}{\pi} = \frac{2 \times 141.4}{\pi} = 90 \text{ V}$$ **Ans.**

(iv) Instantaneous value of voltage for given time, $t = 3 \times 10^{-3}$ sec

$$\therefore \quad v = 141.4 \sin 2\pi \times 50 \times 3 \times 10^{-3} = 114.4 \text{ volt}$$ **Ans.**

(v) For voltage given $v = 100$ time taken

$$v = 141.4 \sin 100\pi t$$

$$100 = 141.4 \sin 100\pi t$$

$$\therefore \quad t = \frac{1}{100\pi} \sin^{-1}\left(\frac{100}{141.4}\right) = \frac{1}{400} \text{sec}$$ **Ans.**

Example 8: An alternating voltage $v = 100 \sin 100t$. Find (*i*) amplitude (*ii*) time period and frequency (*iii*) angular velocity (*iv*) form factor (*v*) peak factor.

[UPTU Sem-II, 2007-08]

Solution: The given instantaneous value of alternating voltage is

$$v = 100 \sin 100 \, t$$

$$\therefore \quad v_m = 100 \text{ V}$$

and $\quad \omega = 100 \text{ rad/sec}$

(i) Amplitude of alternating voltage is

$$V_m = 100 \text{ V}$$ **Ans.**

(ii) Frequency is given by coefficient of time, t divided by 2π,

$$\therefore \quad \text{Frequency, } f = \frac{100}{2\pi} = 15.9 \text{ Hz}$$ **Ans.**

$$\therefore \quad \text{Time period, } T = \frac{1}{f}$$

$$T = \frac{1}{15.9} = 0.063 \text{ seconds}$$ **Ans.**

(iii) Angular velocity

$$\omega = 2\pi f$$

$$\omega = 2\pi \times 15.9 = 100 \text{ rad/sec}$$ **Ans.**

RMS value $\quad V_{rms} = \frac{V_m}{\sqrt{2}} = \frac{100}{\sqrt{2}} = 70.71 \text{ V}$

Average value $\quad V_{avg} = \frac{2V_m}{\pi} = \frac{2 \times 100}{\pi} = 63.7 \text{ volt}$ **Ans.**

(iv) Form factor

$$K_f = \frac{V_{rms}}{V_{avg}} = \frac{70.71}{63.9} = 1.11$$ **Ans.**

(v) Peak factor

$$K_p = \frac{V_m}{V_{rms}} = \frac{100}{70.71} = 1.414 \qquad \textbf{Ans.}$$

Example 9: Find the rms value, average value and form factor of the voltage waveform shown in the figure below. **[UPTU Sem-II, 2002-03]**

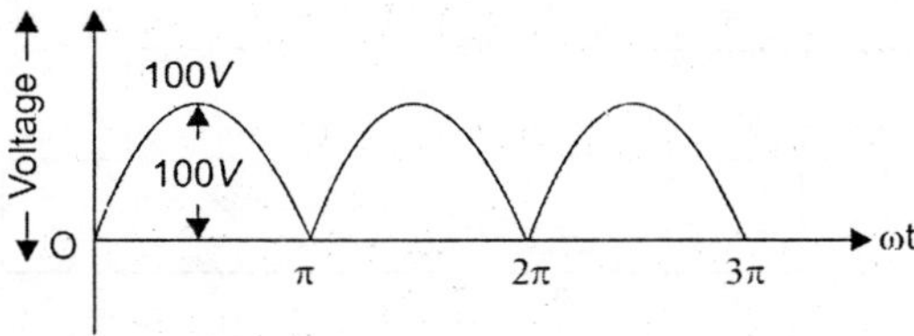

Solution: From a given waveform average value of voltage over one cycle

$$\therefore \quad V_{avg} = \frac{1}{\pi}\int_0^{\pi} v.d\theta$$

$$V = V_m \sin\theta$$

$$V_{avg} = \frac{1}{\pi}\int_0^{\pi} V_m \sin\theta \, d\theta$$

$$= \frac{V_m}{\pi}[-\cos]_0^{\pi} = \frac{V_m}{\pi}\left(-\cos\pi + \cos 0^\circ\right)$$

$$= \frac{2V_m}{\pi} = \frac{2\times 100}{\pi} = 63.66 \text{ V} \qquad (V_m = 100 \text{ V given})$$

RMS value of voltage waveform is

$$\therefore \quad V_{rms} = \sqrt{\frac{1}{\pi}\int_0^{\pi} v^2 \, d\theta}$$

$$v = V_m \sin\theta$$

$$\therefore \quad V_{rms} = \sqrt{\frac{1}{\pi}\int_0^{\pi} (V_m \sin\theta)^2 \, d\theta}$$

$$= \sqrt{\frac{V_m^2}{\pi}\int_0^{\pi}\left(\frac{1-\cos 2\theta}{2}\right)d\theta} = \sqrt{\frac{V_m^2}{2\pi}\left(\theta - \frac{\sin 2\theta}{2}\right)_0^{\pi}}$$

$$= \sqrt{\frac{V_m^2}{2\pi}(\pi - 0)}$$

$$= \frac{V_m}{\sqrt{2}} = \frac{100}{\sqrt{2}} = 70.71 \text{ V} \qquad \textbf{Ans.}$$

Form factor of the waveform shown in the figure.

$$K_{fv} = \frac{V_{rms}}{V_{avg}} = \frac{70.71}{63.66} = 1.11 \qquad \textbf{Ans.}$$

Example 10: Calculate the average and root mean square values, the form factor and peak factor of a periodic current wave having the following values for equal time intervals over half cycle, changing suddenly from one value to the next: 0, 40, 60, 80, 100, 80, 60, 40, 0. **[UPTU 2007-08, NU, 1999]**

Solution: From the given data, we have the following waveform.

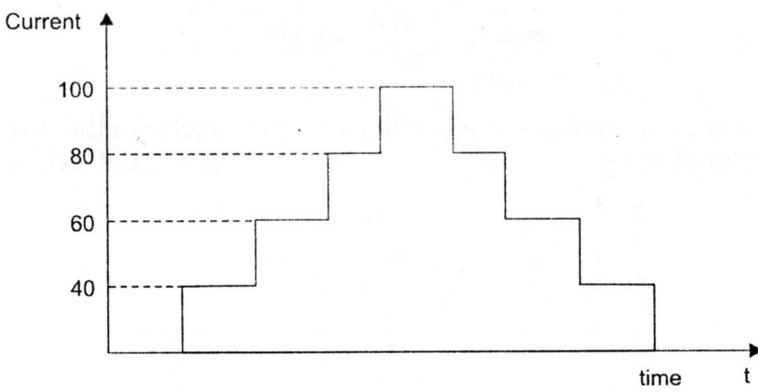

Solution: Since the waveform is symmetrical, so considering one half cycle only. Average value of current from above waveform is

$$I_{avg} = \frac{I_1 + I_2 + I_3 + I_4 + I_5 + I_6 + I_7 + I_8}{8}$$

$$= \frac{0 + 40 + 60 + 80 + 100 + 80 + 60 + 40}{8} = 57.54 \text{ A}$$ **Ans.**

RMS value of current is

$$\therefore \quad I_{rms} = \sqrt{\frac{I_1^2 + I_2^2 + I_3^2 + I_4^2 + I_5^2 + I_6^2 + I_7^2 + I_8^2}{8}}$$

$$= \sqrt{\frac{0 + 1600 + 3600 + 6400 + 10000 + 6400 + 3600 + 1600}{8}}$$

$$I_{rms} = 64.42 \text{ Amp}$$ **Ans.**

From above waveform peak value is

$$I_m = 100 \text{ A}$$

$$\therefore \quad \text{Form factor} = \frac{I_{rms}}{I_{avg}} = \frac{64.42}{57.3} = 1.11$$

$$\text{Peak factor} = \frac{I_m}{I_{rms}} = \frac{100}{64.42} = 1.552$$ **Ans.**

Example 11: An alternating voltage $e = 200 \sin 314t$ is applied to a device which offers an ohmic resistance of 20 Ω to the flow of current in one direction, while preventing the flow of current in opposite direction. Calculate the rms value, average value and form factor for the current over one cycle. **[NU (EE) 1992, 2001; UPTU 2002-03]**

Solution: The given instantaneous voltage applied to the rectifying device is given by the expression.

$$e = 200 \sin 314t$$

∴ Maximum value of applied voltage

$$E_m = 200 \text{ V}$$

Resistance of rectifying device $R = 20$ Ω.

Maximum value of half-wave rectifying alternating current is

$$\therefore \quad I_m = \frac{E_m}{R} = \frac{200}{20} = 10 \text{ A}$$

RMS value of half-wave rectified alternating current,

$$I_{rms} = \frac{I_m}{2} = \frac{10}{2} = 5 \text{ A} \qquad \textbf{Ans.}$$

Average value of the half-wave rectified alternating current

$$I_{avg} = \frac{I_m}{\pi} = \frac{10}{\pi} = 3.18 \text{ A} \qquad \textbf{Ans.}$$

Form factor of the half-wave rectified alternating current

$$= \frac{I_{rms}}{I_{avg}} = \frac{5}{3.18} = 1.57 \qquad \textbf{Ans.}$$

Example 12: A voltage $v(t) = 220\sqrt{2}\sin 100t$ is applied to the circuit shown in figure below. What is the rms value of current through the resistor R of 100 Ω? Derive the formula used. **[PTU EE 2002]**

Diode

V

R = 100Ω

Solution: The given data,

Instantaneous value of voltage

$$v(t) = 220\sqrt{2}\sin 100\,t$$

$$\therefore \quad V_m = 220\sqrt{2} \text{ volt}$$

$$\therefore \quad I_m = \frac{V_m}{R} = \frac{220\sqrt{2}}{100} = 3.11 \text{ A}$$

RMS value of circuit current,

$$I_{rms} = \frac{I_m}{2} = \frac{3.11}{2} = 1.55 \text{ A} \qquad \text{[halfwave rectified wave]}$$

Example 13: Find the average and effective values of voltage for sinusoidal waveform shown in figure below. **[AUEE 1999]**

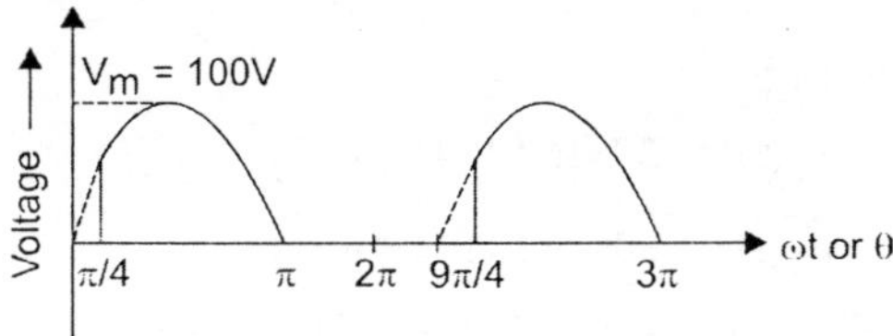

Solution: The equation of the given sinusoidal waveform is $V = 100\sin\theta$

$$\therefore \quad V_{avg} = \frac{1}{2\pi}\int_{\pi/4}^{\pi} v.d\theta = \frac{1}{2\pi}\int_{\pi/4}^{\pi} V\sin\theta\, d\theta$$

$$= \frac{100}{2\pi}[-\cos\theta]_{\pi/4}^{\pi} = 27.17 \text{ V} \qquad \textbf{Ans.}$$

$$\therefore \quad V_{rms} = \sqrt{\frac{1}{2\pi}\int_{\pi/4}^{\pi} v^2.d\theta} = \sqrt{\frac{1}{2\pi}\int_{\pi/4}^{\pi}(V_m\sin\theta)^2\, d\theta}$$

$$= \sqrt{\frac{V_m^2}{2\pi}\int_{\pi/4}^{\pi}\left(\frac{(1-\cos 2\theta)}{2}\right)d\theta} = \sqrt{\frac{V_m^2}{4\pi}\left(\theta - \frac{\sin 2\theta}{2}\right)_{\pi/4}^{\pi}}$$

$$= \sqrt{\frac{2500}{\pi}\left[\pi - \frac{\pi}{4} + \frac{1}{2}\right]} = \sqrt{2273} = 47.67 \text{ V} \qquad \textbf{Ans.}$$

Example 14: The two branches of parallel circuit draws currents i_1 and i_2 such that $i_1 = 10\sqrt{2}\sin\omega t$ and $i_2 = 5\sqrt{2}\sin(\omega t - 60°)$. What is the total current drawn?

[GBTU Sem-II, 2010-11]

Solution: The given branch current

$$i_1 = 10\sqrt{2}\sin\omega t$$

$$i_2 = 5\sqrt{2}\sin(\omega t - 60°).$$

By analytical method

Resolve currents I_{m_1} and I_{m_2} along *x*-axis and *y*-axis.

Algebraic sum of *x*-components $= 10\sqrt{2}\cos 0° + 5\sqrt{2}\cos(-60°)$

$$= 14.1421 + 3.5355 = 14.678$$

Algebraic sum of *y*-components $= 10\sqrt{2}\sin 0° + 5\sqrt{2}\sin(-60°)$

$$= 0 + (-6.124) = -6.124$$

Maximum value of resultant current

$$I_{mr} = \sqrt{(x\text{ comp})^2 + (y\text{ comp})^2} = \sqrt{(17.678)^2 + (6.128)^2}$$

$$\therefore \quad I_{mr} = 18.708 \text{ A}$$

Phase angle

$$\phi_R = \tan^{-1}\left(\frac{y\text{ comp}}{x\text{ comp}}\right) = \tan^{-1}\left(\frac{-6.124}{17.678}\right) = -19.1°$$

$\therefore$ Resultant current $\quad i_r = I_{mr}\sin(\omega t + \theta_2) = 18.708\sin(\omega t - 19.1°)$ **Ans.**

Example 15: Two AC voltages are represented by

$$v_1(t) = 30\sin(314t + 45°)$$

$$v_2(t) = 60\sin(314t + 60°)$$

Calculate the resultant voltage $V(t)$ and express in the form

$V(t) = V_m\sin(314t + \theta)$. **[UPTU 2003-04]**

Solution: The given equations are

$$v_1(t) = 30\sin(314t + 45°)$$

$$v_2(t) = 60\sin(314t + 60°)$$

Resolve voltage V_{m_1} and V_{m_2} along *x*-axis and *y*-axis,

Algebraic sum of *x* components

$$= 30\cos 45° + 60\cos 60°$$

$$= 30 \times \frac{1}{2} + 60 \times \frac{1}{2} = 51.21 \text{ V}$$

Algebraic sum of *y* components

$$= 30\sin 45° + 60\sin 60°$$

$$= 30 \times \frac{1}{\sqrt{2}} + 60 \times \frac{\sqrt{3}}{2} = 73.17 \text{ V}$$

Maximum value of resultant voltage

$$V_{mr} = \sqrt{(x - \text{comp})^2 + (y - \text{comp})^2}$$

$$= \sqrt{(51.21)^2 + (73.17)^2} = 89.31 \text{ V}$$

Phase angle $\theta_r = \tan^{-1}\left(\dfrac{y \text{ comp}}{x \text{ comp}}\right) = \tan^{-1}\left(\dfrac{73.17}{51.21}\right) = 55°$

So expression for resultant voltage is

$$V(t) = V_{m_r} \sin(\omega t + \theta_r) = 89.31 \sin(314t + 55°) \qquad \textbf{Ans.}$$

Example 16: Draw a phasor diagram showing the following voltages:

$v_1 = 100 \sin 500t,$ $\qquad v_2 = 200 \sin\left(500t + \dfrac{\pi}{3}\right)$

$v_3 = -50 \cos 500t,$ $\qquad v_4 = 150 \sin\left(500t - \dfrac{\pi}{4}\right)$

Find rms value of resultant voltage. **[UPTU 2005-06, MTU 2008-09]**

Solution: The given equations

$$v_1 = 100 \sin 500t$$

$$v_2 = 200 \sin\left(500t + \frac{\pi}{3}\right)$$

$$v_3 = -50 \cos 500t$$

$$= 50 \sin\left(500t - \frac{\pi}{2}\right)$$

$$v_4 = 150 \sin\left(500t - \frac{\pi}{4}\right)$$

The phasor diagram is shown in figure below.

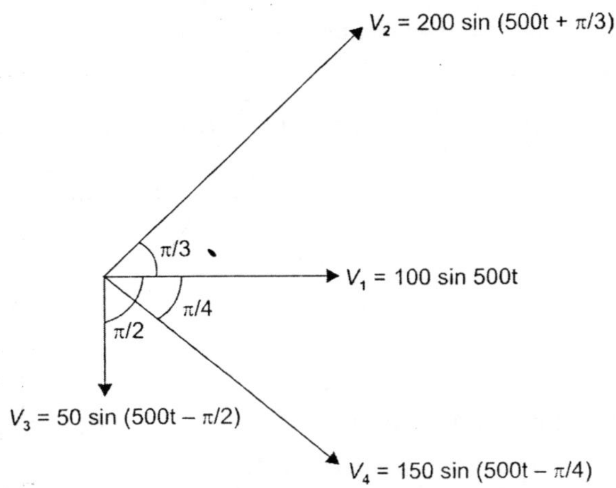

Resolve voltages $V_{m_1}, V_{m_2}, V_{m_3}$ and V_{m_4} along x-axis and y-axis we get.
Algebraic sum of x-components

$$= 100 \cos 0° + 200 \cos\frac{\pi}{3} + 50 \cos\left(-\frac{\pi}{2}\right) + 150 \cos\left(-\frac{\pi}{4}\right)$$

$$= 100 + 200 \times 0.5 + 0 + \frac{150}{\sqrt{2}} = 306.05 \text{ V}$$

Algebraic sum of y-components

$$= 100\sin 0^\circ + 200\sin\frac{\pi}{3} + 50\sin\left(-\frac{\pi}{2}\right) + 150\sin\left(-\frac{\pi}{4}\right)$$

$$= 0 + 200\times 0.866 - 50 - 100 = 17.2 \text{ V}$$

Maximum value of resultant voltage

$$V_{mr} = \sqrt{(x\text{ comp})^2 + (y\text{ comp})^2} = \sqrt{(300)^2 + (17.2)^2} = 306.5 \text{ V}$$

$\therefore$ RMS value of resultant voltage.

$$V_{\text{rms}} = \frac{V_{mr}}{\sqrt{2}} = \frac{306.5}{\sqrt{2}} = 216.72 \text{ V}$$ **Ans.**

Example 17: The instantaneous values of two alternating voltages are represented by $v_1 = 60\sin\theta$ and $v_2 = 40\sin\left(\theta - \frac{\pi}{3}\right)$. Derive an expression for the instantaneous value of (*i*) the sum and (*ii*) the difference of these voltages. **[UTPU July 2002]**

Solution: The give equation are

$$v_1 = 60\sin\theta \text{ and } v_2 = 40\sin\left(\theta - \frac{\pi}{3}\right)$$

(i) Resolve the voltage along x-axis and y-axis

The algebraic sum of x components

$$= 60\cos 0^\circ + 40\cos\left(-\frac{\pi}{3}\right) = 60 + 20 = 80$$

Algebraic sum of y components

$$= 60\sin 0^\circ + 40\sin\left(-\frac{\pi}{3}\right)$$

$$= 0 + (-34.64) = -34.64$$

Maximum value of resultant voltage

$$V_{mr} = \sqrt{(x\text{ comp})^2 + (y\text{ comp})^2}$$

$$= \sqrt{(80)^2 + (-34.64)^2} = 87.178 \text{ volt}$$

Phase angle,

$$\phi = \tan^{-1}\left(\frac{y\text{ comp}}{x\text{ comp}}\right)$$

$$= \tan^{-1}\left(\frac{-34.64}{80}\right) = -23.41^\circ = -0.13\pi \text{ radian}$$

$\therefore$ So expression for the instantaneous value of the sum of given voltages.

$$V_{mr} = 87.17\sin(\theta - 0.13\pi)$$ **Ans.**

(ii) Difference of voltages

Algebraic difference of x components of voltages

$$= 60\cos 0^\circ - 40\cos\left(-\frac{\pi}{3}\right) = 60 - 20 = 40$$

Algebraic difference of voltage of y components

$$= 60\sin 0^\circ - 40\sin\left(-\frac{\pi}{3}\right) = -(-34.64) = -34.64$$

Maximum value of resultant voltage

$$V_{mr} = \sqrt{(x - \text{comp. diff.})^2 + (y - \text{comp. diff})^2}$$

$$= \sqrt{(40)^2 + (34.64)^2} = 52.915 \text{ volt}$$

Phase angle, $$\phi = \tan^{-1}\left(\frac{+34.64}{40}\right) = 40.87°$$

or $$\phi = 0.227\,\pi \text{ radian}$$

∴ So expression for the instantaneous value of the difference of given voltages.

$$V_{mr} = 52.915\sin(\theta + 0.227\pi)$$ **Ans.**

Example 18: Three voltages represented by the equation $e_1 = 15\sin\omega t$, $e_2 = 5\sin\left(\omega t - \frac{\pi}{6}\right)$, and $e_3 = 10\cos\omega t$ act together in an AC circuit, represent these voltage by phasors and calculate an expression for the resultant voltage, check the result graphically. **[GBTU Sem-II, 2009-10]**

Solution: The given equations are

$$e_1 = 15\sin\omega t$$

$$e_2 = 5\sin\left(\omega t + \frac{\pi}{6}\right)$$

$$e_3 = 10\cos\omega t \text{ or } 10\sin\left(\omega t + \frac{\pi}{2}\right)$$

The phasor diagram is shown in figure below.

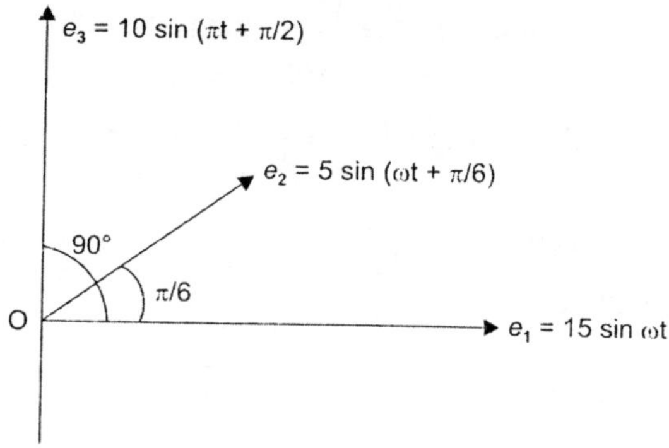

Resolve, e_1, e_2 and e_3 along *x*-axis and *y*-axis we have
Algebraic sum of *x* component

$$= 15\cos 0° + 5\cos\frac{\pi}{6} + 10\cos 90°$$

$$= 15 + \frac{5\sqrt{3}}{2} + 0 = 19.33$$

Algebraic sum of *y* component

$$= 15\sin 0° + 5\cos\frac{\pi}{6} + 10\sin 90°$$

$$= 0 + 25 + 10 = 12.5$$

Maximum of resultant voltage,

$$E_{mr} = \sqrt{(x-\text{comp.})^2 + (y-\text{comp.})^2}$$

$$= \sqrt{(19.33)^2 + (12.5)^2} = 23$$

Phase angle $\phi = \tan^{-1}\left(\frac{y-\text{comp}}{x-\text{comp}}\right) = \tan^{-1}\left(\frac{12.5}{19.33}\right) = 32.9°$

Expression for resultant voltage

$$= E_{mr} \sin(\omega t + \phi)$$

$$e_r = 23 \sin(\omega t + 32.9°)$$

RMS value of resultant voltage

$$E_{rms} = \frac{E_{mr}}{\sqrt{2}} = \frac{23}{\sqrt{2}} = 16.26 \text{ V}$$

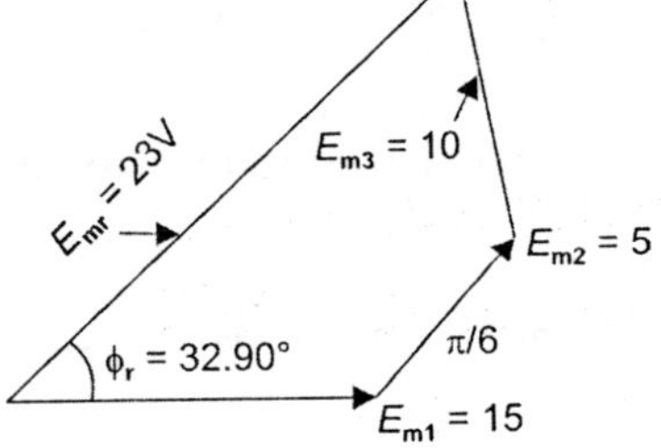

IMPORTANT FORMULAE USED

1. For sinusoidal alternating voltage and current.

(i) $I_{rms} = \frac{I_m}{\sqrt{2}}$ (ii) $V_{rms} = \frac{V_m}{\sqrt{2}}$

(iii) $I_{avg} = \frac{2I_m}{\pi}$ (iv) $V_{avg} = \frac{2V_m}{\pi}$

(v) Form factor for current $K_{fI} = \frac{V_{rm}}{I_{avg}} = 1.11$

(vi) Form factor for voltage $K_{fV} = \frac{V_{rm}}{V_{avg}} = 1.11$

(vii) Peak factor for the voltage $K_{pV} = \frac{V_m}{V_{rms}} = 1.414$

(viii) Similary for current $K_{PI} = \frac{I_m}{I_{rms}} = 1.11$

2. For half-wave rectifier

(i) $I_{rm} = \frac{I_m}{2}$ (ii) $V_{rm} = \frac{V_m}{2}$

(iii) $I_{avg} = \frac{I_m}{\pi}$ (iv) $V_{avg} = \frac{V_m}{\pi}$

(v) $K_{fI} = 1.57$ (vi) $K_{fV} = 1.57$

EXERCISES

Very Short Answer Questions

1. Define the following terms
   (i) Instantaneous value (ii) Maximum value
2. What are the advantages of sinusoidal waveform?
3. What do you mean by form factor?

4. What do you mean by peak factor?
5. What is meant by phase and phase difference?
6. The instantaneous voltage and current for an AC circuit are

$$v = 155.6 \sin 377t$$

$$i = 7.07 \sin(377t - 36.87°) \text{ A}$$

Represent these in a phasor diagram.

Short Answer Questions

1. What is the concept of effectie or RMS value of an alternating quantity? What is the practical significance? **[UPTU 2005-06]**
2. Derive the relationship between
   (i) RMS value and maximum (ii) Average value and maximum
   Value for a purely sinusoidal alternating quantity.
3. How an alternating quantity is represented by a phasor? Explain what is the phase of an alternating quantity?
4. Calculate the average value and RMS value of square wave? **[UPTU 2006-07]**
5. Calculate the average value and RMS value of triangular wave. **[UPTU 2007-08]**
6. The equation of an alternating current $i = 42.42 \sin 628t$. Determine (i) maximum value (ii) frequency (iii) average value (iv) RMS value (v) form factor.

Descriptive Questions

1. Calculate the average value and RMS value of a square wave find the rms value average value, and form factor of the voltage waveform shown in the figure below. **[UPTU 2007-08]**

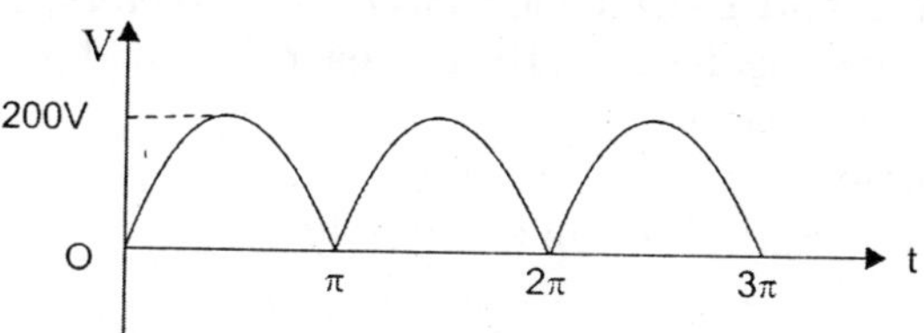

2. Calculate the average value and RMS value of a triangular waveform. Determine the form factor of a voltage waveform as shown in figure below. **[UPTU 2008-09]**

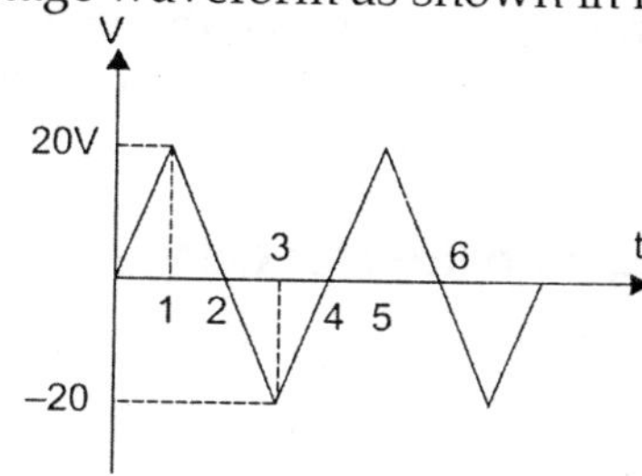

Chapter

4

Steady State Analysis of Single Phase AC Circuits

4.1 INTRODUCTION

We know that an alternating voltage is any voltage that varies both in magnitude and polarity with respect to time. Similarly, an alternating current in any circuit varies in both magnitude and direction with respect to time.

4.2 AC CIRCUIT

Definition: The closed path followed by an alternating current is called an AC circuit. The circuit in which current and voltage vary sinusoidally are called AC circuits. All AC circuits are made up of combination of resistor (R), inductor (L) and capacitor (C). The circuit element R, L and C are called *circuit parameters.* To study a general AC circuits it is necessary to consider the effect of each parameters separately. So we will discuss the following three cases.

(i) AC ciruit containing pure resistor only.
(ii) AC circuit containing pure inductance only.
(iii) AC circuit containing pure capacitor only.

In each case, it is assumed that a purely sinusoidal alternating voltage given by the equation $v = V_m \sin \omega t$ is applied to the circuit. The equation for the current, power and phase shifts are developed in each case. Once the behaviour of pure R, L and C is discussed, then various series and parallel combinations of R, L and C are discussed in this chapter.

4.2.1 AC Circuit Containing Pure Resistor Only

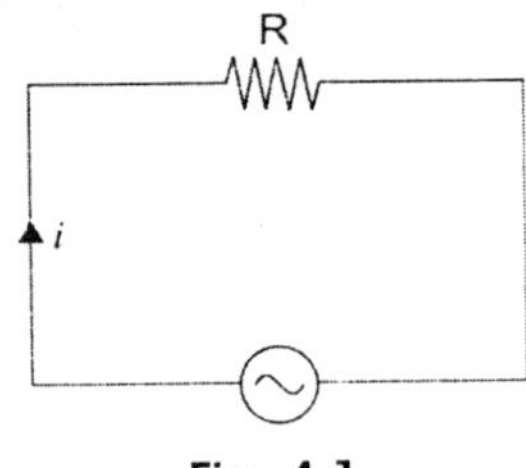

Fig. 4.1

$$v = V_m \sin \omega t \qquad \ldots(4.1)$$

According to ohm's law, we can find the equation for the current I as

$$i = \frac{V}{R} = \frac{V_m \sin \omega t}{R}$$

i.e. $$i = \left(\frac{V_m}{R}\right) \sin \omega t$$

Equation (4.1) gives instantaneous value of the current.

For maximum current, $\sin \omega t = 1$

$\therefore$ $$\omega t = \frac{\pi}{2}$$

$\therefore$ $$I_m = \frac{V_m}{R}$$

Equation (4.1) becomes

$$i = I_m \sin \omega t \quad \text{...(4.2)}$$

Comparing Eqs (4.1) and (4.2), we get there is no phase difference between voltage and current

i.e. $\phi = 0°$

Power factor: It is the cosine of angle between voltage and current.

i.e. $PF = \cos \phi$

where, $\phi = 0°$

$PF = \cos 0° = 1$ (UPF $\rightarrow$ unity power factor)

The waveforms of voltage and current are shown in Fig. 4.2.

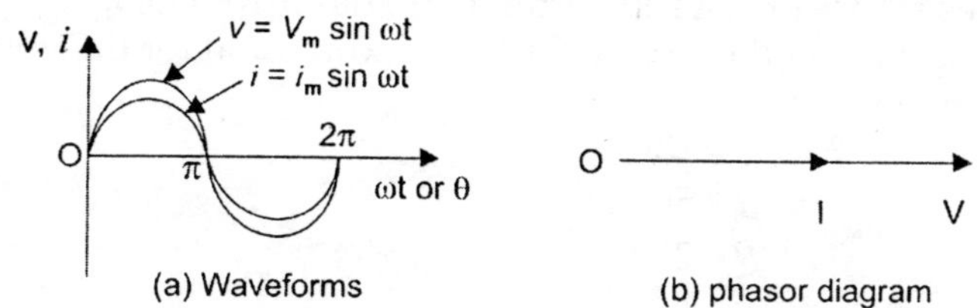

Fig. 4.2: Voltage and current through purely resistive circuit

Power in Pure Resistor

The instantaneous power in AC circuits can be obtained by taking product of the instantaneous values of current and voltage.

$$p = v \times i$$

$$= V_m \sin \omega t \times I_m \sin \omega t = V_m I_m \sin^2(\omega t)$$

$$= V_m I_m \frac{(1 - \cos 2\omega t)}{2}$$

$$p = \underbrace{\frac{V_m I_m}{2}}_{\substack{\text{constant} \\ \text{power} \\ \text{component}}} - \underbrace{\frac{V_m I_m}{2} \cos 2\omega t}_{\substack{\text{fluctuating} \\ \text{power} \\ \text{component}}}$$

Now, the average value of the fluctuating cosine component of double frequency is zero, over one complete cycle.

So, average power consumption over one cycle is equal to the constant power component.

i.e. $$P_{avg} = \frac{V_m I_m}{2}$$

$\therefore$ $$= \frac{V_m I_m}{2} = \frac{V_m}{\sqrt{2}} \times \frac{I_m}{\sqrt{2}}$$

$$= V_{rms} \times I_{rms} \text{ or } P_{avg} = \frac{P_{max}}{2} \text{ W}$$

$\therefore$ $$= I^2 R \text{ W}$$

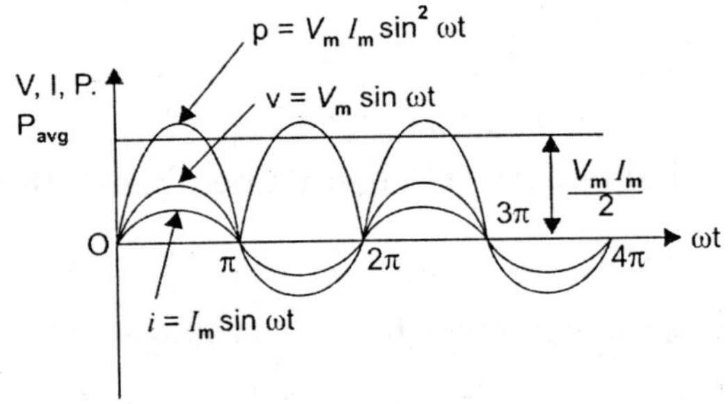

Fig. 4.3: *V*, *I* and *P* for purely resistive circuits

Example: A 250 V (rms), 50 Hz voltage is applied across a circuit consisting of a pure (non inductive) resistance of 20 Ω. Determine (i) The current flowing through the circuit and (ii) power absorbed by the circuit. Give the expression for the voltage and current.

Solution: The given data

$$V = 250 \text{ V}$$
$$f = 50 \text{ Hz}$$
$$R = 20\ \Omega$$

(i) Current flowing through the circuit

$$I = \frac{V}{R} = \frac{250}{20} = 12.5 \text{ A}$$ **Ans.**

(ii) $P = VI = 250 \times 12.5 = 3125$ W **Ans.**

$$V_m = \sqrt{2} \times V_{rms}$$
$$= \sqrt{2} \times 250 = 353.6 \text{ V}$$

$$I_m = \sqrt{2} \times I_{rms}$$
$$= \sqrt{2} \times 12.5 = 17.68 \text{ A}$$

Voltage expression is

$$v = V_m \sin \omega t = 353.6 \sin 314t$$ **Ans.**

Current expression is

$$i = I_m \sin \omega t = 17.68 \sin 314t$$ **Ans.**

4.2.2 AC Circuit Containing Pure Inductor Only

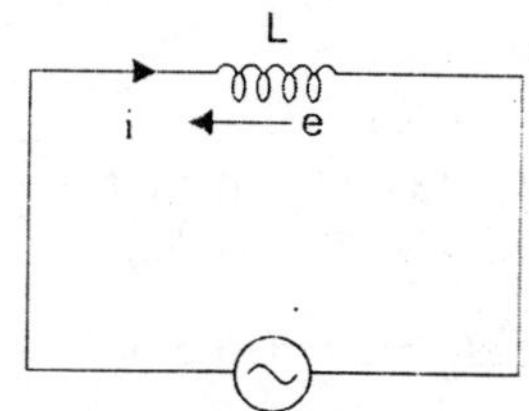

Fig. 4.4: Purely inductive

$$v = V_m \sin \omega t \quad \text{...(4.3)}$$

When alternating current 'I' flows through inductor 'L' it sets up an alternating magnetic field around the inductor. This changing flux links the coil and due to self inductance, emf gets induced in the coil. This emf oppose the applied voltage. The self induced emf in the coil is given by

$$e = -\frac{Ldi}{dt}$$

At all instants, applied voltage V is equal and opposite to the self-induced emf 'e'.

$$v = -e = -\left(-\frac{Ldi}{dt}\right)$$

$$\therefore \quad v = \frac{Ldi}{dt}$$

$$di = \frac{1}{L} v\, dt$$

$$i = \int di = \int \frac{1}{L} v\, dt$$

$$= \frac{1}{L}\int V_m \sin \omega t\, dt = \frac{V_m}{\omega L}\frac{(-\cos \omega t)}{\omega}$$

$$= -\frac{V_m}{\omega L}\cos \omega t = \frac{V_m}{\omega L}\sin\left(\omega t - \frac{\pi}{2}\right)$$

$$= I_m \sin\left(\omega t - \frac{\pi}{2}\right) \quad \text{...(4.4)}$$

where $I_m = \frac{V_m}{\omega L} = \frac{V_m}{X_L}$, $X_L = \omega L = 2\pi f L =$ inductive reactance (Ω), $\omega = 2\pi f$

Comparing Eqs (4.3) and (4.4) current lags behind $\frac{\pi}{2}$ radians from voltage, i.e. $\phi = 90^\circ$ and pf = cos 90°= 0. The waveform and phasor diagram shown in Fig. 4.5.

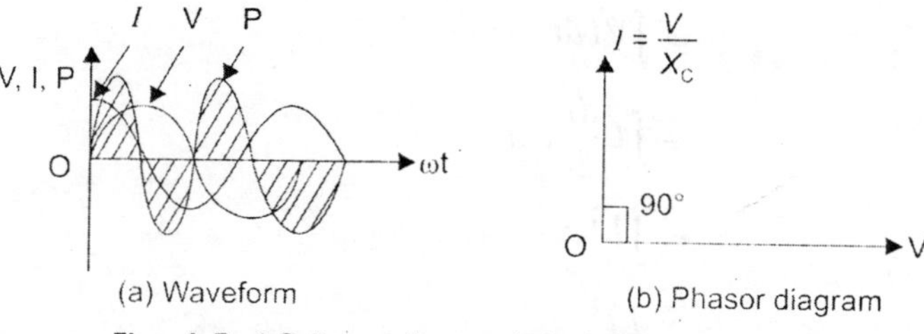

(a) Waveform (b) Phasor diagram

Fig. 4.5: AC through purely inductive circuits

Power in Pure Inductor

We know that instaneous power

$$p = vi$$

or
$$= V_m \sin \omega t \, I_m \sin\left(\omega t - \frac{\pi}{2}\right)$$

$$= V_m I_m \sin \omega t(-\cos \omega t) = -\frac{V_m I_m}{2} 2 \sin \omega t \cos \omega t$$

$$p = -\frac{V_m I_m}{2} \sin 2\omega t$$

$$p = -\frac{V_m I_m}{2} \int_0^{2\pi} \sin 2\omega t \, dt \text{ (for one complete cycle)}$$

$$= -\frac{V_m I_m}{2} \left[\frac{-\cos 2\omega t}{2\omega}\right]_0^{2\pi}$$

$$p = -\frac{V_m I_m}{2} [-1 + 1] = 0$$

Hence
$$p = 0$$

Note: However, it is clear that power consumed in pure inductance AC circuit in one complete cycle is zero. However, the maximum value of instantaneous power is $\frac{V_m I_m}{2}$.

The waveform of power is shown in Fig. 4.6

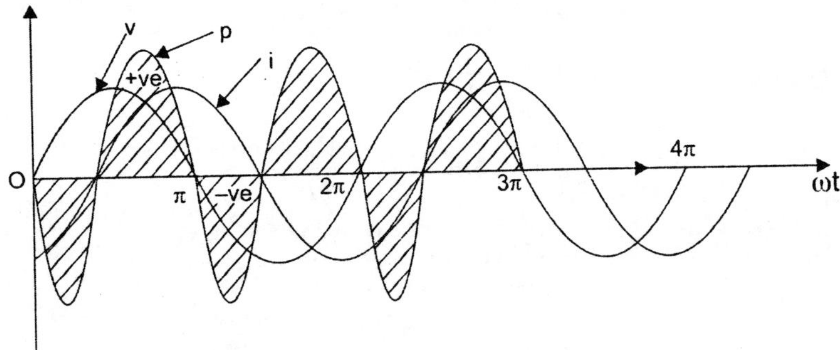

Fig. 4.6: Waveform of voltage, current and power

Energy Stored in Inductor

$$\text{Energy} = \int P \, dt$$

$$= \int VI \, dt$$

$$= \int L \frac{dI}{dt} I \, dt$$

$$= \int LI \, dI$$

$$\text{Energy} = \frac{LI^2}{2}$$

$\therefore$ Energy stored $= \frac{1}{2}LI^2$

Maximum energy stored $= \frac{1}{2}LIm^2$ J

Example: A 0.014 H choke coil with negligible resistance is connected to a 220 V (rms), 50 Hz supply. Determine **[UPTU 2001]**

(i) Inductive reactance of the coil.
(ii) Current flowing through the coil.
(iii) Power consumed by the coil.
(iv) Maximum energy stored in the coil.

Solution: The given data,

$$V = 220 \text{ V}$$
$$L = 0.014 \text{ H}$$
$$f = 50 \text{ Hz}$$

(i) The inductive reactance of coil,

$$X_L = \omega L$$
$$= 2\pi f L = 2\pi \times 50 \times 0.014 = 4.4\ \Omega$$

(ii) Current flowing through the coil,

$$I = \frac{V}{X_L} = \frac{220}{4.4} = 50 \text{ A}$$ **Ans.**

(iii) Power consumed by the coil is zero, $P = 0$ **Ans.**

(iv) Maximum energy stored in the coil

$$W_{\max} = \frac{1}{2}L(I_m)^2$$
$$= \frac{1}{2} \times 0.014 \times \left(\sqrt{2} \times 50\right)^2 = 355 \text{ J}$$ **Ans.**

4.2.3 AC Circuit Containing Pure Capacitance Only

Let, an alternating voltage source is connected across a capacitor of capacitance C farad. Applied voltage is given by

$$V_m \sin \omega t \qquad ...(4.5)$$

When an alternating voltage is applied across a plate of a capacitor, the capacitor is charged first in one direction and then in the opposite direction (Fig. 4.7). Hence charge stored in the capacitor is given by

$$q = Cv$$
$$= CV_m \sin \omega t$$

Now, current i is given by the rate of flow of charge

Hence, $$i = \frac{dq}{dt} = \frac{d(CV_m \sin \omega t)}{dt}$$

$$i = CV_m \frac{d}{dt}(\sin \omega t)$$
$$= CV_m \omega \cos \omega t$$
$$= \frac{V_m}{1/\omega C} \sin\left(\omega t + \frac{\pi}{2}\right)$$

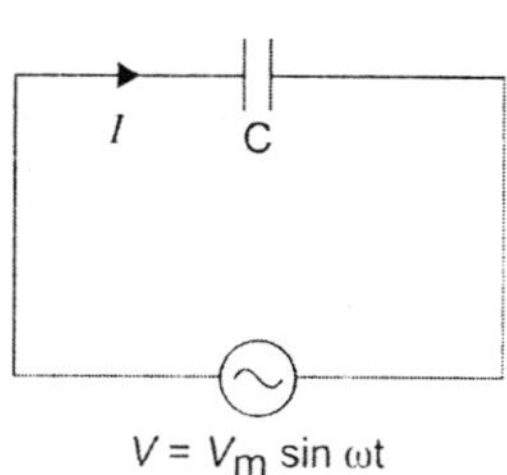

Fig. 4.7

$$= I_m \sin\left(\omega t + \frac{\pi}{2}\right) \qquad ...(4.6)$$

For, the maximum current, $\sin\left(\omega t + \frac{\pi}{2}\right)$ should be unity.

where, $$I_m = \frac{V_m}{X_C}$$

and $$X_C = \frac{1}{\omega C} = \frac{1}{2\pi f C}(\Omega)$$

X_C = capacitive reactance (Ω), $\omega = 2\pi f$

Comparing Eqs (4.5) and (4.6), the current is leading by $\frac{\pi}{2}$ radians from voltage. The waveform is shown in Fig. 4.8

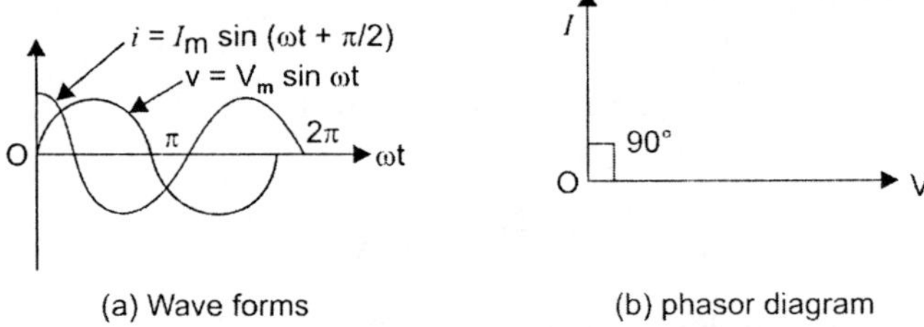

(a) Wave forms (b) phasor diagram

Fig. 4.8: AC circuit through capacitor

Power in Pure Capacitor is

We know that

$$p = vi$$

$$= V_m \sin \omega t \, I_m \sin\left(\omega + \frac{\pi}{2}\right) = \frac{V_m I_m}{2} 2 \sin 2\omega t \cos \omega t$$

$$= \frac{V_m I_m}{2} \sin 2\omega t = \frac{V_m}{\sqrt{2}} \times \frac{I_m}{\sqrt{2}} \sin 2\omega t$$

$\therefore$ Average power $= P_{avg} = \frac{V_m I_m}{2} \times$ average of $\sin^2 \omega t$ over a complete cycle is zero

Hence, $$P_{avg} = 0$$

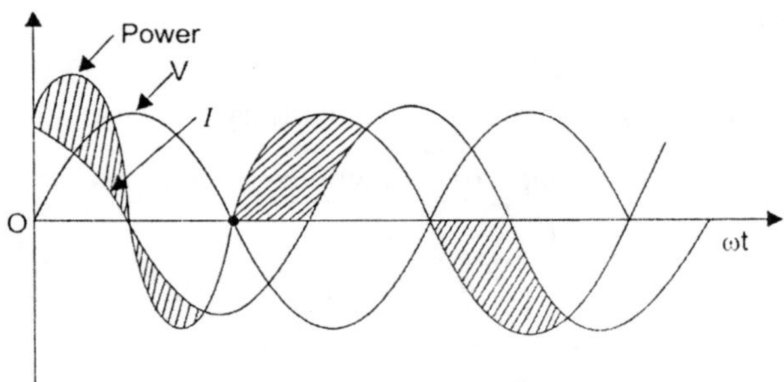

Fig. 4.9: Power waveform

Note: Average power consumed in a pure capacitor is zero.

Proof

$$P = \frac{V_m I_m}{2}\int_0^{2\pi} \sin 2\omega t \, dt$$

$$= \frac{V_m I_m}{2}\left(-\frac{\cos 2\omega t}{2\omega}\right)_0^{2\pi}$$

$$= \frac{V_m I_m}{2}(-1+1) = 0$$

$$P_{avg} = 0$$

Hence proved

Energy Stored in a Capacitor

$$\text{Energy} = \int \rho \, dt = \int V I \, dt$$

$$= \int V \frac{dq}{dt} dt = \int V d(CV) \qquad [\because q = CV]$$

$$= C\int V \, dv = C\frac{V^2}{2}$$

$$\therefore \quad \text{Energy stored} = \frac{1}{2}CV^2. \text{ J}$$

Maximum energy stored in capacitor is

$$W_{max} = \frac{1}{2}CV_m^2 \text{ J}$$

Example: As 318μf capacitor is connected to 200 V, 50 Hz supply determine (i) The capacitive reactance (ii) Maximum current (iii) rms value of the current drawn by the capacitor (iv) Maximum instantaneous charge on the capacitor (v) Maximum energy stored in the capacitor. Write the time equation for the voltage and current. Give the waveform and phasor diagram. **[UPTU 2002]**

Solution: The given data

$$V_{rms} = 200 \text{ V}$$

$$f = 50 \text{ Hz}$$

$$\therefore \quad \omega = 2\pi f = 2\pi \times 50 = 314 \text{ rad/sec}$$

(i) Capacitive reactance offered by the capacitor

$$X_C = \frac{1}{\omega C} = \frac{1}{2\pi f_C} = \frac{1}{314 \times 318 \times 10^{-6}}$$

$$\therefore \quad = 10\ \Omega \qquad \textbf{Ans.}$$

(ii) Maximum value of current drawn by the capacitor

$$I_m = \frac{V_m}{X_C} = \frac{200\sqrt{2}}{10}$$

$$= 28.28 \text{ A} \qquad \textbf{Ans.}$$

(iii) RMS value of current drawn by the capacitor

$$I_{rms} = \frac{V_{rms}}{X_C} = \frac{200}{10}$$

$$= 20 \text{ A} \qquad \textbf{Ans.}$$

(iv) Maximum instantaneous charge on the capacitor

$$Q_{max} = CV_{max}$$
$$= 318 \times 10^{-6} \times 200 \times \sqrt{2}$$
$$= 0.096 \text{ C}$$ **Ans.**

(v) Maximum energy stored in the capacitor is

$$W_{max} = \frac{1}{2}CV_m^2 = \frac{1}{2}318 \times 10^{-6} \times \left(200 \times \sqrt{2}\right)^2$$
$$= 12.72 \text{ J}$$ **Ans.**

Time equation for voltage and current is

$$v = V_m \sin \omega t = 200\sqrt{2} \sin 314t$$ **Ans.**

$$i = I_m \sin\left(\omega t + \frac{\pi}{2}\right) = 28.28 \sin\left(314t + \frac{\pi}{2}\right)$$

Waveform and phase diagram shown in figure below.

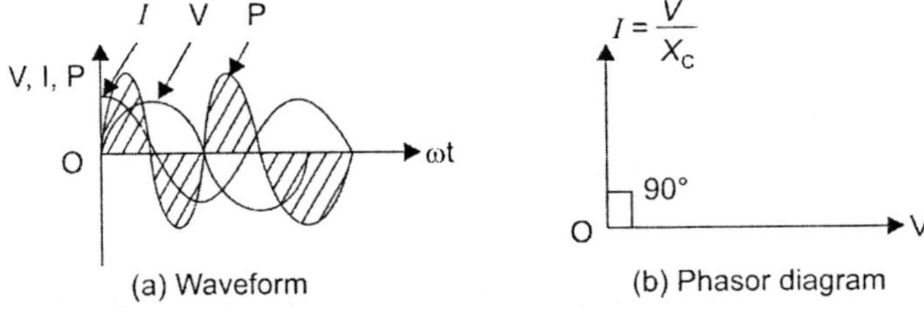

(a) Waveform (b) Phasor diagram

4.3 AC SERIES CIRCUIT

A series combination of circuit elements like *R-L, R-C* and *R-L-C* comes under the category of series AC circuits. Here the sinusoidal voltage is applied across the series circuit and then the behaviour of the circuit is analysed. Now we will discuss three different cases of series circuit.

4.3.1 AC Circuit Containing Resistance and Inductance in Series

[UPTU 2004-05, 2006-07, 2009-10]

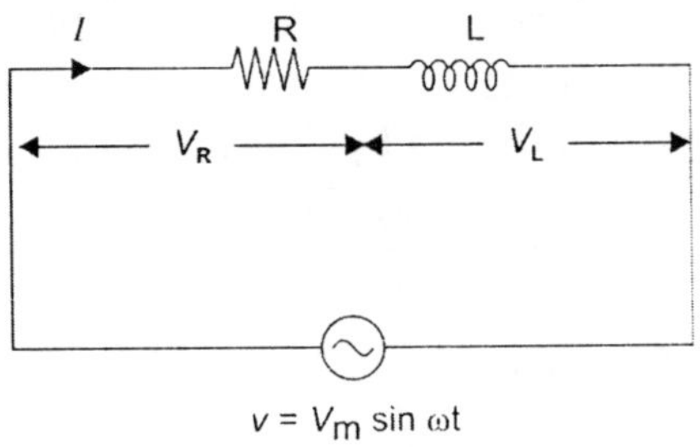

Fig. 4.10: Series RL circuit

Voltage drop across resistance

$$V_R = IR$$

Voltage drop across inductance

$$V_L = IX_L = I\omega L$$

The applied voltage $V = \sqrt{V_R^2 \times V_L^2}$

$$V = \sqrt{(IR)^2 + (IX_L)^2}$$

$$= I\sqrt{R^2 + X_L^2}$$

$$V = IZ$$

Instantaneously current, $i = \dfrac{v}{Z\angle\phi} = \dfrac{V_m \sin \omega t}{Z\angle\phi}$

or $i = \dfrac{V_m}{Z}\sin(\omega t - \phi)$

$$= I_m \sin(\omega t - \phi) \quad ...(4.7)$$

where, $I_m = \dfrac{V_m}{Z}$, $\phi = \tan^{-1}\left(\dfrac{X_L}{R}\right)$

and Z = is known as impedance

$$= \sqrt{R^2 + X_L^2} \quad ...(4.8)$$

Phasor Diagram of R-L-Circuit

Steps to draw phasor diagram

Step I: Take current as a reference phasor because in series circuit, current is same throughout the circuit.

Step II: In case of resistor, voltage and current are in phase, so V_R will be along current phasor as shown in Fig. 4.11

Step III: In case of inductor, current lag voltage by 90°. But as current is reference, so V_L must be shown leading with respect to current by 90°.

Step IV: The supply voltage being vector sum of these two vectors V_L and V_R obtained by law of parallelogram.

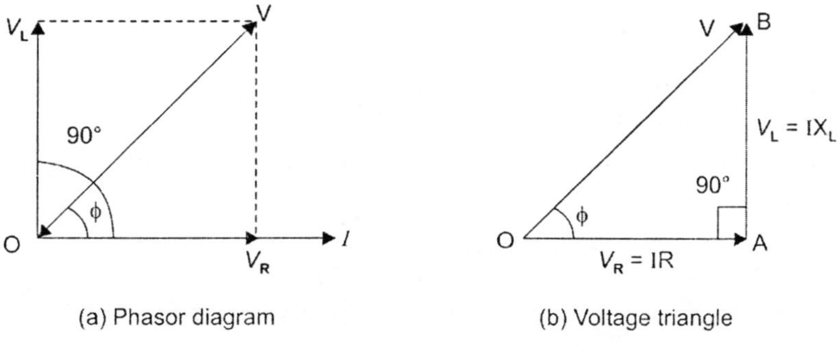

(a) Phasor diagram (b) Voltage triangle

Fig. 4.11

From phasor diagram current lags behind the applied voltage V by angle ϕ

$$\therefore \quad \tan\phi = \frac{V_L}{V_R} = \frac{IX_L}{IR} = \frac{X_L}{R}$$

$$\therefore \qquad \phi = \tan^{-1}\left(\frac{X_L}{R}\right)$$

If the applied voltage $v = V_m \sin \omega t$, then the expression for the circuit current will be

$$i = I_m \sin(\omega t - \phi)$$

Power in R-L-Circuit

We know that

instantaneous power, $i = vi$

$$\therefore \qquad p = V_m \sin \omega t \, I_m \sin(\omega t - \phi)$$

$$= \frac{V_m I_m}{2}\left[2 \sin \omega t \sin(\omega t - \phi)\right]$$

$$= \frac{V_m I_m}{2}\left[\cos \phi - \cos(2\omega t - \phi)\right]$$

$$= \frac{V_m I_m}{2}\cos \phi - \frac{V_m I_m}{2}\cos(2\omega t - \phi)$$

$$\therefore \qquad = \frac{V_m I_m}{2}\cos \phi = \frac{V_m}{\sqrt{2}} \times \frac{I_m}{\sqrt{2}}\cos \phi$$

$$= V_{rms} I_{rms} \cos \phi = VI \cos \phi \text{ watts}$$

Power and power triangle:

$$P = VI \cos \phi$$

where V and I are rms values of voltage and current respectively. We know that the voltage equation is given by

$$\overline{V} = \overline{V_R} + \overline{V_L}$$

If we multiply above voltage equation by current I, we get the power equation.

$$\overline{VI} = \overline{V_R I} + \overline{V_L I}$$

$$= V\overline{\cos \phi I} + V\overline{\sin \phi I}$$

$$= \overline{VI \cos \phi} + \overline{VI \sin \phi}$$

From the above equation, power triangle can be obtained as shown in the Fig. 4.12 So, three sides of this triangle are:

(i) VI (volt ampere), (ii) $VI \cos \phi$ (watts), (iii) $VI \sin \phi$ (volt-ampere reactive)

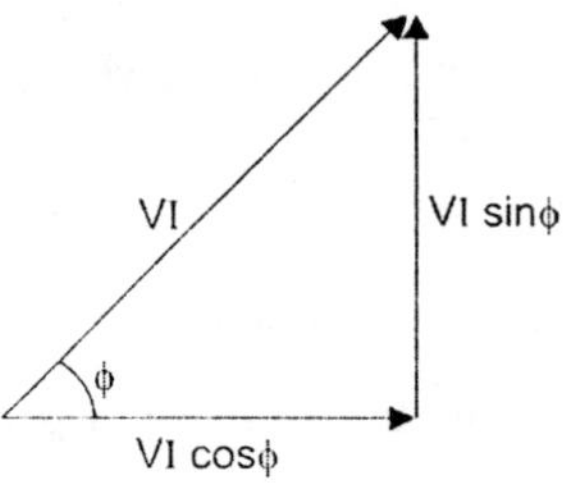

Fig. 4.12: Power triangle

4.3.2 Apparent Power, Real Power and Reactive Power

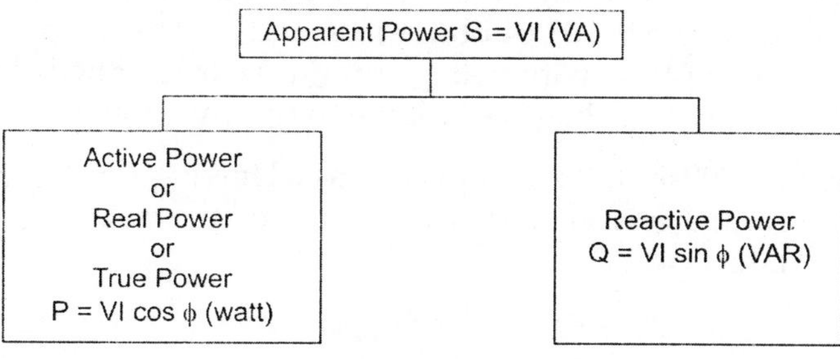

Fig. 4.13

Apparent Power (S)

Definition: It is defined as the product of rms value of voltage V and current I. It is denoted by S.

$$S = VI = (IZ)I = I^2 Z \text{ (VA)}$$

$$\therefore \quad = VI \text{ (VA)}$$

It is measured in volt ampere (VA) or kVA.

Real Power or Active Power (P)

It is the power which is actually dissipated in the circuit resistance.
Definiton: It is the product of apparent power and power factor. It is denoted by P and measured in unit watt or kilo-watt (kW).

$$\therefore \quad P = I^2R = VI\cos\phi \text{ W}$$

Note $\quad P = VI\cos\phi = VI\frac{R}{Z} \quad \left[\because \cos\phi = \frac{R}{Z}\right]$

$$= \left(\frac{V}{Z}\right)IR = I^2R$$

Reactive Power (Q)

It is the power developed in the inductive reactance of the circuit. It is defined as product of the applied voltage and the reactive component ($I\sin\phi$) of the current. It is denoted by Q and is measured in unit volt-ampere reactive (VAR) or kilo-volt ampere reactive (kVAR).

$$Q = I^2 \times L = I^2 Z\sin\phi = I(IZ)\sin\phi$$

$$= VI\sin\phi \text{ volt-ampere-reactive (VAR)}$$

Significance of active power and reactive power: The purpose of passing current through a circuit is to transfer power from the source to the circuit. The power which is actually consumed in the circuits is called true power or active power. We have already seen that power is consumed only in resister since neither pure inductor nor the capacitor consumes any active power. The power consumed (or true power) in L and C is zero because all the power received from the source in half cycle is returned to the source in the next half cycle. This circulating power is called the reactive power and does not do the useful work in the circuit. The reader may recall that current and voltage are in phase in a resistor where as they are 90° of phase in L and C. Therefore, we come to the conclusion that current in phase with voltage produces true or active power whereas current 90° out of phase with voltage contribute to reactive power.

Example: A voltage $v = 200\sin 100\pi t$ is applied to a coil having $R = 200\ \Omega$ and $L = 0.38$ H. Find the expression for the current and power taken by the coil.

Solution: Given data

$$v = 200 \sin 100\pi t$$

$$R = 200\ \Omega$$

$$L = 0.38 \text{ H}$$

$$V_m = 200 \text{ V}$$

$$X_L = \omega L = 100\pi \times 0.38 = 119.38\ \Omega$$

$$Z = \sqrt{R^2 + (X_L)^2}$$

$$= \sqrt{(200)^2 + (119.38)^2} = 232.92\ \Omega$$

$$I_m = \frac{V_m}{Z} = \frac{200}{232.92} = 0.859 \text{ A}$$

$$\phi = \tan^{-1}\left(\frac{X_L}{R}\right) = \tan^{-1}\left(\frac{119.38}{200}\right)$$

$$= 30.8^\circ = 0.174\pi \text{ rad}$$

$$i = I_m \sin(\omega t - \phi) = 0.859\sin(100\pi t - 0.171\pi)$$

Power taken by the coil

$$P = VI\cos\phi$$

$$= \frac{200}{\sqrt{2}} \times \frac{0.859}{\sqrt{2}} \cos 30.8^\circ$$

$$= 73.8 \text{ watts}$$ **Ans.**

4.3.3 AC Circuit Containing Resistance and Capacitance in Series

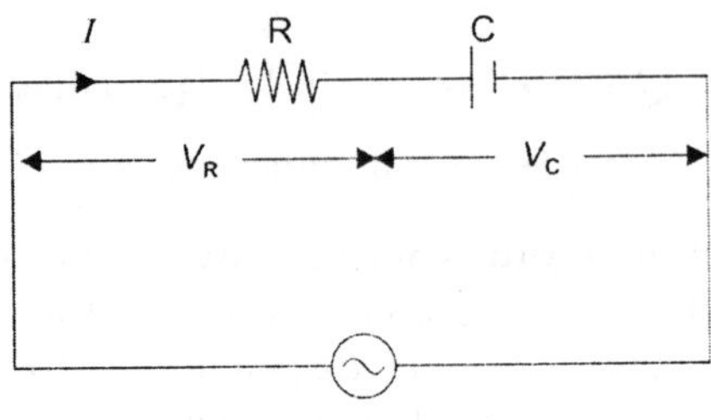

$$v = V_m \sin \omega t \qquad ...(4.9)$$

Fig. 4.14: RC series circuit

Voltage drop across resistance

$$V_R = IR$$

Voltage drop across capacitance

$$V_C = IX_C$$

∴ Total supplied voltage

$$V = \sqrt{(V_R)^2 + (V_C)^2}$$

$$= \sqrt{(I_R)^2 + (V_C)^2} = I\sqrt{R^2 + X_C^2} = IZ$$

Instantaneous current $i = \dfrac{v}{Z} = \dfrac{V_m \sin \omega t}{Z\angle\phi}$

$$= \frac{V_m}{Z}\sin(\omega t + \phi)$$

$$= I_m \sin(\omega t + \phi) \qquad ...(4.10)$$

where $I_m = \dfrac{V_m}{Z}$

$$Z = \sqrt{R^2 + X_C^2} = \text{impedance } (\Omega)$$

$$\phi = \tan^{-1}\left(\frac{X_C}{R}\right)$$

$$z = R - J\,X_C$$

Now let us draw the phasor diagram.

Steps for Drawing Phasor Diagrams

Step I: Take current as a reference phasor because it is common throughout the circuit.

Step II: In case of resistor, voltage and current are in phase, so V_R will be drawn along with current as shown in Fig. 4.15a.

Step III: In case of pure capacitor, current leads voltage by 90°, i.e. voltage lag current by 90°. So V_C is shown downwords, i.e. lagging by 90° as shown in Fig. 4.15a.

Step IV: The supply voltage being vector sum of these two voltage V_C and V_R obtained by completing parallelogram.

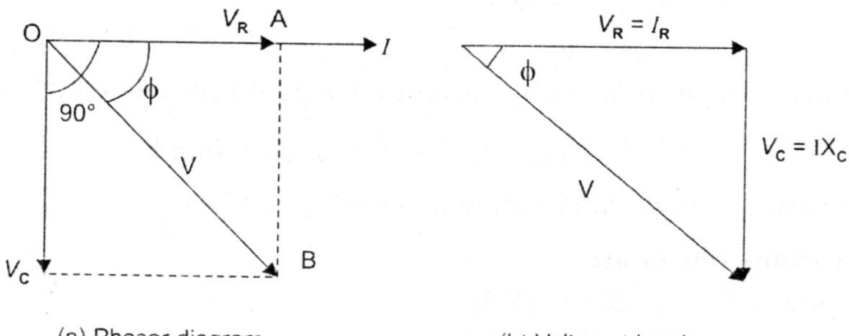

(a) Phasor diagram (b) Voltage triangle

Fig. 4.15

From voltage triangle

$$V = \sqrt{(V_R)^2 + (V_C)^2}$$

$$= I\sqrt{R^2 + X_C^2} = IZ$$

Impedance triangle is shown in Fig. 4.16

From impedance triangle

$$Z = \sqrt{R^2 + X_C^2}$$

$$\cos\phi = \frac{R}{Z} \text{ and } \sin\phi = \frac{X_C}{Z}$$

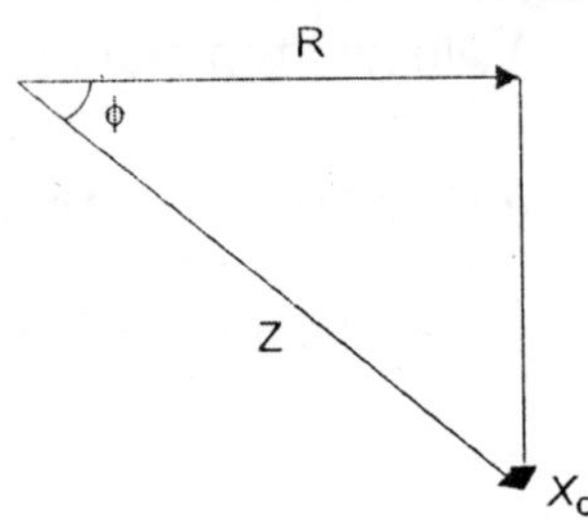

Fig. 4.16: Impedance triangle

Power and Power Triangle

The current leads voltage by angle ϕ hence its expression is

$$i = I_m \sin(\omega t + \phi)$$

and

$$v = V_m \sin \omega t$$

$\therefore$ Instanteous power = Product of instantaneous values of voltage and current.

$$p = v \times i = V_m \sin \omega t \times I_m \sin(\omega t + \phi)$$

$$= V_m I_m (\sin(\omega t)\sin(\omega t + \phi)$$

$$= V_m I_m \left[\frac{\cos(-\phi) - \cos(2\omega t + \phi)}{2}\right]$$

$$= \underbrace{\frac{V_m I_m}{2}\cos\phi}_{\text{Part (I)}} - \underbrace{\frac{V_m I_m}{2}\cos(2\omega t + \phi)}_{\text{Part (II)}}$$

[since $\cos(-\phi) = \cos\phi$]

Now, second term (π) is cosine term whose average value over a cycle is zero. Hence, average power consumed by the circuit is

$$P_{avg} = \frac{V_m I_m}{2}\cos\phi$$

$$P = \frac{V_m}{\sqrt{2}} \times \frac{I_m}{\sqrt{2}}\cos\phi$$

$$= VI\cos\phi \text{ watts}$$

We know that total supply voltage is

$$\overline{V} = \overline{V_R} + \overline{V_C}$$

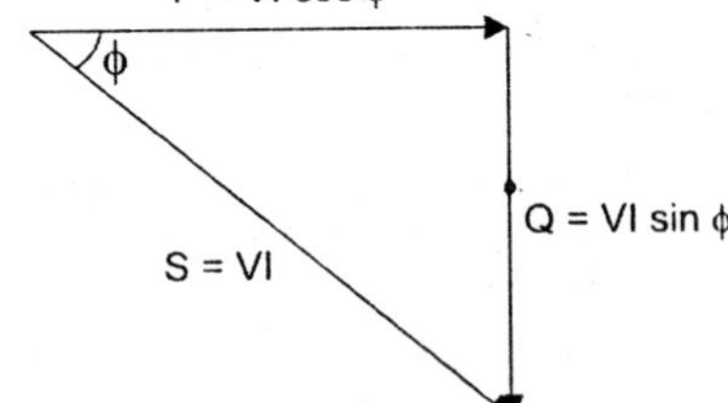

Fig. 4.17: Power triangle

If we multiply voltage equation by current I, we get the power equation.

$$\therefore \quad \overline{V}\overline{I} = \overline{V_R}\overline{I} + \overline{V_C}I = \overline{V}\,\overline{I}\cos\phi + \overline{V}\overline{I}\sin\phi$$

Hence the power triangle can be shown in the Fig. 4.17

Thus the various power are

Apparent power $S = VI(VA)$

True or average power $= VI\cos\phi\,(W)$

Reactive power $Q = VI\sin\phi\,(VAR)$

Note

X_L term appears positive in Z.

$$\therefore \quad Z = R + jX_L = Z\angle\phi, \ \phi \text{ is the positive for inductive loads.}$$

X_C terms appears negative in Z.

$$\therefore \quad Z = R - jX_C = Z\angle -\phi$$

Average power is given by

$$P = VI\cos\phi \text{ W}$$

where V and I are rms values.

SOLVED EXAMPLE ON ABOVE THEORY

Example: A resistance of 100 Ω is connected in series with a 56 μF capacitor to a supply at 230 V, 50 Hz. Find (i) the impedance, (ii) current (iii) the phase angle (iv) the pf (v) the voltage across the resistor and the voltage across the capacitor. Draw the phasor diagram.

Solution: The given data

$$R = 100\ \Omega$$

$$C = 56\ \mu\text{F} = 56 \times 10^{-6}\ \text{F}$$

$$f = 50\ \text{Hz},\ V = 230\ \text{V}$$

$$\therefore \quad X_C = \frac{1}{\omega C} = \frac{1}{2\pi f C} = \frac{1}{2\pi \times 50 \times 56 \times 10^{-6}}$$

$$\therefore \quad = 56.89\ \Omega$$

(i) The circuit impedance

$$Z = \sqrt{R^2 + X_C^2}$$

$$= \sqrt{(100)^2 + (56.89)^2} = 115\ \Omega \qquad \textbf{Ans.}$$

(ii) Circuit current $\quad I = \dfrac{V}{Z} = \dfrac{230}{115} = 2\ \text{A}$ **Ans.**

(iii) The phase angle $\quad \phi = \tan^{-1}\left(\dfrac{X_C}{R}\right) = \tan^{-1}\left(\dfrac{56.89}{100}\right) = 29.6°$ **Ans.**

(iv) Power factor (PF)

$$\therefore \quad \text{PF} = \cos\phi = \cos 29.6° = 0.87 \text{ (lead)}$$

(v) Voltage across resistor

$$V_R = 1\text{R} = 2 \times 100 = 200\ \text{V} \qquad \textbf{Ans.}$$

$$\therefore \quad V_C = IX_C = 2 \times 56.84 = 113.7 \text{ volt} \qquad \textbf{Ans.}$$

The phasor diagram

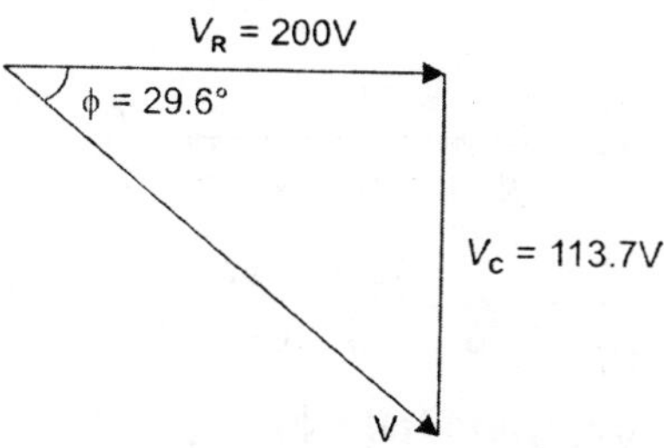

4.4 AC CIRCUIT CONTAINING RESISTANCE, INDUCTANCE AND CAPACITANCE IN SERIES (R-L-C SERIES)

The AC supply is given by

$$v = V_m \sin \omega t \qquad ...(4.11)$$

The circuit drawn a current I.

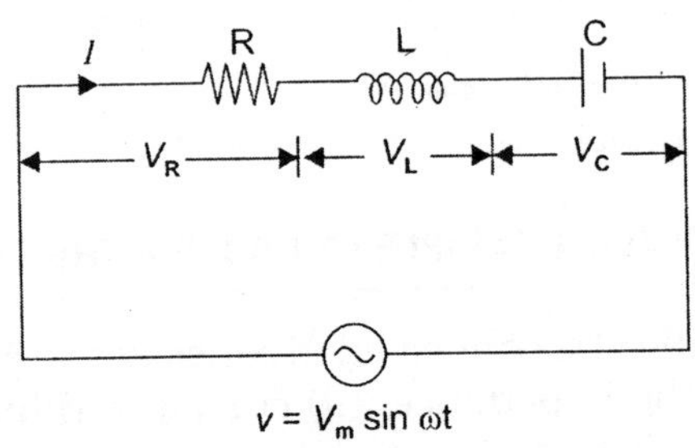

Fig. 4.18

Due to current I, there are different voltage drops across R, L and C.

Voltage drop across resistance R is

$$\therefore \quad V_R = IR$$

Voltage drop across inductance L is

$$\therefore \quad V_L = IX_L$$

Voltage drop across capacitance C is

$$\therefore \quad V_C = IX_C$$

The values of I, V_R, V_L and V_C are rms values.

The characteristics of three drops are

V_R is in phase with current I.

V_L leads current I by 90°.

V_C lags current I by 90°.

The total supply voltage according to kirchhoff's laws are

$$\overline{V} = \overline{V_R} + \overline{V_L} + \overline{V_C}$$

Let us consider the case when V_L is greater than V_C. The applied voltage V is

$$\therefore \quad V = \sqrt{(V_R)^2 + (V_L - V_C)^2}$$

$$= \sqrt{(IR)^2 + (IX_L - IX_C)^2}$$

$$= I\sqrt{R^2 + (X_L - X_C)^2}$$

$$\therefore \quad I = \frac{V}{\sqrt{R^2 + (X_L - X_C)^2}} = \frac{V}{Z}$$

$$\text{instantaneous current } i = \frac{v}{Z\angle\phi} = \frac{V_m \sin \omega t}{Z\angle\phi}$$

$$I = I_m \sin(\omega t - \phi)$$

where, $I_m = \frac{V_m}{Z}$

$$Z = \sqrt{R^2 + (X_L - X_C)^2}$$

(impedance of *R-L-C* series circuit (Ω)

Phase angle (ϕ)

$$\phi = \tan^{-1}\left(\frac{X_L - X_C}{R}\right)$$

$X_L > X_C \rightarrow$ Current lags behind the voltage

$X_C > X_L \rightarrow$ Current leads the voltage

Phasor Diagram: Case I: If $X_L > X_C$.

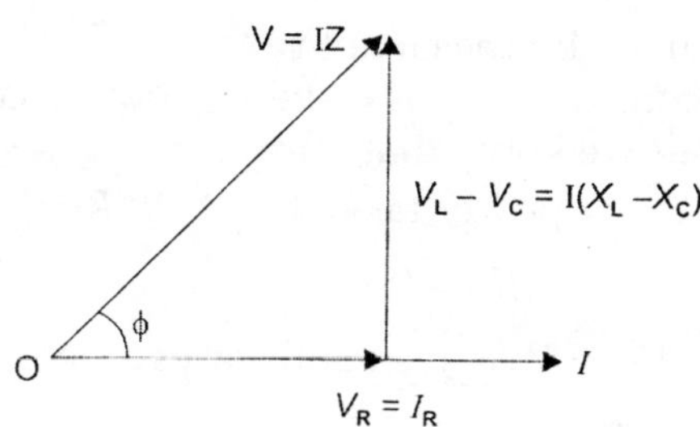

Fig. 4.19: Phasor diagram of R-L-C series circuit

Case II: $X_C > X_L$

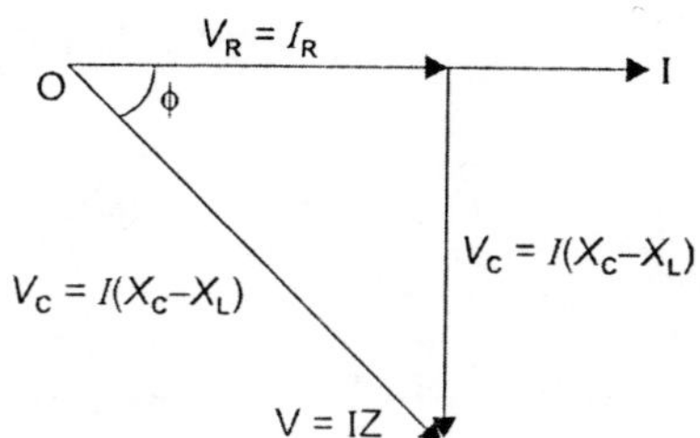

Fig. 4.20: Phasor diagram ($X_L < X_C$)

4.4.1 Impedance Triangle

As the expression of impedance

$$Z = \sqrt{R^2 + (X_L - X_C)^2}$$

∴ Impedance triangle becomes

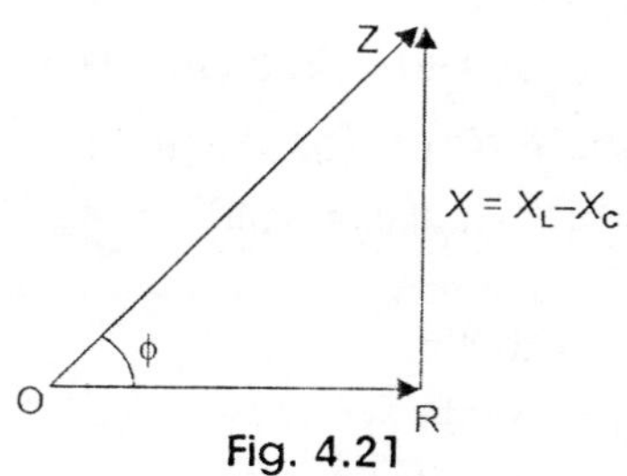

Fig. 4.21

X is the total reactance (net reactance)

$$\therefore \quad X = X_L - X_C$$

$$\phi = \tan^{-1}\left(\frac{X_L - X_C}{R}\right)$$

$$\cos\phi = \frac{R}{Z};\ \sin\phi = \frac{X}{Z}$$

Note

If $X_L > X_C, X$ is positive and circuit is inductive in nature.
If $X_C > X_L, X$ is negative and circuit is capacitive in nature.
If $X_L = X_C, X$ is zero and circuit is purely resistive.

4.4.2 Power and Power Triangle

The average power consumed by the circuit is

P_{avg} = average power consumed by R + average power consumbed by L + average power consumed by C. But we know that pure L and C never consume any power.

$$\therefore \quad P_{avg} = \text{power taken by } R = I^2 R$$

$$= I(IR) = IV_R$$

But $\quad V_R = V\cos\phi$ in both cases

$$\therefore \quad P = VI\cos\phi \text{ W}$$

Now the power triangle can be obtained as shown in Fig. 4.24a and 4.24b.

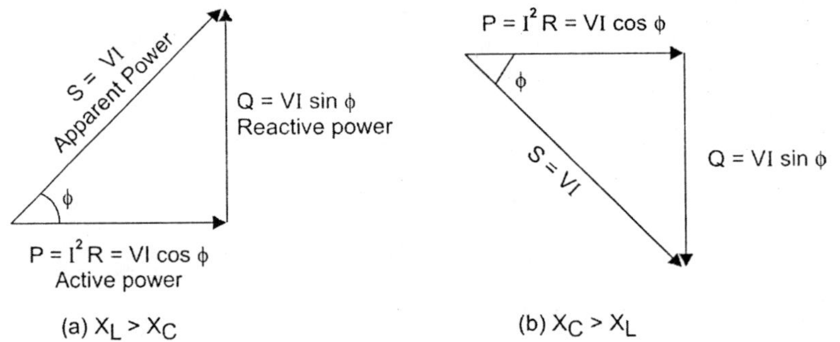

Fig. 4.22: Power triangle

Example: Find an expression for the instantaneous value of the current through an R-L-C series circuit in which $R = 80\ \Omega$, $L = 41.3$ mH and $C = 0.79\ \mu$F. When applied voltage is $1\sin 2000\pi t$ volt. **[UPTU 2006-07]**

Solution: Given data

$$R = 80\ \Omega$$

$$L = 41.3 \text{ mH} = 41.3\times10^{-3} \text{ H}$$

$$C = 0.797\,\mu\text{F} = 0.797\times10^{-6} \text{ F}$$

$$V = 1.\sin 2000\pi t \text{ volt}$$

$$V_m = 1 \text{ volt}$$

$$\omega = 2000\pi$$

$$\therefore \quad 2\pi f = 2000\pi$$

$$f = 1000 \text{ Hz}$$

$$X_L = \omega L$$
$$= 2000\pi \times 41.3 \times 10^{-3} = 259.5\ \Omega$$

$$X_C = \frac{1}{\omega C} = \frac{1}{2000\pi \times 0.797 \times 10^{-6}} = 199.7\ \Omega$$

∴ Impedance
$$Z = \sqrt{R^2 + (X_L - X_C)^2}$$
$$= \sqrt{80^2 + (259.5 - 199.7)^2} = 99.88\ \Omega$$

∴
$$I_m = \frac{V_m}{Z} = \frac{1}{99.88} = 0.01\text{ A}$$

Phase angle (ϕ)

$$\phi = \tan^{-1}\left(\frac{X_L - X_C}{R}\right) = \tan^{-1}\left(\frac{259.5 - 199.7}{80}\right)$$
$$= 36.8° \text{ or } 0.209\pi\text{ rad}$$

∴ Current expression

$$i = I_m \sin(\omega t - \phi)$$
$$I = 0.01 \sin(2000t - 0.209\pi)$$ **Ans.**

4.5 AC PARALLEL CIRCUIT

A parallel circuit is one in which two or more branches are connected in parallel across the supply voltage. The voltage is the same for each branch but the branch current may differ in magnitude and phase depending on the branch impedance. Each branch of the circuit is analysed separately and voltage is taken as the reference phasor.

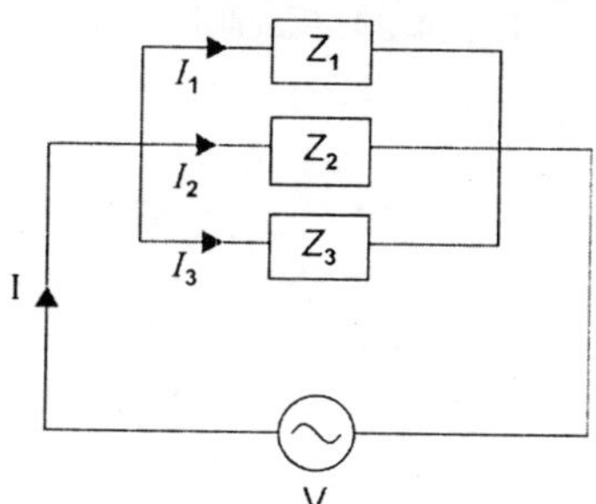

Fig. 4.23: Parallel circuit

Figure 4.23 shows a parallel circuit consisting of three impedances in parallel across AC supply of V volts. The voltage across all the impedance is same as supply voltage of V volts. From Fig. 4.23

$$\overline{I} = \overline{I_1} + \overline{I_2} + \overline{I_3}$$

$$\frac{\overline{V}}{Z} = \frac{\overline{V}}{Z_1} + \frac{\overline{V}}{Z_2} + \frac{\overline{V}}{Z_3} \Rightarrow \frac{1}{Z} = \frac{1}{Z_1} + \frac{1}{Z_2} + \frac{1}{Z_3}$$

where Z is called equivalent impedance.

There are two principal reason for it: The operation of each device become independent of the other. Therefore it is possible to turn ON or OFF any device without disturbing the operation of other device. Most of the electrical appliances require different current at the same voltage from the same power source.

Notes: In parallel circuit, the voltage across all the impedances is same as supply voltage. Total line current is the phasor sum of branch currents. Always voltage is taken reference phasor as it is same across all branches. Parallel circuits are used more frequently in electrical system as compared to series circuit because electrical devices and equipment are connected in parallel across AC mains.

4.6 METHOD OF SOLVING AC PARALLEL CIRCUIT

- By phasor diagram method
- By impedance method
- By phasor algebra method
- By admittance method

4.6.1 By Phasor Diagram Method

The phasor diagram method is suitable only when the parallel circuit is simple and contains two branches. Consider a parallel circuit consisting of two branches and connected to an alternating voltage of V volts as shown in Fig. 4.24.

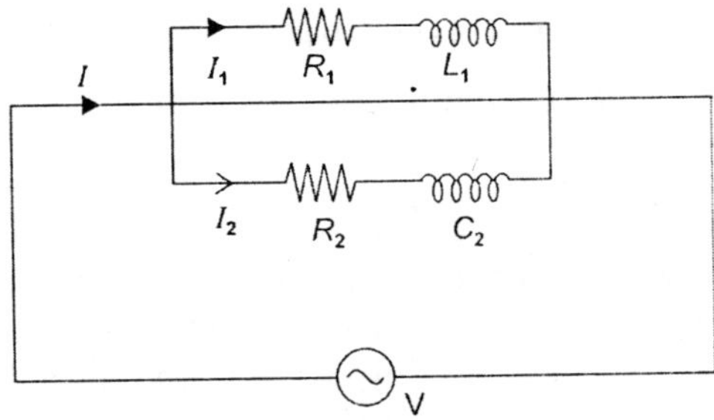

Fig. 4.24: Parallel circuit

Draw the phasor diagram

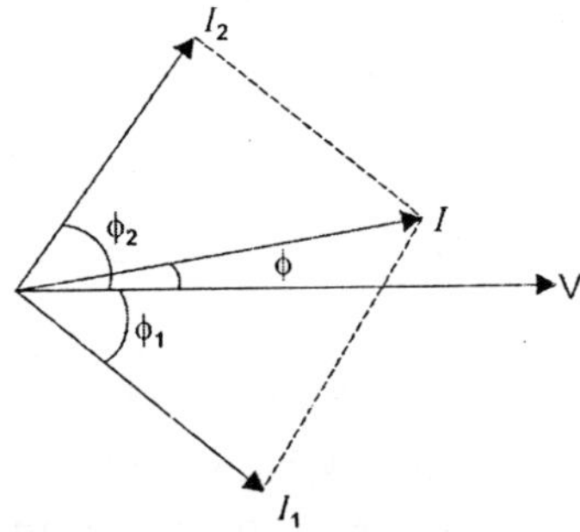

Fig. 4.25: Phasor diagram

Branch 1: Impedance

$$Z_1 = \sqrt{R_1^2 + (X_{L_1})^2}$$

Current

$$I_1 = \frac{V}{Z_1}$$

$$\phi_1 = \tan^{-1}\left(\frac{X_{L_1}}{R_1}\right)$$

Current I_1 lags behind V by ϕ_1.

Branch 2: Impedance

$$Z_2 = \sqrt{R_2^2 + (X_{C_2})^2}$$

Current $$I_2 = \frac{V}{Z_2}$$

$$\phi_2 = \tan^{-1}\left[\frac{X_{C_2}}{R_2}\right]$$

Current I_2 leads the voltage V by ϕ_2

To Calculate Current

From phasor diagram, the value of I and ϕ can be determined by resolving the current into rectangular components.

⇒ Algebraic sum of component of I_1 and I_2 along x-axis.

$$= I_1 \cos\phi_1 + I_2 \cos\phi_2$$

⇒ Algebraic sum of component of I_1 and I_2 along y-axis.

$$= I_1 \sin\phi_1 + I_2 \sin\phi_2$$

Resultant of current

∴ $$I = \sqrt{(x\text{ comp})^2 + (y\text{ comp})^2}$$

Phase angle

$$\phi = \tan^{-1}\left(\frac{y\text{ comp}}{x\text{ comp}}\right)$$

4.6.2 By Phasor Algebra

In this method, voltage, current and impedances are expressed in the complex form i.e. either in the rectangular or polar form. Since complex from includes both magnitude and phase angle.

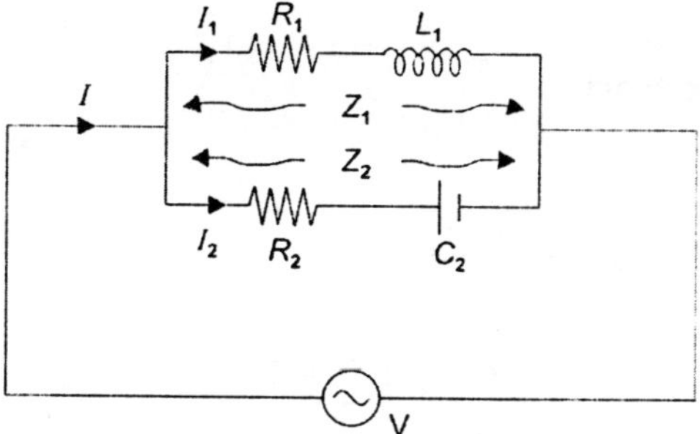

Fig. 4.26: Parallel circuit

Given

$$V = V + j0 = V$$

$$Z_1 = R_1 + jX_{L_1}$$

$$Z_2 = R_2 - jX_{C_2}$$

Rectangular form:

$$I_1 = \frac{V}{Z_1} = \frac{V}{R_1 + jX_{L_1}}$$

$$I_2 = \frac{V}{Z_2} = \frac{V}{R_2 - jX_{C_2}}$$

$$\cdot\ I = I_1 + I_2 = \frac{V}{R_1 + jX_{L_1}} + \frac{V}{R_1 - jX_{C_2}}$$

Polar form:

$$V = V\angle 0°$$
$$Z_1 = |Z_1| \angle \phi_1$$
$$Z_2 = |Z_2| \angle -\phi_2$$

where $|Z_1| = \sqrt{R_1^2 + XL_1^2}, \phi_1 = \tan^{-1}\left(\frac{X_{L_1}}{R_1}\right)$

$$|Z_2| = \sqrt{R_2^2 + XC_2^2}, \phi_2 = \tan^{-1}\left(\frac{X_{C_2}}{R_2}\right)$$

Total current $I = I_1 + I_2$

$$I_1 = \frac{V}{Z_1} = \frac{V\angle 0°}{|Z_1| \angle +\phi_1} = \left|\frac{V}{Z_1}\right| \angle -\phi_1$$

$$I_2 = \frac{V}{Z_2} = \frac{V\angle 0°}{|Z_2| \angle -\phi_2} = \left|\frac{V}{Z_2}\right| \angle \phi_2$$

$$\therefore \quad I = I_1 + I_2 = \left[\frac{V}{Z_1}\right] \angle -\phi_1 + \left[\frac{V}{Z_2}\right] \angle \phi_2$$

Note: The reader is strongly advised to use polar form for multiplication and division of complex quantities. However, for addition and subtraction, rectangular form should be prefrerred.

4.6.3 Impedance Method

The total impedance is

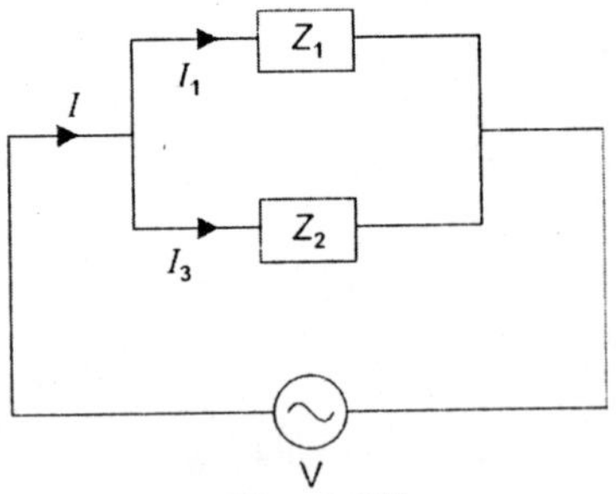

$$Z_T = \frac{Z_1 Z_2}{Z_1 + Z_2}$$

Total current $I = \frac{V}{Z_T} = V\frac{(Z_1 + Z_2)}{Z_1 Z_2}$

Fig. 4.27

Branch current $I = I\frac{Z_2}{Z_1 + Z_2}$ (by current division rule)

Similarly $I_2 = I\frac{Z_1}{Z_1 + Z_2}$

Note: The reader may note that finding the equivalent impedance in complex form involves lengthy calculation. Such an approach to solve parallel AC circuit is not recommended particularly when there are more than two branches in the circuit.

Multiplication and Division of Impedance

In AC circuit analysis the addition, subtraction, multiplication and division of impedance is required to be done frequently. All the impedance can be represented either in polar form or rectangular form. Thus, if $Z_1 = a \pm jb\,\Omega$ and $Z_2 = c \pm jd\,\Omega$ then $Z_1 \pm Z_2 = (a + c) \pm j(b + d)\,\Omega$, While doing multiplication and division both must be represented in polar form.

$$Z_1 Z_2 = |Z_1|\,|Z_2|\angle(\phi_1 + \phi_2)$$

While division,

$$\frac{Z_1}{Z_2} = \frac{|Z_1|\angle\phi_1}{|Z_2|\angle\phi_2} = \left|\frac{Z_1}{Z_2}\right|\angle\phi_1 - \phi_2$$

Note: For addition and subtraction → **Use Rectangular**
For multiplication and division → **Use Polar form**

4.6.4 Admittance Method

Admittance: It is defined as the reciprocal of impedance or admittance is the inducement of current flow.

Component of admittance: Consider an impedance,

$$Z = R \pm jX$$

Here positive sign is taken for inductive and negative sign for capacitive circuit.

∴ **Admittance**

$$Y = \frac{1}{Z} = \frac{1}{R \pm jX}$$

Rationalising the above expression, we have

$$Y = \frac{R \mp jX}{(R \pm jX)(R \mp jX)} = \frac{R \mp jX}{R^2 + X^2}$$

$$= \frac{R}{R^2 + X^2} \mp j\frac{X}{R^2 + X^2} = \frac{R}{Z^2} \mp j\frac{X}{Z^2}$$

∴ From the above expression

$$Y = G \mp jB$$

where, G = Conductance $= \dfrac{R}{R^2 + X^2}$ and $B = \dfrac{X}{Z^2}$ = susceptance

Conductance (G): It is defined as the ratio of the resistance to the square of the impedance." It is measured in the unit siemens.

Susceptance (B): It is defined as the ratio of the reactance to the square of the impedance." It is measured in the unit siemens.

Admittance triangle: The side of the triangle representing conductance, susceptance and admittance of the circuit, it is known as admittance triangle.

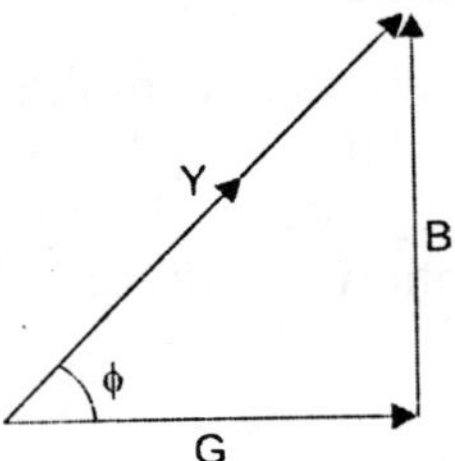

Fig. 4.28: Admittance triangle

$$|Y| = \sqrt{G^2 + B^2} \text{ or } \phi = \tan^{-1}\left(\frac{B}{G}\right)$$

Method: Consider the parallel circuit.

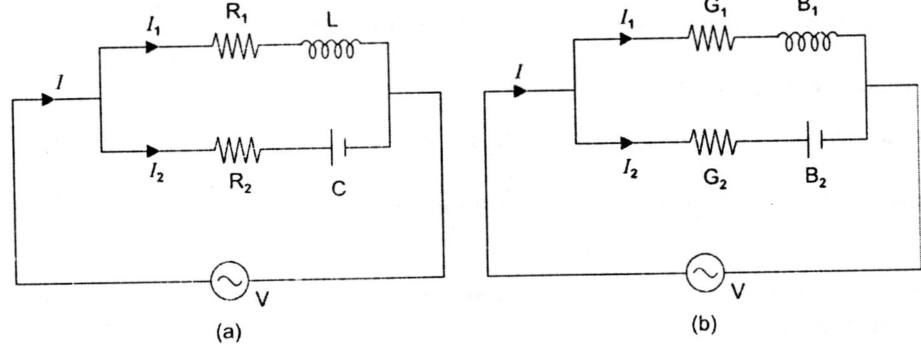

Fig. 4.29

From Fig. 4.29 $\quad Y_1 = \dfrac{1}{Z_1} = \dfrac{1}{R_1 + jX_L} = \dfrac{R_1 - jX_L}{R_1^2 + X_L^2}$

[after rationalising the denominator]

$$= \frac{R_1}{R_1^2 + X_L^2} - j\frac{X_L}{R_1^2 + X_L^2} = G_1 - JB_1$$

Similarly $\quad Y_2 = \dfrac{1}{Z_2} = \dfrac{1}{R_2 - JX_C} = \dfrac{R_2 - jX_C}{R_2^2 + X_C^2}$

$$= \frac{R_2}{R_2^2 + X_C^2} + j\frac{X_C}{R_2^2 + X_C^2} = G_2 + jB_2$$

Total admittance $\quad Y = Y_1 + Y_2 = G_1 + G_2 + j(B_2 - B_1)$

$$= \sqrt{(G_1 + G_2)^2 + (B_2 - B_1)^2}$$

Line current $\quad I = VY$

Phasor angle $\quad \phi = \tan^{-1}\dfrac{B_2 - B_1}{G_1 + G_2}$

Power consumed $\quad P = VI\cos\phi$ W

SOLVED EXAMPLES FOR PRACTICE

Example 1: The following circuit shows a parallel *R-L* arrangement connected across 200 V, 50 Hz AC supply calculate:

(i) The current drawn from the supply. **[UPTU 2002-03]**
(ii) Apparent power
(iii) Real power and
(iv) Reactive power

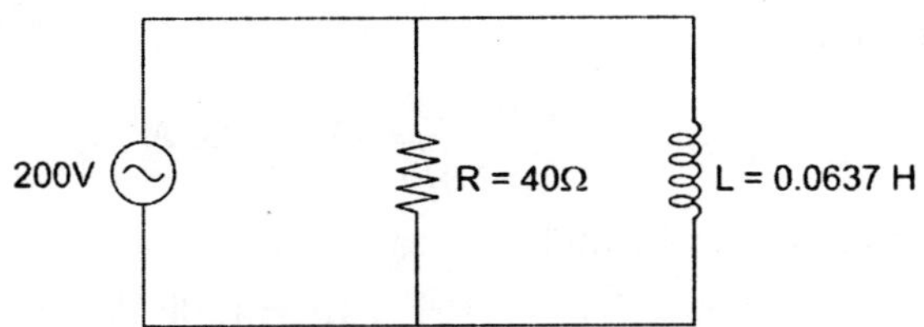

Solution: Given data

$$R = 40\ \Omega$$
$$L = 0.0637\ \text{H}$$
$$V = 200\ \text{V}$$
$$\therefore \quad X_L = \omega L = 2\pi f L = 2\pi \times 50 \times 0.637$$
$$X_L = 20\ \Omega$$

Current drawn by resistive branch

$$I_R = \frac{V}{R} = \frac{200}{40} = 5\ \text{A}$$

Current drawn by inductive branch

$$I_L = \frac{V}{X_L} = \frac{200}{20} = 10\ \text{A}$$

(i) Current drawn form the supply

$$I = \sqrt{I_R^2 + I_L^2} = \sqrt{5^2 + 10^2} = 11.18\ \text{A}$$ **Ans.**

(ii) Apparent power

$$S = V \times I$$
$$= 200 \times 11.18$$
$$= 2.236\ \text{kVA}$$ **Ans.**

(iii) Real power

$$P = V \times I_R = 200 \times 5 = 1000\ \text{W}$$ **Ans.**

(iv) Reactive power

$$Q = V \times I_L = 200 \times 10 = 2\ \text{kVAR}$$ **Ans.**

Example 2: Consider an electric circuit shown in figure below. Determine (i) the current and power consumed in each branch (ii) supply current and power factor.

[UPTU 2001]

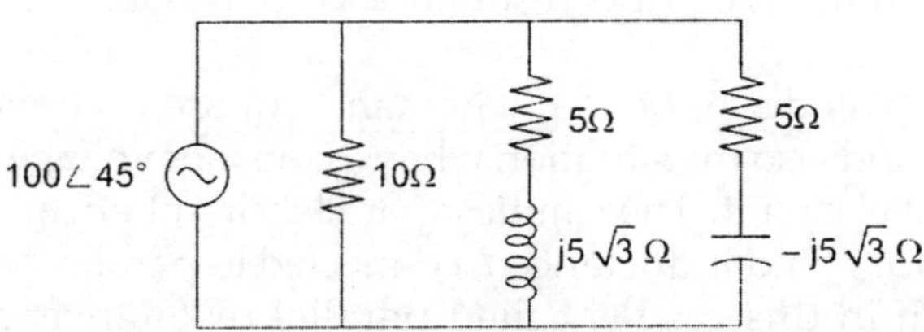

Solution: (i) Current in 10 Ω, branch I_1

$$\therefore \quad I_1 = \frac{V}{R} = \frac{100\angle 45^\circ}{10\angle 0^\circ} = 10\angle 45^\circ \text{A} \qquad \textbf{Ans.}$$

Current in inductive branch, I_2

$$\therefore \quad I_2 = \frac{V}{Z_2} = \frac{100\angle 45^\circ}{5 + j5\sqrt{3}} = \frac{100\angle 45^\circ}{10\angle 60^\circ} = 10\angle -15^\circ \text{A} \qquad \textbf{Ans.}$$

Current in capacitive branch

$$\therefore \quad I_3 = \frac{V}{Z_3} = \frac{100\angle 45^\circ}{5 - j5\sqrt{3}} = 10\angle 105^\circ \text{A} \qquad \textbf{Ans.}$$

Power consumed in resistive branch,

$$P_1 = I_1^2 R_1 = (10)^2 \times 10 = 1000 \text{ W} \qquad \textbf{Ans.}$$

Power consumed in inductive branch,

$$P_2 = I_2^2 R_2 = (10)^2 \times 5 = 500 \text{ W} \qquad \textbf{Ans.}$$

Power consumed in capacitive branch,

$$P_3 = I_3^2 R_3 = (10)^2 \times 5 = 500 \text{ W} \qquad \textbf{Ans.}$$

(ii) Supply current

$$\begin{aligned} I &= I_1 + I_2 + I_3 \\ &= 10\angle 45^\circ + 10\angle -15^\circ + 10\angle 105^\circ \\ &= 7.071 + j7.071 + 9.659 - j2.588 - 2.588 + j9.659 \\ &= 14.142 + j14.142 \\ I &= 20\angle 45^\circ \text{ A} \end{aligned} \qquad \textbf{Ans.}$$

Power factor, $\phi = 45^\circ - 45^\circ = 0^\circ$

$$\text{PF} = \cos 0^\circ = 1 \qquad \textbf{Ans.}$$

4.7 RESONANCE IN R-L-C CIRCUITS

4.7.1 Introduction

Resonance is identified with engineering situations which involves energy-storing elements subjected to a forcing function of varying frequency. Specially resonance is the term employed for describing the steady-state operation of a circuit or system at that frequency for which the resultant response is in time phase with the source function despite the presence of energy-storing elements. If we have an AC circuit having a resistance *R*, an inductance *L* and a capacitance *C*, connected in series and apply voltage *V* from a variable frequency source.

We find that the magnitude of current drawn from the source of supply varies with the variation in frequency of supply source. There will be a value of frequency at which the current is maximum. Electrical resonance is said to exist when this condition is reached.

In this topics we will discuss this phenomanon (more precisely called the series or voltage resonance) and also the situation when a constant voltage of variable frequency is applied to a parallel circuit. The simplest parallel circuit encountered in practice is a coil having resistance *R* and inductance *L* connected in parallel with a capacitor *C*. The resonant condition in this case is called parallel resonance, and sometimes antiresonance. The latter name is prompted due to the fact that at resonance the input current in the parallel circuit is minimum.

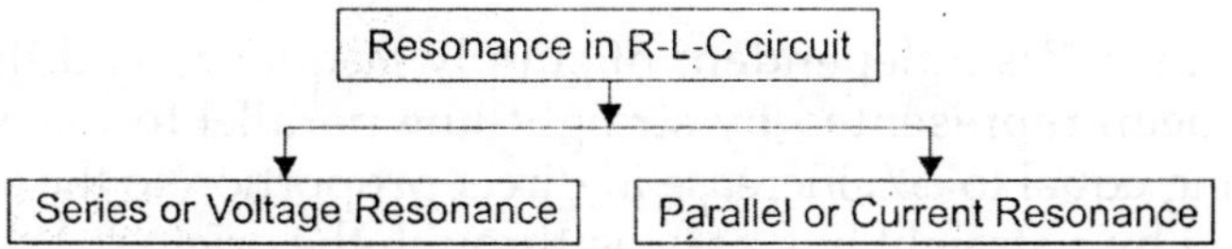

Fig. 4.30: Block diagram of resonance

Under the conditions of resonace such a network becomes purely resistive in its effects, and the voltage and the current in the network are in phase. For this to occurs, the inductive reactance and the capacitive reactance should be made equal.

4.7.2 Series or Voltage Resonance

Consider an AC circuit containing a resistance R, an inductance L and a capacitance C connected in series, as shown in Fig. 4.31

Impedance of the circuit $Z = \sqrt{R^2 + (X_L - X_C)^2}$

$$\therefore \quad Z = \sqrt{R^2 + \left(\omega L - \frac{1}{\omega C}\right)^2}$$

If for some frequency of applied voltage, $X_L = X_C$ in magnitude then

Net reactance is zero, i.e. $X = 0$. Impedance of the circuit $Z = R$.The current flowing through the circuit is maximum and in phase with the applied voltage,

$$\therefore \quad I_m = \frac{V}{R}$$

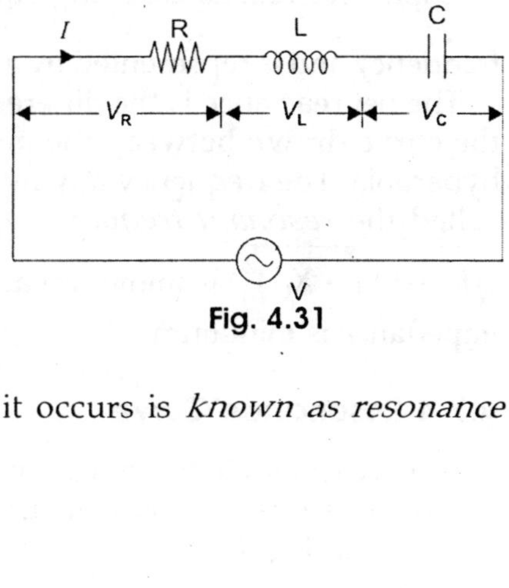

Fig. 4.31

The power factor is unity.

⇒ When this condition exists, the circuit is said to be in resonance and the frequency at which it occurs is *known as resonance frequency*.

It is denoted by f_r, then

$$X_L = \omega L = \omega_r L = 2\pi f_r L$$

$$X_C = \frac{1}{\omega C} = \frac{1}{\omega_r C} = \frac{1}{2\pi f_r C}$$

Since for resonance

$$X_L = X_C$$

$$\omega_r L = \frac{1}{\omega_r C}$$

$$\omega_r = \frac{1}{\sqrt{LC}}$$

$$2\pi f_r = \frac{1}{\sqrt{LC}}$$

$$\therefore \quad f_r = \frac{1}{2\pi\sqrt{LC}}$$

4.7.3 Graphical Representation of Resonance in an R-L-C Series Circuits

Explanation

The circuit resistance R is independent of supply frequency and therefore remains constant. It has been represented by straight-line parallel to the x-axis. Inductive reactance X_L, being equal to ωL, increase in direct proportion to the supply frequency and is represented by a straight line passing through the origin.

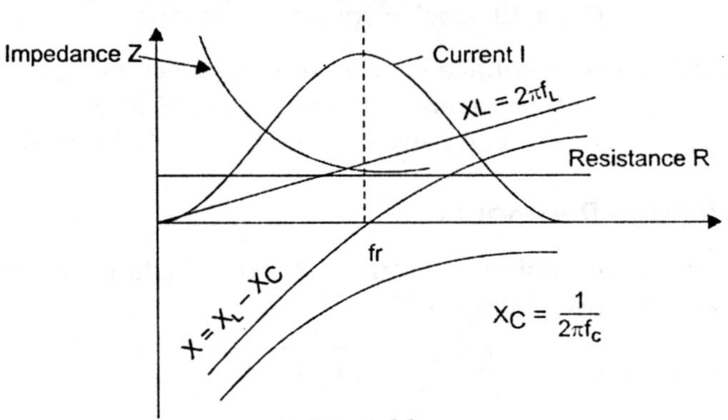

Fig. 4.32

Capacitive reactance, being equal to $\frac{1}{\omega C}$ decreases inversely with the increase in frequency and is represented by a rectangular hyperbolla lying in the fourth quadrant.

The net reactance is the difference of inductive reactance X_L and capacitive X_C and the curve drawn between the net reactance $(X = X_L - X_C)$ and frequency will be a hyperbola. The frequency at which the reactance curves crosses the frequency axis is called the *resonant frequency* f_r. The impedance of the circuit, Z being equal to $\sqrt{R^2 + (X_L - X_C)^2}$ is minimum at resonant frequency f_r. Current is maximum where impedance is minimum.

4.7.4 Resonance Curve

The curve drawn between circuit currents and the frequency of the applied voltage is called the resonance curve and its shape depends upon the value of circuit resistance R as shown in Fig. 4.33.

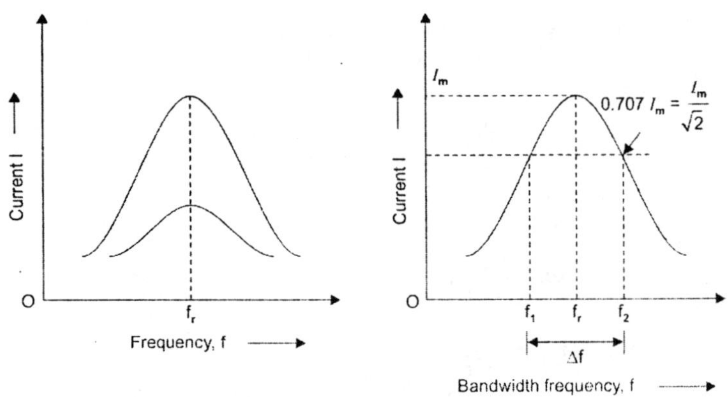

Fig. 4.33: Resonace curve

4.7.5 Determination of Bandwidth and Edge Frequencies

Bandwidth is the band of frequencies between upper and lower half power frequencies (between f_2 and f_1). The impedance of the circuit at half power frequencies (f_2 and f_1) must be $\sqrt{2}$ times its impedance at resoance so that the current is $\frac{I_m}{\sqrt{2}}$. But the impedance resonance is $Z = R$ so at half-power points the impedance is $\sqrt{2}R$.

Since
$$Z = \sqrt{R^2 + X^2} \quad \text{or } Z = \frac{V}{I} = \frac{V}{\frac{I_m}{\sqrt{2}}}$$

$$\sqrt{2}R = \sqrt{R^2 + X^2}$$

or
$$X = \pm R \Rightarrow \sqrt{2}\frac{V}{I_m} = \sqrt{2}R$$

This information can now be used to obtain an expression for the bandwidth in term of the series circuit parameters. Reactance at lower-half power frequency $X_1 = -R$

$$X_1 = -R, \; X_1L - X_1C = -R, \; \omega_1 L - \frac{1}{\omega_1 C} = -R$$

or
$$\omega_1^2 LC - 1 = -\omega_1 CR$$

or
$$\omega_1^2 + \frac{R}{L}\omega_1 - \frac{1}{LC} = 0$$

$\therefore$
$$\omega_1 = -\frac{R}{2L} \pm \sqrt{\left(\frac{R}{2L}\right)^2 + \left(\frac{1}{\sqrt{LC}}\right)^2}$$

or
$$= -\alpha \pm \sqrt{\alpha^2 + \omega_r^2} \qquad \text{...(4.12)}$$

where
$$\alpha = \frac{R}{2L}$$

$$\omega_r = \frac{1}{\sqrt{LC}}$$

Similarly the upperhalf-power frequency

$$X_2 = +R, \; X_2L - X_2C = R$$

$$\omega_2 L - \frac{1}{\omega_2 C} = R$$

or
$$\omega_2^2 - \frac{R}{L}\omega_2 - \frac{1}{LC} = 0$$

$$\omega_2 = \alpha \pm \sqrt{\alpha^2 + \omega_r^2} \qquad \text{...(4.13)}$$

From Eqs (4.12) and (4.13), we get the bandwidth.

$$\Delta\omega = \omega_2 - \omega_1$$

$$= 2\alpha = 2 \cdot \frac{R}{2L}$$

$$= \frac{R}{L} \quad \text{or} \quad 2\pi\Delta f = \frac{R}{L}$$

$$\therefore \quad \Delta f = \frac{R}{2\pi L} \text{ Hz (bandwidth)}$$

From Fig. 4.34 lower half-power frequency

$$f_1 = f_r - \frac{\Delta f}{2} = f_r - \frac{R}{4\pi L} \text{Hz}$$

Upper half-power frequency

$$f_2 = f_r + \frac{\Delta f}{2} = f_r + \frac{R}{4\pi L} \text{Hz}$$

⇒ By multiplying Eqs (4.12) and (4.13), we get

$$\text{or} \quad \omega_1 \omega_2 = \omega_r^2$$

$$f_1 f_2 = f_r^2$$

$$\therefore \quad f_r = \sqrt{f_1 f_2} \text{ Hz}$$

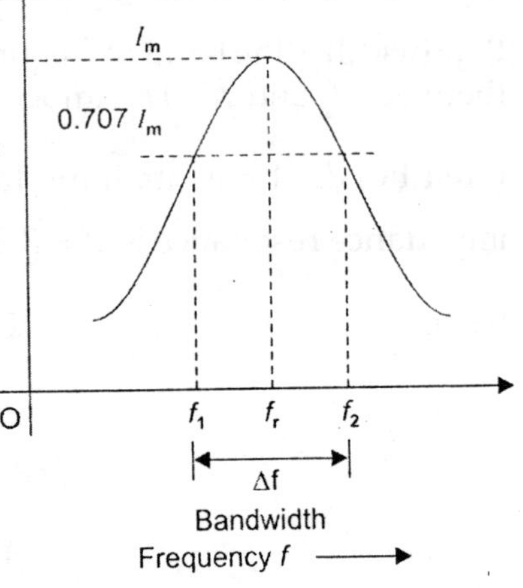

Fig. 4.34: Resonance curve

4.7.6 Quality Factor of a Series Resonant Circuit

At series resonance, the potential difference across L or C (the two drops being equal and opposite) builds up to a value many times greater than the applied voltage V. This voltage magnification produced by resonance is termed as Q-factor of the series resonant circuit (Q stands for quality).

$$\therefore \quad Q\text{-factor} = \frac{V_L}{V_R} = \frac{IX_L}{I_R} = \frac{X_L}{R}$$

$$= \frac{\omega_r L}{R} = \frac{1}{\sqrt{LC}} \cdot \frac{L}{R} = \frac{1}{R}\sqrt{\frac{L}{C}}$$

$$\therefore \quad = \frac{1}{R}\sqrt{\frac{L}{C}}$$

OR

$$Q\text{-factor} = \frac{1}{R}\sqrt{\frac{L}{C}} \frac{\sqrt{L}}{\sqrt{L}} = \frac{L}{R}\frac{1}{\sqrt{LC}} = \frac{2\pi L}{R}\frac{1}{2\pi\sqrt{LC}}$$

$$Q\text{-factor} = \frac{f_r}{\Delta f}$$

Example: Voltage across resistance, inductance and capacitance connected in series are 3 V, 4 V and 5 V respectively. If supply voltage has 50 Hz frequency, what is magnitude of supply voltage. Find the resonant frequency of this series R-L-C circuit.

[UPTU 2006-07]

Solution: Given:

Voltage across resistance

$$V_R = 3 \text{ V}$$

Voltage across inductance

$$V_L = 4 \text{ V}$$

Voltage across capacitane

$$V_C = 5 \text{ V}$$

$\therefore$ Supply voltage $\quad V = \sqrt{V_R^2 + (V_L - V_C)^2} = \sqrt{3^2 + (4-5)^2}$

$$V = \sqrt{10} = 4.162 \text{ V}$$ **Ans.**

$\because \quad V_L = 4 = IX_L$ ...(1)

and $\quad V_C = 5 = IX_C$ ...(2)

$\Rightarrow$ From Eqs (1) and (2), we get

$$\frac{4}{5} = 4\pi^2 f^2 LC \qquad f = 50 \text{ Hz}$$

or $$LC = \frac{0.8}{4\pi^2 \times 50} = 8.1051 \times 10^{-6}$$

resonant frequency

$$f_r = \frac{1}{2\pi\sqrt{LC}} = \frac{1}{2\pi\sqrt{8.10 \times 10^{-6}}}$$

$$= 55.9 \text{ Hz}$$ **Ans.**

4.7.7 Parallel or Current Resonance

When an inductive reactance and capacitive reactance are connected in parallel, as shown in Fig. 4.35, conditions may reach under which current resonance will take place.

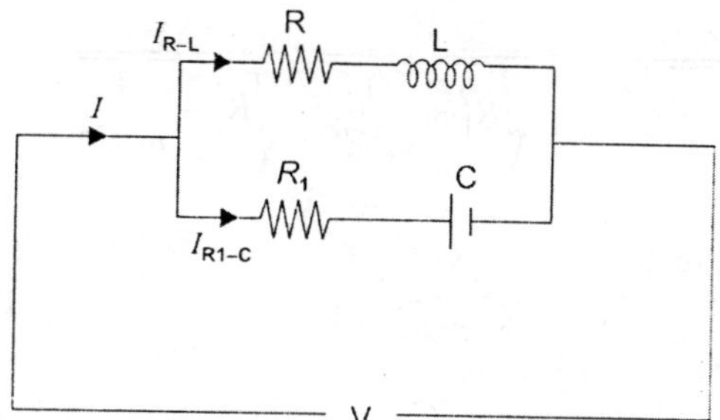

Fig. 4.35: Parallel resonance

Such a circuit is said to be in electrical resonance when the reactive (or wattless) component of line current becomes zero. The frequency at which this happen is known as resonant frequency. Circuit will be in electrical resonance if reactive component of $R–L$ branch current = Reactive component of $R_1–C$ branch current.

$$\therefore \quad I_{R-L} \sin\phi_{R-L} = I_{R_1-C} \cdot \sin\phi_{R_1-C}$$

Now, since $$I_{R-L} = \frac{V}{Z_{R-L}} = \frac{V}{\sqrt{R^2 + (\omega_r L)^2}}$$

and $$\sin\phi_{R-L} = \frac{\omega_r L}{\sqrt{R^2 + (\omega_r L)^2}} = \frac{X_L}{Z_{R-L}}$$

$$I_{R_1-C} = \frac{V}{Z_{R_1-C}} = \frac{V}{\sqrt{R_1^2 + \left(\frac{1}{\omega_r C}\right)^2}} \qquad (4.14)$$

$$\sin\phi_{R_1-C} = \frac{X_C}{Z_{R_1-C}} = \frac{\frac{1}{\omega_r C}}{\sqrt{R_1^2 + \left(\frac{1}{\omega_r C}\right)^2}} \tag{4.15}$$

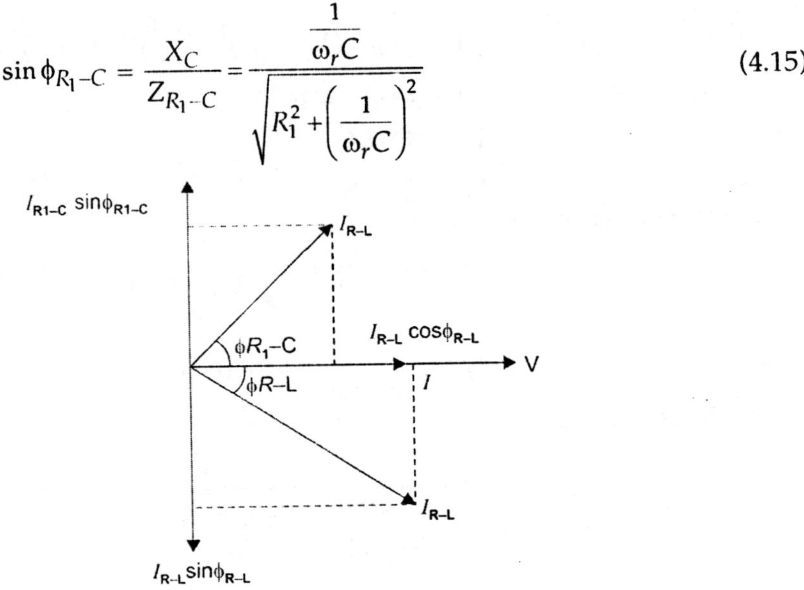

Fig. 4.36

Putting all values in Eq (4.14) we have

$$\frac{V}{\sqrt{R^2+\omega_r^2 L^2}} \times \frac{\omega_r L}{\sqrt{R^2+\omega_r^2 L^2}} = \frac{V}{\sqrt{R_1^2+\frac{1}{\omega_r^2 C^2}}} \times \frac{\frac{1}{\omega_r C}}{\sqrt{R_1^2+\frac{1}{\omega_r^2 C^2}}}$$

or
$$\frac{\omega_r L}{R^2+\omega_r^2 L} = \frac{\omega_r C}{R_1^2 \omega_r^2 C^2 + 1}$$

or
$$\frac{L}{R^2+\omega_r^2 L^2} = \frac{C}{R_1^2 \omega_r^2 C^2 + 1}$$

or
$$L\left(\omega_r^2 R_1^2 C^2 + 1\right) = C\left(R^2 + \omega_r^2 L^2\right)$$

or
$$\omega_r^2 LC\left(R_1^2 C - L\right) = CR^2 - L$$

$\therefore$
$$\omega_r = \frac{1}{\sqrt{LC}}\sqrt{\frac{CR^2-L}{CR_1^2-L}}$$

$\therefore$
$$f_r = \frac{1}{2\pi\sqrt{LC}}\sqrt{\frac{CR^2-L}{CR_1^2-L}}$$

Case I: If resistance of capacitor is negligible, i.e. $R_1 = 0$

$\therefore$
$$f_r = \frac{1}{2\pi\sqrt{LC}}\sqrt{1-\frac{CR^2}{L}}$$

Case II: If resistance of coil is also zero, i.e. $R = 0$

$$\therefore \qquad f_r = \frac{1}{2\pi\sqrt{LC}}$$

equivalent impedance of parallel resonance circuit is

$$Z = \frac{L}{CR}$$

4.7.8 Q-Factor or Current Magnification Factor for Parallel Resonance Circuit

Q-factor of a parallel circuit is defined as the ratio of the circulating current to the line current, it also represents current magnification.

$$\therefore \qquad Q\text{-factor} = \frac{\text{Circulating current between } L \text{ and } C}{\text{Line current}}$$

Circulating current $\quad I_C = 2\pi f_r CV$

The line current $\quad I = \dfrac{V}{Z} = \dfrac{V}{\frac{L}{CR}} = \dfrac{VCR}{L}$

$$\therefore \qquad Q\text{-factor} = \frac{I_C}{I} = \frac{2\pi frCV}{\frac{VCR}{L}} = \frac{2\pi frL}{R}$$

$$f_r = \frac{1}{2\pi\sqrt{LC}} \text{ (neglecting } R\text{)}$$

$$Q\text{-factor} = 2\pi \times \frac{1}{2\pi\sqrt{LC}} \times \frac{L}{R} = \frac{1}{R}\sqrt{\frac{L}{C}}$$

Example: Find the resonant frequency for the circuit shown in figure below.

[UPTU 2004-05]

Solution: The given data

$R = 5\,\Omega$
$L = 10 \times 10^{-3}$ H
$R_1 = 2\,\Omega$
$C = 40 \times 10^{-6}$

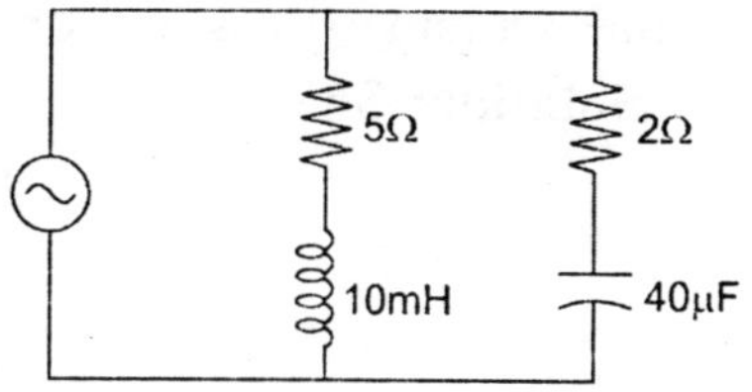

5Ω 2Ω 10mH 40μF

$\therefore$ The resonant frequency is

$$= \frac{1}{2\pi\sqrt{LC}}\sqrt{\frac{CR^2 - L}{CR_1^2 - L}}$$

$$= \frac{1}{2\pi\sqrt{10\times10^{-3}\times40\times10^{-6}}}\sqrt{\frac{40\times10^{-6}\times5^2 - 10\times10^{-3}}{40\times10^{-6}\times2^2 - 10\times10^{-3}}}$$

$= 263$ Hz **Ans.**

SOLVED EXAMPLES FOR PRACTICE

Example 1: A 100 Ω resistance is carrying a sinusoidal current given by $3\cos\omega t$. Determine (i) Instantaneous power taken by resistance (ii) Average power.

[UPTU 2003-04]

Solution: The given instantaneous equation of current is $I = 3\cos\omega t$

Resistance $R = 100\ \Omega$

(i) The instantaneous power taken by the resistance

$$p = vi = iR \times i$$

$$= i^2R = (3\cos\omega t)^2 \times 100$$

$$= 900\frac{(1+\cos\omega t)}{2} = 450(1+\cos\omega t)$$ **Ans.**

(ii) Average power = 450 watts. **Ans.**

Example 2: A 100 V, 60 watt bulb is to be operated from 220 V supply. What resistance must be connected in series with the bulb to glow normally? **[MTU 2011-12]**

Solution: Given

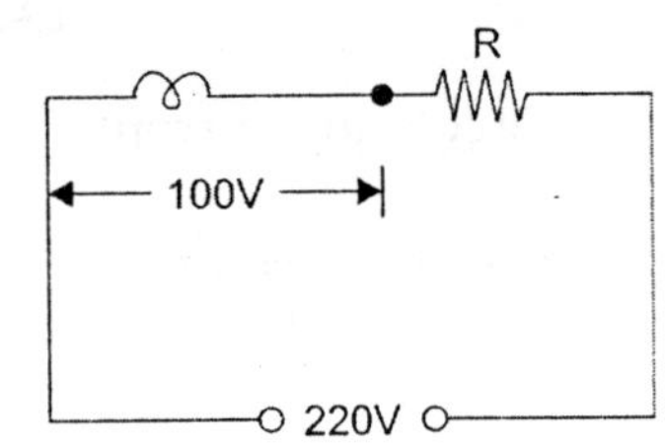

$$V = 100\text{ V}$$

$$P = 60\text{ watts}$$

Current drawn by lamp, $I = \frac{P}{V} = \frac{60}{100}$

$$I = 0.6\text{ A}$$

$$V_R + 100\text{ V} = 220\text{ V}$$

$$V_R = 120\text{ V}$$

$\therefore$ Resistance $R = \frac{V_R}{I} = \frac{120}{0.6} = 200\ \Omega$ **Ans.**

Example 3: The voltage and current through a circuit element are

$$v = 100\sin(314t + 45^\circ)\text{ V}$$

$$i = 10\sin(314t + 315^\circ)\text{ A}$$

(i) Identify the circuit element.

(ii) Find the value.

(iii) Obtain expression for power. **[UPTU 2001]**

Solution: Given

$$v = 100\sin(314t + 45^\circ)\text{ volts}$$

$$i = 10\sin(314t + 315^\circ)\text{ A}$$

$\therefore$ $\phi = 315^\circ - 45^\circ = 270^\circ$

$\therefore$ $\phi_R = 270^\circ - 360 = -90^\circ$

(i) From the equation for voltage and current it is observed that the circuit current I lags behind the applied voltage V by 90°. It means the circuit elements is an inductor. **Ans.**

(ii) Inductive reactance of the inductor

$$X_L = \frac{V_{rms}}{I_{rms}} = \frac{\frac{100}{\sqrt{2}}}{\frac{10}{\sqrt{2}}} = 10\ \Omega$$

$$L = \frac{X_L}{\omega} = \frac{10}{314} = 0.0318\text{ H}$$ **Ans.**

(iii) Power

$$p = -\frac{V_m I_m}{2}\sin 2\omega t$$

$$= -500\sin 628t$$

Ans.

Example 4: An alternating current of 1.5 A flows in a circuit when applied voltage is 300 V. The power consumed is 225 W. Find resistance and reactance of the circuit.

[UPTU 2004-05]

Solution: Given

$$I = 1.5\text{ A},\ V = 300\text{ V},\ P = 225\text{ W}$$

The circuit resistance $R = \frac{P}{I^2} = \frac{225}{(1.5)^2} = 100\ \Omega$

Circuit impedance $Z = \frac{V}{I} = \frac{300}{1.5} = 200\ \Omega$

Circuits reactance $X = \sqrt{Z^2 - R^2}$

$$= \sqrt{(200)^2 - (100)^2} = 173.2\ \Omega$$

Ans.

Example 5: The voltage and current through a circuit element are

$$v = 50\sin(314t + 55^\circ)\text{ V}$$

$$i = 10\sin(314t + 325^\circ)\text{ A}$$

Find the value of power drawn by the element. **[UPTU 2006-07]**

Solution: The given voltage and current equation are

$$V = 50\sin(314t + 55^\circ)\text{ V}$$

$$I = 10\sin(314t + 325^\circ)\text{ A}$$

∴ The phase angle difference between voltage and current

$$\phi = 325^\circ - 55^\circ = 270^\circ$$

∴ Power $= VI\cos\phi$

$$= \frac{V_m}{\sqrt{2}} \times \frac{I_m}{\sqrt{2}}\cos\phi$$

$$= \frac{50}{\sqrt{2}} \times \frac{10}{\sqrt{2}}\cos 270^\circ = 0$$

Ans.

Example 6: If load draws current of 10 A at 0.8 pf lagging when connected to 100 V supply, calculate the value of real, reactive and apparent power. Also find out the resistance of the load.

Solution: Given

$$V = 100\text{ V}$$

$$I = 10\text{ A}$$

$$\text{PF} = \cos\phi = 0.8\text{ (lagging)}$$

∴ $\phi = \cos^{-1}(0.8) = 36.87^\circ$

Real power $P = VI\cos\phi$

$$= 100 \times 10\cos 36.87^\circ = 800\text{ watt}$$

Ans.

Reactive power $Q = VI\sin\phi$

$= 100 \times 10 \sin 36.87° = 600$ VAR **Ans.**

Apparent power $S = \sqrt{P^2 + Q^2}$

$= \sqrt{(800)^2 + (600)^2} = 100$ VA **Ans.**

Load impedance $Z = \dfrac{V}{I}$

$Z = \dfrac{100}{10} = 10\ \Omega$

Load resistance $R = Z\cos\phi$

$= 10 \times 0.8 = 8\ \Omega$ **Ans.**

Example 7: We have, $v = 200\sin 377t$ V and $i = 8\sin(377t - 30°)$ A for an AC circuit. Deter-mine (i) power factor (ii) true power (iii) apparent power (iv) reactive power. **[UPTU 2008-09]**

Solution: Given

$$v = 200\sin 377t \text{ V};$$

$$i = 8\sin(377t - 30°) \text{ A}$$

∴ Phase angle $\phi = 30°$ (lagging)

RMS value of applied voltage

$$V = \frac{V_m}{\sqrt{2}},\ \frac{200}{\sqrt{2}} = 141.42 \text{ V}$$

RMS value of current

$$I = \frac{I_m}{\sqrt{2}} = \frac{8}{\sqrt{2}} = 5.657 \text{ A}$$

(i) The power factor $= \cos\phi = \cos 30° = 0.866$ (lagging) **Ans.**

(ii) True power $P = VI\cos\phi$

$= 141.2 \times 5.657 \times 0.866 = 682.82$ Watt **Ans.**

(iii) Apparent power $S = VI$

$= 141.42 \times 5.657 = 800$ VA **Ans.**

(iv) Reactive power $Q = VI\sin\phi$

$= 141.42 \times 5.657 \sin 30° = 400$ VAR **Ans.**

For an AC circuit, the voltage and current are given by

$$V = 200\sin 377t \text{ V and}$$

$$I = 8\sin(377t - 30°) \text{ A}$$

Example 8: Determine the power factor, true power, apparent power and reactive power of the circuit. Also cross verify form power triangle.

Solution: Refer to Example 7

From power triangle $S = \sqrt{P^2 + Q^2}$

$= \sqrt{(692.8)^2 + (400)^2} = 800$ VA

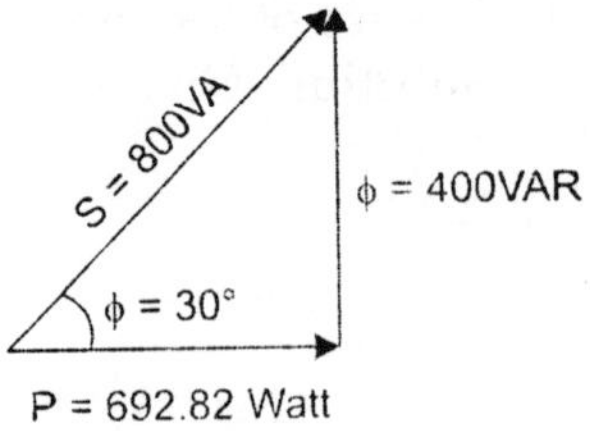

S = 800VA
ϕ = 400VAR
ϕ = 30°
P = 692.82 Watt

Phase angle $\phi = \tan^{-1}\left(\dfrac{Q}{P}\right) = \tan^{-1}\left(\dfrac{400}{692.8}\right)$

$= 30°$ (verified) **Ans.**

Example 9: A noninductive resistance of 10 Ω is connected in series with an inductive coil across 200 V, 50 Hz AC supply. The current drawn by the series combination is 10 A. The resistance of the coil is 2 Ω. Determine (i) inductance of the coil (ii) power factor (iii) voltage across the coil. **[UPTU 2005-06]**

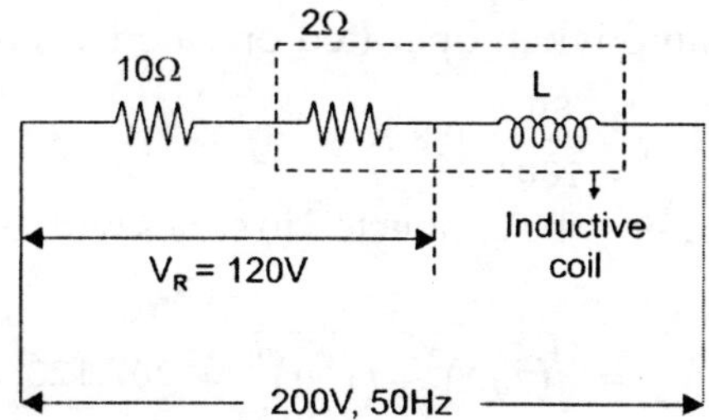

Solution: From the given data, draw the circuit.

Total resistance of the circuit

$$R = \text{Noninductive resistance} + \text{resistance of coil}$$
$$= 10 + 2 = 12\ \Omega$$

Voltage drop across the resistance of the whole circuit,

$$V_R = IR = 10 \times 12 = 120\ \text{V}$$

Let the voltage drop across the inductance of the coil be V_L volt

$$\therefore \quad V = \sqrt{V_R^2 + V_L^2}$$

or $$V_L = \sqrt{V^2 - V_R^2} = \sqrt{(200)^2 - (120)^2} = 160\ \text{V}$$ **Ans.**

Inductive reactance of the coil

$$X_L = \frac{V_L}{I} = \frac{160}{10} = 16\ \Omega$$

(*i*) Inductance of coil

$$L = \frac{X_L}{2\pi f} = \frac{16}{2\pi \times 50} = 0.051\ \text{H}$$ **Ans.**

(*ii*) Power factor of the coil

$$= \cos\left[\tan^{-1}\left(\frac{X_L}{R}\right)\right]$$
$$= \cos\left[\tan^{-1}\left(\frac{16}{2}\right)\right] = 0.124\ \text{(lagging)}$$

Power factor of the circuit

$$\cos\phi = \frac{R}{Z} = \frac{12}{\sqrt{12^2 + 16^2}}$$
$$= 0.6\ \text{(lagging)}$$

(*iii*) Voltage across the coil

$$V_{coil} = I\sqrt{2^2 + 16^2} = 10 \times \sqrt{260}$$
$$= 161.245\ \text{V}$$ **Ans.**

Example 10: A 100 V, 80 W lamp is to be operated on 230 V, 50 Hz AC. Calculate the inductance to be connected in series with the lamp. Lamp can be taken as a pure resistance. **[UPTU 2004-05]**

Solution: The given data

$$V = 230 \text{ V}$$
$$f = 50 \text{ Hz}$$
$$P = 80 \text{ W}$$
$$100 \text{ V} \rightarrow \text{Lamp}$$

Current drawn by the lamp when operated on rated voltage

$$\therefore \quad I = \frac{80}{100} = 0.8 \text{ A}$$

Let pure inductance of L henry be connected in series with the lamp, the voltage across inductace

$$V_L = \sqrt{(230)^2 - (100)^2} = 207.123 \text{ V}$$

and $$L = \frac{V_L}{2\pi f I} = \frac{207.123}{2\pi \times 50 \times 0.8} = 0.824 \text{ H}$$ **Ans.**

Example 11: A 120 V, 60 W lamp is to be operated on 220 V, 50 Hz supply mains. In order that lamp should operated on correct voltage calculate value of
(a) noninductive resistance (b) pure inductance. **[UPTU 2005-06]**

Solution:

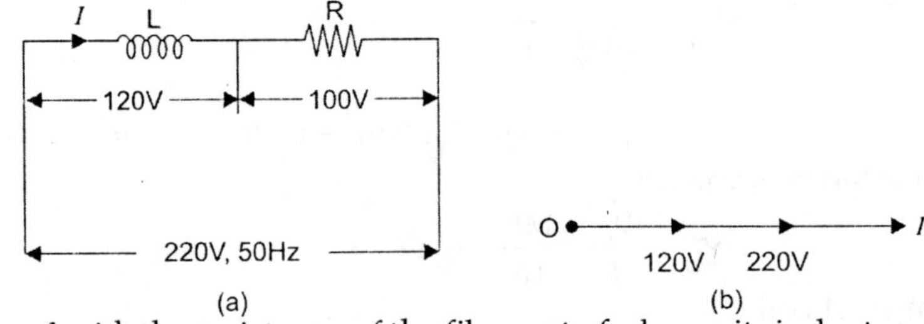

(a) (b)

As compared with the resistance of the filament of a lamp, its inductance is negligible. As such a lamp is considered to be a noninductive resistance. Rated power of lamp $P = 60$ W. Rated voltage of lamp $V = 120$ V. Current drawn by the lamp is

$$I = \frac{P}{V} = \frac{60}{120} = 0.5 \text{ A}$$

(a) $$V_R + 120 = 220$$

or $$V_R = 220 - 120 = 100 \text{ V}$$

Resistance $$R = \frac{V_R}{I} = \frac{100}{0.5} = 200 \ \Omega$$ **Ans.**

(b)

60W lamp
L
120V
V_L = 184.4V
220V, 50Hz

$$(120)^2 + (V_L)^2 = (220)^2$$

or $$V_L = \sqrt{(220)^2 - (120)^2} = 184.4 \text{ V}$$

or $$2\pi f IL = 184.4$$

$$L = \frac{184.4}{2\pi \times 50 \times 0.5} = 1.174 \text{ H}$$ **Ans.**

Example 12: Three coils are connected in series across a 100 V, 50 Hz supply. Values of their resistances and inductances are as follows:

$R_1 = 15\ \Omega,\ L_1 = 0.01$ H
$R_2 = 10\ \Omega,\ L_2 = 0.03$ H
$R_3 = 3\ \Omega,\ L_3 = 0.06$ H

Calculate the potential drop and phase angle for each coil.

Solution: Total resistance in the circuit are

$$R = R_1 + R_2 + R_3 = 15 + 10 + 3 = 28\ \Omega$$

Total inductance in the circuit

$$L = L_1 + L_2 + L_3 = 0.01 + 0.03 + 0.06 = 0.1 \text{ H}$$

Impedance of first coil

$$Z_1 = \sqrt{R_1^2 + (X_{L_1})^2}$$

$$= \sqrt{(15)^2 + (2\pi \times 50 \times 0.01)^2} = 15.325\ \Omega$$

Impedance of second coil,

$$Z_2 = \sqrt{R_2^2 + (X_{L_2})^2}$$

$$= \sqrt{(10)^2 + (2\pi \times 50 \times 0.03)^2} = 13.742\ \Omega$$

Impedance of third coil

$$Z_3 = \sqrt{R_3^2 + (2\pi f L_3)^2}$$

$$= \sqrt{3^2 + (2\pi \times 50 \times 0.06)^2} = 19.087\ \Omega$$

Impedance of whole circuit

$$Z = \sqrt{R^2 + (2\pi f_L)^2}$$

$$= \sqrt{(28)^2 + (2\pi \times 50 \times 0.1)^2} = 42.083\ \Omega$$

Current through the circuit

$$I = \frac{V}{Z} = \frac{100}{42.083} = 2.376 \text{ A}$$ **Ans.**

Potential drop across first coil

$$V_1 = IZ_1 = 2.376 \times 15.325 = 36.417 \text{ V}$$ **Ans.**

Potential drop across second coil

$$V_2 = IZ_2 = 2.376 \times 13.742 = 32.65 \text{ V}$$ **Ans.**

Potential drop across third coil

$$V_3 = IZ_3 = 2.376 \times 19.087 = 45.35 \text{ V}$$ **Ans.**

Phase angle of first coil

$$\phi_1 = \cos^{-1}\left(\frac{R_1}{Z_1}\right) = \cos^{-1}\left(\frac{15}{15.325}\right) = 11.82° \quad \textbf{Ans.}$$

Phase angle of second coil

$$\phi_2 = \cos^{-1}\left(\frac{R_2}{Z_2}\right) = \cos^{-1}\left(\frac{10}{13.742}\right) = 43.18°$$

Phase angle of third coil

$$\phi_3 = \cos^{-1}\left(\frac{R_3}{Z_3}\right) = \cos^{-1}\left(\frac{3}{19.087}\right) = 80.57° \quad \textbf{Ans.}$$

Example 13: An iron cored coil takes a current of 4 A when connected to a 20 V dc supply and takes 5 A from 65 V, 50 Hz AC supply, determine

(i) The resistance and inductance of the coil.

(ii) The power drawn by the coil.

(iii) The power factor **[UPTU 2001]**

Solution:

(i) Resistance of coil

$$R = \frac{V_{dc}}{I_{dc}} = \frac{20}{4} = 5\ \Omega$$

Impedance of coil $\quad Z = \frac{V_{ac}}{I_{rms}} = \frac{65}{5} = 13\ \Omega$

Inductive reactance of coil

$$X_L = \sqrt{Z^2 - R^2}$$

$$= \sqrt{13^2 - 5^2} = 12\ \Omega$$

Inductance of coil, $\quad L = \frac{X_L}{2\pi f} = \frac{12}{2\pi \times 50} = 382\ \text{mH}$ **Ans.**

(ii) Power drawn by the coil,

$$P = (I_{rms})^2 \times R$$

$$= (5)^2 \times 5 = 125\ \text{watt} \quad \textbf{Ans.}$$

(iii) Power factor, $\quad \cos\phi = \frac{R}{Z} = \frac{5}{13} = 0.3846$ (lagging) **Ans.**

Example 14: An iron cored coil has a dc resistance of 8 Ω. When it is connected to 230 volt, 50 Hz mains the current taken is 3.4 A at a power factor of 0.5. Determine (i) The effective resistance of the coil (ii) Inductance of this coil (iii) The resistance which represents the effect of the iron loss.

Solution: Total power consumed by an iron-cored choke coil

$$\frac{P}{I^2} = R + \frac{P_i}{I^2}$$

where $\frac{P}{I^2}$ is the effective resistance of the coil.

(i) Now, since power consumed

$$P = VI\cos\phi = 230 \times 3.4 \times 0.5 = 391 \text{ watts}$$

Current $I = 3.4$ A

$$R_e = \frac{P}{I^2} = \frac{391}{(3.4)^2} = 33.8\ \Omega$$ **Ans.**

(ii) Impedance of choke coil

$$Z = \frac{V}{I} = \frac{230}{3.4} = 67.65\ \Omega$$ **Ans.**

Inductive reactance of coil

$$X_L = \sqrt{Z^2 - R_e^2}$$

$$= \sqrt{(67.65)^2 - (33.8)^2} = 58.6\ \Omega$$ **Ans.**

Inductance of choke coil

$$L = \frac{X_L}{2\pi f} = \frac{58.6}{2\pi \times 50} = 0.8165 \text{ H}$$ **Ans.**

(iii) Since $\frac{P}{I^2} = R + \frac{P_i}{I^2}$

$\therefore$ Iron loss resistance $= R_e - R = 33.8 - 8 = 25.8\ \Omega$ **Ans.**

Example 15: A circuit consists of 20 Ω resistance in series with capacitance of 200 μf, connected across 50 Hz supply. The current through the circuit is 10.8 sin 314*t* amperes. Determine the voltage across each component and across the circuit.

Solution: The given data

Maximum value of current

$$I_m = 10.8 \text{ A}$$

$$\therefore \quad I_{rms} = \frac{I_m}{\sqrt{2}} = \frac{10.8}{\sqrt{2}} = 7.637 \text{ A}$$

Voltage across 20 Ω resistance

$$V_R = IR = 7.637 \times 20 = 152.74 \text{ V}$$ **Ans.**

Voltage across 200μf capacitor is

$$V_C = IX_C = 7.637 \times \frac{1}{2\pi \times 50 \times 200 \times 10^{-6}} = 121.55 \text{ V}$$ **Ans.**

Voltage across the circuit

$$V = \sqrt{V_R^2 + V_C^2}$$

$$= \sqrt{(152.74)^2 + (121.55)^2} = 195.2 \text{ V}$$ **Ans.**

Example 16: The voltage applied to a circuit is $v = 100\sin(\omega t + 30°)$ and current flowing in the circuit $i = 20\sin(\omega t + 60°)$. Determine the impedance, resistance, reactance, power and power factor of the circuit. **[GBTU 2011-12]**

Solution: The given data

$$v = 100\sin(\omega t + 30°);\ i = 20\sin(\omega t + 60°)$$

$\therefore$ The current leads the applied voltage by $\phi = 60° - 30° = 30°$

Circuit impedance $Z = \frac{V_m}{I_m} = \frac{100}{20} = 5\ \Omega$

Circuit resistance $R = Z\cos\phi$

$= 5 \times \cos 30° = 3.33\ \Omega$ **Ans.**

Circuit reactance $X_C = Z\sin\phi = 5 \times \sin 30° = 2.5\ \Omega$ **Ans.**

Power factor of the circuit $= \cos\phi$

$pf = \cos 30° = 0.866$ (leading) **Ans.**

Power of the circuit

$$P = VI\cos\phi = \frac{100}{\sqrt{2}} \times \frac{20}{\sqrt{2}} \cos 30° = 862 \text{ watts}$$ **Ans.**

Example 17: A supply of 400 V, 50 Hz is applied to a series *R-C* circuit. Find the valve of *C* if the power absorbed by the resistor be 500 W at 150 V. What is the energy stored in the capacitor. **[RGPV 2005]**

Solution: The given data

$$V_R = 150 \text{ V},\ V = 400 \text{ V},\ P = 500 \text{ W}$$

$$I = \frac{P}{V_R} = \frac{500}{150} = 3.33 \text{ A}$$

I R C
V_R = 150V V_C
V = 400V

Voltage drop across capacitor is

$$V_C = \sqrt{V^2 - V_R^2}$$

$$= \sqrt{400^2 - (150)^2} = 370.8 \text{ V}$$

$$\therefore \quad X_C = \frac{V_C}{I} = \frac{370.8}{3.33} = 111.25\ \Omega$$

Capacitance of circuits

$$C = \frac{1}{2\pi f X_C} = \frac{1}{2\pi \times 50 \times 1112.5} = 28.6\ \mu f$$ **Ans.**

Energy stored in capacitor$= \frac{1}{2} C V_m^2$

$$= \frac{1}{2} 28.6 \times 10^{-6} \times \left(370.8\sqrt{2}\right)^2 = 3.934 \text{ J}$$ **Ans.**

Example 18: A metal-filament lamp rated at 750 W, 100 V is to be connected in series with a capacitance across 230 V, 50 Hz supply calculate the value of capacitance required draw phasor diagram. **[UPTU 2002, GBTV 2011-12]**

Solution: Given

$$V_C = \sqrt{(230)^2 - (100)^2} = 207 \text{ V}$$

$$I = \frac{P}{V_R} = \frac{750}{100} = 7.5 \text{ A}$$

$$X_C = \frac{V_C}{I} = \frac{207}{7.5} = 27.6\ \Omega$$

and

$$C = \frac{1}{2\pi f X_C} = \frac{1}{2\pi \times 50 \times 27.6}$$

$$= 115.33\ \mu f$$ **Ans.**

750W C
207V 100V $= V_R$
230V, 50Hz

Phasor diagram is given below

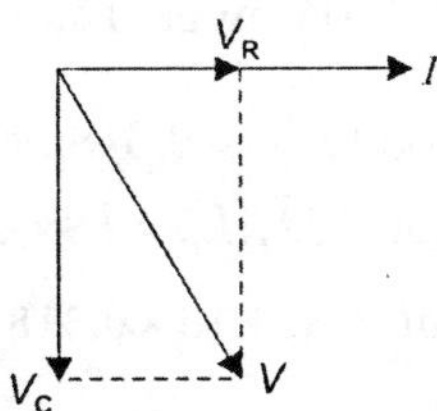

Example 19: A coil having resistance of 6 Ω and inductance of 0.0255 H is connected across a 230 V, 50 Hz AC supply. Calculate (i) current (ii) power factor (iii) active power (iv) reactive power (v) appearent power. (vi) It is desired to improve power factor of 0.8. What value of capacitance is to be connected in series with R and what is the magnitude of reduction in reactive power? **[GBTU Sem-I 2011-12]**

Solution: The given data

$$R = 6\ \Omega;\ L = 0.0255\ \text{H};\ V = 230\ \text{V};\ f = 50\ \text{Hz}$$

Inductive reactance $X_L = 2\pi fL = 2\pi \times 10 \times 0.0255 = 8\ \Omega$

Impedance $Z = \sqrt{R^2 + X_L^2} = \sqrt{6^2 + 8^2} = 10\ \Omega$

(i) Current $I = \dfrac{V}{Z} = \dfrac{230}{10} = 23$ A **Ans.**

(ii) Power factor $\cos\phi = \dfrac{R}{Z} = \dfrac{6}{10} =$ (0.6 lagging) **Ans.**

(iii) Active power $P = VI\cos\phi$

$= 230 \times 23 \times 0.6 = 3174$ watts **Ans.**

(iv) Reactive power $Q = VI\sin\phi$

$= 230 \times 23 \times 0.8 = 4232$ VAR **Ans.**

(v) Appearent power $S = VI$

$= 230 \times 23 = 5290$ VA **Ans.**

(vi) New power factor, $\cos\phi^1 = 0.8$ (lagging) **Ans.**

New impedance $Z' = \dfrac{R}{\cos\phi^1} = \dfrac{6}{0.8} = 7.5\ \Omega$

Reactance of circuit $X = \sqrt{(Z')^2 - R^2}$

$$= \sqrt{(7.5)^2 - (6)^2} = 4.5\ \Omega$$

$$X = X_L - X_C \therefore X_C = X_L - X = 8 - 4.5$$

$$X_C = 3.5\ \Omega$$

Capacitance to be connected in series with R to improve pf 0.8 (lagging)

$$C = \frac{1}{2\pi f X_C} = \frac{1}{2\pi \times 50 \times 3.5} = 910\ \mu\text{f}$$

New current $I^1 = \dfrac{V}{Z^1} = \dfrac{230}{7.5} = 30.667$ A

New reactive power, $Q = VI^1\sin\phi$

$= 230 \times 30.667 \times 0.6 = 4232$ VAR **Ans.**

Reduction in reactive power = 4243 – 4232 = 0 VAR

Example 20: A series R-L-C circuit has 100 Ω resistor, 0.318 H, $v = 230 \times \sqrt{2}\sin\omega t$ V, $i = 2.3\sqrt{2}\sin\omega t$ A. Find (i) C (ii) V_L (iii) power. Take $\omega = 314.15$ rad/sec. **[UPTU 2007-08]**

Solution: The given data

$$R = 100\ \Omega;\ L = 0.318\ \text{H}$$

$$V_m = 230\times\sqrt{2},\ I_m = 2.3\times\sqrt{2},\ \omega = 314.5\ \text{radian/sec}$$

$$X_L = \omega L = 314.15\times 0.318 = 100\ \Omega$$

$$Z = \frac{V_m}{I_m} = 100\ \Omega$$

Also impedance

$$Z = \sqrt{R^2 + X^2}$$

$$X = \sqrt{Z^2 - R^2}$$

∴

$$X = \sqrt{(100)^2 - (100)^2} = 0$$

$$X = X_L - X_C = 0\ \therefore X_L = X_C = 100\ \Omega$$

(i) Capacitance of the capacitor

$$C = \frac{1}{\omega X_C} = \frac{1}{314.15\times 100} = 31.8\ \mu\text{F}$$ **Ans.**

(ii) Voltage across inductor

$$V_L = I\cdot X_L = \frac{2.3\sqrt{2}}{\sqrt{2}}\times 100 = 230\ \text{V}$$ **Ans.**

(iii) Total power consumed

$$P = VI\cos\phi \qquad (\text{As } X_L = X_C,\ \cos\phi = 1)$$

$$= \frac{230\sqrt{2}}{\sqrt{2}}\times\frac{2.3\sqrt{2}}{\sqrt{2}} = 529\ \text{watts}$$

Example 21: A resistance R, an inductance $L = 0.01$ H, and a capacitance C are connected in series. When a voltage $v = 400\cos(3000t - 10°)$ V is applied to the series combination, the current flowing is $10\sqrt{2}\cos(3000t - 55°)$. Find R and C. **[MTU 2009-10]**

Solution: The given voltage and current equation are

$$v = 400\cos(3000t - 10°)$$

$$= 400\sin(3000t - 10° + 90°)$$

$$= 400\sin(3000t + 80°)\ \text{V}$$

$$i = 10\sqrt{2}\cos(3000t - 55°)\ \text{A}$$

$$= 10\sqrt{2}\sin(3000t - 55° + 90°)$$

$$= 10\sqrt{2}\sin(3000t + 35°)\ \text{A}$$

∴

$$\phi = 80° - 35° = 45°$$

$$\omega = 3000$$

Inductive reactance

$$X_L = \omega L$$

$$= 3000\times 0.01 = 30\ \Omega$$

Circuit impedance, $Z = \frac{V_m}{I_m} = \frac{400}{10\sqrt{2}}$

$= 28.28\ \Omega$

$R = Z\cos\phi = 28.28 \times 6545 = 20\ \Omega$ **Ans.**

Net reactance, $X = X_L - X_C = Z\sin\phi$

$= 28.28 \sin 45° = 20\ \Omega$

Capacitive reactance, $X_C = X_L - X$

$= 30 - 20 = 10\ \Omega$

Circuit capacitance, $C = \frac{1}{\omega X_C} = \frac{1}{3000 \times 10} = 33.33\ \mu F$ **Ans.**

Example 22: A coil of 0.8 pf is connected in series with 110 μF capacitor. Supply frequency is 50 Hz. The potential difference across the coil is found to be equal to that across the capacitor. Calculate the resistance and inductance of the coil. Calculate the net power factor. **[NU 1997]**

Solution: Given

$$X_C = \frac{1}{\omega C} = \frac{1}{2\pi \times 50 \times 110 \times 10^{-6}}$$

$= 28.94\ \Omega$

R L 110μF

50Hz, A.C. Supply

Since the voltage drop across the coil is equal to that across the capacitor which are connected in series, impedance of the coil will be equal to that of capacitor, thus

$Z = X_C = 28.94\ \Omega$

Coil resistance $R = Z\cos\phi$

$= 28.94 \times 0.8 = 23.1\ \Omega$ **Ans.**

Coil reactance $X_L = \sqrt{Z^2 - R^2}$

$= \sqrt{(28.90)^2 - (23.15)^2}$

$= 17.36\ \Omega$

Coil inductance $L = \frac{X_L}{2\pi f} = \frac{17.36}{2\pi \times 50}$

$= 0.0553$ H **Ans.**

Total impedance of circuit

$$Z_T = \sqrt{R^2 + (X_L - X_C)^2}$$

$= \sqrt{(23.15)^2 + (17.36 - 28.94)^2}$

$= 25.88\ \Omega$ **Ans.**

Hence power factor, $\cos\phi = \frac{R}{Z_T} = \frac{23.15}{25.883}$

pf $= 0.8443$ (leading, as $X_C > X_L$) **Ans.**

Example 23: Find applied voltage and power loss in a circuit shown in figure below. The value of C is 20 μF, current $I = 0.345$ A. **[UPTU 2007-08]**

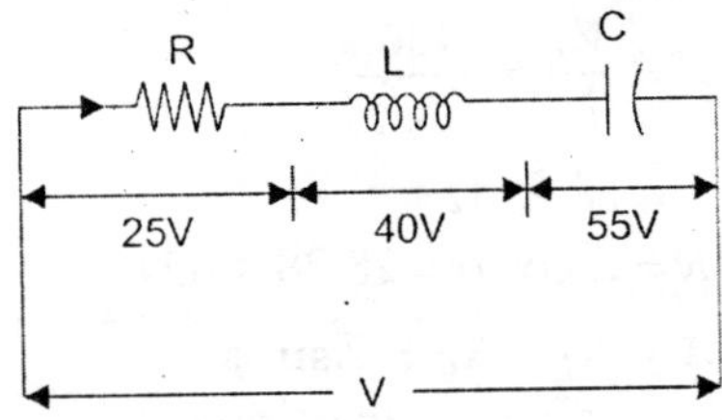

Solution: From the circuit diagram we have

$$R = \frac{V_R}{I} = \frac{25}{0.345} = 72.46\ \Omega$$

Power loss $= I^2R$

$= (0.345)^2 \times 72.96 = 8.625$ watt **Ans.**

Applied voltage $V = \sqrt{(V_R)^2 + (V_L - V_C)^2}$

$= \sqrt{25^2 + (40-55)^2} = 29.155$ V **Ans.**

Example 24: A load having impedance of $1 + j1\ \Omega$ is connected to an AC voltage represented as $v = 20\sqrt{2}\cos(\omega t + 10°)$ volt.

(i) Find the current in load, express in the form of $I = I_m \sin(\omega t + \phi)$ A.

(ii) Find real power consumed by the load. **[UPTU 2004-05]**

Solution: The given data

$$Z = 1 + j1 = \sqrt{2}\angle 45°\ \Omega,\ V_m = 20\sqrt{2}\ \text{V}$$

$$V_{rms} = \frac{V_m}{\sqrt{2}} = \frac{20\sqrt{2}}{\sqrt{2}} = 20\ \text{V}$$

$$v = 20\sqrt{2}\cos(\omega t + 10°)$$

$$= 20\sqrt{2}\sin(\omega t + 10° + 90°)$$

$$= 20\sqrt{2}\sin(\omega t + 100°) = 20\angle 100°$$

Load current $I = \frac{V}{Z} = \frac{40\angle 100°}{\sqrt{2}\angle 45°} = 10\sqrt{2}\angle 55°$ A **Ans.**

$I_m = \sqrt{2} \times I_{rms} = \sqrt{2} \times 10\sqrt{2} = 20$ A **Ans.**

∴ Current equation $I = 20\sin(\omega t + 55°)$ A **Ans.**

Real power consumed $= VI\cos\phi = 20 \times 10\sqrt{2} \times \cos(45) = 200$ W **Ans.**

Example 25: In a given *R-L* circuit, $R = 35\ \Omega$ and $L = 0.1$ H. Find (i) current through the circuit and (ii) power factor if a 50 Hz frequency, voltage $V = 220\angle 30°$ is applied across the circuit. **[RGTU 2001]**

Solution: Given

$$R = 35\ \Omega;\ L = 0.1\ \text{H};\ V = 220\angle 30°$$

Inductive reactance $X_L = \omega L = 2\pi f L = 2\pi \times 50 \times 0.1 = 31.42\ \Omega$ **Ans.**

∴ Impedance $Z = \sqrt{R^2 + X_L^2}$

$= \sqrt{(35)^2 + (31.42)^2} = 47.03\ \Omega$ **Ans.**

Phase angle $\phi = \tan^{-1}\left(\frac{X_L}{R}\right)$

$= \tan^{-1}\left(\frac{31.42}{35}\right) = 41.91°$

Hence $Z = R + jX_L = 35 + j31.42$

$V = 220\angle 30°$

(i) Current $I = \frac{220\angle 30°}{47.03\angle 41.91°}$

$I = 4.678\angle -11.9°\text{A}$ **Ans.**

(ii) Power factor $\cos\phi = \cos(41.9°)$

$= 0.7403$ (lagging) **Ans.**

Example 26: A coil of resistance 8 Ω and inductance 0.1 H is connected in series with a condenser of 160 μF across 230 V, 50 Hz supply. Calculate complex impedance, current and power factor. **[MTU 2011-12]**

Solution: The given data

$R = 8\ \Omega,\ L = 0.1;\ C = 160 \times 10^{-6}\text{ F};\ V = 230\text{ V};\ f = 50\text{ Hz}$

Inductive reactance $X_L = 2\pi fL = 2\pi \times 50 \times 0.1$

$= 31.42\ \Omega$

Capacitive reactance $X_C = \frac{1}{2\pi fC} = \frac{1}{2\pi \times 50 \times 160 \times 10^{-6}} = 19.39\ \Omega$

Impedance $Z = \sqrt{R^2 + (X_L - X_C)^2} = \sqrt{8^2 + (31.42 - 19.89)^2} = 14.03\ \Omega$

In complex form $Z = R + j(X_L - X_C), Z = (8 + j11.53)\ \Omega$ **Ans.**

Current $I = \frac{V}{Z} = \frac{230}{8 + j11.53} = (9.343 - j13.5)\text{ A}$

$= 16.42\angle -55.31°\text{ A}$ **Ans.**

Power factor $\cos\phi = \cos -55.31° = 0.569$ (lagging) **Ans.**

Example 27: A coil of resistance 10 Ω and inductance 0.1 H is connected in series with a condenser of capacitance 150μ*F* across a 200 V, 50 Hz supply. Determine the following:

(i) Impedance (ii) current (iii) power factor (iv) voltage across the coil and (v) voltage across the condensor.

Solution: The given data

$R = 10\ \Omega;\ L = 0.1\text{ H};\ C = 150\mu F;\ V = 200\text{ V};\ f = 50\text{ Hz}$

$X_L = 2\pi fL$

$= 2\pi \times 50 \times 0.1 = 31.42\ \Omega$

$X_C = \frac{1}{\omega C} = \frac{1}{2\pi fC} = \frac{1}{2\pi \times 50 \times 150 \times 10^{-6}}$

$= 21.22\ \Omega$

$Z = \sqrt{R^2 + (X_L - X_C)^2}$

$= \sqrt{10^2 + (31.42 - 21.22)^2} = 14.28\ \Omega$

Phase angle $\phi = \tan^{-1}\left(\frac{X_L - X_C}{R}\right)$

$$= \tan^{-1}\frac{(31.42 - 21.22)}{10} = 45.57°$$

(i) Hence, impedance in complex form

$$Z = R + j(X_L - X_C)$$
$$= 10 + j(31.42 - 21.22)$$
$$= 10 + j10.2\ \Omega$$

or $= 14.28\angle 45.57°\ \Omega$ **Ans.**

(ii) Current $I = \frac{V}{Z} = \frac{200\angle 0°}{14.28\angle 45.57°}$

$= 14\angle -45.57°\text{A}$ **Ans.**

(iii) Power factor $=$ pf $= \cos 45.5 = 0.7$ (lagging)

(iv) Voltage across the coil $= I(R + jX_L) = 14\angle -45.57(10 + j31.42)$

$= 14\angle -45.57° \times 32.97\angle 72.34°$

$= 461.58\angle 26.77°$ volt **Ans.**

(v) Voltage across the condensor

$$V_C = IX_C = 14\angle -45.57° \times 21.22\angle -90°$$
$= 297.08\angle -135.570$ volts **Ans.**

Example 28: In a circuit, the applied voltage is found to lag the current by 30°. (a) Is the power factor lagging or leading? (b) What is the value of power factor (c) Is the circuit inductive (or) capacitive?

In the figure below the voltage drop across Z_1 is $(10 + j0)$ volts. Find out (i) The current in the circuit, (ii) The voltage drop across Z_2 and Z_3 (iii) The voltage of the generator.

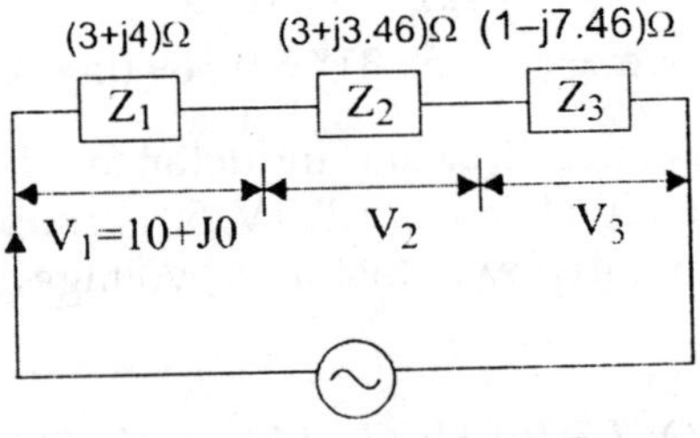

(3+j4)Ω (3+j3.46)Ω (1−j7.46)Ω

Z_1 Z_2 Z_3

V_1=10+J0 V_2 V_3

Solution: (a) Since the applied voltage lags behind the current, current leads the applied voltage. It means that power factor is leading.

(b) Power factor $= \cos\phi$

$$\text{pf} = \cos 30° = 0.866 \text{ (leading)}$$

(c) Since the current leads the applied voltage, the circuit is capacitive.

(i) Circuit current I = current through impedance Z_1.

$$I = \frac{V_1}{Z_1} = \frac{10\,j0}{3 + j4} = \frac{10\angle 0°}{5\angle 55.13} = 2\angle -53.13°$$

(ii) Voltage drop across Z_2

$$V_2 = I \times Z_2 = 2\angle -53.13 \times (2 + j3.46)$$
$$= 2\angle -53.13 \times 3.996\angle 59.97^\circ$$
$$= 7.993\angle 6.84^\circ \text{ volts}$$

Voltage drop across Z_3

$$V_3 = I \times Z_3 = 2\angle -53.13 \times (1 - J7.46)$$
$$= 2\angle -53.13 \times 7.527\angle -82365^\circ$$
$$= 15.05\angle -135.495^\circ \text{ volts}$$

(iii) Generator voltage

$$V = V_1 + V_2 + V_3$$
$$= (10 + j0) + 7.936 + j0.952 + (-10.74 - j10.55)$$
$$= 7.196 - j9.598 = 10\angle -53.13^\circ \text{ V}$$

Ans.

Example 29: A voltage source of $e(t) = 141 \sin 377t$ is applied to two parallel branches. The time expression for the current in the first branches $i_1(t) = 7.07 \sin\left(\omega t - \frac{\pi}{3}\right)$. In the second branch it is $i_2(t) = 10 \sin\left(\omega t + \frac{\pi}{6}\right)$. Compute the total power supplied by the source. **[UPTU 2008-09]**

Solution: The given equation for voltage and current are

$$V(t) = 141 \sin 377t$$

$$i_1(t) = 7.07 \sin\left(\omega t - \frac{\pi}{3}\right)$$

$$i_2(t) = 10 \sin\left(\omega t + \frac{\pi}{6}\right)$$

$\therefore$ RMS value of applied voltage,

$$V_{rms} = \frac{V_m}{\sqrt{2}} = \frac{141}{\sqrt{2}} = 99.7 \text{ V}$$

$$I_{1rms} = \frac{I_{m_1}}{\sqrt{2}} = \frac{7.07}{\sqrt{2}} = 5 \text{ A}$$

$$\phi_1 = -\frac{\pi}{3} = -60^\circ \text{ (lagging)}$$

$$I_{2rms} = \frac{I_{m_2}}{\sqrt{2}} = \frac{10}{\sqrt{2}} = 7.071 \text{ A}$$

$$\phi_2 = \frac{\pi}{6} = 30^\circ \text{ (leading)}$$

$\therefore$ Total power supplied by the source is,

$$= V_{rms} \times I_{1rms} \cos\phi_1 + V_{rms} \times I_{2rms} \cos\phi_2$$
$$= 99.7 \times 5 \cos 60^\circ + 99.7 \times 7.071 \cos 30^\circ$$
$$= 249.257 + 610.55 = 859.0 \text{ W}$$

Ans.

Example 30: The following circuit shows a parallel *R-L* arrangment connected across 200 volts, 50 Hz AC supply, calculate (i) the current drawn from the supply; (ii) apparent power; (iii) real power and (iv) reactive power.

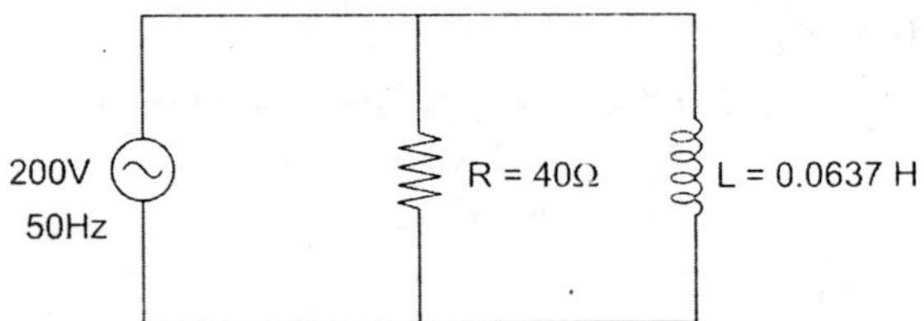

Solution: Given

$$R = 40\ \Omega;\ L = 0.06367\ \text{H}$$

Inductive reactance of inductive branch,

$$X_L = 2\pi f L = 2\pi \times 50 \times 0.0637$$
$$= 20\ \Omega$$

Current drawn by the resistive branch

$$I_R = \frac{V}{R} = \frac{200}{40} = 5\ \text{A}$$

Current drawn by inductive branch

$$I_L = \frac{V}{X_L} = \frac{200}{20} = 10\ \text{A}$$

(i) The current drawn from the supply

$$I = \sqrt{I_R^2 + I_L^2} = \sqrt{5^2 + 10^2} = 11.18\ \text{A}$$ **Ans.**

(ii) Apparent power

$$S = V \times I = 200 \times 11.18 = 2.236\ \text{kVA}$$ **Ans.**

(iii) Real power and

$$P = V \times I_R = 200 \times 5 = 1000\ \text{W, or 1 kW}$$ **Ans.**

(iv) Reactive power

$$Q = V \times I_L = 200 \times 10 = 2000\ \text{VAR} = 2\ \text{kVAR}$$ **Ans.**

Example 31: A series AC circuit has a resistance of 15 Ω and inductive reactance of 10 Ω. Calculate the value of a capacitor which is connected across the series combination so that system has unity power factor. The frequency of AC supply is 50 Hz.

[UPTU 2005-06]

Solution: The given data

$$R = 15\ \Omega;\ X = 10\ \Omega$$

Series circuit conductance

$$G = \frac{R}{R^2 + X^2} = \frac{15}{15^2 + 10^2} = \frac{15}{325}\ \text{siemens}$$

Series circuit susceptance

$$B_L = \frac{X}{R^2 + X^2} = \frac{10}{15^2 + 10^2} = \frac{10}{325}\ \text{siemens}$$

At unity pf

$$B_L = B_C$$

$$\therefore \quad X_C = \frac{1}{B_C} = \frac{1}{\frac{10}{325}} = 32.5\ \Omega$$

Capacitance of required capacitor

$$C = \frac{1}{2\pi f X_C} = \frac{1}{2\pi \times 50 \times 32.5} = 98\ \mu\text{F}$$ **Ans.**

Example 32: Two impedances $Z_1 = 10 + j5$ and $Z_2 = 8 + j6$ are connected in parallel across a voltage of $V = 200 + j0$. Calculate the circuit current, power factor and reactive power. **[UPTU 2004-05]**

Solution: Equivalent impedance of parallel combination

$$Z_{eq} = \frac{Z_1 Z_2}{Z_1 + Z_2} = \frac{(10 + j5)(8 + j6)}{10 + j5 + 8 + j6}$$

$$= \frac{11.18\angle 26.56° \times 10\angle 36.87°}{18 + j11}$$

$$= \frac{11.18\angle 26.56 \times 10\angle 36.87°}{21.095\angle 31.43°}$$

$$= 5.3\angle 32°\ \Omega$$

Circuit current $$I = \frac{V}{Z_{eq}} = \frac{200\angle 00}{5.3\angle 32°}$$

$$= 37.736\angle -32°\ \text{A}$$

∴ The circuit current $I = 37.736$ A **Ans.**

Phase angle $\phi = -32°$

∴ $\text{pf} = \cos\phi = \cos(-32°) = 0.848\ (\text{lagging})$ **Ans.**

Reactive power $Q = VI\sin\phi$

$$= 200 \times 37.736 \sin(-32°)$$

$$= -4000\ \text{VAR} = 4\ \text{kVAR (lagging)}$$ **Ans.**

Example 33: Two impedance $Z_1\ (10 + j15)\ \Omega$ and $Z_2\ (6 - j8)\ \Omega$ are connected in parallel. The total current supplied is 15 A. What is power taken by each impedance? **[GBTU 2009-10]**

Solution: The given total current supplied is

$$I = 15\ \text{A}$$

Current through impedance, Z_1 by current division rule:

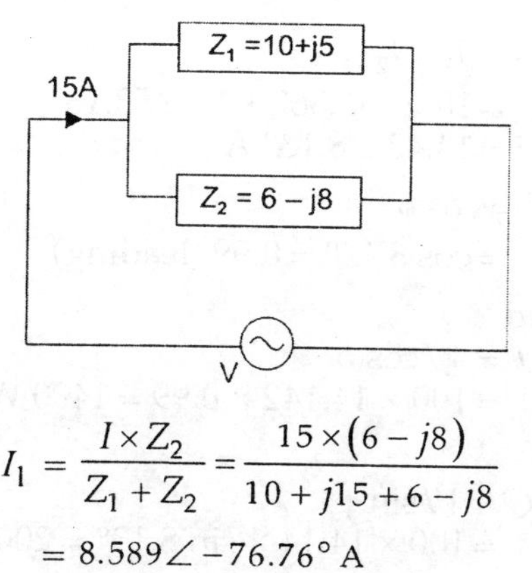

$$I_1 = \frac{I \times Z_2}{Z_1 + Z_2} = \frac{15 \times (6 - j8)}{10 + j15 + 6 - j8}$$

$$= 8.589\angle -76.76°\ \text{A}$$ **Ans.**

Current through impedance Z_2 by current division rule:

$$I_2 = \frac{I.Z_1}{Z_1 + Z_2} = \frac{15 \times (10 + j15)}{10 + j15 + 6 - j8}$$

$$= \frac{15(10 + j15)}{16 + j7} = 15.489\angle 32.68° \text{ A}$$ **Ans.**

Power absorbed in branch 1,

$$P_1 = I_1^2 \times R_1$$

$$= (8.589)^2 \times 10 = 738 \text{ W}$$ **Ans.**

Power absorbed in branch 2,

$$P_2 = I_2^2 \times R_2$$

$$= (15.489)^2 \times 6 = 1438 \text{ W}$$ **Ans.**

Example 34: The parallel circuit shown in Fig. 4.56 is connected across a single phase 100 V, 50 Hz AC supply, calculate (i) branch currents, (ii) total current (iii) supply power factor, (iv) active and reactive power supplied by the supply. **[UPTU 2006-07]**

Solution: The given data,

$$Z_1 = (8 + j6)\,\Omega$$

$$Z_2 = (6 - j8)\,\Omega$$

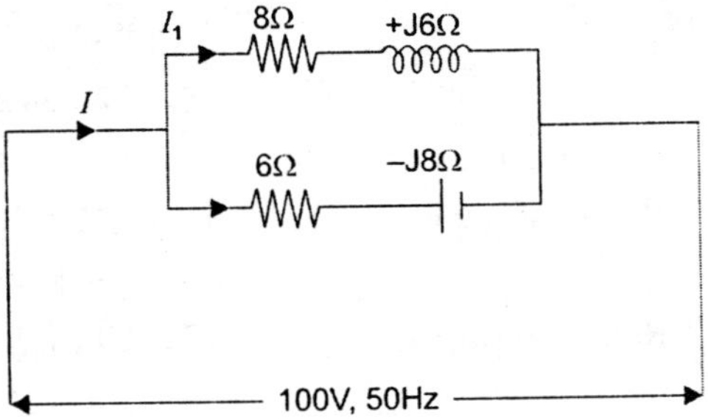

I_1 8Ω +J6Ω
I
6Ω –J8Ω
100V, 50Hz

(i) The 1st branch current

$$I_1 = \frac{V}{Z_1} = \frac{100}{8 + j6}$$

$$= \frac{100}{10\angle 36.86°}$$

$$= 10\angle -36.86° \text{ A}$$ **Ans.**

The 2nd branch current

$$I_2 = \frac{V}{Z_2}$$

$$= \frac{100}{6 - j8} = 10\angle 53.13° \text{ A}$$ **Ans.**

(ii) Total current $I = I_1 + I_2$

$$= 10\angle -36.86° + 10\angle 53.13°$$

$$= 14.42\angle 8.13° \text{ A}$$ **Ans.**

(iii) Supply power factor $= \cos\phi$

$$= \cos 8.13° = 0.99 \text{ (leading)}$$ **Ans.**

(iv) Active power supplied

$$P = VI\cos\phi$$

$$= 100 \times 14.142 \times 0.99 = 1400 \text{ W}$$ **Ans.**

Reactive power supplied

$$Q = VI\sin\phi$$

$$= 100 \times 14.14 \times \sin 8.13° = 200 \text{ VAR}$$ **Ans.**

Example 35: Determine the power factor for the circuit given in figure below.

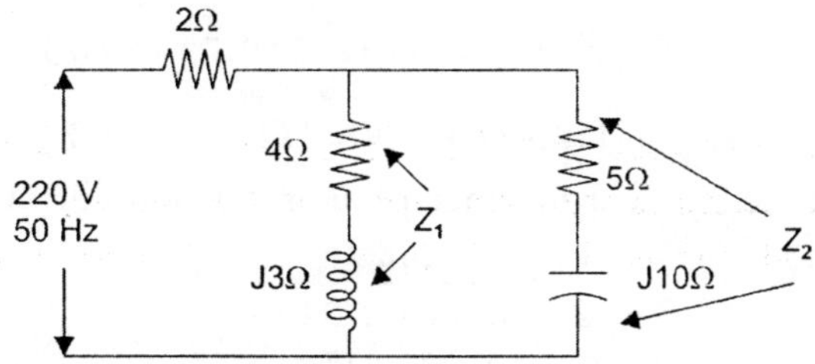

Solution: The equivalent impedance

$$Z_{eq} = Z + \frac{Z_1 Z_2}{Z_1 + Z_2}$$

$$= (2 + j0) + \frac{(4 + j3)(5 - j10)}{(4 + j3) + (5 - j10)} = \frac{885 + j125}{130}\,\Omega$$

∴ Phase angle $\phi = \tan^{-1}\left[\frac{\frac{125}{130}}{\frac{885}{130}}\right] = -8.039° \text{ (lag)}$

∴ Power factor $pf = \cos(+8.039°) = 0.99 \text{ (lagging)}$ **Ans.**

Example 36: Determine the following in the circuit shown in figure below.

(i) The current phasors I, I_1 and I_2.

(ii) Active power dissipated in the three resistive branches.

(iii) Power factor of the circuit. **[UPTU 2007-08]**

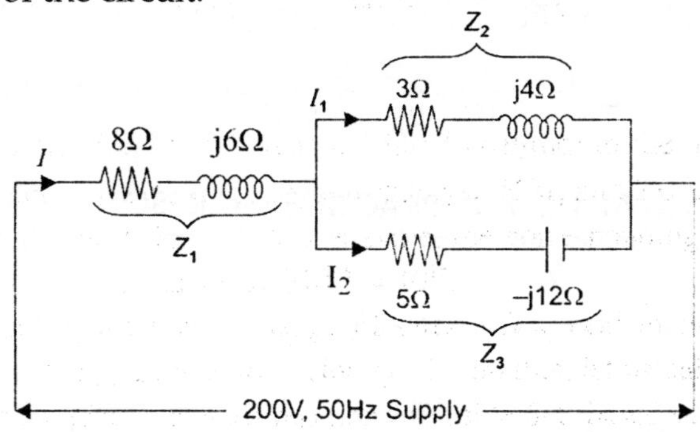

Solution: Given

$$Z_1 = (8 + j6)\,\Omega,\ Z_2 = (3 + j4)\,\Omega = 10\angle 36.87°$$

$$Z_2 = 5\angle 53.13°\,\Omega$$

and $Z_3 = (5 - j12)\,\Omega = 13\angle -67.38°\,\Omega$

Equivalent impedance of parallel circuit

$$Z_P = \frac{Z_2 Z_3}{Z_2 + Z_3} = \frac{5\angle 53.13° \times 13\angle -67.38°}{3 + j4 + 5 - j12}$$

$$= \frac{65\angle -14.25°}{8 - j8} = \frac{65\angle -14.25°}{11.314\angle -45°}$$

$$= 5.745\angle 30.75° = (4.937 + j^2.937)\,\Omega$$

Total impedance of the circuit

$$Z = Z_S + Z_P = 8 + j6 + \left(4.937 + j^2.937\right)$$

$$= \left(12.937 + j8.937\right)\Omega = 15.7237\angle 34.64°\,\Omega$$

Let the supply voltage by the reference phasor, i.e. $V = 200\angle 0°$ V

(i) Circuit current, $I = \dfrac{V}{Z} = \dfrac{200\angle 0°}{15.7237\angle 34.64°}$

$$I = 12.72\angle -34.64°\text{ A}$$ **Ans.**

(ii) $P_1 = I^2 R_1 = (12.72)^2 \times 8 = 1294$ watts **Ans.**

$$I_2 = I \times \frac{Z_3}{Z_2 + Z_3} = \frac{12.72\angle -34.64° \times 13\angle -67.60°}{(3 + j4) + (5 - j12)}$$

$$= 14.616\angle -57.0°\text{ A}$$

$P_2 = I_2^2 R_2 = (14.616)^2 \times 3 = 641$ watts **Ans.**

$$I_3 = I \times \frac{Z_2}{Z_2 + Z_3} = \frac{12.72\angle -34.69 \times 5\angle 53.13°}{11.314\angle -45°}$$

$$= 5.62\angle 63.99°\text{ A}$$

$P_3 = I_3^2 \times R_3 = (5.6)^2 \times 5 = 158$ watts **Ans.**

∴ Total power $P = P_1 + P_2 + P_3$

$= 1294.4 + 641 + 158 = 2093.4$ watts **Ans.**

(iii) Power factor of the circuit

$$\cos\phi = \frac{P}{VI} = \frac{2093.4}{200 \times 12.72} = 0.8228\ (\text{lagging})$$ **Ans.**

SOLVED EXAMPLES FOR PRACTICE ON RESONANCE CIRCUITS

Example 1: Voltage across *R-L-C* connected in series are 5, 8 and 10 V respectively. Calculate the value of supply voltage at 50 Hz. Also find the frequency at which this circuit would resonance. **[GBTU 2001-02]**

Solution: Given

Voltage across *R*, $V_R = 5$ V; voltage across *L*, $V_L = 8$ V; voltage across *C*, $V_C = 10$ V

Supply voltage $V = \sqrt{V_R^2 + (V_L - V_C)^2}$

$$= \sqrt{5^2 + (8 - 10)^2} = \sqrt{29} = 5.39\text{ V}$$ **Ans.**

Inductance $L = \dfrac{V_L}{2\pi f\, I} = \dfrac{8}{2\pi \times 50 \times I} = \dfrac{8}{1000\pi\, I}$

Capacitance $C = \dfrac{I}{2\pi f\, V_C} = \dfrac{I}{2\pi \times 50 \times 10} = \dfrac{I}{1000\pi}$

∴ Resonant frequency $f_r = \dfrac{1}{2\pi\sqrt{LC}} = \dfrac{1}{2\pi}\sqrt{\dfrac{100\pi I}{8} \times \dfrac{1000\pi}{I}} = 55.9$ Hz **Ans.**

Example 2: A 10 mH coil is connected in series with a loss free capacitor to a variable frequency source of 20 V. The current in the circuit has maximum value of 0.2 A at a frequency of 100 kHZ. Calculate (i) Value of capacitance (ii) *Q*-factor of the coil (iii) half power frequencies. **[UPTU 2006-07]**

Solution: Given

Supply voltage $V = 20$ V,

Supply frequency $f = 100\ \text{kHz} = 10^5\ \text{Hz}$

Maximum current at resonance

$$I_m = \frac{V}{R}$$

So circuit resistance $R = \frac{V}{I_m} = \frac{20}{0.2} = 100\ \Omega$

Resonant frequency = Supply frequency

$$f_r = f$$

$$10^5 = f$$

and $\omega L = \frac{1}{\omega C}$

$$C = \frac{1}{(2\pi \times 10^5)^2 \times 10 \times 10^{-3}} = 253.3\ \text{pf} \quad \textbf{Ans.}$$

(ii) *Q*-factor of the coil $= \frac{\omega_r L}{R} = \frac{2\pi \times 10^5 \times 10 \times 10^{-3}}{100} = 62.83$ **Ans.**

(iii) Lower half power frquency

$$f_1 = f_r - \frac{R}{4\pi L}$$

$$= 10^5 - \frac{100}{4\pi \times 10 \times 10^{-3}} = 99.204\ \text{kHz} \quad \textbf{Ans.}$$

Upper half power frquency

$$f_2 = f_r + \frac{R}{4\pi L}$$

$$= 10^5 + \frac{100}{4\pi \times 10 \times 10^{-3}} = 100.796\ \text{kHz} \quad \textbf{Ans.}$$

Example 3: A series circuit has $R = 10\ \Omega$, $L = 0.01$ H and $C = 10\ \mu\text{F}$. Calculate *Q*-factor of the circuit.

Solution: Q-factor of the circuit at resonance

$$= \frac{1}{R}\sqrt{\frac{L}{C}} = \frac{1}{10}\sqrt{\frac{0.01}{10 \times 10^6}} = 3.162 \quad \textbf{Ans.}$$

Example 4: A series *R-L-C* circuit has $R = 10\ \Omega$, $L = 0.01$ H and $C = 8\ \mu F$. Determine

(i) Resonant frequency

(ii) Q-factor of the circuit at resonance

(iii) The half power frequencies **[UPTU 2005-06]**

Solution: Given

$$R = 10\ \Omega,\ L = 0.01\ \text{H} \text{ and } C = 8\mu F.$$

(i) Resonant frequency

$$= \frac{1}{2\pi\sqrt{LC}} = \frac{1}{2\pi\sqrt{0.1\times 8\times 10^{-6}}}$$

$$= 177.99\ \text{Hz}$$ **Ans.**

(*ii*) Q-Factor of the circuit at resonance

$$= \frac{1}{R}\sqrt{\frac{L}{C}} = \frac{1}{10}\sqrt{\frac{0.1}{10\times 10^{-6}}} = 11.18$$ **Ans.**

(*iii*) The half power frequencies

Lower $$f_1 = f_r - \frac{R}{4\pi L} = 177.94 - \frac{10}{4\pi\times 0.1} = 170\ \text{Hz}$$ **Ans.**

Upper $$f_2 = f_r + \frac{R}{4\pi L} = 177.94 + \frac{10}{4\pi\times 0.1} = 185.9\ \text{Hz}$$ **Ans.**

Example 5: If the bandwidth of a resonant circuit is 10 kHz and the lower half power frequency is 120 kHz, find out the value of upper half-power frequency and quality factor of the circuit. **[UPTU 2003-04]**

Solution: Given

$$\Delta f = 10\ \text{kHz};\ f_1 = 120\ \text{kHz}$$

We know that

$$f_1 = f_r - \frac{\Delta f}{2}$$

$\therefore$ $$f_r = f_1 + \frac{\Delta f}{2}$$

$$= 120 + \frac{10}{2} = 125\ \text{kHz}$$ **Ans.**

Upper half power frequency

$$f_2 = f_r + \frac{\Delta f}{2} = 125 + \frac{10}{2} = 130\ \text{kHz}$$ **Ans.**

Quality factor of the circuit at resonance

$$Q_r = \frac{f_r}{\Delta f} = \frac{125}{10} = 12.5$$ **Ans.**

Example 6: A 20 Ω resistor is connected in series with an inductor and a capacitor across a variable frequency of 25 V supply. When the frequency is 400 Hz, the current is at its maximum value of 0.5 A and the potential difference across the capacitor is 150 V. Calculate the resistance and inductance of the inductor. **[UPTU 2003]**

Solution: Given data

$$V = 25\ \text{V};\ f_r = 400\ \text{Hz};\ I_m = 0.5\ \text{A};\ V_C = 150\ \text{V}$$

So circuit resistance $$R = \frac{V}{I_m} = \frac{25}{0.5} = 50\ \Omega$$ **Ans.**

We know that $$V_C = \frac{I_m}{2\pi f_C}$$

$$\therefore \quad C = \frac{I_m}{2\pi f V_C} = \frac{0.5}{2\pi \times 400 \times 150}$$
$$= 1.3263 \mu F$$ **Ans.**

At resonance condition

$$X_L = X_C$$

and $$2\pi f_L = \frac{1}{2\pi f C}$$

$$L = \frac{1}{4\pi^2 f^2 C} = \frac{1}{4\pi^2 \times 400^2 \times 13263 \times 10^{-6}}$$
$$= 0.119 \text{ H}$$ **Ans.**

Example 7: A voltage $v(t) = 10 \sin \omega t$ is applied to a series *R-L-C* circuits. At resonant frequency of the circuit the maximum voltage acorss the capacitor is found to be 500 V. Moveover the bandwidth is known to be 400 rad/s and impedance at resonance is 100 Ω. Find the value of

(i) Resonant frequency
(ii) Upper and lower half power frequency
(iii) Value of *L* and *C* **[MTU 2011-12]**

Solution: Given

$R = 100\ \Omega = Z$ (at resonance); $\Delta_{\omega b} = 400$ rad/sec; $V_{Cm} = 500$ V; $v = 10 \sin \omega t$

We know that bandwidth is

$$\Delta_{\omega b} = \frac{R}{L}$$

So, $$400 = \frac{100}{L}$$

$$L = \frac{100}{400} = 0.25 \text{ H}$$ **Ans.**

$$\therefore \quad V_m = 10 \text{ V (given)}$$

$$I_m = \frac{V_m}{R} = \frac{10}{100} = 0.1 \text{ A}$$

At resonance $$V_C = V_L = 500 \text{ V} = 2\pi f_L I_m$$ **Ans.**
$$= 500 \text{ V} = 2\pi f L I_m$$

or $$f_r = \frac{500}{2\pi L I_m} = \frac{500}{2\pi \times 0.25 \times 0.1}$$
$$= 3.183 \text{ kHz}$$ **Ans.**

(i) Resonant frequency

$$f_r = 3.183 \text{ kHz}$$ **Ans.**

(ii) Lower half power frequency

$$f_1 = f_r - \frac{\Delta f}{2}$$

$$= f_r - \frac{\Delta\omega b}{4\pi}$$

$$= 3183 - \frac{400}{4\pi} = 3151.17 \text{ Hz}$$ **Ans.**

Upper half power frequency

$$f_r + \frac{\Delta f}{2} = f_r + \frac{\Delta\omega b}{4\pi}$$

$$= 3183 + \frac{\Delta\omega}{4\pi} = 3214.83 \text{ Hz}$$ **Ans.**

(iii) Capacitance $$C = \frac{1}{\omega r^2 L} = \frac{1}{(2\pi \times 3183)^2 \times 0.25} = 0.01 \ \mu\text{F}$$ **Ans.**

Example 8: For the circuit below determine (i) resonant frequency; (ii) total impedance of the circuit at resonance (iii) bandwidth (iv) quality factor. **[UPTU 2005-06]**

Solution: The given data from the given figure.

$R = 25\ \Omega$; $L = 0.5$ H; $C = 5 \times 10^{-6}\ \mu$F

(i) Resonant frequency $$f_r = \frac{1}{2\pi}\sqrt{\frac{1}{LC} - \frac{R^2}{L^2}}$$

$$= \frac{1}{2\pi}\sqrt{\frac{1}{0.5 \times 5 \times 10^{-6}} - \frac{(25)^2}{(0.5)^2}}$$

$$= 100.34 \text{ Hz}$$

(ii) Impedance of the circuit at resonance

$$Z = \frac{L}{CR} = \frac{0.5}{5 \times 10^{-6} \times 25} = 4000\ \Omega$$ **Ans.**

(iii) Bandwidth $$= \frac{R}{2\pi L} = \frac{25}{2\pi \times 0.5} = 7.958 \text{ Hz}$$ **Ans.**

(iv) Quality factor $$Q = \frac{1}{R}\sqrt{\frac{L}{C}} = \frac{1}{25}\sqrt{\frac{0.5}{5 \times 10^{-6}}} = 12.65$$ **Ans.**

Example 9: Calculate the resonance frequency of the circuit shown in figure below. **[GBTU 2011-12]**

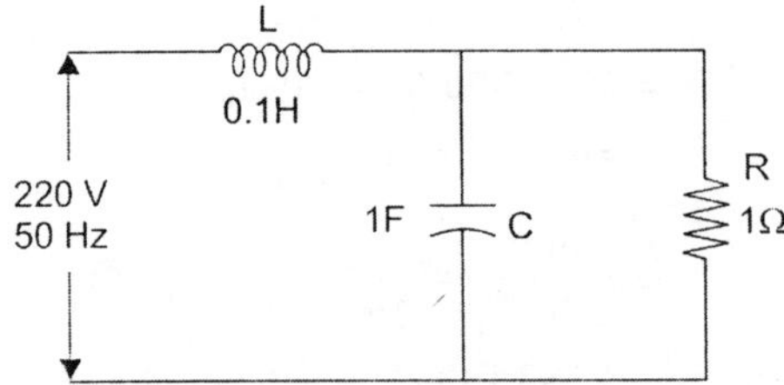

Solution: The impedance of the given circuit is given by,

$$Z = j\omega L + \frac{1}{\frac{1}{R} + j\omega C} = j\omega L + \frac{R}{1 + J\omega RC}$$

$$= j\omega L + \frac{R(1 - j\omega RC)}{1 + \omega^2 R^2 C^2}$$

$$= \frac{J\omega L + J\omega^3 R^2 LC^2 + R - J\omega R^2 C}{1 + \omega^2 R^2 C^2}$$

For resonance, sum of J parts must be equal to zero $\omega \rightarrow \omega_r$

So, $\omega_r L + \omega_r{}^3 LR^2C^2 - \omega_r R^2 C = 0$

$$\omega_r \left(L + \omega_r^2 LR^2C^2 - R^2C\right) = 0$$

or $L + \omega r^2 LR^2C^2 - R^2C = 0$

or $$\omega_r = \sqrt{\frac{R^2C - L}{LR^2C^2}} = \sqrt{\frac{1}{LC} - \frac{1}{R^2C^2}}$$

⇒ Substituting L = 0.1 H, C = 1 F and R = 1, we get

$$\omega_r = \sqrt{\frac{1}{0.1 \times 1} - \frac{1}{1 \times (1)^2}} = \sqrt{10 - 1} = 3$$

and resonant frequency

$$f_r = \frac{3}{2\pi} = 0.4775 \text{ Hz}$$ **Ans.**

POWER FACTOR IMPROVEMENT

Concept of Power Factor

1. It is cosine angle between voltage and current, i.e. $pf = \cos\phi$.

2. Power factor $= \frac{\text{Resistance}}{\text{Impedance}} = \frac{R}{Z}$

3. Power factor $= \frac{\text{Active power}}{\text{Apparent power}} = \frac{\text{watt}}{\text{volt-ampere}} = \frac{P}{S}$

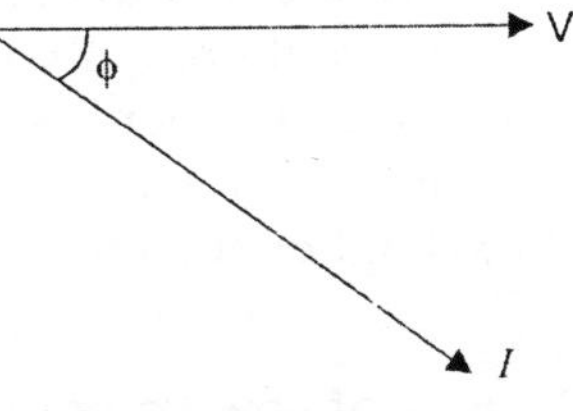

Fig. 4.37

We know that the electrical energy is generated and transmitted in the form of alternating current and hence the question of power factor immediately arises.

The low power factor is undesirable and for better and economical conditions of supply system, it is necessity to have power factor as close to unity, as possible. For sinusoidal wave forms the power factor is defined as the consine of phase angle between voltage and current.

i.e. $$\text{PF} = \cos\phi$$

Note: The value of power factor can not be greater than one.

Importance of Power Factor

We know that

$$\text{Power factor} = \cos\phi$$

$$\cos\phi = \frac{P}{V\,I}$$

$$I = \frac{P}{V\cos\phi} \qquad \text{...(4.16)}$$

Equation 4.16 shows that current is affected by the power factor. The supply voltage V is kept fairly constant. Hence for a given power 'P' required by the load, the current I taken by the load varies inversely as the load power factro, $\cos\phi$. Thus a given load take more current at a low power factor than it does at a high power factor.

Disadvantage of Low Power Factor

The undersirable effects of operating a load at a low power are due to large current required at low power factor.

Example: Let a load of 100 kW is to be supplied from 230 V, single phase supply at 0.8 PF lagging then the current drawn becomes.

Solution: The given

$$V = 230\text{ V};\ PF = \cos\phi = 0.8$$

$$I = \frac{100\times10^3}{230\times0.8} = 543.4\text{ A}$$

Now, if the same load is to be supplied with power factor of 0.6.

$$I = \frac{100\times10^3}{230\times0.6} = 724.6\text{ A}$$

So as power factor decreases, current drawn from the supply increases to supply the same load power. As against this if power factor is improved to unity in this case

$$I = \frac{100\times10^3}{230\times1} = 434.7\text{ A}$$

This is the minimum current drawn from the supply. In general, lower is the power factor, higher is load current, and vice-versa.

Disadvantages

(i) **Greater conductor size:** The conductor size depends on the current, for higher current greater conductor size is required. This increase the cost.

(ii) **Large copper loss:** The large current at low power factor causes more I^2R losses in all elements of power supply. Thus result in poor efficiency.

(iii) **Higher current produce** larger voltage drop in cables and other apparatus. This result in poor voltage regulation.

Causes of Low Power Factor

The usual cause of low power factor is due to inductive loads. The current in an inductive load lags behind the voltage. The power factor is therefore lagging. The important inductive loads responsible for low power factor are as follows.

(i) A transformer draws magnetising current from the supply. At normal load, this current does not affect the power factor much but at light loads the primary current power factor is low.

(ii) Most of the AC motors are of induction type. Three phase induction motors operate at a power factor of about 0.8 lag, at full load. At light loads these motors work at a very small power factor of the order of 0.2 to 0.3 lagging.

(iii) Arc lamps, electric discharge lamps, industrial heating furness, welding equipment operate at low lagging *PF*.

Power Factor Improvement

If the power factor is low (or poor) it is necessary to improve (or correct) it. The basic principle of power factor improvement is to inject a leading current into the circuit. So as to neutralize the effect of lagging current. The power factor may be improved by the following methods.

1. By using static capacitors.
2. By using synchronous motors.

1. Power Factor Correction Using Static Capacitor

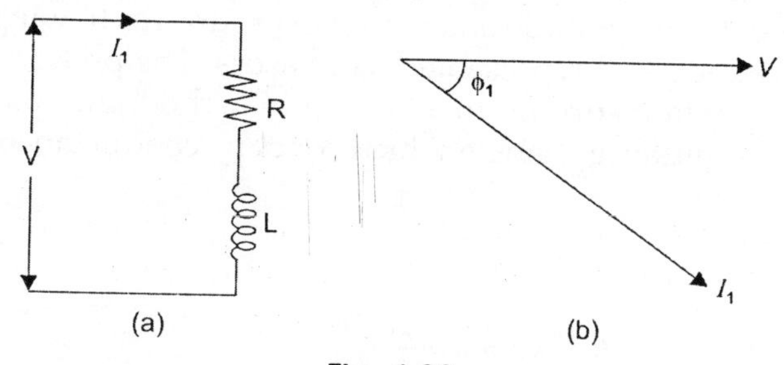

Fig. 4.38

Consider an inductaive load consisting of a resistor R and an inductors of L connected to an AC supply.

Let
V = supply voltage
I_1 = load current
ϕ_1 = Phase angle by which the current I_1 lags behind the voltage V.
$\cos\phi_1$ = original power factor.

- Let a capacitor C be connected in parallel with the load.
- It will take leading current I_C from the supply. The circuit and phasor diagram are shown in Fig. 4.39.

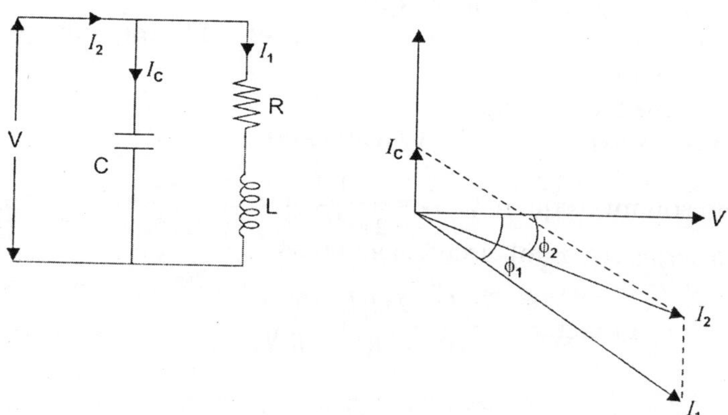

Fig. 4.39

The phase angle of I_2 is ϕ_2. It is seen from the phasor diagram that ϕ_2 is less than ϕ_1 and hence $\cos\phi_2 > \cos\phi_1$. In other words, the power factor is improved from $\cos\phi_1$ and $\cos\phi_2$.

2. Power Factor Correction by Synchronous Motor

Power factor correction can be achieved by operating over excited synchronous motor in parallel with inductive loads.

SUMMARY

AC Parallel Circuits: An AC circuit having two or more branches, each branch having different components in series, is known as an AC parallel circuit.

AC parallel circuits can be solved by the following methods:

1. Phasor method
2. Admittance method
3. Symbolic or *j* method.

In phasor method, the magnitude and direction of currents flowing through different branches are determined and represented as phasors. The phasor sum of the branch currents gives the resultant current. In admittance method, the component values are determined as per admittance triangle which contains conductance and susceptance.

Conductance, $$G = Y\cos\phi = \frac{R}{Z^2}$$

Susceptance, $$B = Y\sin\phi = \frac{X}{Z^2}$$

Admittance, $$Y = \sqrt{G^2 + B^2},$$

where $G = G_1 + G_2 + ... + G_n$ and $B = B_1 + B_2 + ... + B_n$

Current, $$I = V \times Y$$

1. An R-L-C series circuit is said to be in electrial resonance when

   $X_L = X_C$ *i.e.* the net reactance $X = 0$

   Under resonant conditions

   (i) Circuit impedance, $Z = R$

   (ii) The current flowing through the circuit is maximum and is in phase with the applied voltage and will be equal to V/R

   (iii) The voltage drop across inductance is equal to the voltage drop across capacitance and is maximum.

   (iv) The power factorisunity.

   (v) The power expended, $P = VI$ watts and

   (vi) The resonant frequency, $f_r = \dfrac{1}{2\pi\sqrt{LC}}$ Hz

Q-factor of a series resonant circuit is given as

$$\text{Q-factor} = \frac{\omega_r L}{R} = \frac{2\pi f_r L}{R} = \frac{1}{R}\sqrt{\frac{L}{C}}$$

$$\text{Bandwidth (BW)} = \frac{R}{2\pi L} = \frac{f_r}{\text{Q-factor}}$$

2. A parallel circuit is said to be in resonance when it draws no reactive current. Under resonant condition of parallel as circuit

$$\text{Impedance } Z = \frac{L}{CR}$$

$$\text{The maximum current } I = \frac{V}{L/CR}$$

The maximum power factor = Unity

$$\text{Resonant frequency } f_r = \frac{1}{2\pi}\sqrt{\frac{1}{LC} - \frac{R^2}{L^2}} = \frac{1}{2\pi\sqrt{LC}} \quad \text{(if } R \text{ is negligibly small)}$$

$$\text{Q-factor} = \frac{1}{R}\sqrt{L/C} \text{ and bandwidth} = \frac{R}{2\pi L}\text{Hz}$$

EXERCISES

1. Define the terms: Impedance, admittance, power factor, active power and reactive power.
[Punjab Technical Univ; Elec. Engineering, June 2000; December 2000; May 2001]
2. Derive the sinusoidal response of parallel R-C circuit.
[GB Technical Univ; Electrical Engineering, First Semester 2010-11]
3. Write the expression of currents in different branches and the total current of a circuit consisting of an inductance, a capacitance and a non-inductive resistance connected in parallel. Draw also the phasor diagram.
4. Derive the expression of impedance, admittance, conductance and susceptance of R-L series circuit. **[RGPV Bhopal; Basic Electrical Engineering, Jan-Feb 2006]**
5. Derive the response of R-L-C series circuit ot sinusoidal input. Also derive the condition for resonance.
[GB Technical Univ; Electrical Engineering, First Semester, 2010-11]
6. Explain the concept of bandwidth and quality factor for a series R-L-C circuit. Derive their expressions.
[UP Technical Univ; Electrical Engineering, Second Semester, 2007-08]
7. Derive the quality factor Q of the series R-L-C circuit at resonance. Define the bandwidth for the same.
[GB Technical Univ; Electrical Engineering, First Semester, 2011-12]
8. Explain the following terms:
Bandwidth and quality factors. **[GB Technical Univ; Electrical Engineering, First Semester, 2010-11]**
9. Deduce the formula for half-power frequencies for a series R-L-C circuit under resonance. Why are they called "half-lower frequencies"?
[GB Technical Univ; Electrical Engineering, Second Semester, 2011-12]
10. For an LCR series circuit derive an expression for resonant frequency, bandwidth and quality factor.
[UP Technical Univ; Electrical Engineering, First Semester, 2004-05]
11. Explain series resonance in R-L-C circuit. What are bandwidth and quality factor of the circuit? **[UP Technical Univ; Electrical Engineering, Second Semester, 2006-07]**
12. Explain the selectivity of a series RLC resonance circuit. Prove that selectivity is reciprocal of quality of the circuit.
[UP Technical Univ; Electrical Engineering, Second Semester, 2004-05]

13. Show that for an RLC series circuit the resonant frequency $\omega_0 = \sqrt{\omega_1 \omega_2}$, where ω_1 and ω_2 are the lower and upper half power frequencies respectively.
[UP Technical Univ; Electrical Engineering, Second Semester, 2004-15]
14. Derive an expression for parallel resonance and mention its salient features.
[UP Technical Univ; Electrical Engineering, First Semester, 2006-07]
15. Explain parallel resonance. Why is parallel resonance called the current resonance? Show the graphical representation of current in parallel resonance.
[UP Technical Univ; Electrical Engineering, Second Semester, 2005-06]
16. Define parallel resonance. Calculate at resonance the resultant current and quality factor in terms of the parameters of a circuit.
[UP Technical Univ; Electrical Engineering, First Semester, 2007-08]
17. Derive an expression for the resonance frequency of the parallel resonance circuit, one branch consisting of inductor L, resistance R and other branch contain capacitor C. Also draw the phasor for the same.
[Mahamaya Technical Univ; Electrical Engineering, Second Semester, 2010-11]
18. Explain parallel resonance and draw graphs of Z, X_L and X_C against frequency.
[GB Technical Univ; Electrical Engineering, First Semester, 2009-10]
19. Show that the condition for resonance in a parallel R-L-C circuit is same as that in a series R-L-C circuit. State the application of series as well as parallel resonance.
[GB Technical Univ; Electrical Engineering, Second Semester, 2006-07]
20. Derive the quality factor Q_P of the parallel RLC circuit at resonance. Define bandwidth for the same.
[UP Technical Univ; Electrical Engineering, First Semester, 2005-06]
21. Derive the expression for Q-factor in the R-L-C parallel circuit.
[GB Technical Univ; Electrical Engineering, Second Semester, 2007-08]
22. A series R-L-C circuit has R = 10 Ω, L = 0.1 Hand C = 8 μF. Determine (i) resonant frequency (ii) Q-factor of the circuit at resonance and (iii) the half-power frequencies. **[UP Technical Univ; Electrical Engineering, September 2001]**
[**Ans.:** (*i*) 177.94 Hz (*ii*) 11.18 (*iii*) 170 Hz, 185.8 Hz]
23. A 20 Ω resistor is connected in series with an inductor and a capacitor, across a variable frequency 25 V supply. When the frequency is 400 Hz, the current is at its maximum value of 0.5 A and the potential difference across the capacitor is 150 V. Calculate the resistance and inductance of the inductor.
[UP Technical Univ; Electrical Engineering, January 2003] [**Ans.:** 50 Ω; 0.119 Ω]
24. An inductive coil of resistance 10 Ω and inductance 0.1 H is connected in parallel with a 150 μF capacitor to a variable frequency, 200 V supply. Find the resonant frequency at which the total current taken from the supply is in phase with the supply voltage. Also find the value of this current.
[GGSIP Delhi Univ; Electrical Science, June 2006]
[**Ans.:** 37.886 Hz; 3 A]
25. A series RLC circuit with R = 250 Ω, and L = 0.6 H results in a leading phase angle of 60° at a frequency of 40 Hz. At what frequency will the circuit resonate?
[Punjab Technical Univ; Basic Electrical Engineering December 2006]
[**Ans.:** 81.2 Hz]
26. An R-L-C series circuit consists of a resistance of 1,000 Ω, an inductance of 100 mH and a capacitance of 10 μF. If the voltage of 100 V is applied across the combination, find (*i*) the resonance frequency (*ii*) Q-factor of the circuit and (*iii*) the half-power points. **[Bombay Univ; Nov. 1971]**
[**Ans.:** (*i*) $10^6/2\pi$ Hz; (*ii*) 100; (*iii*) 158.4 kHz and 160 kHz]

27. An inductive coil when connected across 500 V, 50 Hz supply draws 1.0 A at 0.8 pf. What capacitance is connected in parallel with the coil to make the power factor of the combination unity? What will be the current (*i*) drawn from the supply; and (*ii*) in each branch with this new capacitor.

[**Ans.:** 3.82 μF; (*i*) 0.8 A (*ii*) 1.0 A, 0.6 A]

28. An inductive circuit of resistance 2 Ω and inductance 0.01 H is connected to 250-V, 50 Hz supply. What capacitance placed in parallel will produce resonance? Find the total current taken from the supply and the current in the branch circuits.

[Kerala Univ; Electrical Engineering 1987]

[**Ans.:** 72 μF; 36.05 A; 125 A; 67.13 A $\angle -57.52°$ A; 56.63 $\angle 90°$ A]

29. In the circuit given below, if the value of $R = \sqrt{\dfrac{L}{C}}$, then prove that the impedance of the entire circuit is equal to *R* only and is independent of the frequency of supply. Find the value of impedance for *L* = 0.02 H and *C* = 10011 F.

[Hyderabad Univ; Communication System 1991]

[**Ans.:** 14.142 Ω]

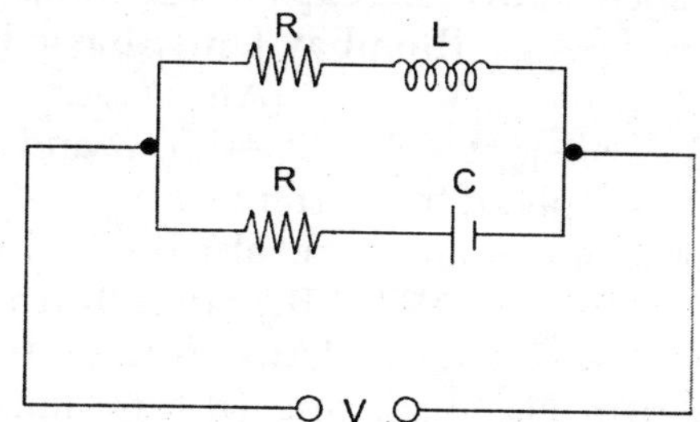

30. A circuit containing a resistance of 40 Ω in parallel will an inductive reactance of 30 Ω is connected across 240 V AC mains. Calculate (*i*) the current in each branch and the total current drawn from the mains (*ii*) the power factor of each branch and power factor of the whole circuit (*iii*) the power drawn by each branch and the total power drawn from the mains.

[**Ans.:** (*i*) 6A, 8A, 10A, (*ii*) 1.0, zero, 0.6 (lag) (*iii*) 1,440 watts, zero 1,440 watts]

31. An inductance of 0.6 H, a resistor of 100 Ω and a 30 μF capacitor are connected in parallel across a 230 V, 50 Hz supply. Calculate the line current, circuit phase angle, power dissipated, total circuit impedance and parameters of equivalent series circuit. [**Ans.:** 2.49 A, 22.39° (lead), 529 W, 92.53 W, 80.51°, 35.25°]

32. A resistance of 100 Ω, an inductance of 0.1 H and a capacitance of 150 μF are connected in parallel across 200 V, 50 Hz AC supply. Determine the branch currents, total current and the total power taken from the supply.

[**Ans.:** 2A, 6.366 A, 9.42A, 3.655 A; 400 watts]

33. A series combination of *R* and *C* is in parallel with a 20 Ω resistor across 50 Hz source results in a total current of 7 A, a current through the 20 Ω resistor of 5 A and a current in the R-C branch of 3 A. Determine R and C.

[Punjab Univ; Electrical Circuits and Systems, December 1988]

[**Ans.:** R = 16.667 Ω; X_C = 28.8675 Ω]

34. An inductor of 0.5 H inductance and 90 Ω resistance is connected in parallel with a 2 μF capacitor. A voltage of 230 V at 50 Hz is maintained across the circuit. Determine the total power taken form the source [**Ans.:** 146 watts]

35. Two parallel circuits comprise respectively of (*i*) a coil of resistance 20 Ω and inductance 0.07 H and (*ii*) a capacitor or capacitance 60 mF in series with resistance

of 50 Ω. Calculate the current in each branch and the current taken from the supply and power factor when connected to 220 V, 50 Hz supply.

[**Ans.:** 7.4 A, 3A, 7.8 A, 0.907 (lag)]

36. Two circuits having the same numerical ohmic impedances are joined in parallel. The power factor of one circuit is 0.8 (lag) and other is 0.6 (lead). What is the power factor of the combination? [**Ans.:** $1.4/\sqrt{2}$ lead]

37. Two circuits, the impedances of which are given by $Z_1 = (15 + j12\ \Omega)$ and $Z_2 = (8 - j5)\Omega$ are connected in parallel. If the potential difference across one of the impedances is (250 + j) V, calculate (*i*) total current and branch currents (*ii*) total power and power consumed in each branch and (*iii*) overall power factor and power factor of each branch. **[Nagpur University, November 1998]**

[**Ans.:** (*i*) 33.15 ∠10.36° A; 13 ∠–38.6° A; 26.5 ∠32° A
(*ii*) 8.153 kW; 2.535 kW, 5.618 kW,
(*iii*) 0.984 lead; 0.78 lag; 0.848 lead]

38. Two impednaces $Z_1 = (6 - j8)$ ohms and $Z_2 = (16 + j12)$ ohms are in parallel. If the total current of the combination is (20 + j 10) amperes, find the complexor power taken by each impedance. Draw and explain the complete phasor diagram.

[Bombay Univ; Basic Electricity, October 1971]

[**Ans.:** (2,400 + j 3,200), (1,600 – j 1,200)]

39. Three impedances $Z_1 = (8 + j6)\ \Omega$, $Z_2 = (2 - j1.5)\ \Omega$ and $Z_3 = 2\ \Omega$ are connected in parallel across a 50 Hz supply. If the current through Z_1 is (3 + j4) A, calculate the current through the other impedances and also the power absorbed by this parallel circuit. **[VTU Belgaum, Karnataka Univ; Winter 2004]**

[**Ans.:** (–12 + j 16) A, (0 + j 25) A, 2.25 kW]

40. For the circuit shown in Fig. 4.65, find (*i*) total impedance (*ii*) total current (*iii*) total power absorbed and power factor. Draw a phasor diagram.

[Osmania Univ; Electrical Technology Jan./Feb. 1992]

[**Ans.:** (*i*) 14.12∠29.2° Ω (*ii*) 7.08∠–29.2° (*iii*) 618.2 W (*iv*) 0.873 (lag)]

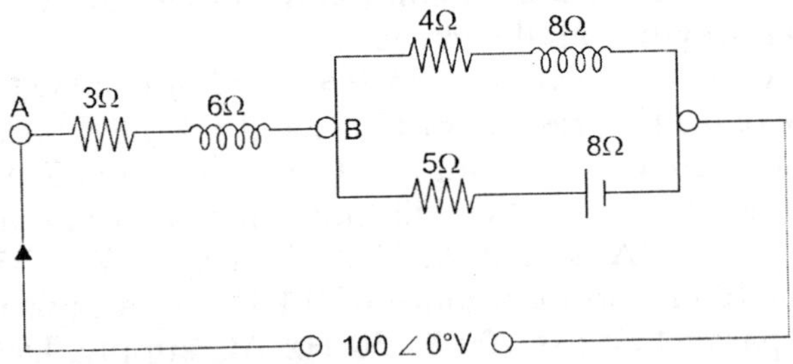

41. In the circuit shown in Fig. 4.66, determine the voltage at 50 Hz to be applied across AB in order that a current of 10 A flows in the capacitor.

[UP Technical Univ; Electrical Engineering, June 2001]

[**Ans.:** 288.62 ∠22.15° V]

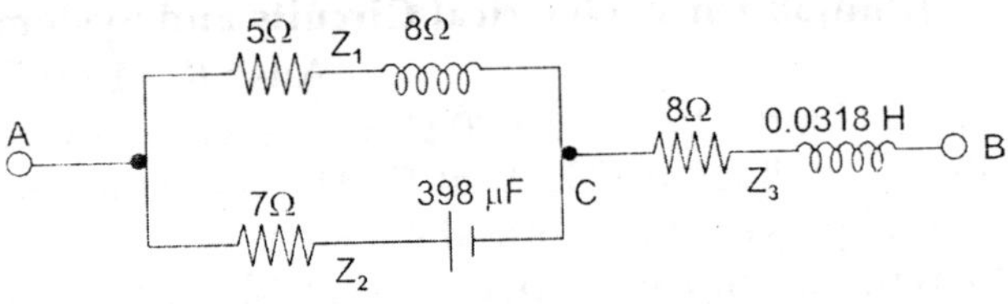

Chapter

5 DC Network Theorems

5.1 INTRODUCTION

Generally, any network problem may be solved by the three basic laws such as ohm's law, KVL and KCL. However, in a large and complex network, these methods are laborious and time consuming. Certain techniques have been developed which are used to solve complex electric network. These special techniques are called network theorems. In this chapter, we shall study five basic theorems.

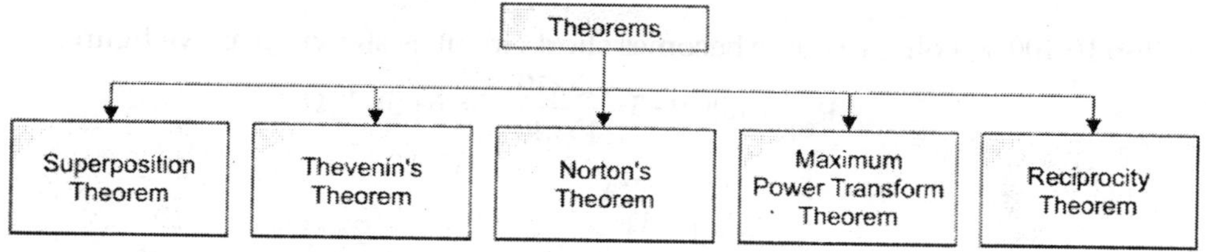

5.2 SUPERPOSITION THEOREM

If a number of voltage and current sources are acting simultaneously in a linear networks, then the resultant current in any branch is the algebric sum of the currents that will be produced in it when each source acting alone replacing all the other independent sources by their internal resistance.

The superposition theorem states that in any linear network containing two or more sources, the response (current) in any element is equal to the algebraic sum of the responses (current) caused by individual sources acting alone, while the other sources remain inactive.

Note: The superposition theorem is an important concept in the circuit analysis. This theorem is useful when a network contains more than one energy sources. It helps us to determine a voltage across a component or branch current by calculating the effect of each source individually and determining the combined effect of these sources.

5.2.1 Steps to Solve Problems on Superposition Theorem

Step I: Select any one energy source.

Step II: Replace all other energy sources by their internal resistances.

Step III: With only one energy source calculate the voltage drops or branch current paying attention to the voltage polarities and current direction.

Step IV: Repeat steps I, II and III for each source individually.

Step V: Add algebraically the voltage drops or currents obtain due to individual source obtain the combined effect of all the sources.

SOLVED EXAMPLES ON SUPERPOSITION THEOREM

Example 1: Find the current in 10 Ω resistor by using superposition theorem.

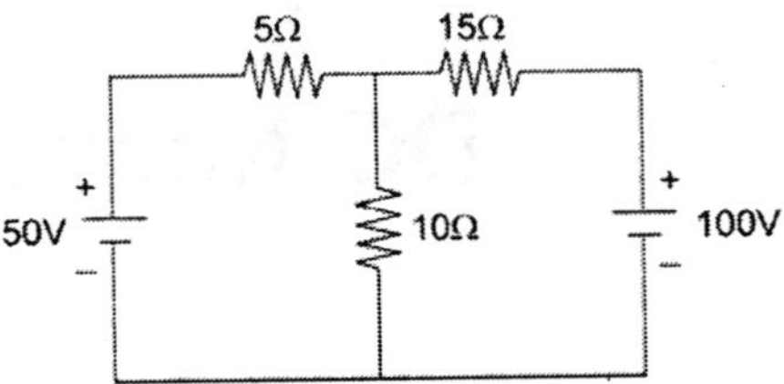

Solution: Step I: We select the 50 V source first.

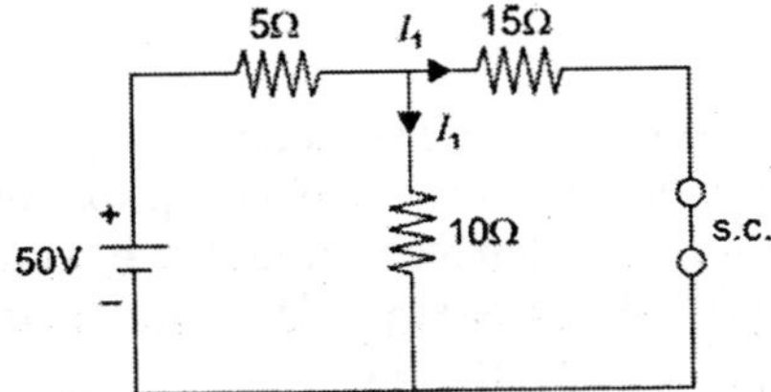

Step II: 100 V, voltage source becomes short circuit as shown in above figure.

$$R_{eq} = 15||10+5 = \frac{15\times10}{15+10}+5 = 6+5 = 11\,\Omega$$

$$I_1 = \frac{V_1}{R_{eq1}} = \frac{50}{11}\text{A}$$

$$I_1' = I_1 \times \frac{15}{10+15}$$

$$I_1' = \frac{50}{11}\times\frac{15}{25} = \frac{30}{11}\text{ A} \qquad \text{(By current division rule)}$$

Step III: Current flowing through 10 Ω is $\frac{30}{11}$ due to 50 V source.

Step IV: Now, we have to repeat the above steps for the other voltage source, i.e. with 100 V.

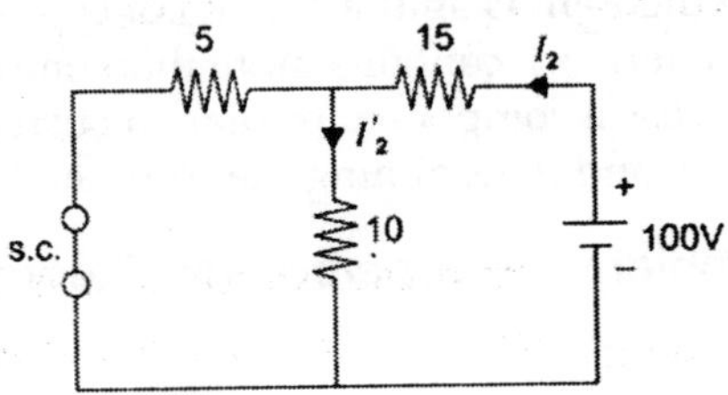

$$I_2 = \frac{100}{Req_2} = \frac{100}{15+\frac{5\times10}{15}} = \frac{60}{11}$$

$$I_2' = \frac{60}{11}\times\frac{5}{5+10} = \frac{20}{11}\text{ A (by current division rule)}$$

Step V: Total current flow through 10 Ω equation

$$I_1' + I_2' = \frac{30}{11}+\frac{20}{11} = \frac{50}{11} = 4.54\text{ A}$$ **Ans.**

Example 2: Calculate the current I using superposition theorem. **[MTU 2009-10]**

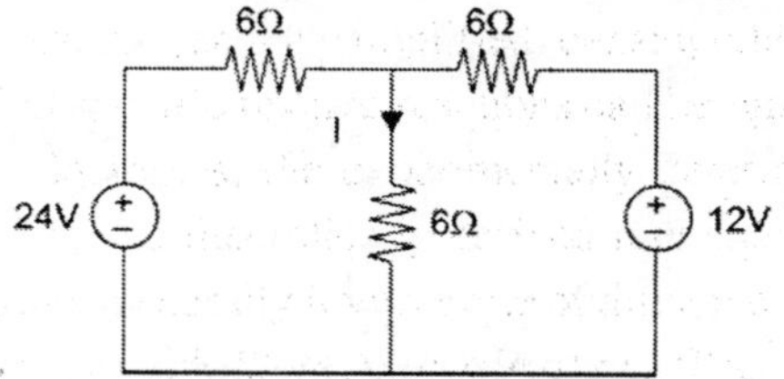

Solution: Step I: Select 24 V voltage source

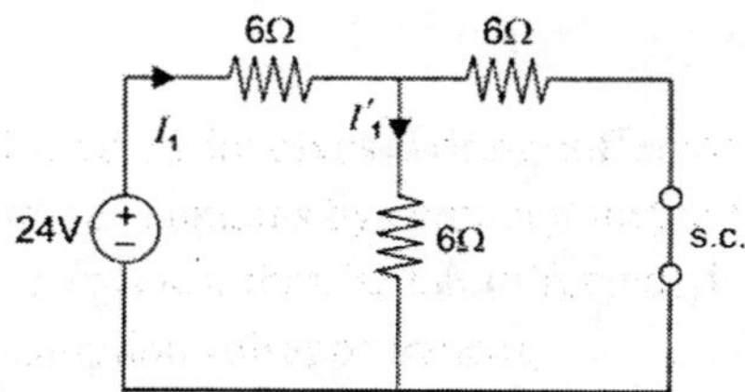

Step II: Short the terminal 12 V voltage source.

$$R_{eq} = (6\|6) + 6 = 9\ \Omega$$

$$I_1 = \frac{24}{9}$$

and $$I_1' = \frac{24}{9}\times\frac{6}{6+6} = 1.333\text{ A}$$ (by current division rule)

Step III: $I_1' = 1.333$ A

Step IV: Now select 12 V voltage source.

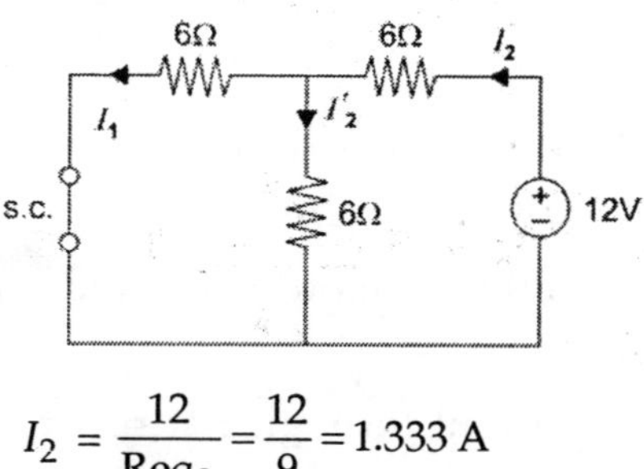

$$I_2 = \frac{12}{Req_2} = \frac{12}{9} = 1.333\text{ A}$$

$$I_2' = \frac{12}{9} \times \frac{6}{6+6} = 0.666 \text{ A} \qquad \text{(by current division rule)}$$

Step V: The total current through 6 Ω resistance.

$$I = I_1' + I_2'$$

$$= 1.333 + 0.666$$

$$I = 1.999 = 2 \text{ A}$$

Ans.

Example 3: Use the superposition theorem to calculate the current in branch AB of the circuit shown in figure below.

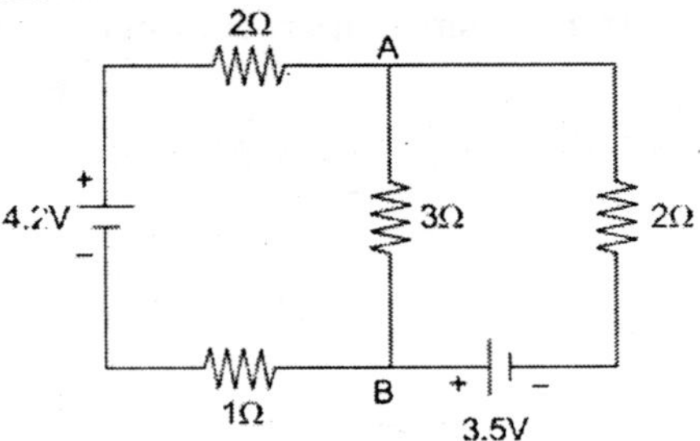

Solution: Step I: Select 4.2 V voltage source and short 3.5 V source.

Step II:

$$R_{eq} = (2+1)+(3 \| 2)$$

$$= 3 + \frac{6}{5} = 4.2 \ \Omega$$

$$I_1 = \frac{4.2}{4.2} = 1 \text{ A}$$

Step III:

$$I_1' = 1 \times \frac{2}{3+2}$$

$$= \frac{2}{5} = 0.4 \text{ A} \qquad \text{(by current division rule)}$$

Step IV: Now, select 3.5 V source and short 4.2 V source.

$$I_2 = \frac{3.5}{(2+1) \| 3 + 2}$$

$$= \frac{3.5}{3.5} = 1 \text{A}$$

$$I_2' = 1 \times \frac{3}{3+3} = 0.5 \text{ A}$$

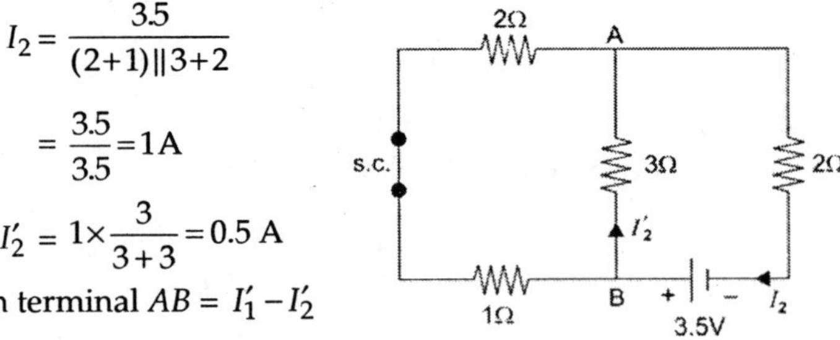

Step V: Total current I in terminal $AB = I_1' - I_2'$

$$= 0.4 - 0.5 = -0.1 \text{ A}$$

or $I = 0.1 \text{ A}(\uparrow)$ flowing upward **Ans.**

Example 4: Determine the current through 8 Ω resistor in the circuit shown in figure using superposition theorem.

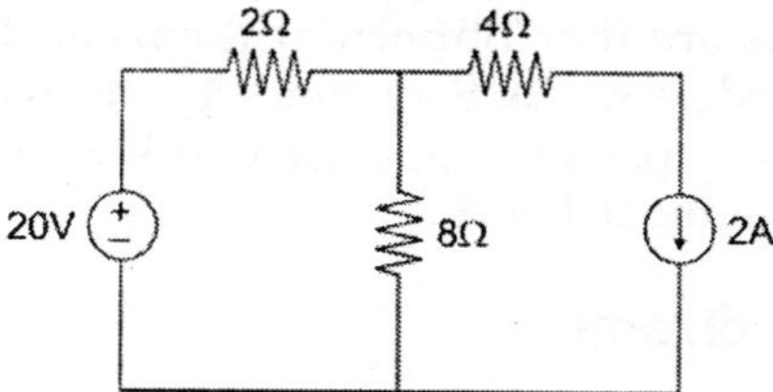

Solution: Step I: Select 20 V voltage source and open the 2 A current source.

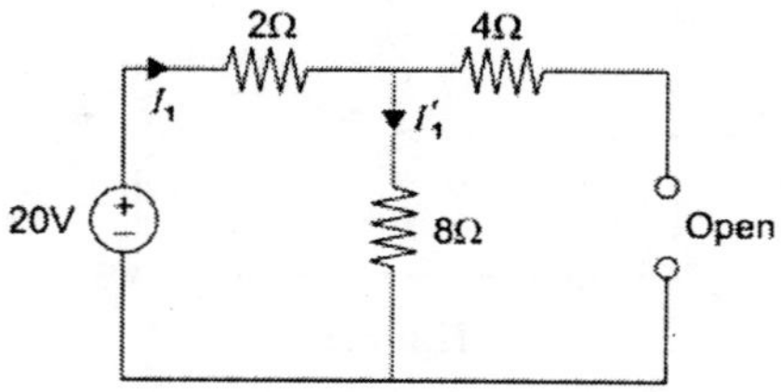

Step II: $I_1 = \frac{20}{10} = 2\text{ A}$

Step III: $I_1' = I_1 = 2\text{ A}$

Step IV: Now, select 2 A current source and short 20 V source.

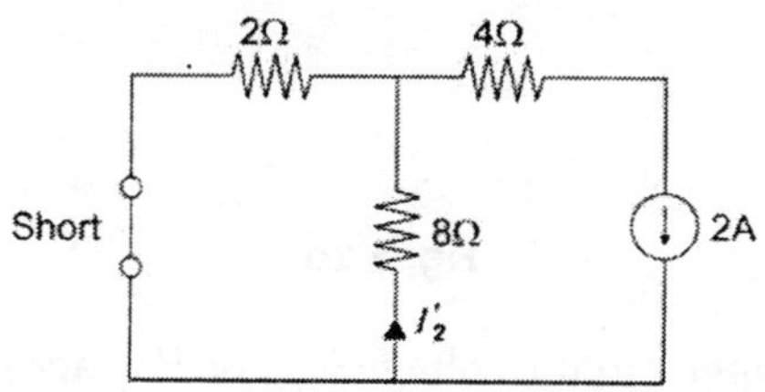

$$I_2' = 2 \times \frac{2}{2+8} = 0.4\text{ A} \quad \text{(by current division rule).}$$

Step V: Current through

$$I = I_1' - I_2'$$
$$= 2 - 0.4 = 1.6\text{ A}$$

Ans.

5.3 THEVENIN'S THEOREM

Statement: Any two terminal bilateral linear DC circuit consisting of independent and/or dependent voltage and current sources and resistors can be replaced by an equivalent circuit consisting of a DC voltage source and series resistor.

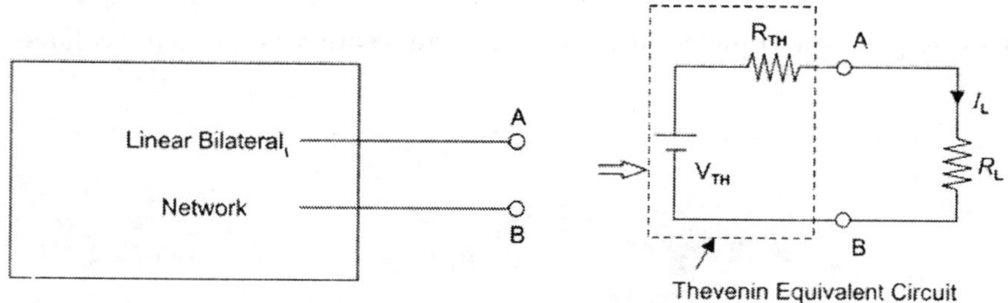

Fig. 5.1

Thevenin's theorem is another important theorem that can be used for the simplification of complicated networks. Sometimes it is desired to determine the current through or voltage across any one branch in a network without calculating current or voltage in other branches of the network.

5.3.1 Steps for Solving Problems

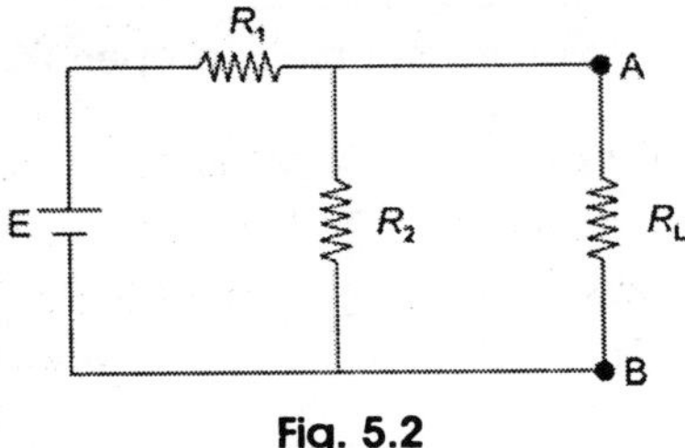

Fig. 5.2

Step I: Remove the load resistance (R_L).

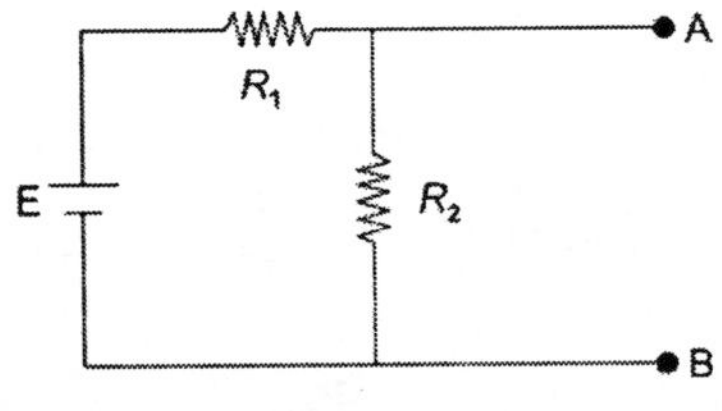

Fig. 5.2a

Step II: Calculate the open circuit voltage V_{TH} or V_{AB} across terminal AB (By using KVL and KCL).

Step III: Short circuit the voltage source and open circuit the current source. Find the equivalent resistance looking across AB.

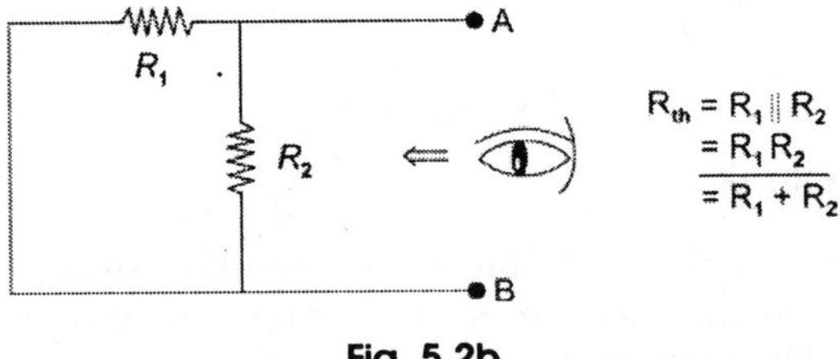

Fig. 5.2b

Step IV: Replace the voltage source and the current source and find the voltage across AB.

$$I = \frac{E}{R_1 + R_2} \qquad \therefore IR_2 = \frac{ER_2}{R_1 + R_2} = V_{th}$$

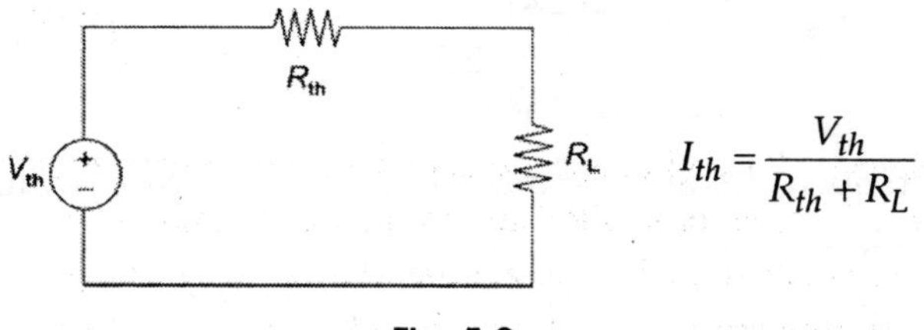

$$I_{th} = \frac{V_{th}}{R_{th} + R_L}$$

Fig. 5.2c

5.3.2 Applications

Thevenin's theorem is applicable to a linear circuit and a bilateral network only.

5.3.3 Advantages

- It reduces a complex circuit into a simpler one.
- It is useful in finding current in a particular branch of a network.
- It is possible to apply this theorem at any two points of a given network.

5.3.4 Disadvantages

Thevenin's theorem is not applicable to the network containing unilateral elements, e.g. diode, etc. nonlinear elements, e.g. diode, transistor etc. and also to magnetic coupling between load and any other circuit element.

SOLVED EXAMPLES ON THEVENIN'S THEOREM

Example 1: Find the current in 10 Ω resistor by using Thevenin's theorem.

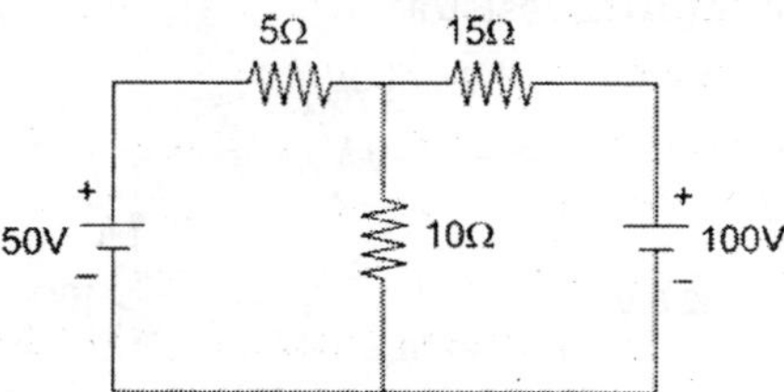

Solution: Step I: Remove 10 Ω resistor and marked terminal *AB* shown in figure below.

Step II: To find voltage across terminal *AB* i.e., $V_{AB} = V_{TH}$.

Applying KVL in above loop

$$50 - 5I - 15I - 100 = 0$$

$$I = -2.5 \text{ A}$$

$$\therefore \quad V_{AB} = V_{TH} = 50 - 5I$$
$$= 50 - 5(-2.5)$$
$$V_{TH} = 62.5 \text{ V}$$

Step III: To find open circuit resistance $(R_{AB} = R_{TH})$ across terminal AB when 50 V and 100 V voltage sources are shorted.

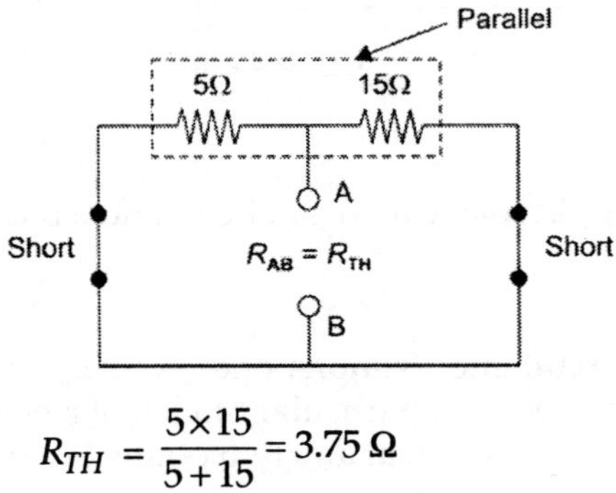

$$R_{TH} = \frac{5 \times 15}{5 + 15} = 3.75 \ \Omega$$

Step IV: Draw Thevenin's equivalent circuit.

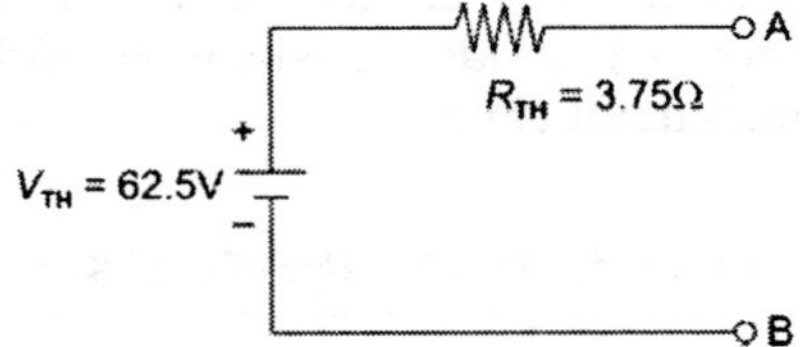

Step V: To find current in 10 Ω resistor.

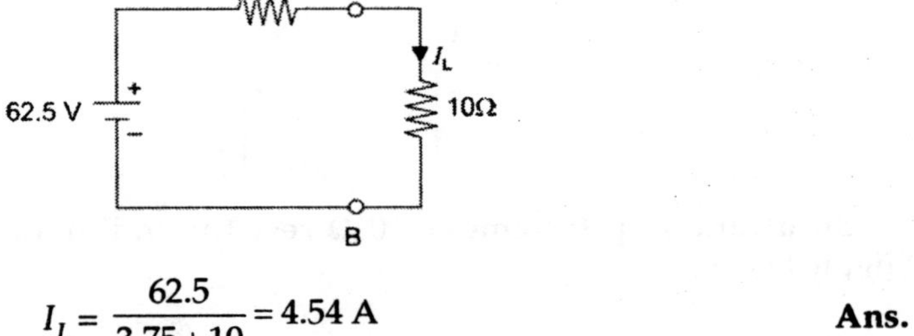

$$I_L = \frac{62.5}{3.75 + 10} = 4.54 \text{ A}$$ **Ans.**

Example 2: Find the current across 12 Ω resistor for a given network shown in the figure below by using Thevenin's theorem.

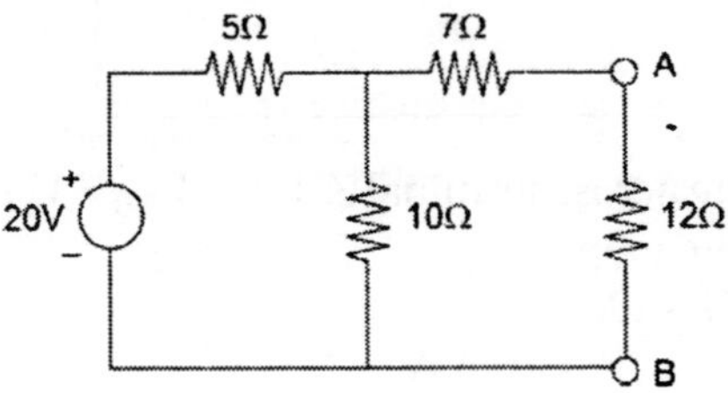

Solution: Step I: Remove 12 Ω resistor

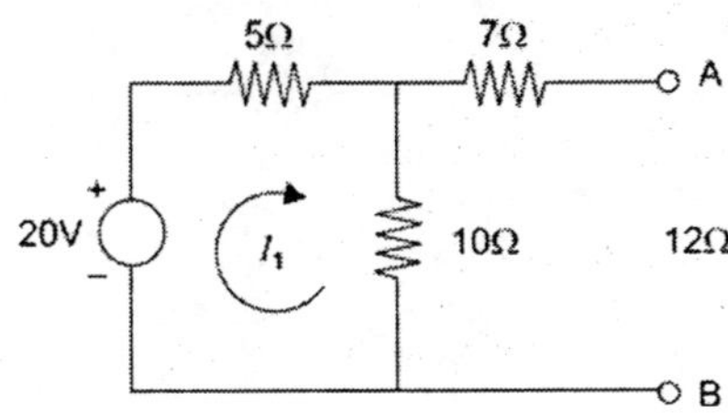

Step II: To find V_{TH}, i.e. V_{AB}.

Applying KVL in above loop

$$20 - 5I_1 - 10I_1 = 0$$

$$\therefore \quad I_1 = \frac{20}{15} = \frac{20}{15} \text{A}$$

$$\therefore \quad V_{TH} = V_{AB} = 10 \times \frac{20}{15} = \frac{200}{15}$$

$$= 13.33 \text{ V}$$

Step III: To find R_{TH} or R_{AB}.

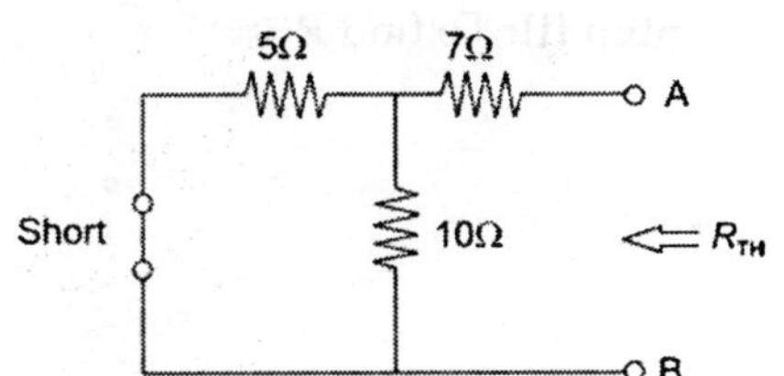

$$\therefore \quad R_{TH} = (5 \| 10) + 7$$

$$R_{TH} = 10.33 \ \Omega$$

Step IV: Draw Thevenin's equivalent circuits.

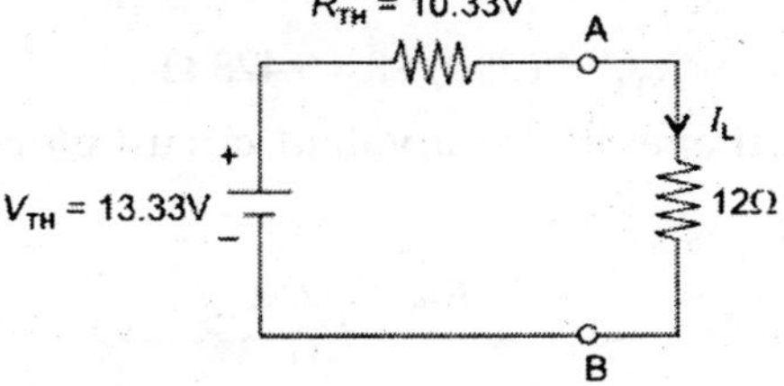

Step V: Current through 12 Ω is I_L

$$\therefore \quad I_L = \frac{V_{TH}}{R_{TH} + R_L}$$

$$= \frac{13.33}{10.33 + 12} = 0.59 \text{ A}$$

Example 3: Find the current in the 10 Ω resistance by using Thevenin's theorem.

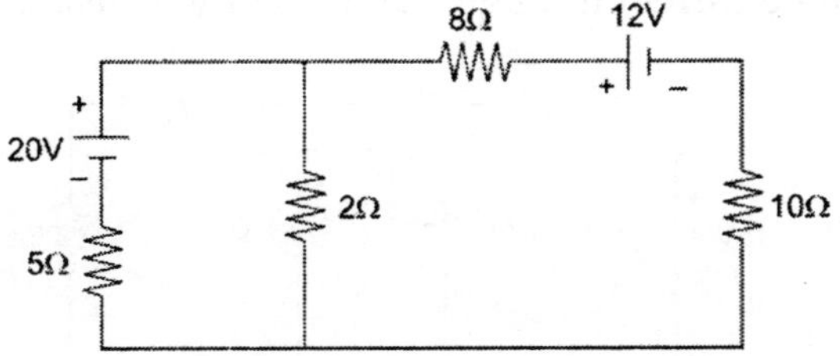

Solution: Step I: Remove 10 Ω resistance, mark terminal AB.

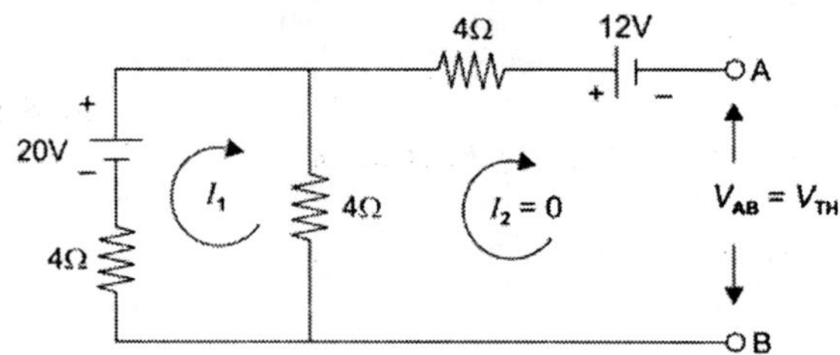

Step II: To find V_{TH}.
Applying KVL

$$20 - 2I_1 - 5I_1 = 0$$

$$I_1 = \frac{20}{7} A$$

$$\therefore \quad V_{TH} = +2 \times \frac{20}{7} - 12 = -6.285 \text{ V}$$

Step III: To find R_{TH}.

$$R_{TH} = (5 \| 2) + 8 = 9.428 \ \Omega$$

Step IV: Draw the thevenin's equivalent circuit by connecting V_{TH}, R_{TH} and $(R_L = 10\Omega)$ in series.

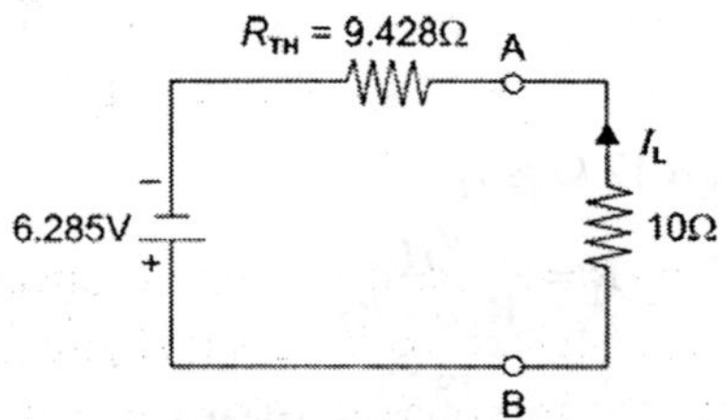

Step V: $$I_L = \frac{V_{TH}}{R_{TH} + R_L} = \frac{6.285}{9.428 + 10} = 0.323 \text{ A}$$ **Ans.**

Example 4: Determine current through 5 Ω resistance by using Thevenin's theorem.

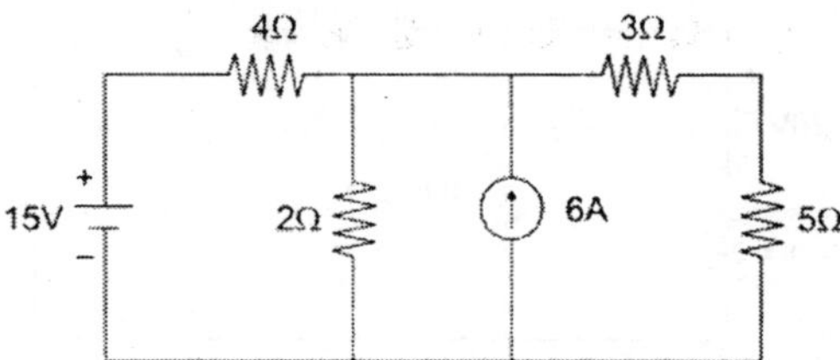

Solution: Step I: Remove the 5 Ω resistor.

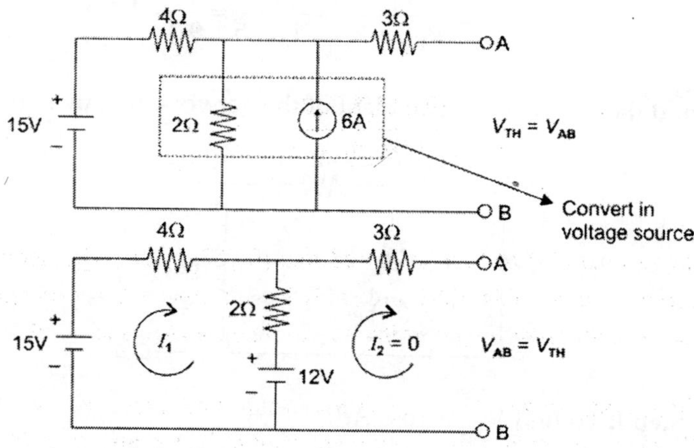

Step II: To find V_{TH}, apply KVL

$$15 - 4I_1 - 2I_1 - 12 = 0$$

$$I_1 = \frac{3}{6} = \frac{1}{2} = 0.5 \text{ A}$$

$$V_{TH} = V_{AB} = 2I_1 + 12 = 2 \times 0.5 + 12$$

$$V_{TH} = 13 \text{ V}$$

Step III: To find R_{TH},

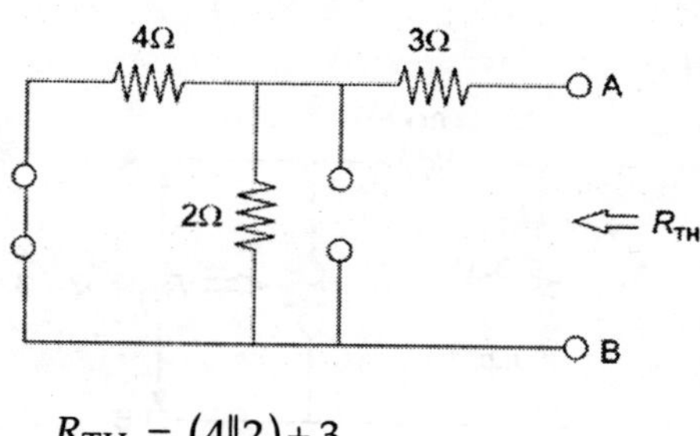

$$R_{TH} = (4 \| 2) + 3$$

$$= \frac{8}{6} + 3 = 4.3\ \Omega$$

Step IV: Draw the Thevenin's equivalent circuit.

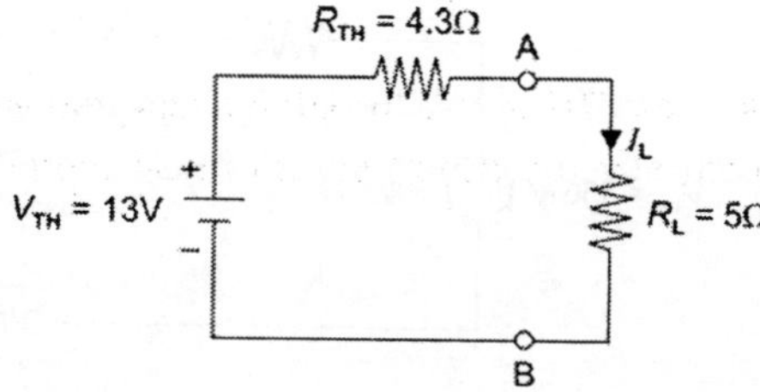

Step V: To find current through 5 Ω resistance.

$$I_L = \frac{V_{TH}}{R_{TH}+R_L} = \frac{13}{4.3+5} = \frac{13}{9.3} = 1.4 \text{ A}$$ **Ans.**

Example 5: Find the Thevenin's equivalent of the network as shown in figure below.

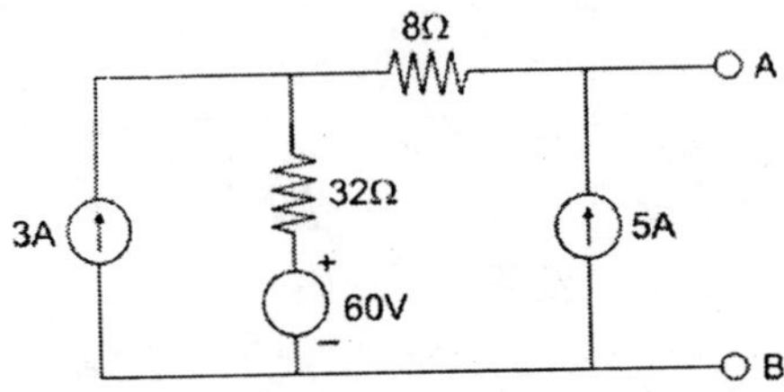

Solution: Step I: To find V_{TH} across AB.

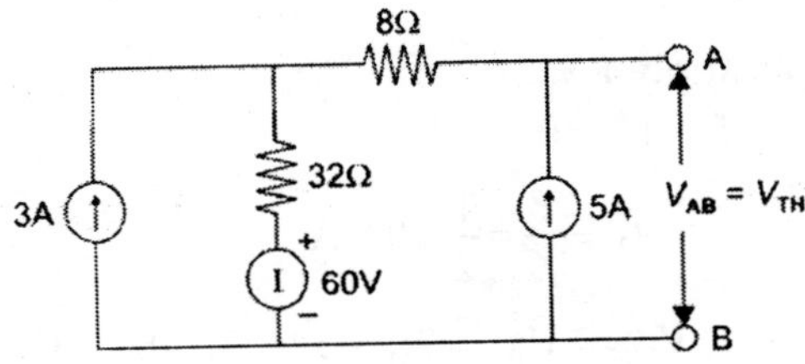

Step II: $V_{TH} = 8 \times 5 + 32(5+3) + 60 = 356$ volt

Step III: To find R_{TH}

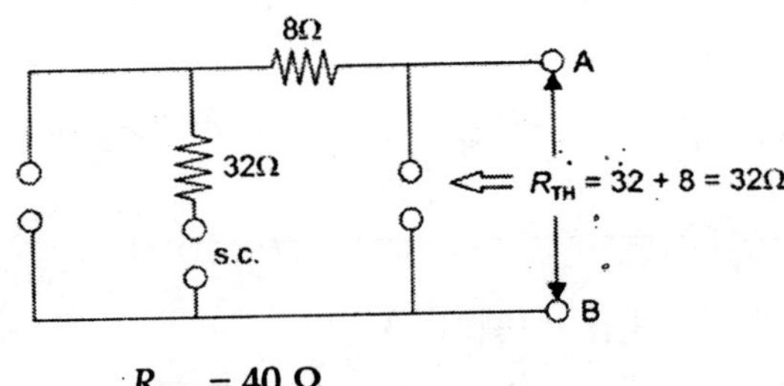

∴ $R_{TH} = 40\ \Omega$

Step IV: Draw Thevenin's equivalent circuits diagram.

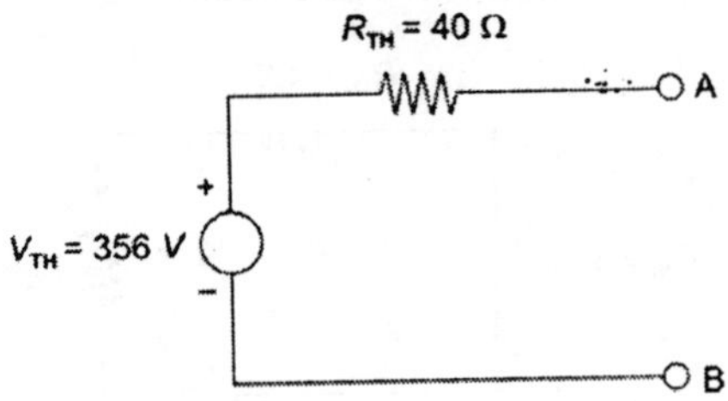

5.4 NORTON'S THEOREM

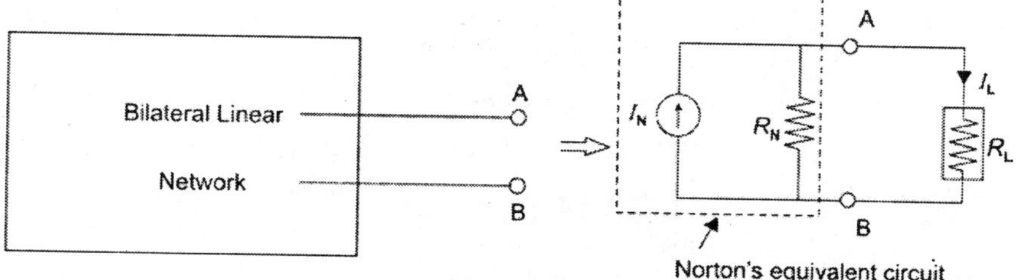

Fig. 5.3: Norton circuit

Statement: Norton's theorem is the converse of Thevenin's theorem. A linear active networks consisting of independent and/or dependent current or voltage sources and bilateral network elements can be replaced by an equivalent circuit consisting of a current source and a parallel resistance, with current source being the short circuit current of the source terminals and the resistance being the internal resistance of source network looking through the open circuited load terminals.

$$I_L = I_N \times \frac{R_N}{R_N + R_L}$$

where I_N is short circuited current and R_N is resistance of network when viewed from load terminals with all energy sources replaced by their internal resistances.

Norton theorem is the dual of Thevenin's theorem, is applicable to linear circuit and to to bilateral network.

5.4.1 Steps for Solving Problems on Norton's Theorem

Step I: Remove the load resistance (R_L) mark terminal A-B, if not marked and short terminal AB.

Step II: Find short circuit current (I_N) in terminal AB, by using KVL and KCL.

Step III: Find the open circuit resistance (R_N) similar to the Thevenin's theorem (R_{TH}), i.e.

$$R_{TH} = R_N$$

Step IV: Draw the Norton's equivalent circuit.

Step V: To find the current through load resistor (R_L).

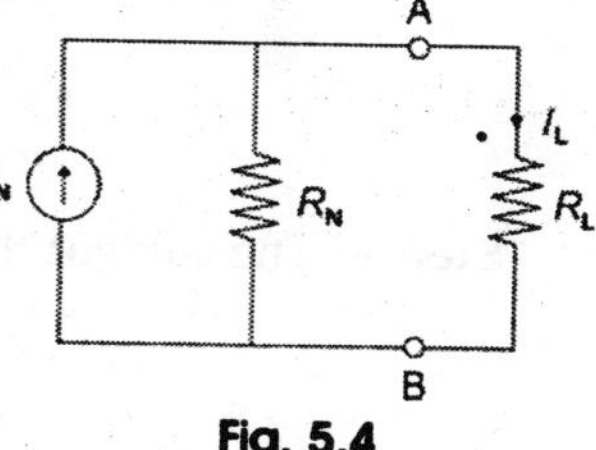

Fig. 5.4

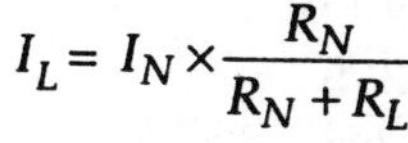

$$I_L = I_N \times \frac{R_N}{R_N + R_L}$$

SOLVED EXAMPLES BASED ON NORTON'S THEOREM

Example 1: Find the current in 10 Ω resistor by using Norton's theorem.

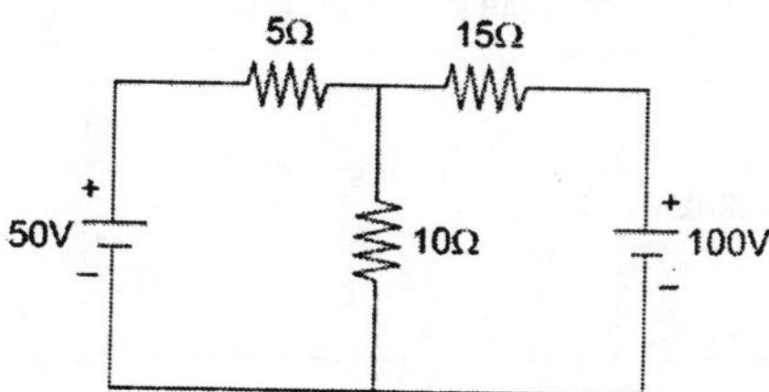

Solution: Step I: Remove 10 Ω resistance, marked terminal *AB* and short.

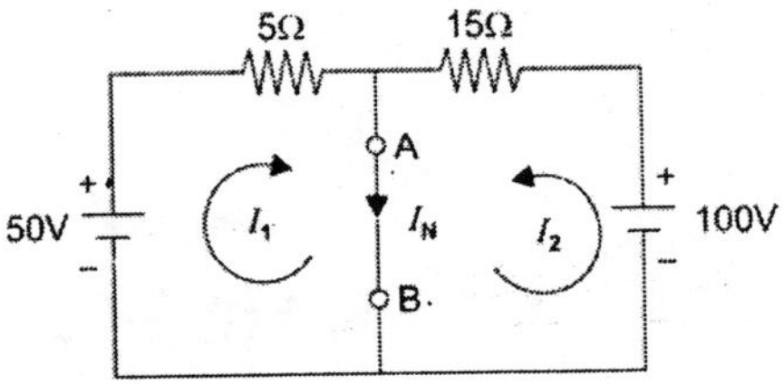

Step II: To find I_N as shown in figure below.

$$I_1 = \frac{50}{5} = 10 \text{ A} \quad I_2 = \frac{100}{15} = 6.66 \text{ A}$$

$$\therefore \quad I_N = I_1 + I_2 = 10 + 6.66 = 16.66 \text{ A}$$

Step III: To find R_N across terminal *AB*.

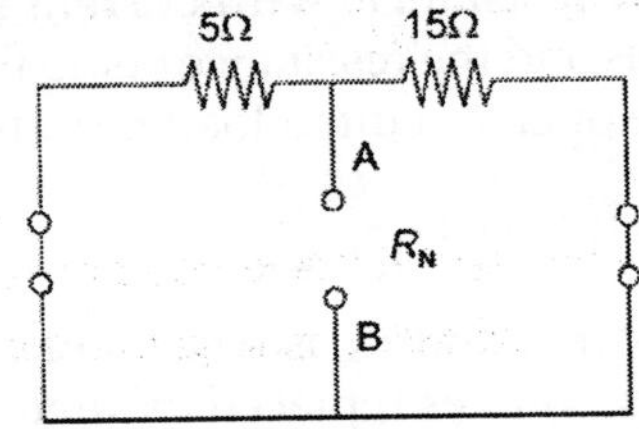

$$R_N = \frac{5 \times 15}{5 + 15} = 3.75 \ \Omega$$

Step IV: Draw the Norton's equivalent circuit.

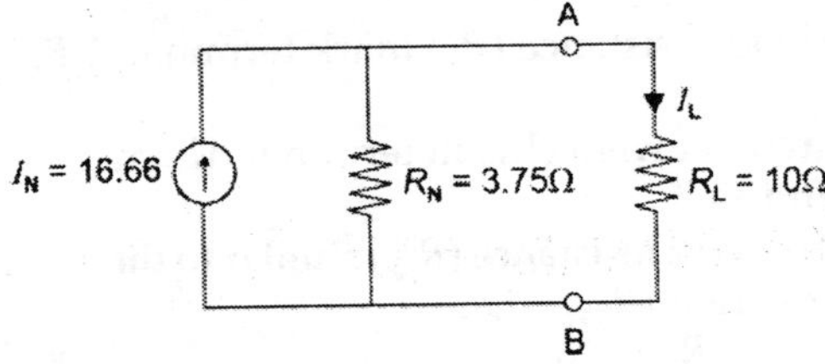

Step V: The current through 10 Ω resistor.

$$I_L = I_N \times \frac{R_N}{R_N + R_L}$$

$$= \frac{16.66 \times 3.75}{3.75 + 10} = 4.54 \text{ A} \qquad \textbf{Ans.}$$

Example 2: Find the current in 12 Ω resistor for a given network as shown in figure below by using Norton's theorem.

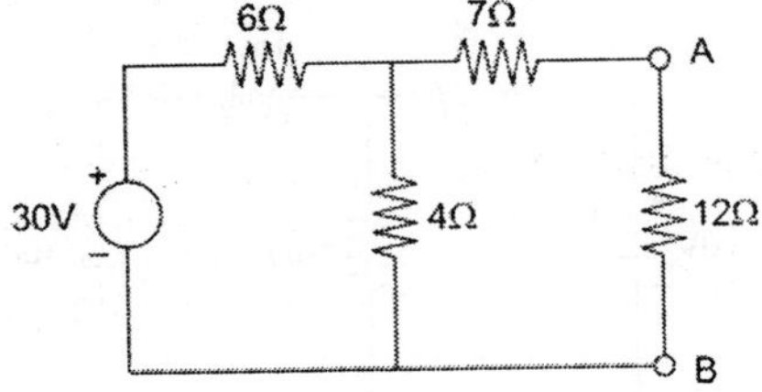

Solution: Step I: Remove 12 Ω resistance and short terminal *AB*.

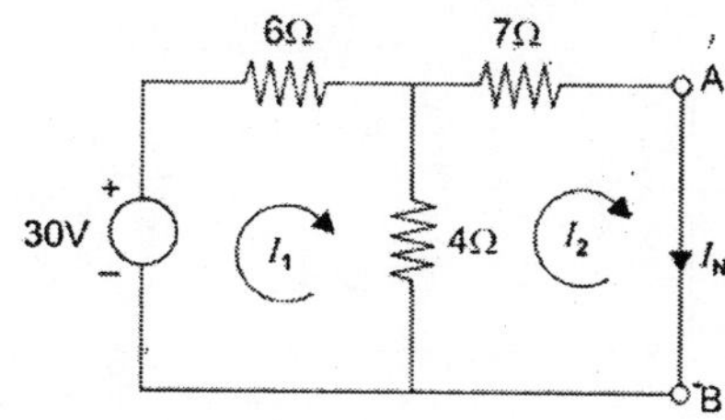

Step II: To find I_N through terminal *AB*.

Applying KVL **in loop 1**

$$30 - 6I_1 - 4(I_1 - I_2) = 0$$

$$30 - 10I_1 + 4I_2 = 0 \qquad ...(1)$$

In loop 2

$$-4(I_2 - I_1) - 7I_2 = 0$$

$$-11I_2 + 4I_1 = 0 \qquad ...(2)$$

Solving Eqs (1) and (2), we get

$$I_2 = 1.27 \text{ A}$$

$$\therefore \quad I_N = I_2 = 1.27 \text{ A}$$

Step III: To find R_N.

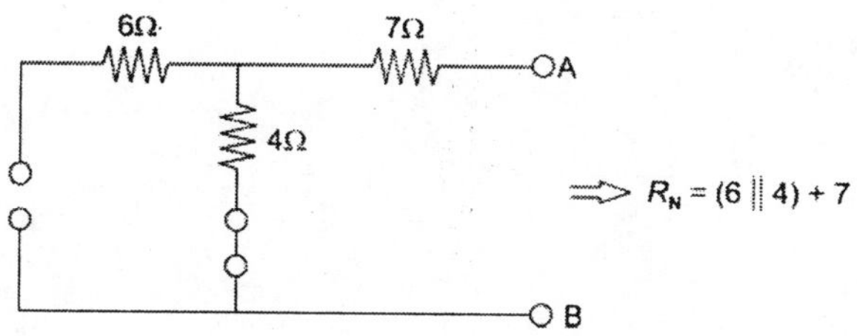

$$R_N = 2.4 + 7 = 9.4\ \Omega$$

Step IV: Draw Norton equivalent circuit.

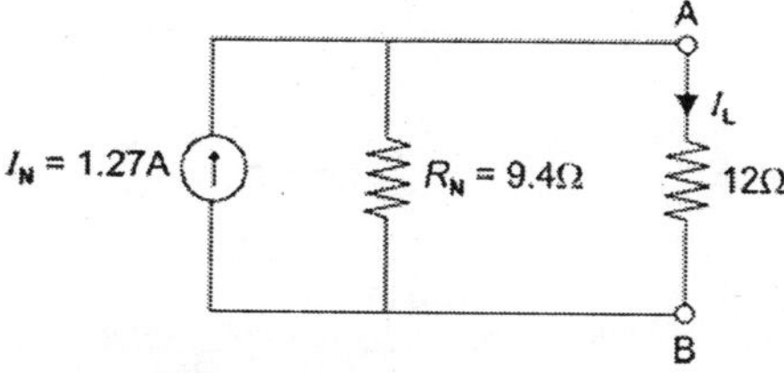

Step V: To find current in 12 Ω resistor

$$I_L = 1.27 \times \frac{9.4}{9.4 + 12} = 0.557 \text{ A}$$ **Ans.**

Example 3: Find the current in 6 Ω resistor using Norton's theorem.

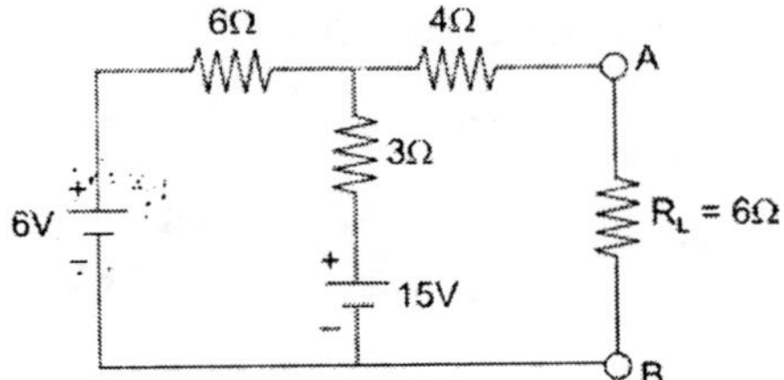

Solution: Step I: Remove load resistor 6 Ω and short terminal *AB*.

Step II: To find I_N

Applying KVL in loop 1.

$$6 - 6I_1 - 3(I_1 - I_2) - 15 = 0$$

$$-9I_1 + 3I_2 = 9$$

$$3I_1 - I_2 = -3 \quad ...(1)$$

Applying KVL in loop 2.

$$15 - 3(I_2 - I_1) - 4I_2 = 0$$

$$3I_1 - 7I_2 = -15 \quad ...(2)$$

Solving Eqs (1) and (2), we get

$$I_2 = 2 \text{ A}$$

$$\therefore \quad I_N = I_2 = 2 \text{ A}$$

Step III: To find R_N

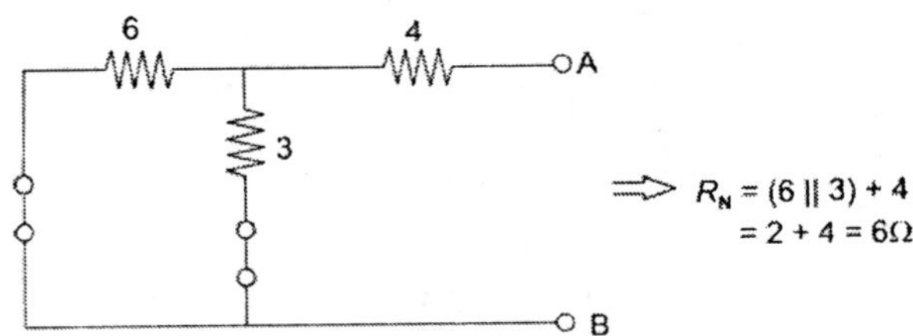

Step IV: Draw Norton's equivalent circuit.

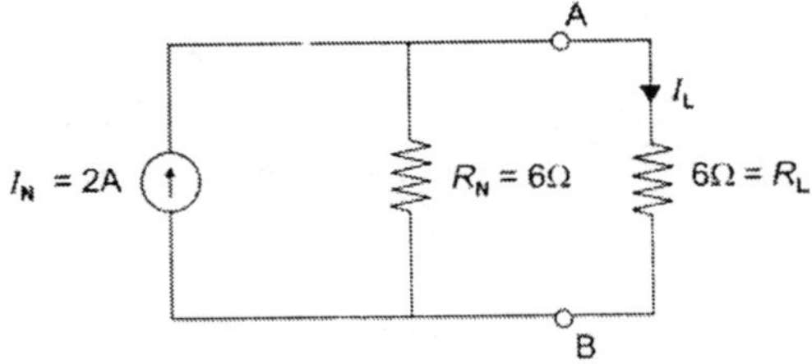

Step V: To find the current in 6 Ω

$$I_N = 2 \times \frac{6}{6+6} = 1 \text{ A}$$ **Ans.**

5.5 MAXIMUM POWER TRANSFER THEOREM

Maximum power transfer theorem deals with transfer of maximum power from a source to load. This theorem is particularly useful for analysing communication network because it is usually desirable to deliver maximum power to load.

Notes: This theorem is applicable to linear circuit only. The efficiency at maximum power transfer is only 50%.

Statement: Power through a load resistance will be maximum when the load resistance is equal to the internal resistance (Thevenin's equivalent resistance) of the source networks a seen from the load terminals, i.e. $R_L = R_i$

5.5.1 Proof of Maximum Power Transfer Theorem

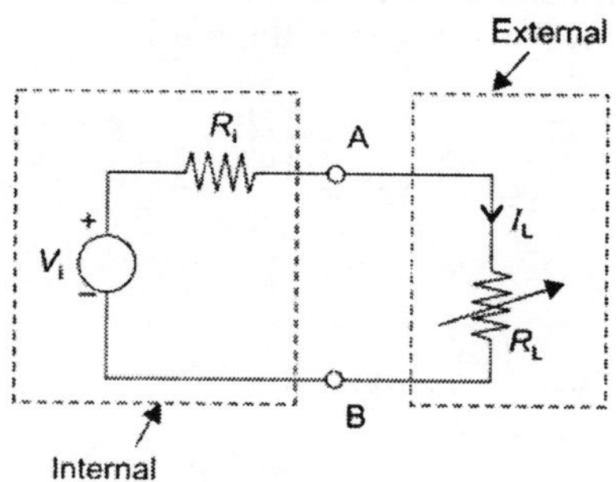

Fig. 5.5

when, V_i= input supply voltage; R_i = internal resistance; R_L = variable load resistance and I_L = load current

The power supplied to load P_L

$$= I_L^2 . R_L$$

$$I_L = \frac{V_i}{R_i + R_L}$$

$$\therefore \quad P_L = \frac{V_i^2}{R_i + R_L{}^2} \times R_L$$

For the power transfer to load to be maximum, the condition is

$$\frac{\partial P_L}{\partial R_L} = 0$$

$$\frac{\partial P_L}{\partial R_L} = \frac{v_i^2\{(R_i + R_L)^2 - R_L . 2(R_i + R_L)\}}{(R_i + R_L)^4} = 0$$

$$V_i = 0$$

$$\therefore \quad (R_i + R_L)^2 - 2R_iR_L - 2R_L^2 = 0$$

$$R_i^2 + 2R_iR_L + R_L^2 - 2RiR_L - 2R_L^2 = 0$$

$$R_i^2 - R_L^2 = 0$$

$$\therefore \quad R_L = R_i$$

As $V_i = V_{TH}$ and $R_i = R_{TH}$, hence for maximum power transfer $R_L = R_{TH}$.

$$\therefore \quad P_{L\max} = \frac{V_{TH}^2 R_{TH}}{(R_{TH} + R_L)^2}$$

$$= \frac{V_{TH}^2}{4R_{TH}} = \frac{V_{TH}^2}{4R_L}$$

Under the condition of maximum power transfer, efficiency is 50%.

We know that source power

$$P_s = V_i I_L$$

$$= V_{TH} \frac{V_{TH}}{R_{TH} + R_{TH}} = \frac{V_{TH}^2}{2R_{TH}}$$

The efficiency of power transfer is defined as the ratio of the average power consumed by the load and the total power supplied to the load.

$$\eta = \frac{P_{L\max}}{P_s} = \frac{\frac{V_{TH}^2}{4R_{TH}}}{\frac{V_{TH}^2}{2R_{TH}}} = \frac{1}{2}$$

$$\% \ \eta = \frac{1}{2} \times 100 = 50\%$$

5.5.2 Steps for Solving Problems on Maximum Power Transfer Theorems

Step I: Remove the load resistance from the network leaving behind the two terminal *A* and *B*.

Step II: Replace the network by Thevenin's equivalent circuit with terminal *A-B*.

Step III: For maximum power to be delivered, select $R_L = R_{TH}$ (or R_i).

Step IV: Maximum power can now be calculated using.

$$P_{L\max} = \frac{V_{TH}^2}{4R_{TH}}$$

5.6 RECIPROCITY THEOREM

Statement: In any linear bilateral network if a source of emf *E* in any branch produces a current *I* in any other branch, then the same emf *E* acting on the second branch would produce the same current *I* as in the first branch.

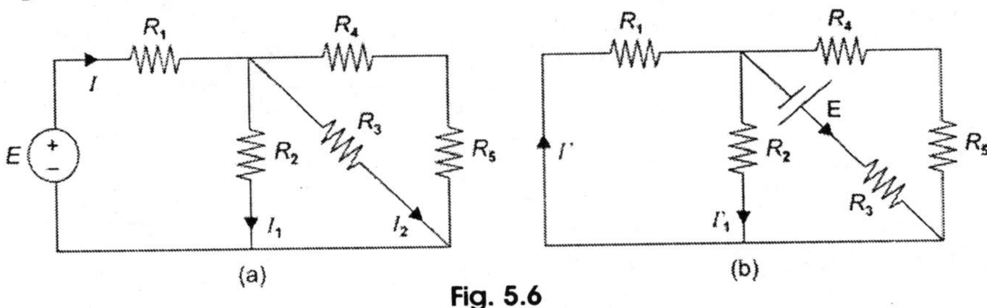

Fig. 5.6

$$\therefore \quad I_2 = I'$$

SOLVED EXAMPLES BASED ON RECIPROCITY THEOREM

Example 1: In the network of figure (a), find the (i) ammeter current battery at A and (ii) when battery is at B and ammeter at point A. Values of various resistances are as shown in the figure below. Also, calculate the transfer for resistance.

Solution: (i) Equivalent resistance between point *C* and *B* in figure below

$$= 12 \times \frac{4}{16} = 3\ \Omega$$

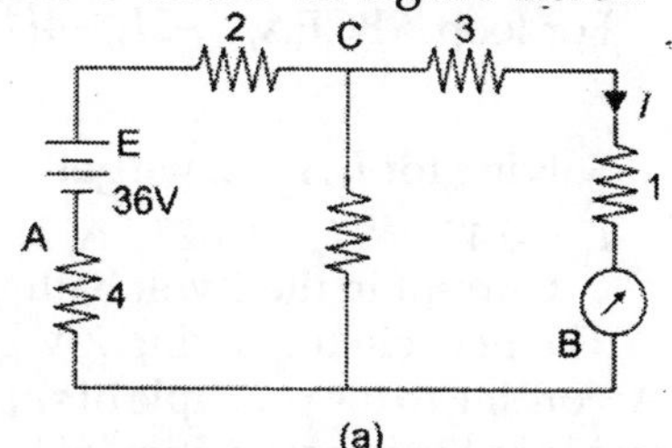

Total circuit resistance = 2 + 3 + 4 = 9 Ω

$$\text{Battery current} = \frac{36}{9} = 4\text{ A}$$

$$\text{Ammeter current} = 4 \times \frac{12}{16} = 3\text{ A}$$

(b) Equivalent resistance between point *C* and *D* in figure (b)

$$= 12 \times \frac{6}{18} = 4\ \Omega$$

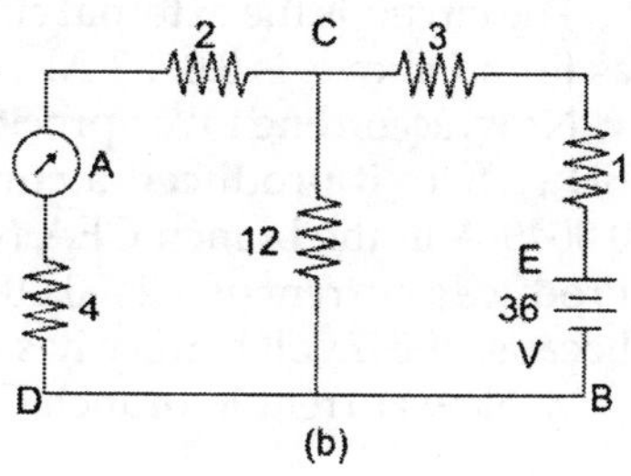

Total current resistance = 4 + 3 + 1 = 8 Ω

Battery current = 36/8 = 4.5 A

$$\text{Ammeter current} = 4.5 \times \frac{12}{18} = 3\text{ A}$$

Hence ammeter current in both cases is the same.

$$\text{Transfer resistance} = \frac{36}{3} = 12\ \Omega$$

Example 2: Calculate the currents in various branches of the network as shown in figures (a) and (b) below and then utilize the principle of superposition and reciprocity theorem together to find the value of the current in the 1-volt battery circuit when an emf of 2 volts is added is branch BD opposing the flow of original current is that branch.

Solution: Let the currents in various branches be as shown in the figures (a) and (b).

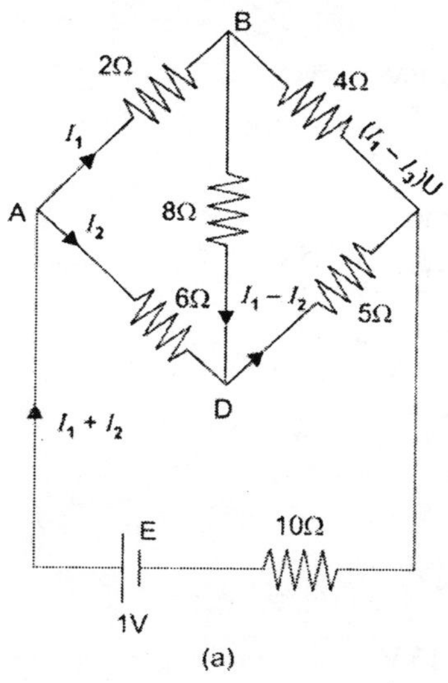

(a)

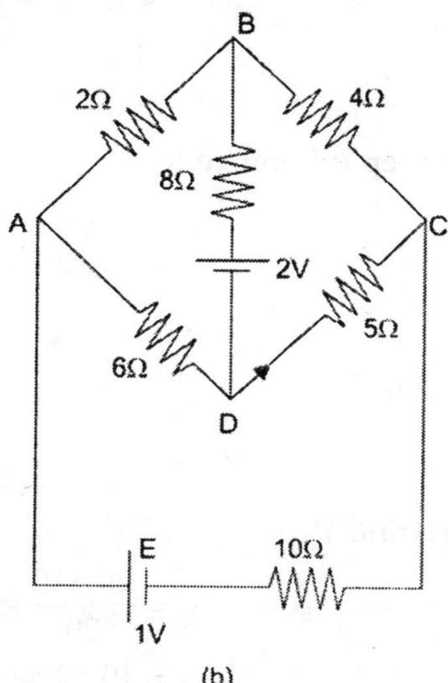

(b)

Applying Kirchhoff's second law, we have

For loop ABDA, $-2I_1 - 8I_3 + 6I_2 = 0$

$$I_1 - 3I + 4I_3 = 0 \quad \text{...(1)}$$

For loop BCDB, $BCDB - 4(I_1 - I_3) + 5(I_2 - I_3) + 8I_3 = 0$

$$4I_1 - 5I_2 - 17I_3 = 0 \quad \text{...(2)}$$

For loop ABCEA, $-2I_1 - 4(I_1 - I_3) - 10(I_1 + I_2) + I_0 = 0$

$$16I_1 + 10I_2 - 4I_3 = 1 \quad \text{...(3)}$$

Solving for I_1, I_2, I_3, we get

$I_1 = 0.494$ A, $I_2 = 0.0229$ A, $I_3 = 0.0049$ A

∴ Current in the 1 volt battery circuit is $I_1 + I_2 = 0.0723$ A

The new circuit having 2-V battery connected in the branch BD is shown in figure. According to the principle of superposition. The new current is the 1-volt battery current is due to the superposition of two currents, one due to 1-volt battery and the other due to the 2-volt battery when each acts independently.

The circuit is the external circuit due to 1-volt battery when 2-volt battery is not there as found above, is 0.0723 A.

Now, according to reciprocity theorem, if 1-volt battery were transferred to the branch BD (where it produced a current of 0.0049 A), then it would produce a current of 0.0049 A in the branch CEA (where it was before). Hence, a battery of 2-volts would produce a current of (–2 × 0.0049) = – 0.0098 A (by product in), the negative sign is used because the 2-volt battery has been so connected as to oppose the current is branch BD.

∴ New current in branch CEA = 0.0723 – 0.0098 = 0.0625 A.

SOLVED EXAMPLES BASED ON MAXIMUM POWER TRANSFER THEOREM

Example 1: For the network shown in figure below. Calculate the value of R for maximum power transfer and also calculate the value of maximum power.

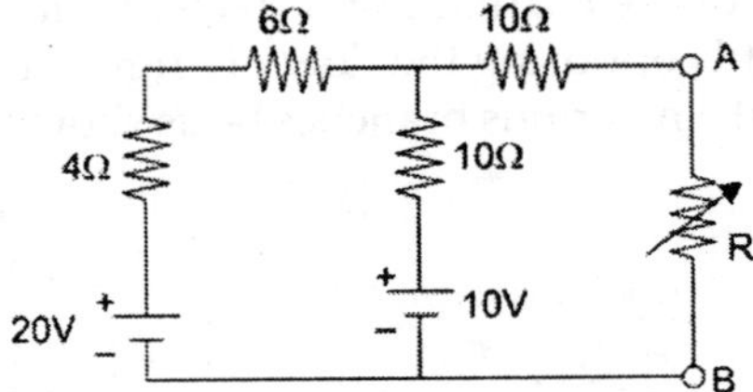

Solution: Step I: Remove R

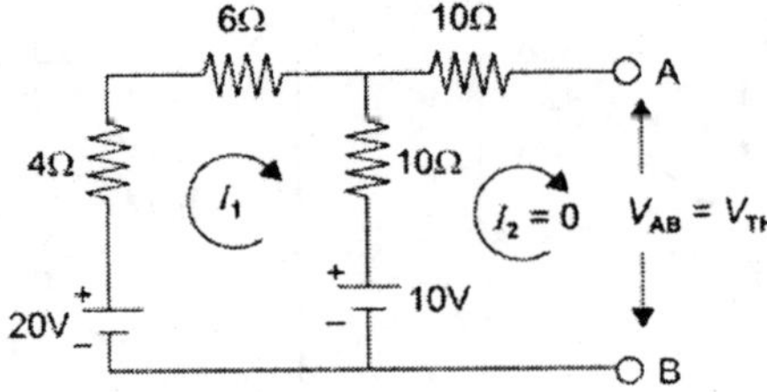

Step II: To find V_{TH}.

$$I_1 = \frac{20-10}{20} = 0.5\ A$$

$$V_{TH} = 10 \times 0.5 + 10 = 15\ V$$

Step III: To find R_{TH}.

$\Rightarrow R_{TH} = \{(4 + 6) \,||\, (10)\} + 10$
$= 5 + 10 = 15\Omega$

$$R_{TH} = 10\ \Omega$$

$\therefore$ For maximum power transfer

$$R = R_{TH} = 15\ \Omega$$ **Ans.**

Step IV: Calculate maximum power

$$\therefore \quad P_{L\max} = \frac{V_{TH}^2}{4R_{TH}} = \frac{(15)^2}{4 \times 15} = 3.65\text{ W}$$ **Ans.**

Example 2: Find the value of load resistor, R_L for maximum power transfer and the magnitude of maximum power in the circuit shown in figure below.

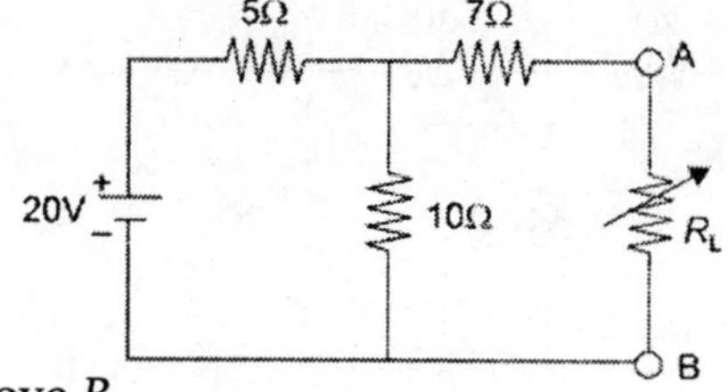

Solution: Step I: Remove R_L

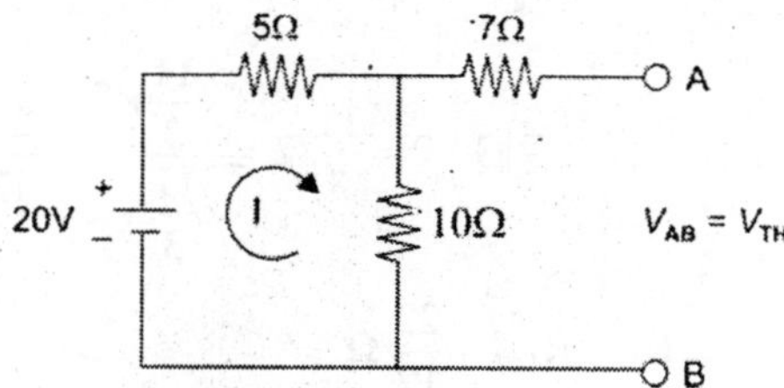

Step II: Find V_{TH}.

$$I = \frac{20}{15}$$

$$V_{TH} = 10 \times \frac{20}{15} = \frac{200}{15}\text{ V}$$

Step III: To find R_{TH}.

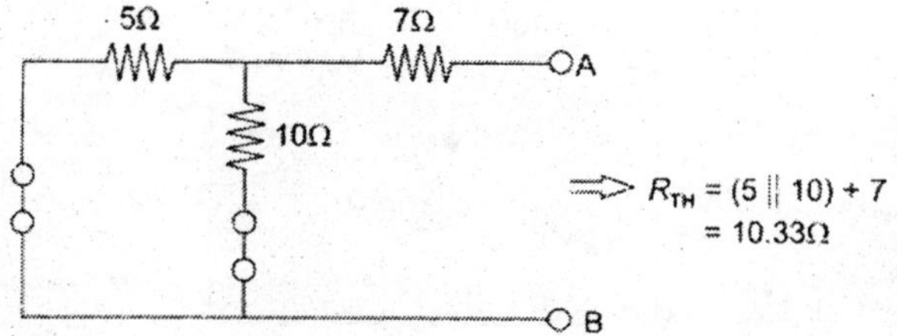

$\Rightarrow R_{TH} = (5 \,||\, 10) + 7$
$= 10.33\Omega$

Select $R_L = R_{TH} = 10.33\ \Omega$ for maximum power transfer. **Ans.**

Step IV: To find maximum power

$$P_{L\max} = \frac{V_{TH}^2}{4R_{TH}} = \frac{\left(\frac{200}{15}\right)^2}{4\times 10.33} = 4.30\ \text{W}$$ **Ans.**

Example 3: Find the value of R such that maximum power transfer take place.

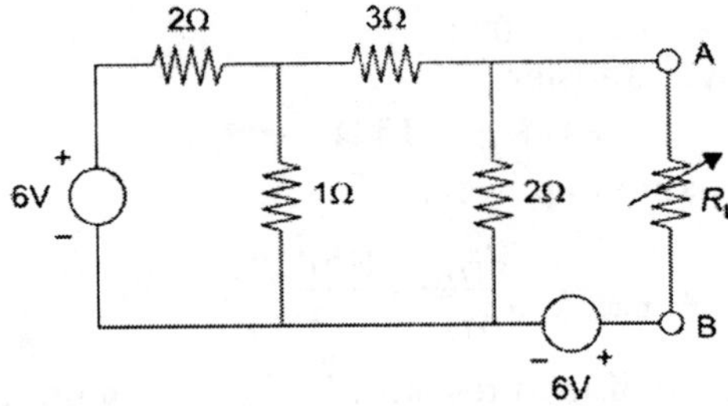

Solution: Step I: Remove R_L.

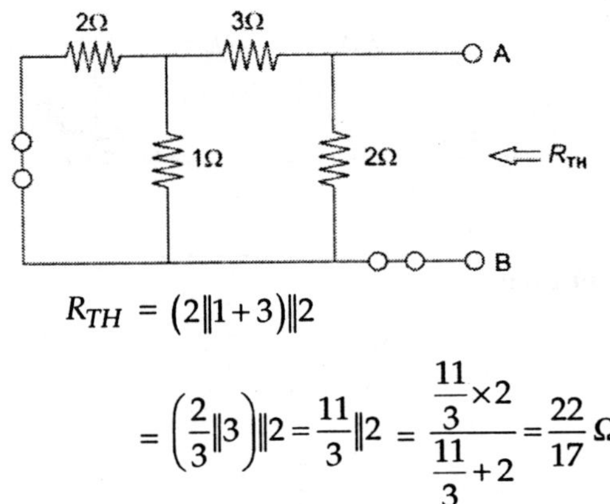

$$R_{TH} = (2\|1+3)\|2$$

$$= \left(\frac{2}{3}\|3\right)\|2 = \frac{11}{3}\|2 = \frac{\frac{11}{3}\times 2}{\frac{11}{3}+2} = \frac{22}{17}\ \Omega$$

For maximum power $\quad R_L = R_{TH} = \frac{22}{17}\ \Omega$

SOLVED EXAMPLES ON NETWORK THEOREMS

Based on Superposition Theorem

Example 1: Find I for the circuit shown in figure below using superposition theorem. **[MTU Sem. II 04-05]**

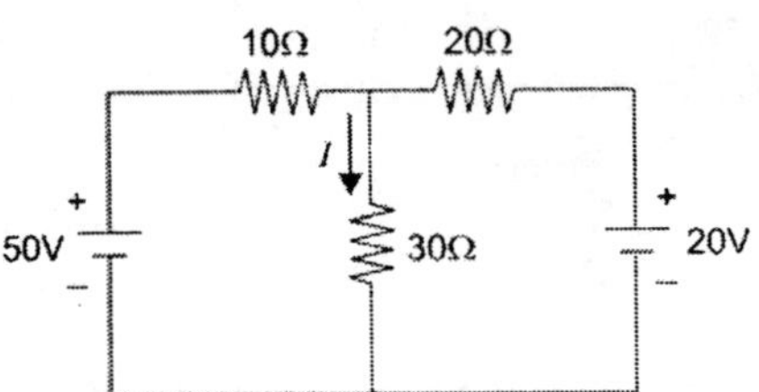

Solution: Step I: According to superposition theorem, select a single source in the circuit. Consider 50 V source active alone and short 20 V source as shown in figure below.

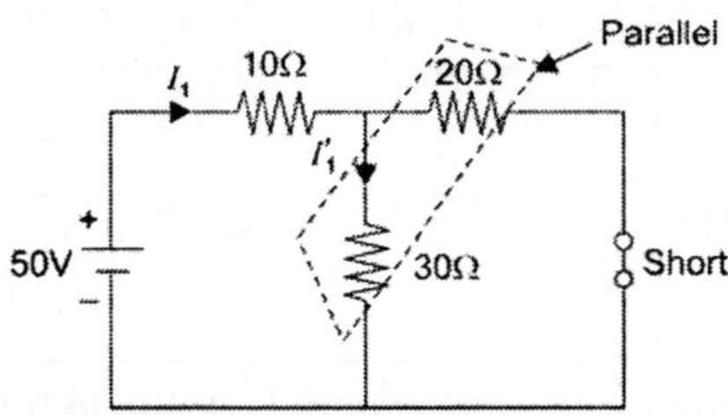

Step II: Calculate the equivalent resistance and total curent in the above figure. Resistance 20 Ω and 30 Ω are in parallel.

$$\therefore \quad R_{eq1} = \frac{20\times 30}{20+30} + 10 = 22\ \Omega$$

$$I_1 = \frac{V_1}{R_{eq1}}$$

$$\therefore \quad \text{Total current } I_1 = \frac{50}{22} = 2.27\ \text{A}$$

Step III:

$$\therefore \quad I'_1 = 2.27\times\frac{20}{20+30} \qquad \text{(by current division rule)}$$

$$\therefore \quad I'_1 = 0.909\ \text{A} \qquad ...(1)$$

Step IV: Now consider 20 V source alone and 50 V source short. Now calculate total resistance and total current from figure below.

Parallel

10 20

I_2 I'_2

$\frac{10\times 30}{10+30} = \frac{300}{40}$ 30 + 20V −

$$R_{eq_2} = \frac{30}{4} + 20 = 27.5\ \Omega$$

$$I_2 = \frac{V_2}{Req_2} = \frac{20}{27.5} = 0.72\ \text{A}$$

$$\therefore \quad I'_2 = 0.72\times\frac{10}{10+30} = 0.181\ \text{A} \qquad \text{(by current division rule)}$$

Step V: Calculate the current through 30 Ω.

$$I = I'_1 + I'_2$$

$$= 0.909 + 0.181$$

$$= 1.09\ \text{A}$$

Ans.

Example 2: Using superposition theorem find the current through 8 Ω for the given network figure below. **[MTU 2008-09]**

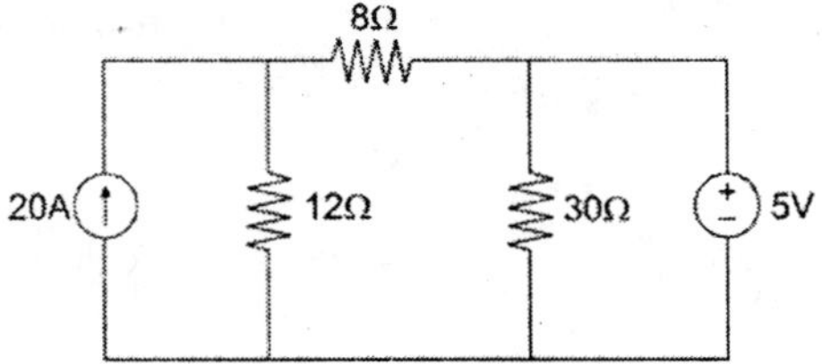

Solution: Step I: Calculate current through 8 Ω due to 5 V source only.
Open circuit 20 A current source and active only 5 V source.

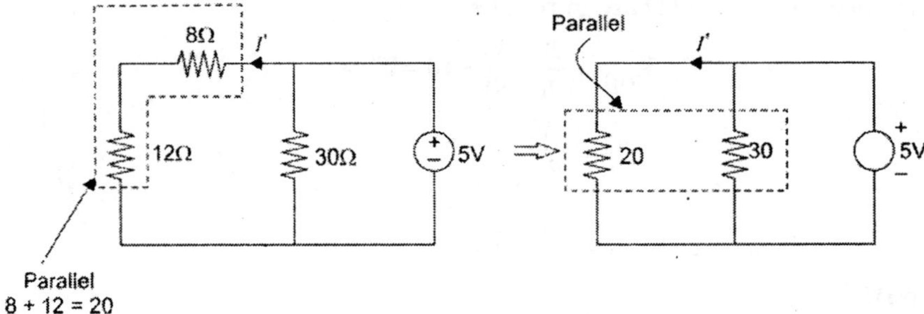

In parallel voltage is same, i.e.

$$\therefore \qquad I' = \frac{5}{20} = 0.25 \text{ A} \qquad \text{...(1)}$$

Step II: Calculate current through 8 Ω due to 20 A source only.

As 5 V source is shorted, the 30 Ω is by passed, so it is not shown in figure below.

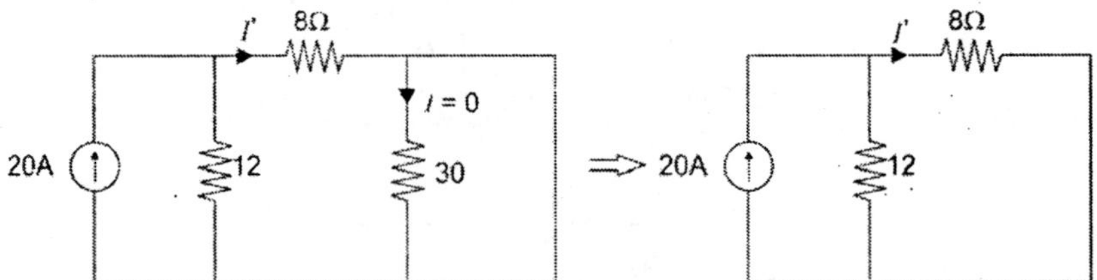

Using current division rule

$$I'' = \frac{20 \times 12}{12 + 8} = 12 \text{ A} \qquad \text{...(2)}$$

Step III: Calculate total current through 8 Ω resistance is

From Eqs (1) and (2) we get

Total current through 8 Ω resistance is

$$= I'' - I'$$
$$= 12 - 0.25$$
$$= 11.75 \text{ A (from left to right)}$$

Ans.

Example 3: Find the voltage V_{AB} using superposition theorem.

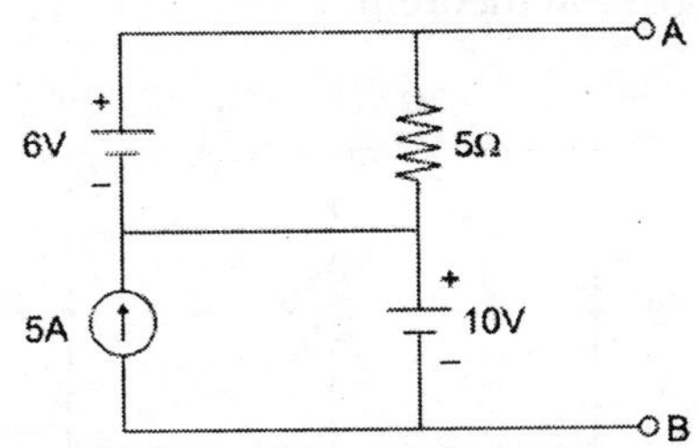

Solution: Step I: Select 6 V source, find the current in 5 Ω resistance.
All other soures are deactive. 5 A current source is open. 10 V source is shorted.

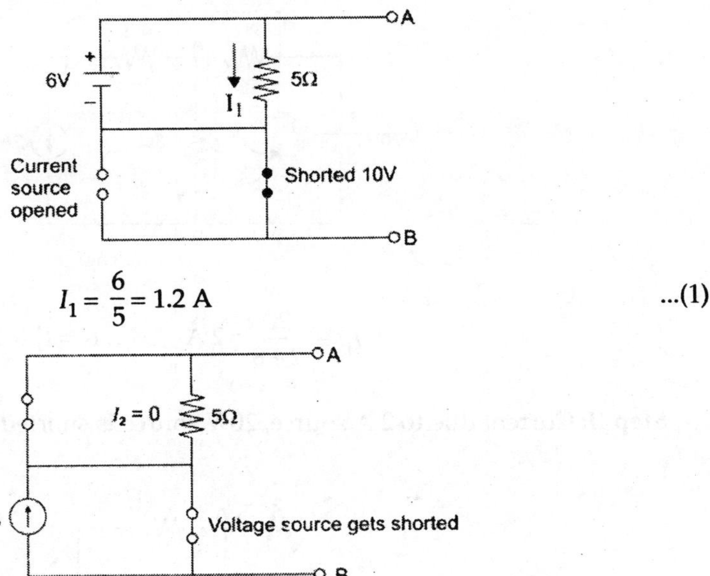

$$I_1 = \frac{6}{5} = 1.2 \text{ A} \qquad ...(1)$$

Step II: Current through 5 Ω due to only 5 A source.

$$I_2 = 0$$

Step III: Current due to only 10 V source.

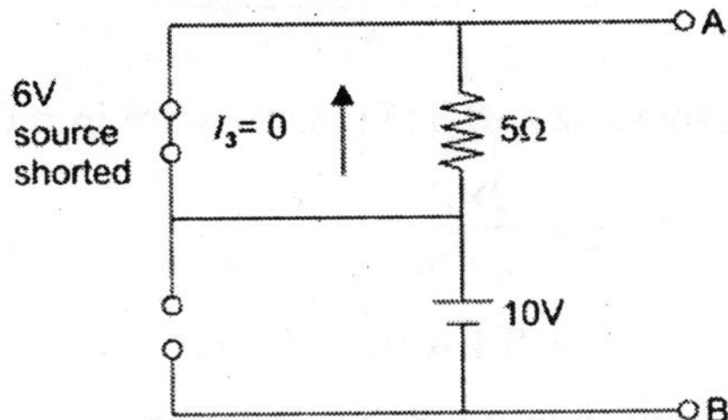

Since there is no return path for I_3.

$$\therefore \quad I_3 = 0$$

Step IV: Total current through 5 Ω resistance is

$$I = I_1 + I_2 + I_3$$

$$\therefore \quad = 1.2 + 0 + 0 = 1.2 \text{ A}$$

$$\therefore \quad V_{AB} = 5 \times I + 10 = 5 \times 1.2 + 10 = 16 \text{ V}$$ **Ans.**

Example 4: Determine the current through 8 Ω resistor in the network shown in figure below using superposition theorem.

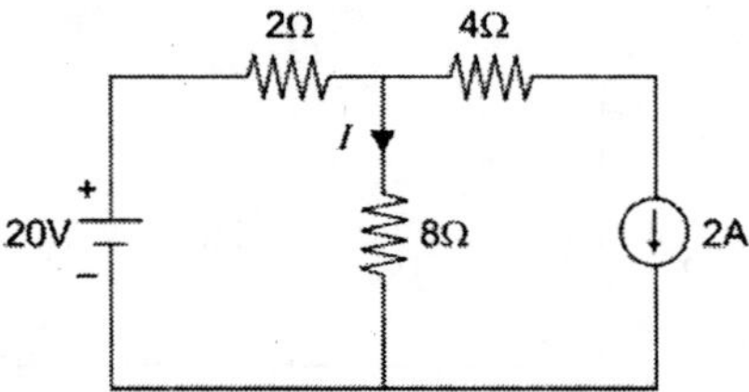

Solution: Step I: Current due to 20 V source, 2 A current source in opened.

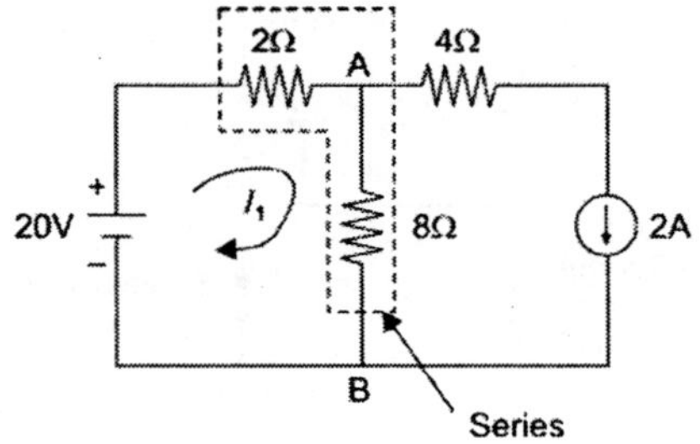

∴ $$I_1 = \frac{20}{2+8} = 2\text{ A} \qquad \therefore I_1 = I_1' = 2\text{ A (from A to B)} \qquad ...(1)$$

Step II: Current due to 2 A source, 20 V source is shorted.

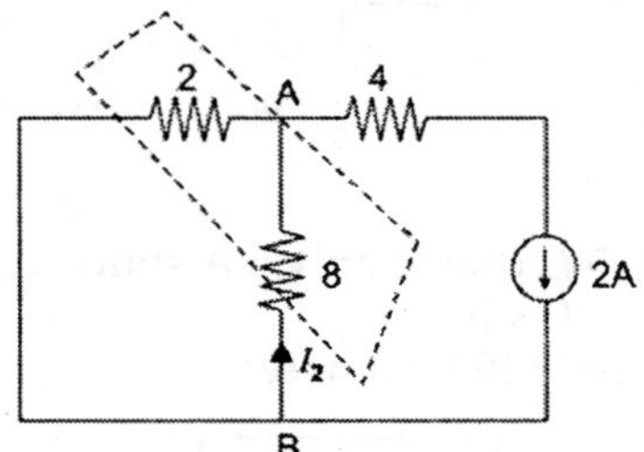

As shown in figure above 2 Ω and 8 Ω resistors are in parallel.

∴ $$I_2' = \frac{2 \times 2}{2+8} \qquad \text{(current division rule)}$$

$$I_2' = 0.4\text{ A from } B \text{ to } A \qquad ...(2)$$

Step III: Calculate current through 8 Ω resistance.
From Eqs (1) and (2)

$$I = I_1' + I_2'$$
$$= 2 - 0.4 = 1.6\text{ A}$$

Example 5: Using superposition theorem, determine currents in all the resistance of the network as shown in figure below. **[UPTU Sem-I, 05-06, 07-08]**

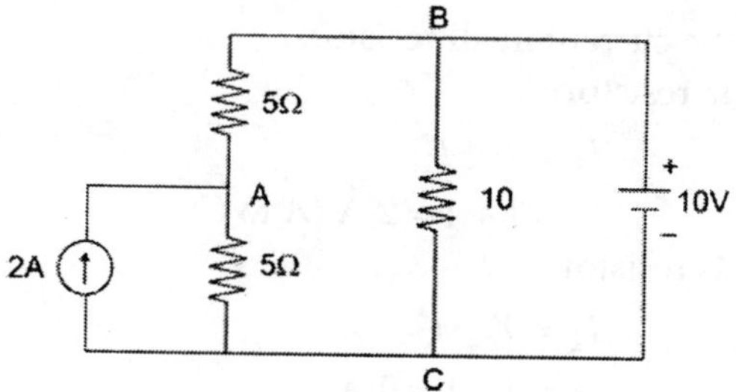

Solution: Step I: Currents due to 2 A source.

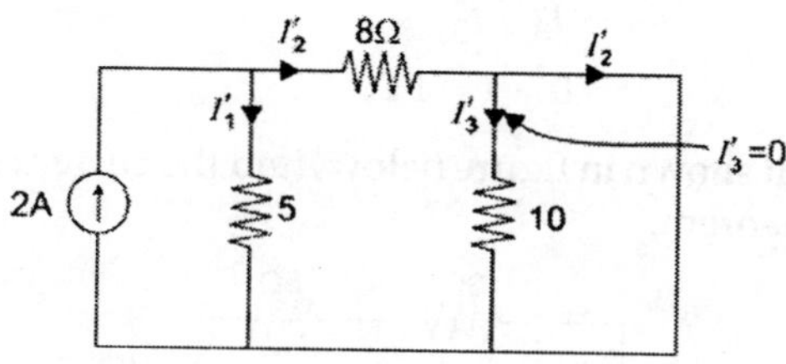

$$I_1' = I_2' = 2 \times \frac{5}{5+5} = 1\text{ A (by current division rule)} \qquad ...(1)$$

$$I_3' = 0$$

By current division rule

$$I_1' = 1\text{ A}$$

$$I_2' = 1\text{ A}$$

Step II: Current due to 10 V source.

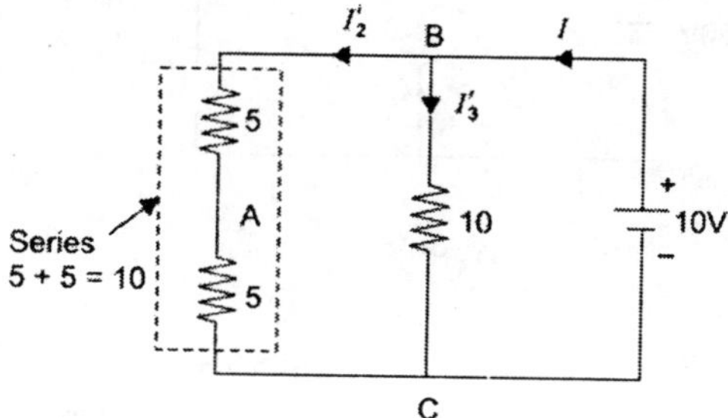

$$R_{eq} = (10\Omega \| 10\Omega) = 5\ \Omega$$

$$I = \frac{V}{R_{eq}} = \frac{10}{5} = 2\text{ A}$$

By current division rule

$$I_1'' = \frac{10 \times 2}{10+10} = 1\text{ A}$$

$$I_3'' = \frac{10 \times 2}{10+10} = 1\text{ A} \qquad ...(2)$$

Step III: Calculate the current in all resistors.

Current through 5 Ω resistor

$$I_1 = I_1' + I_1''$$
$$= 1 + 1 = 2 \text{ A } (A \text{ to } C)$$ **Ans.**

Current through 5 Ω resistor

$$I_2 = I_2' - I_2''$$
$$= 1 - 1 = 0 \text{ A}$$ **Ans.**

Current through 10 Ω resistor

$$I_3 = I_3' + I_3''$$
$$= 0 + 1 = 1 \text{ A}$$ **Ans.**

Example 6: In the circuit shown in figure below, find the current through the 6 Ω resistor using superposition theorem. **[Sem-1, 07-08]**

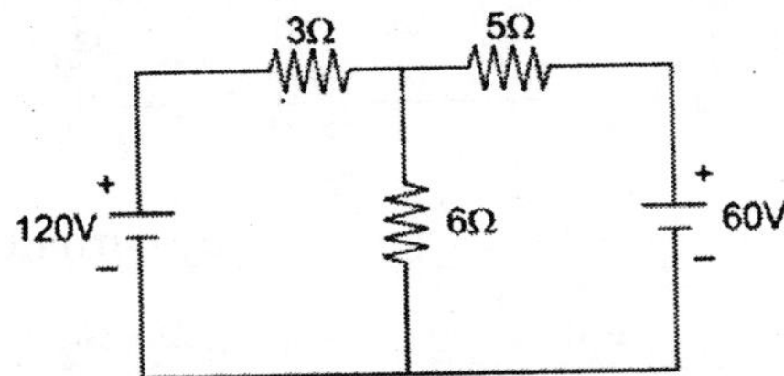

Solution: Step I: Current due to only 120 V source.

60 V source is short circuited.

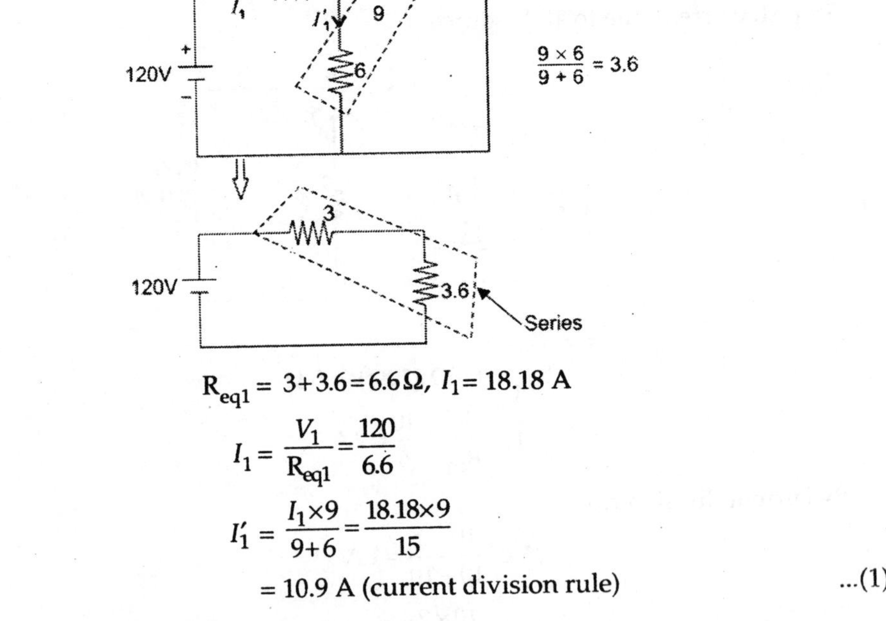

$$R_{eq1} = 3 + 3.6 = 6.6\,\Omega,\ I_1 = 18.18 \text{ A}$$

$$\therefore \quad I_1 = \frac{V_1}{R_{eq1}} = \frac{120}{6.6}$$

$$\therefore \quad I_1' = \frac{I_1 \times 9}{9+6} = \frac{18.18 \times 9}{15}$$

$$= 10.9 \text{ A (current division rule)} \qquad \text{...(1)}$$

Step II: Current due to 60 V source only:

120 V source is shorted

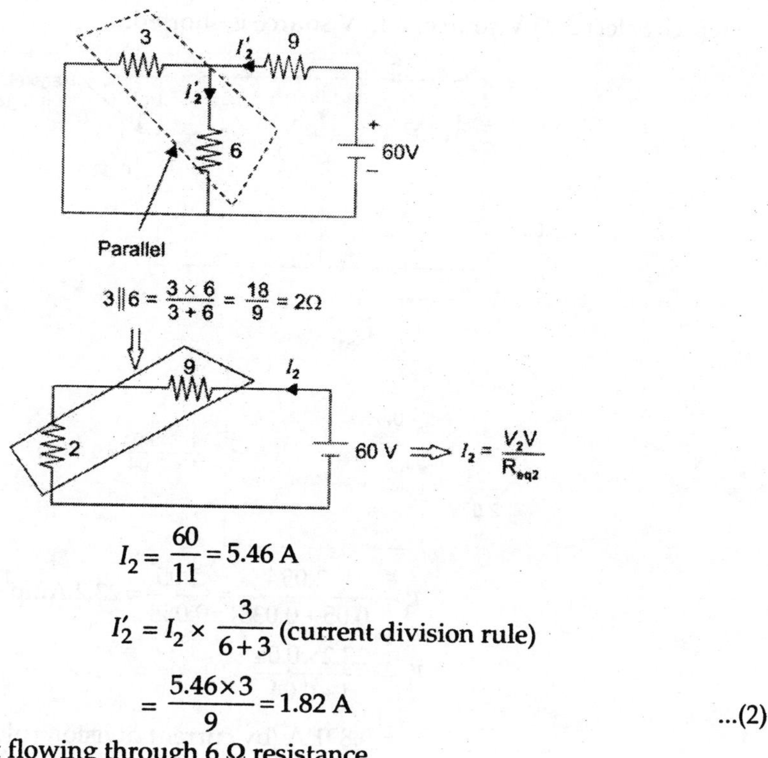

$$I_2 = \frac{60}{11} = 5.46 \text{ A}$$

$$I_2' = I_2 \times \frac{3}{6+3} \text{ (current division rule)}$$

$$= \frac{5.46 \times 3}{9} = 1.82 \text{ A} \qquad \text{...(2)}$$

Step III: Current flowing through 6 Ω resistance,
From Eqs (1) and (2), we get

$$I = I_1' + I_2'$$

$$= 10.9 + 1.82 = 12.72 \text{ A}$$

Ans.

Example 7: By superposition theorem, find the current in resistance 'R' shown in figure below. **[UPTU Sem-I, 2004-05]**

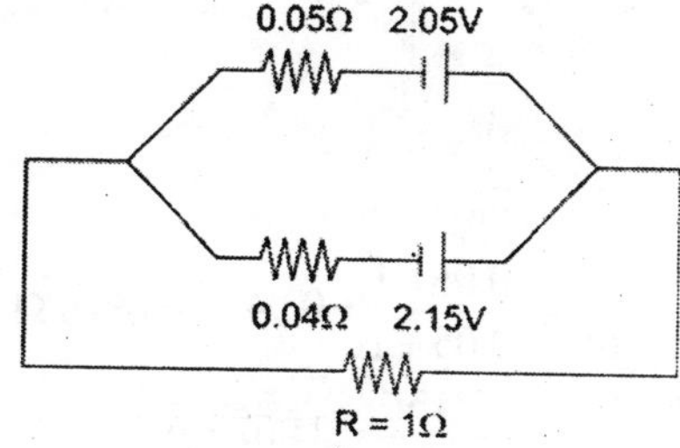

Solution: Step I: Redraw the above given figure.

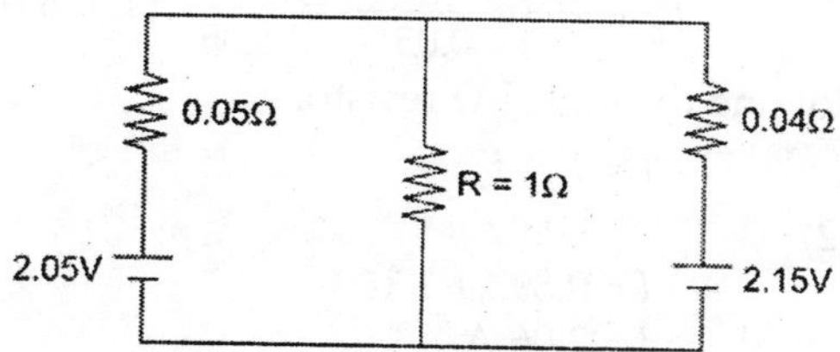

Step II: Select 2.05 V source, 2.15 V source is shorted.

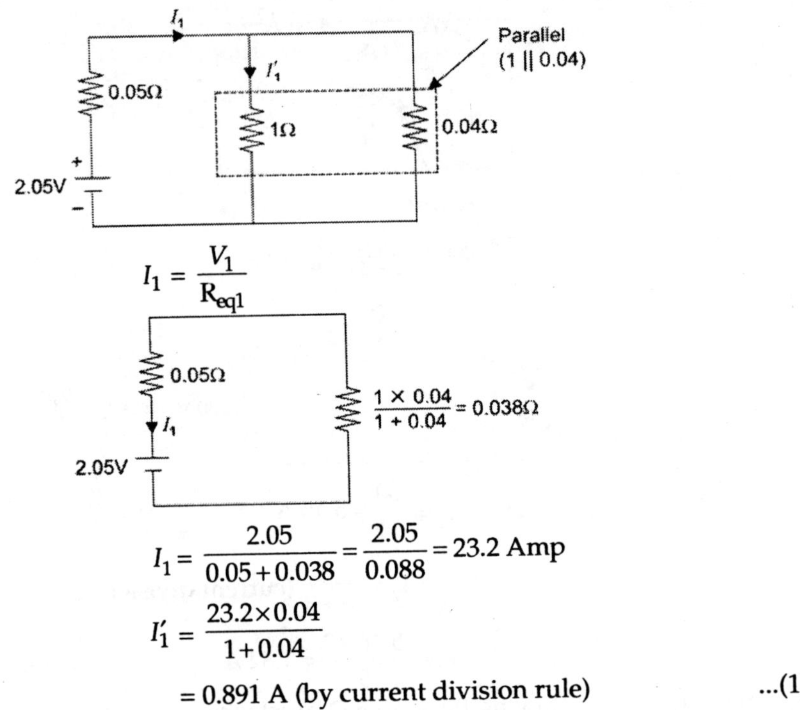

$$I_1 = \frac{V_1}{R_{eq1}}$$

$$\therefore \qquad I_1 = \frac{2.05}{0.05+0.038} = \frac{2.05}{0.088} = 23.2 \text{ Amp}$$

$$I'_1 = \frac{23.2 \times 0.04}{1+0.04}$$

$$= 0.891 \text{ A (by current division rule)} \qquad \text{...(1)}$$

Step III: Select 2.15 V source, 2.05 V source is shorted.

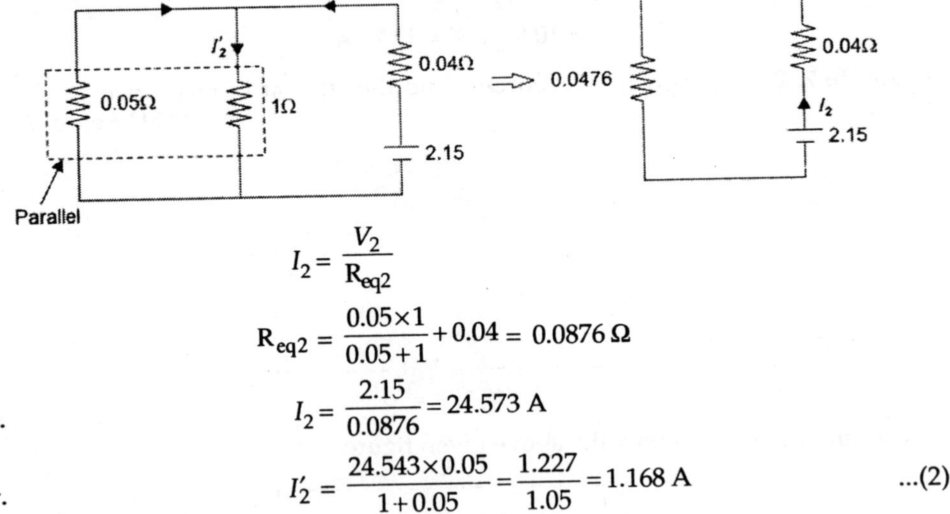

$$I_2 = \frac{V_2}{R_{eq2}}$$

$$R_{eq2} = \frac{0.05 \times 1}{0.05+1} + 0.04 = 0.0876\ \Omega$$

$$\therefore \qquad I_2 = \frac{2.15}{0.0876} = 24.573 \text{ A}$$

$$\therefore \qquad I'_2 = \frac{24.543 \times 0.05}{1+0.05} = \frac{1.227}{1.05} = 1.168 \text{ A} \qquad \text{...(2)}$$

Step IV: Current flowing through 1 Ω resistor

$$\therefore \qquad I = I'_1 + I'_2$$

From Eqs (1) and (2)

$$I = 0.892 + 1.169$$

$$I = 2.06 \text{ A}$$

Ans.

Example 8: Determine current through 8 Ω resistor in the following network figure below using superposition theorem.

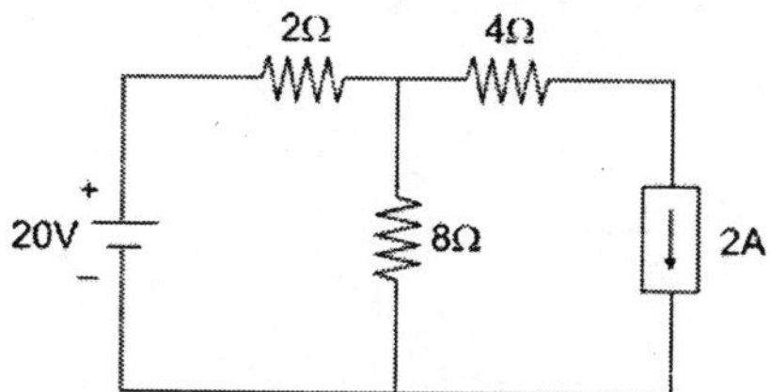

Solution: Step I: Select 20 V source, 2 A current source is open.

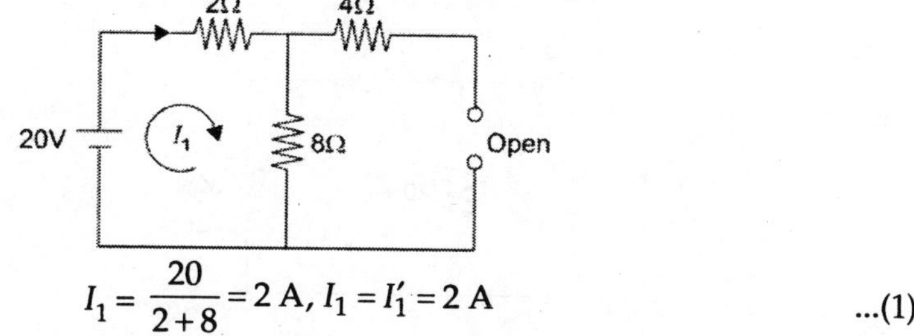

$$I_1 = \frac{20}{2+8} = 2\text{ A},\ I_1 = I_1' = 2\text{ A} \qquad ...(1)$$

Step II: Select 2 A current source, 20 V source is shorted.

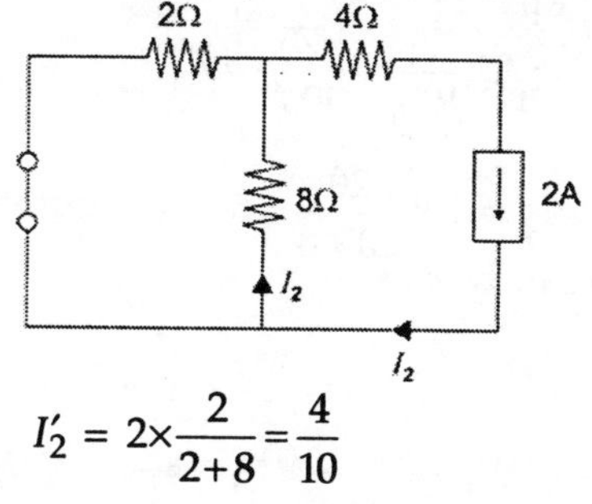

$\therefore$

$$I_2' = 2\times\frac{2}{2+8} = \frac{4}{10}$$

$= 0.4$ A (by current division rule) ...(2)

Step III: Calculate current through 8 Ω resistance is

From Eqs (1) and (2), we get

$$I = I_1' - I'_2$$

$$= 2 - 0.4$$

$= 1.6$ A (from top to bottom)

Example 9: For the circuit of figure below, find I using superposition theorem.

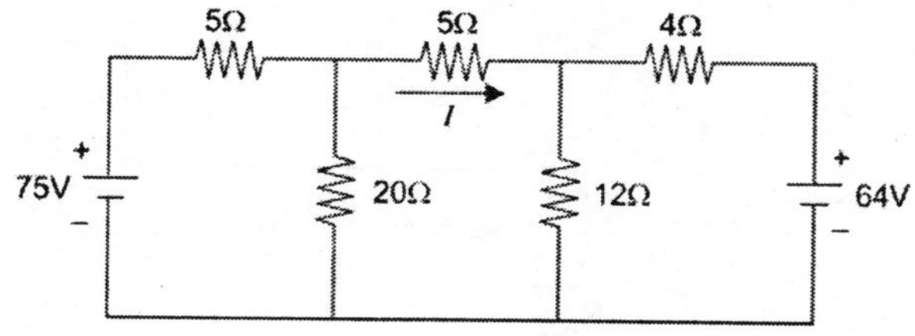

Solution: Step I: Select 75 V source, 64 source is shorted.

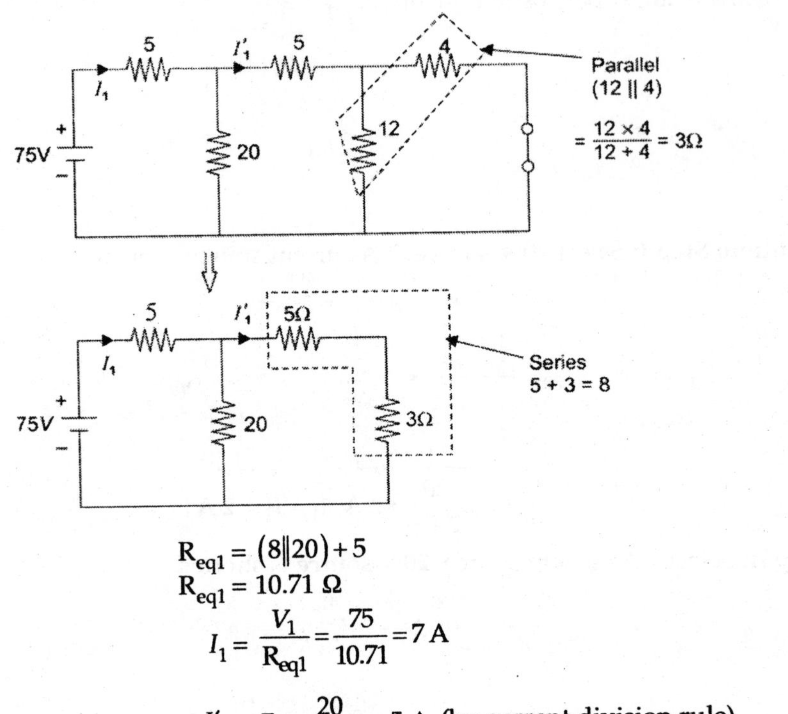

$$R_{eq1} = (8\|20) + 5$$
$$R_{eq1} = 10.71\ \Omega$$

$\therefore$ $$I_1 = \frac{V_1}{R_{eq1}} = \frac{75}{10.71} = 7\text{ A}$$

$\therefore$ $$I_2' = 7 \times \frac{20}{20+8} = 5\text{ A (by current division rule)} \qquad ...(1)$$

Step II: Select 64 V source only.
75 V source is shorted.

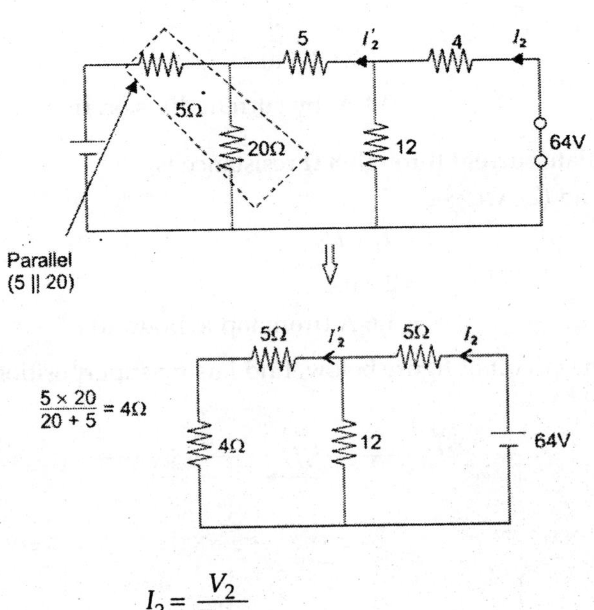

$\therefore$ $$I_2 = \frac{V_2}{R_{eq2}}$$

$$\therefore \quad R_{eq2} = (9\|12) + 4$$

$$= \frac{12 \times 9}{12 + 9} + 4 = 9.142\ \Omega$$

$$I_2 = \frac{64}{9.142} = 7\ \text{A}$$

$$\therefore \quad I_2' = 7 \times \frac{12}{12 + 9} = 4\ \text{A} \qquad \text{...(2)}$$

Step III: Calculate the current 'I'.
From Eqs (1) and (2), we get

$$I = I_1' - I_2'$$

$$= 5 - 4 = 1\ \text{A}$$

Ans.

EXAMPLES BASED ON THEVENIN THEOREM

Example 1: Find current through branch AB using Thevenin's theorem shown in figure below. **[Sem-1, 2003-04]**

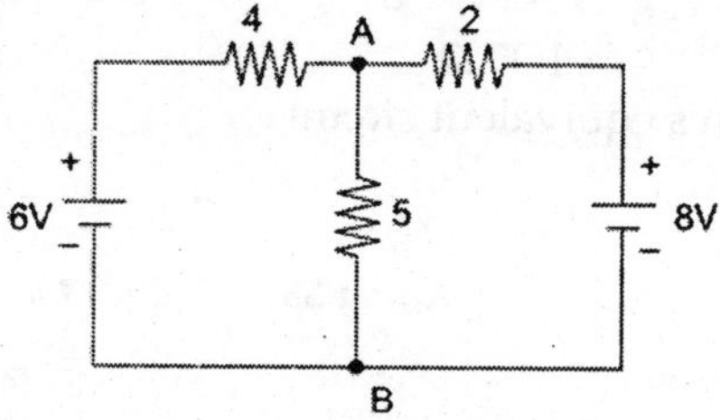

Solution: Step I: Remove the load resistance 5 Ω

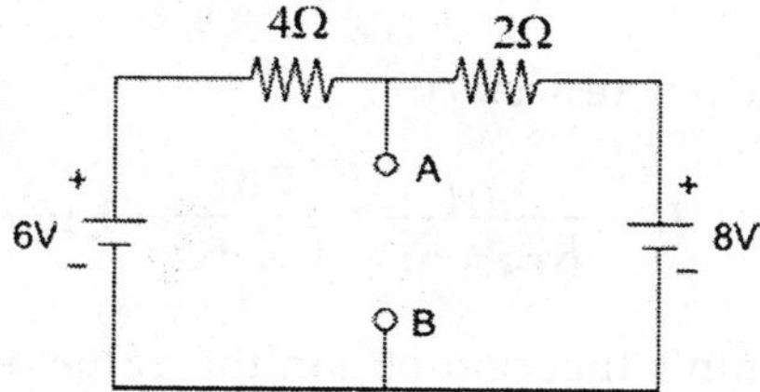

Step II: To find open circuit voltage V_{AB} or V_{TH}.

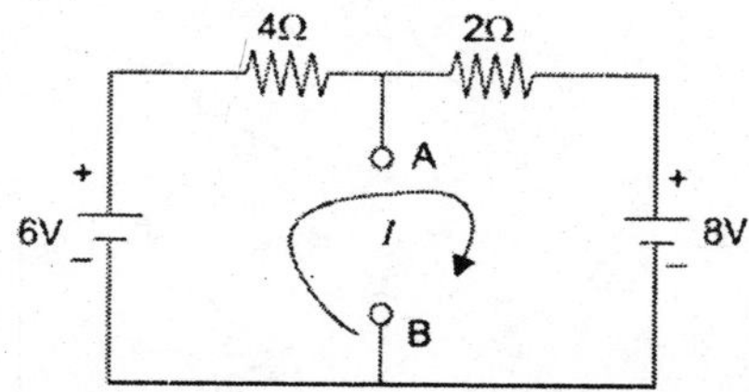

Apply KVL in loop.

$$6 - 4I - 2I - 8 = 0$$

$$I = -\frac{2}{6} = -0.33\ \text{A}$$

Open circuit voltage V_{AB} or V_{TH}

$$V_{TH} = 6 - 4I$$
$$= 6 - 4 \times (-0.333)$$
$$= 6 + 1.332$$
$$= 7.33 \text{ V}$$

Step III: To find open circuit resistance across terminal *AB* when 6 V and 8 V are shorted, i.e. R_{TH}.

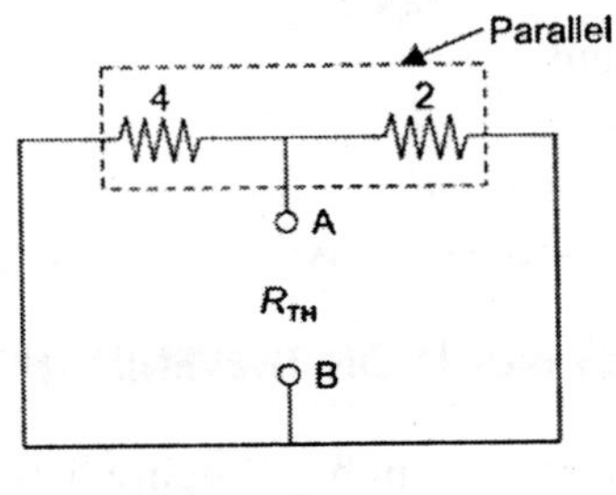

$$R_{TH} = \frac{4 \times 2}{4+2} = \frac{8}{6}$$
$$= 1.33\ \Omega$$

Step IV: Draw Thevenin's equivalent circuit.

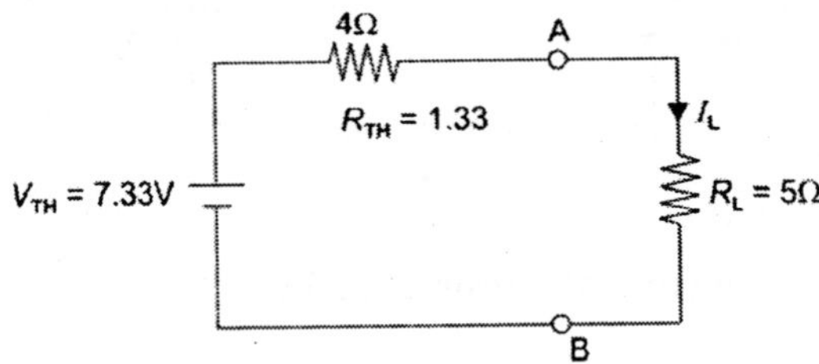

Step V: Current through 5 Ω resistance

$$I_L = \frac{V_{TH}}{R_{TH} + R_L} = \frac{7.33}{1.33+5} = 1.16 \text{ A}$$ **Ans.**

Example 2: Using Thevenin's theorem obtain the value of current flowing in the galvanometer branch. Assume that the resistance of galvanometer is 50 Ω.

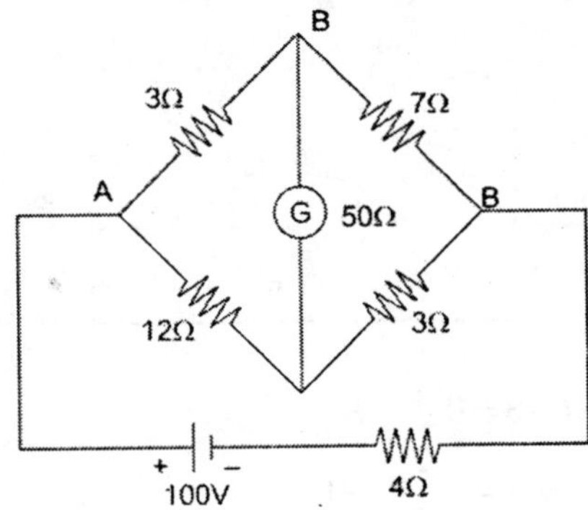

Solution: Step I: Remove the galvanometer from the source, the given circuit gets modified as shown in figure below.

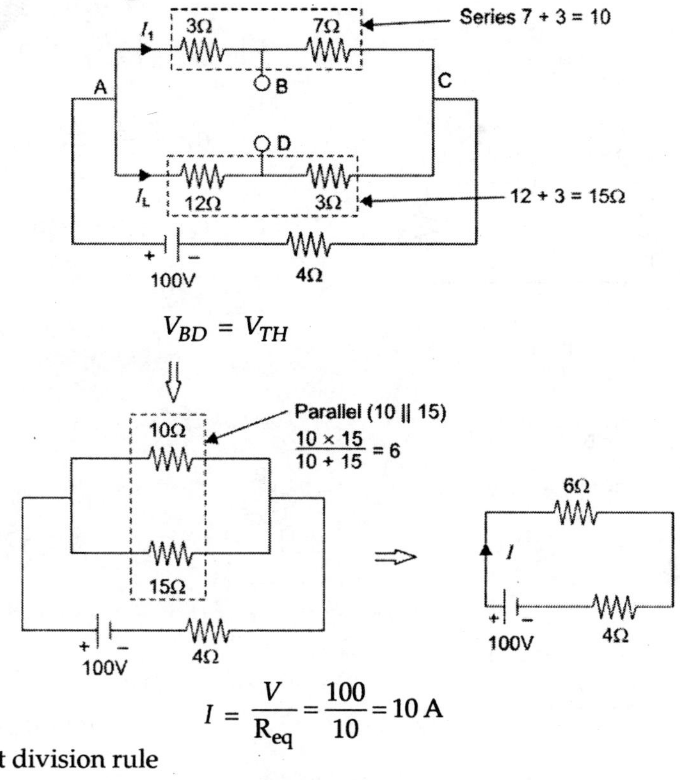

$$I = \frac{V}{R_{eq}} = \frac{100}{10} = 10 \text{ A}$$

By current division rule

$$I_1 = \frac{10 \times (12+3)}{15+10} = 6 \text{ A}$$

$$I_2 = \frac{10 \times 10}{15+10} = 4 \text{ A}$$

From above figure

Voltage drop across $AB = 3 \times I_1 = 3 \times 6 = 18$ V

Voltage drop across $AD = 12 I_2 = 12 \times 4 = 48$ V

$$V_{BD} = (100 - 18) - (100 - 48) = 82 - 52 = 30 \text{ V}$$

$$V_{TH} = V_{BD} = 30 \text{ V}$$

Step II: Calculate Thevenin's equivalent resistance.

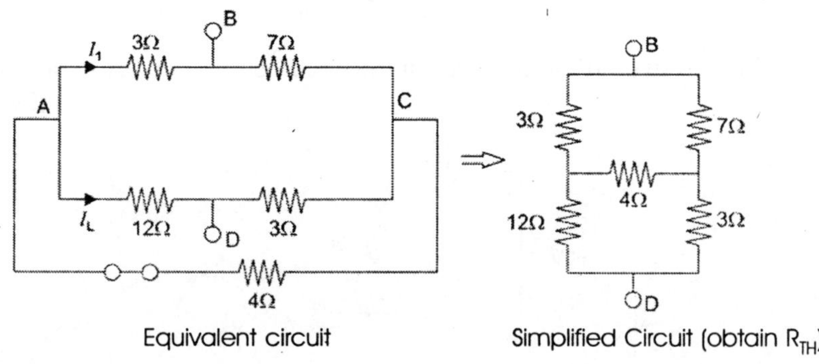

Equivalent circuit

Simplified Circuit (obtain R_{TH})

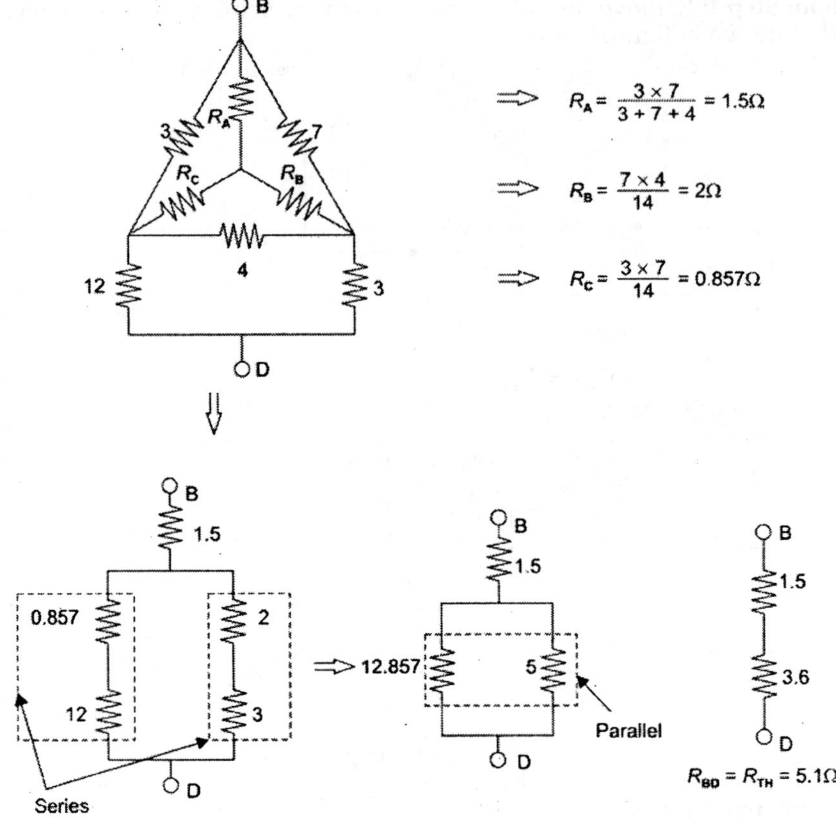

Step III: Draw Thevenin's equivalent circuit and obtain current.

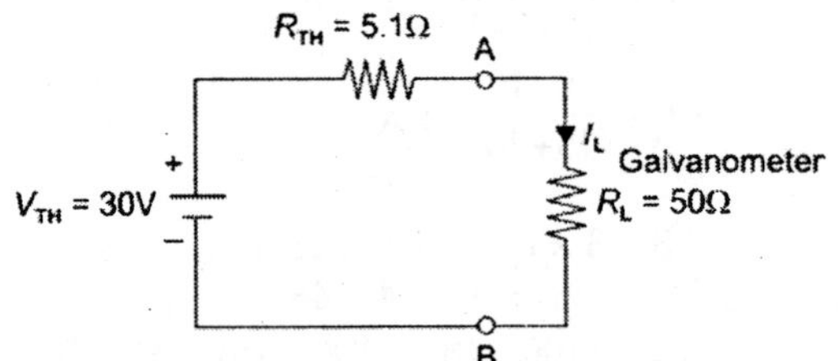

Step V: Calculate galvanometer current.

$$\therefore \quad I_L = \frac{V_{TH}}{R_{TH} + R_L} = \frac{30}{5.1+50} = 0.54 \text{ A} \qquad \textbf{Ans.}$$

Example 3: Find Thevenin's equivalent of the circuit shown in figure below.

[Sem-I, 04-05].

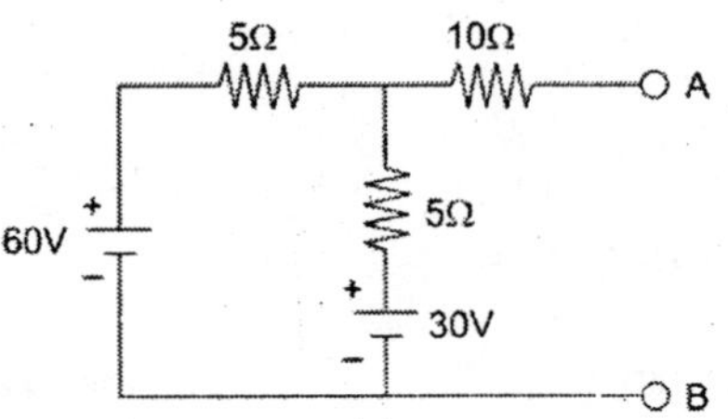

Solution: Step I: Calculate the open circuit voltage across *AB* terminals.

Current in 10 Ω resistance is zero. Apply KVL to the loop.

$$60 - 5I - 5I - 30 = 0$$

$$I = \frac{30}{10} = 3 \text{ A}$$

$$V_{AB} = V_{TH} = 30 + 5I$$

$$= 30 + 5 \times 3 = 45 \text{ V}$$

Step II: Calculate equivalent Thevenin resistance (60 V and 30 V source is shorted).

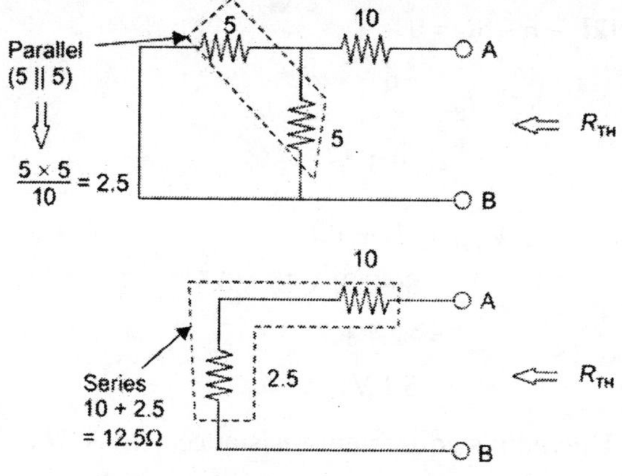

$R_{TH} = 12.5\ \Omega$

Step III: Draw Thevenin's equivalent circuit.

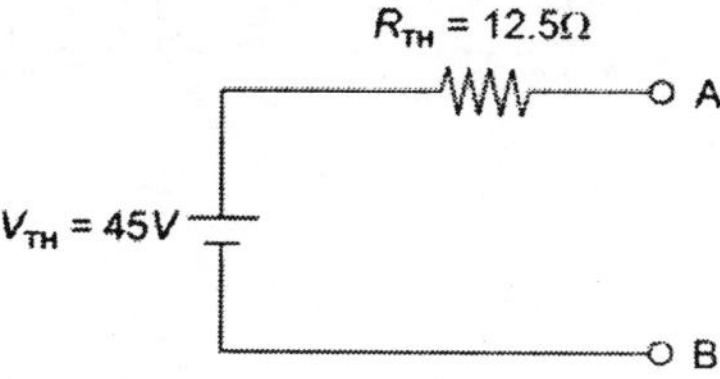

Example 4: Find current *I* in figure below by using of Thevenin's theorem.

[Sem-II, 05-06]

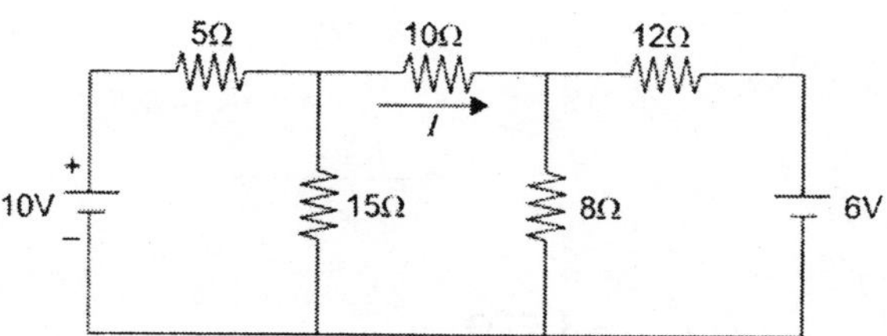

Solution: Step I: Remove 10 Ω resistance marked terminal *AB*.

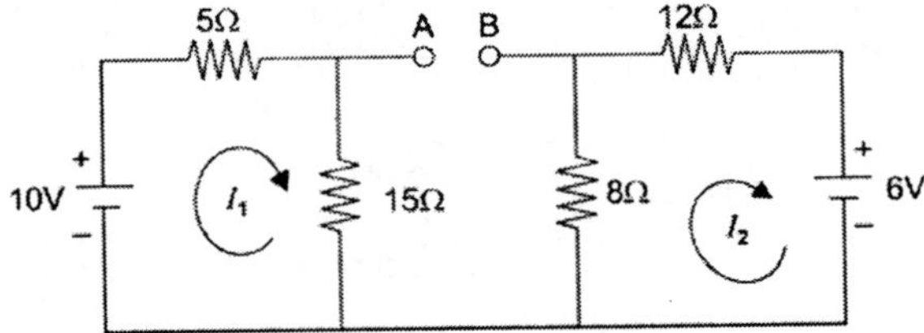

Calculate $V_{AB} = V_{TH}$.

Apply KVL in loop 1.

$$10 - 5I_1 - 15I_1 = 0$$

$$I_1 = \frac{10}{20}$$

$$= 0.5 \text{ A}$$

Apply KVL in loop 2.

$$-12I_2 - 6 - 8I_2 = 0$$

$$I_2 = \frac{-6}{20}$$

$$= -0.3 \text{ A}$$

For V_{TH}

$$V_{TH} = 8I_2 + 15I_1$$

$$= 8(-0.3) + 15 \times 0.5$$

$$= -2.4 + 7.5$$

$$= 5.1 \text{ V}$$

Step II: To find Thevenin's equivalent resistance across *AB*.

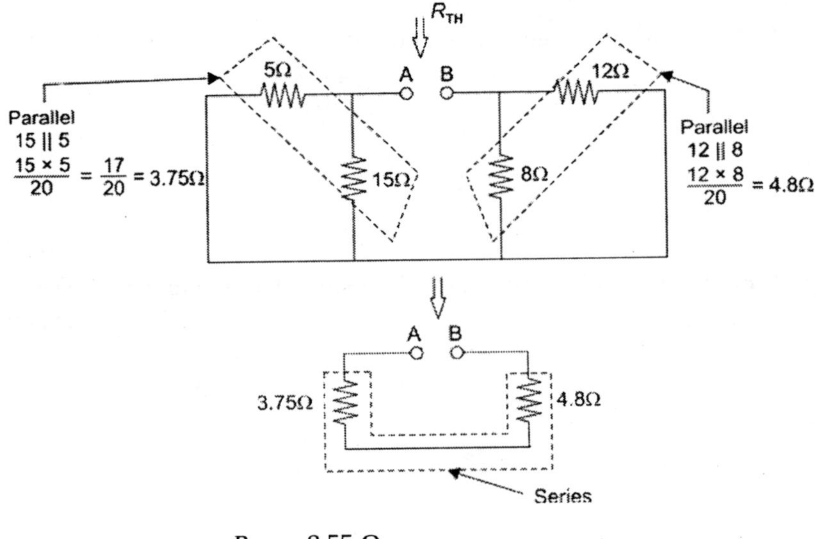

$$R_{TH} = 8.55 \ \Omega$$

Step III: Draw Thevenin's equivalent circuit diagram

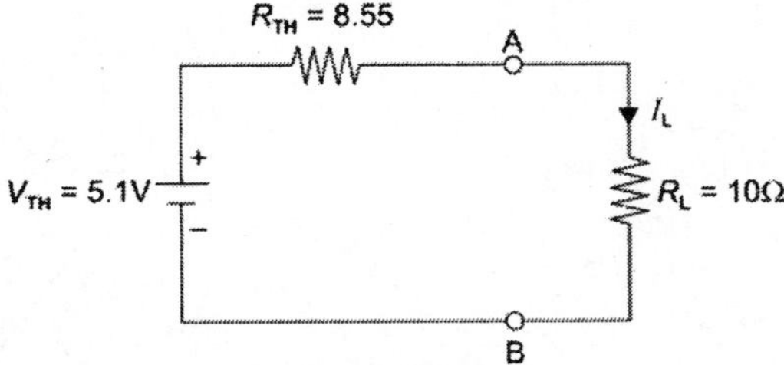

Step IV: Calcualte current in load resistance

$$I_L = \frac{5.1}{8.55+10} = \frac{5.1}{18.55} = 0.275 \text{ A}$$ **Ans.**

Example 5: Use Thevenin's theorem to find the current in the branch '*BD*' of the network shown in figure below.

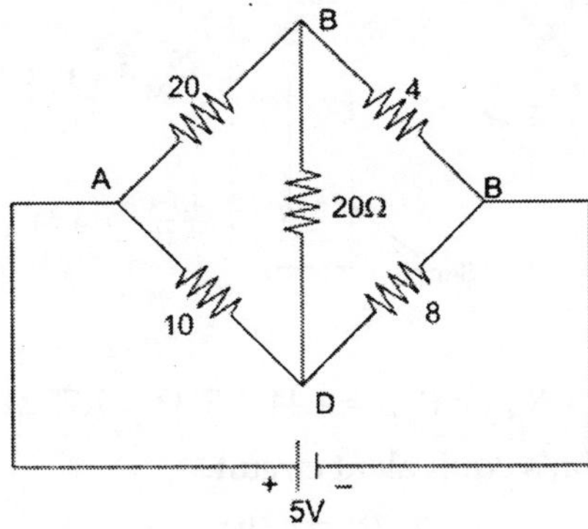

Solution: Step I: Remove the load resistance 20 Ω. Calculate the open circuit voltage.

$$V_{BD} = V_{TH}$$

$$V_{BD} = V_{TH} = V_B - V_D$$

$$= \left(5 - \frac{20\times 5}{20+4}\right) - \left(5 - \frac{10\times 5}{10+5}\right) \quad \text{(by voltage division rule)}$$

$$V_{TH} = -1.38 \text{ V} \quad \text{(i.e. } V_D \text{ is at higher potential than } V_A)$$

Step II: Calculate Thevenin's equivalent resistance across BD terminal when 5 V source is shorted.

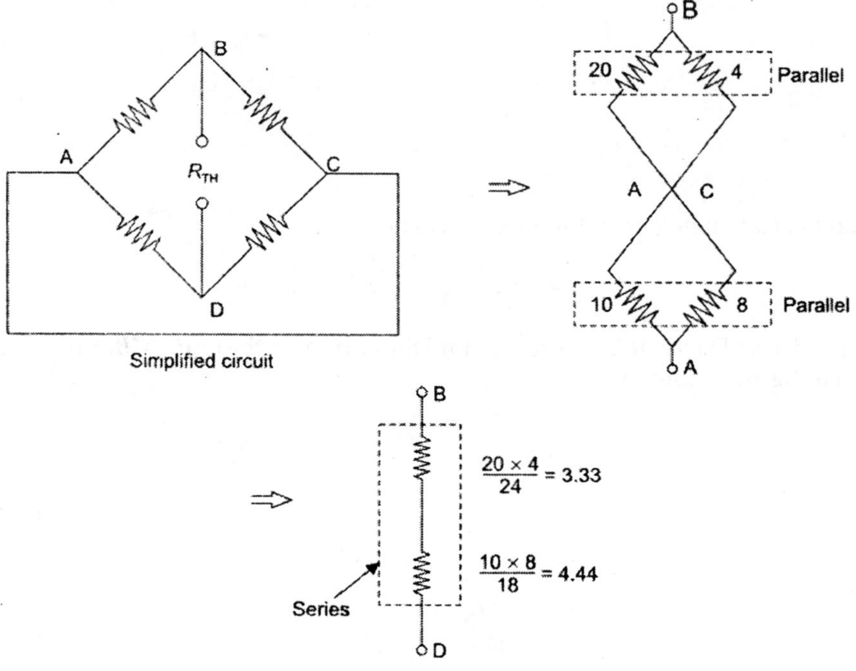

$$R_{BD} = R_{TH} = 4.44 + 3.33 = 7.77\ \Omega$$

Step III: Draw Thevenin's equivalent circuit.

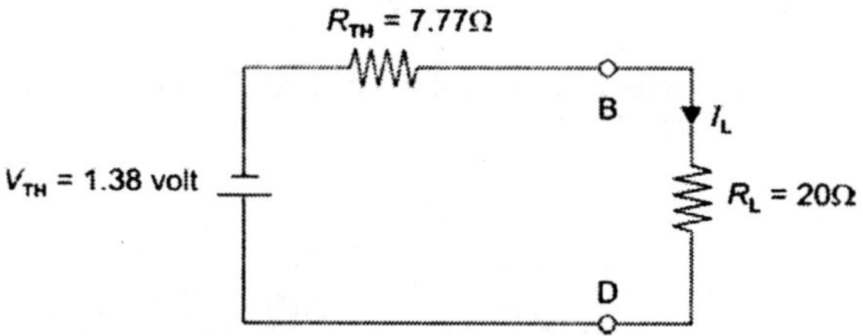

Step IV: Calculate current through 20 Ω resistance.

$$\therefore \qquad I_L = \frac{V_{TH}}{R_{TH} + R_L} = \frac{1.38}{7.77 + 20} = 0.05 \text{ A}$$ **Ans.**

Example 6: Find the Thevenin's equivalent of the network shown in figure below between terminal 'a' and 'b'. **[Sem-II, 04-05]**

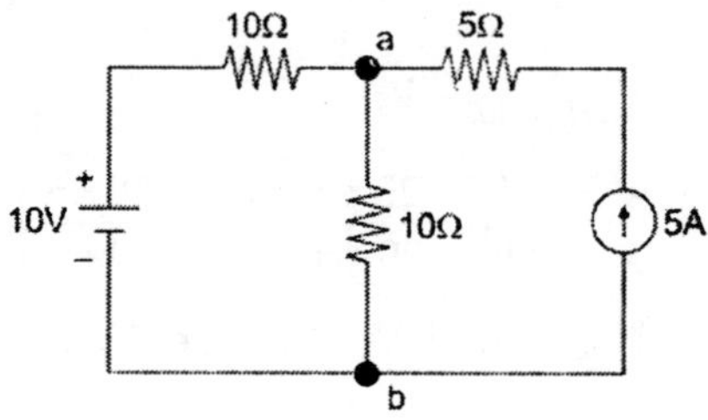

Solution: Step I: Remove the load resistance 10 Ω.

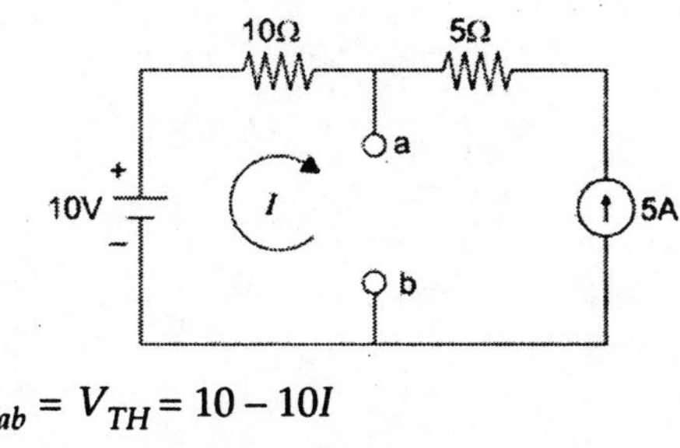

$$V_{ab} = V_{TH} = 10 - 10I$$
$$= 10 - 10 \times -5$$
$$= 60 \text{ V}$$

Step II: To find open circuit resistance when 10 V source is shorted and 5 A current source is opened.

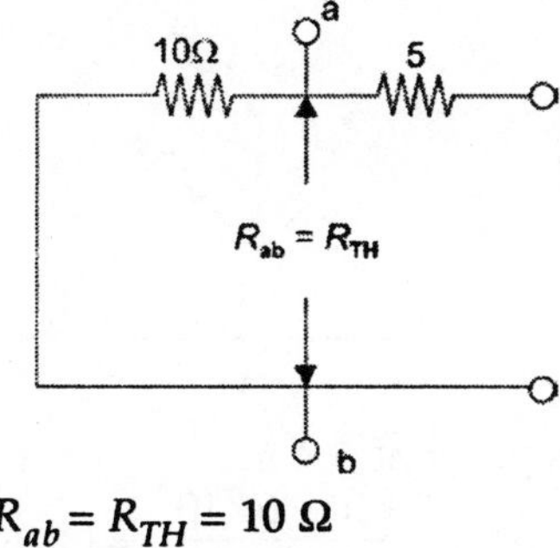

$$R_{ab} = R_{TH} = 10\ \Omega$$

Step III: Draw Thevenin's equivalent circuit.

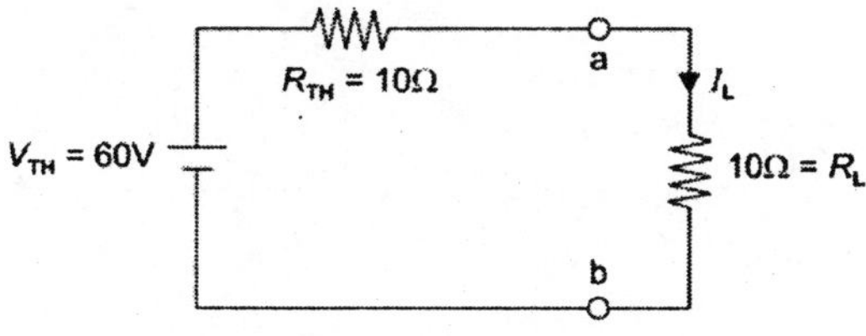

Thevenin's equivalent circuit

Step IV: Calculate current through 10 Ω.

$$\therefore \qquad I_L = \frac{V_{TH}}{R_{TH} + R_L}$$

$$= \frac{60}{10+10}$$

$$= 3 \text{ A}$$ **Ans.**

Example 7: Using Thevenin's theorem find the current *I* shown in figure below. **[Sem-I, 02-03]**

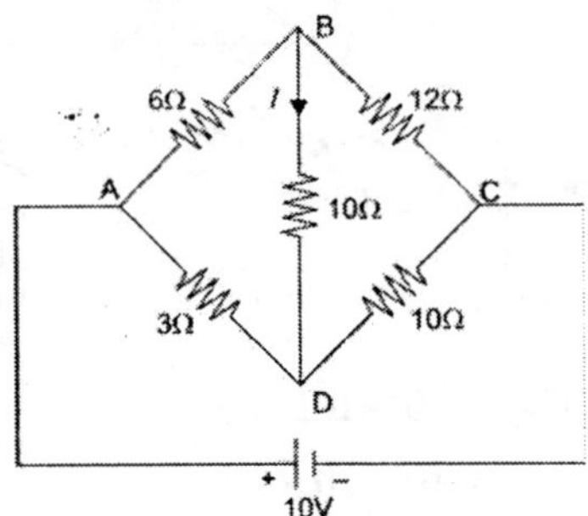

Solution: Step I: Remove the 10 Ω resistance from branch *BD*.
Calculate open circuit voltage, i.e. $V_{BD} = V_{TH}$.

$$V_{TH} = V_{AD} - V_{AB}$$

$$= \frac{3\times10}{13} - \frac{6\times10}{18} = -1.025 \text{ V} \quad \text{(by voltage division rule)}$$

(i.e. point D is at higher potential than point B)

Step II: To find open circuit resistance across terminal *BD*, when 10 V source as shorted.

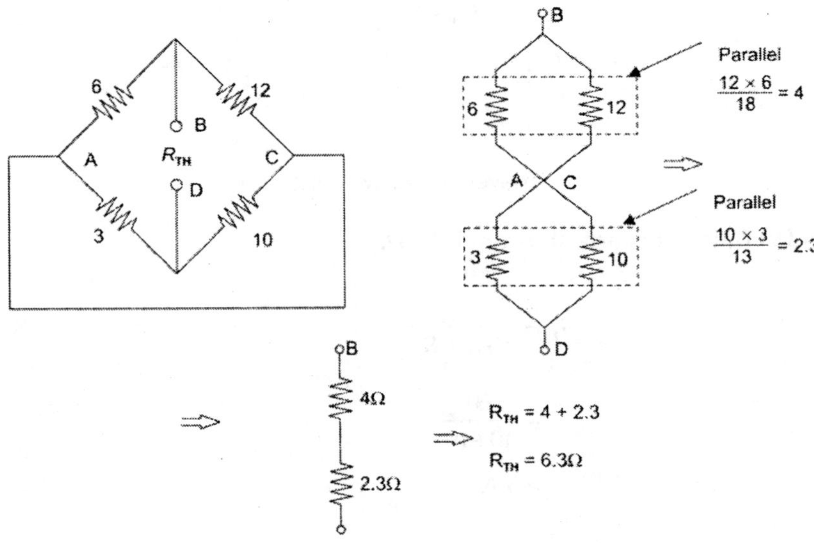

Step III: Draw Thevenin's equivalent circuit.

Step IV: Calculate current in *BD* branch.

$$\therefore \qquad I_L = \frac{-1.022}{6.3+10} = 1.0627 \text{ A} \qquad \textbf{Ans.}$$

Example 8: Find Thevenin's equivalent circuit across *AB* shown in figure below.

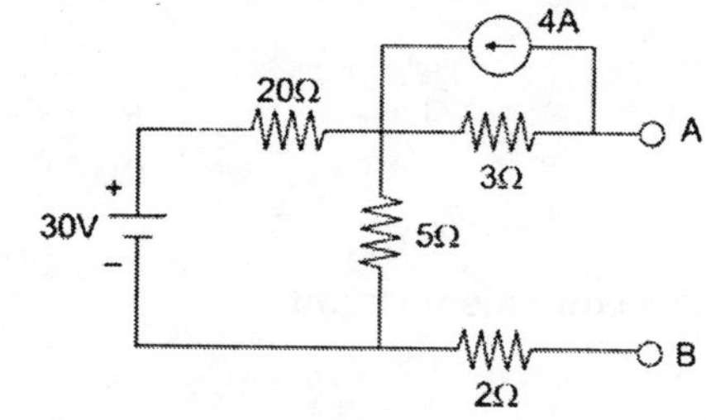

Solution: Step I: Convert current source 4 A to voltage source.

$$V = 4 \times 3 = 12 \text{ V}$$

Redraw the circuit

Step II: Find V_{TH} across terminal '*AB*'

Apply KVL

$$30 - 20I - 5I = 0$$

$$I = \frac{30}{25} = \frac{6}{5} = 1.2 \text{ A}$$

$$V_{AB} = 5 \times 1.2 - 12$$

$$V_{TH} = -6 \text{ V}$$

Step III: Find R_{TH} (when all voltage source are shorted).

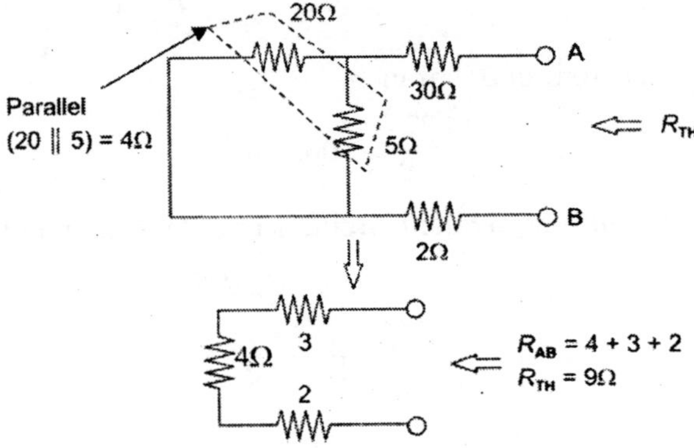

Step IV: Draw Thevenin's equivalent circuit.

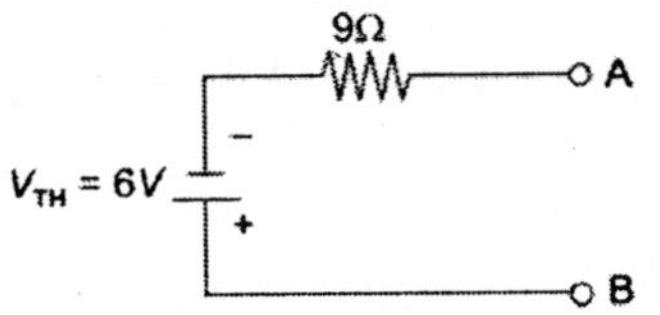

EXAMPLES BASED ON NORTON'S THEOREM

Example 1: For the circuit shown in figure below, draw the Norton's equivalent circuit.

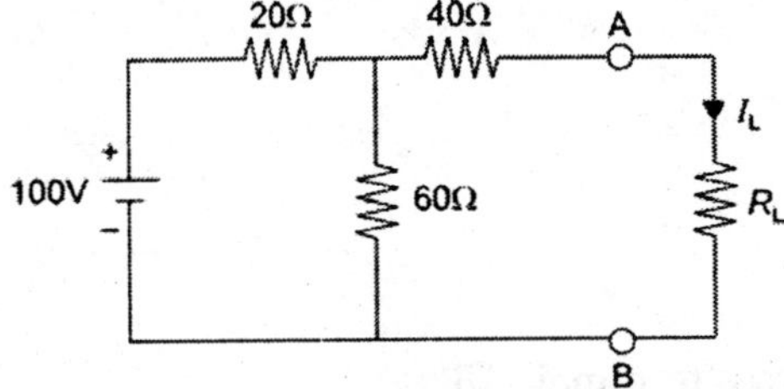

Solution: Step I: Remove the R_L and short terminal AB.

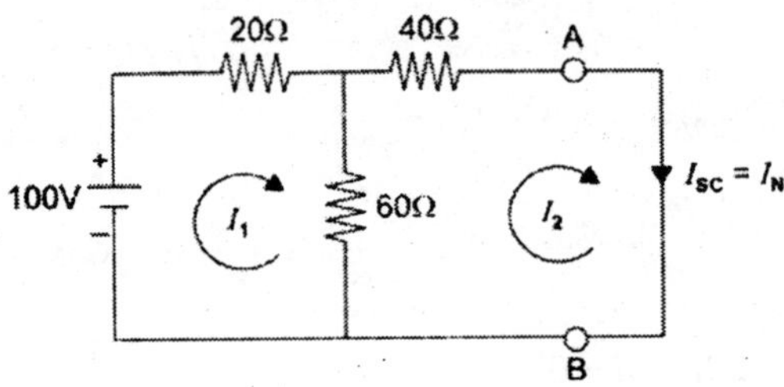

Step II: Calculate short circuit current (i.e. $I_{SC} = I_N$)
Apply KVL in loop 1.

$$100 - 20I_1 - 60(I_1 - I_2) = 0$$

$$100 - 80I_1 + 60I_2 = 0$$

$$8I_1 - 6I_2 = 10 \quad \text{...(1)}$$

Apply KVL in loop 2.

$$-60(I_2 - I_1) - 40I_2 = 0$$

$$-60I_2 + 60I_1 - 40I_2 = 0$$

$$100I_2 = 60I_1$$

$$I_1 = \frac{100}{60}I_2 = \frac{5}{3}I_2 \quad \text{...(2)}$$

From Eqs (1) and (2), we get

$$I_2 = 1.363 \text{ A}$$

$$I_2 = I_N = 1.363 \text{ A}$$

Step III: To find R_N (when voltage source 100 V is shorted)

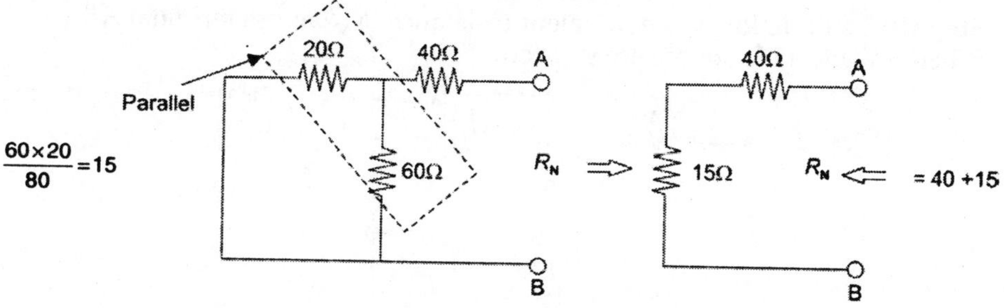

$$R_N = 55\ \Omega$$

Step IV: Draw Norton's equivalent circuit.

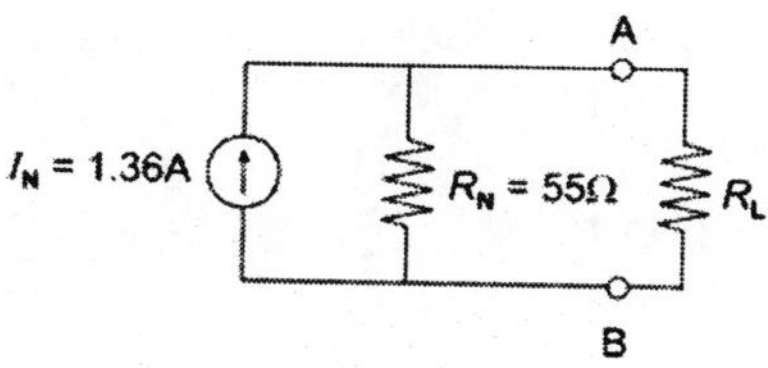

Example 2: Using Norton's theorem calculate current flowing in 2 Ω resistance from the network shown in figure below. **[Sem-I, 2001-02]**

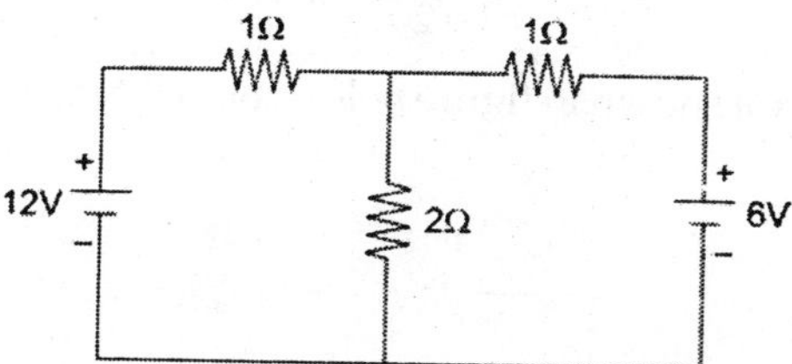

Solution: Step I: Remove the 2 Ω resistance, marked terminal *AB* and shorted the branch *AB*.

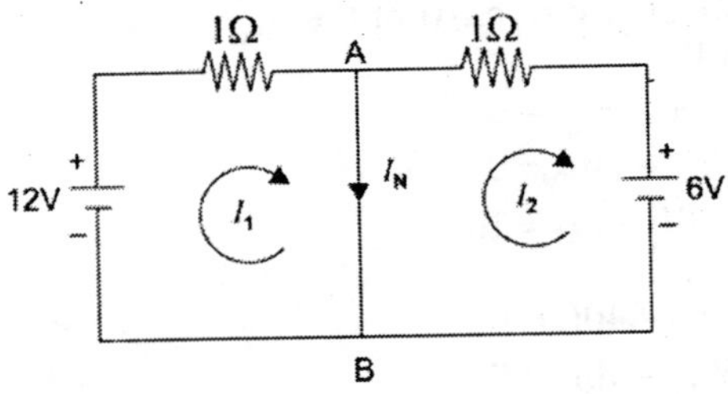

Step II: Calculate the current 'I_N' in branch AB.
Apply KVL in loop 1

$$12 - 1I_1 = 0$$
$$I_1 = 12 \text{ A}$$

Apply KVL in loop 2.

$$-1I_2 - 6 = 0$$
$$I_2 = -6 \text{ A}$$
$$I_N = I_1 - I_2$$
$$= 12 - (-6) = 18 \text{ A}$$

Step III: To find Norton's equivalent resistance 'R_N' across terminal AB.
When 6 V and 12 V source are shorted.

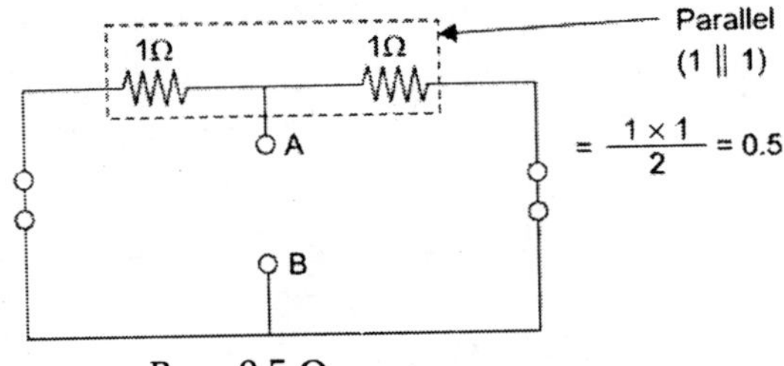

$$R_N = 0.5 \ \Omega$$

Step IV: Draw Norton's equivalent circuit.

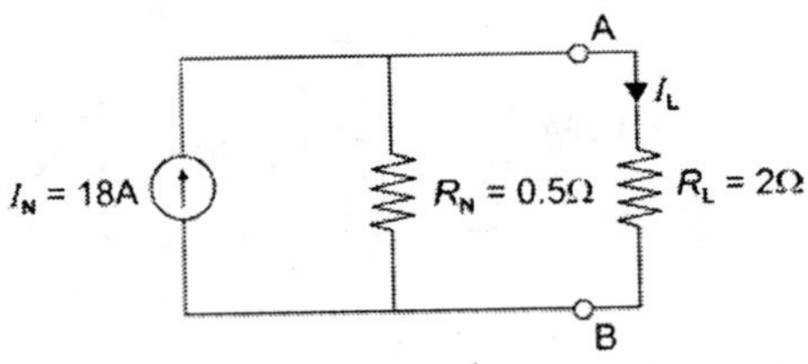

Step V: Calculate current in 2 Ω.

$$I_N = \frac{18 \times 0.5}{0.5 + 2} = 3.6 \text{ A}$$ **Ans.**

Example 3: For the circuit shown in figure below, obtain Norton's current and equivalent resistance seen from 'ab'. **[Sem-I, 2003-04]**

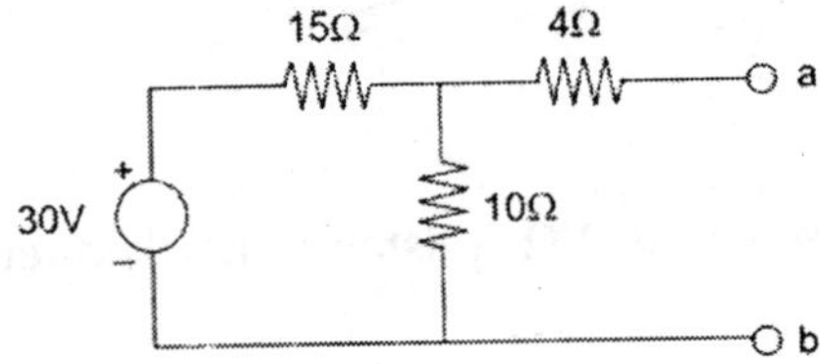

Solution: Step I: Short terminal *'ab'*.
To find short circuit current in *'ab'* (I_N).

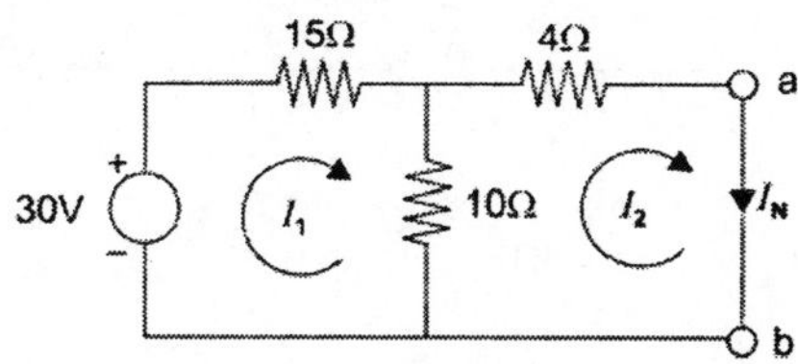

Apply KVL in loop 1.

$$30-15I_1-10(I_1-I_2)=0$$
$$30-25I_1+10I_2=0$$
$$25I_1-10I_2=30$$
$$5I_1-2I_2=6 \qquad ...(1)$$

Apply KVL in loop 2.

$$-10(I_2-I_1)-4I_2=0$$
$$-14I_2+10I_1=0$$
$$7I_2=5I_1 \qquad ...(2)$$

Solving Eqs (1) and (2), we get

$$I_2=1.2\text{ A}$$
$$I_N=I_2=1.2\text{ A}$$

Step III: To find Norton's equivalent resistance across terminal 'ab'.
When voltage source 30 V is shorted.

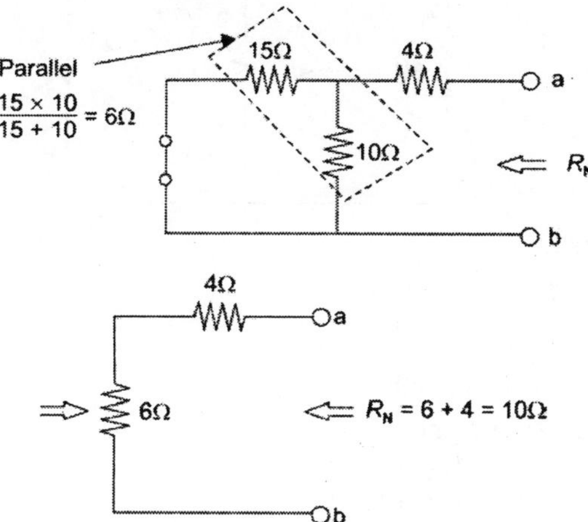

Step III: Draw Norton's equivalent circuit.

a

$I_N = 1.2\text{A}$ $R_N = 10\Omega$

b

Example 4: Draw Norton's equivalent across *AB* and determine current flowing through 12 Ω resistor. **[Sem-II, 03-04]**

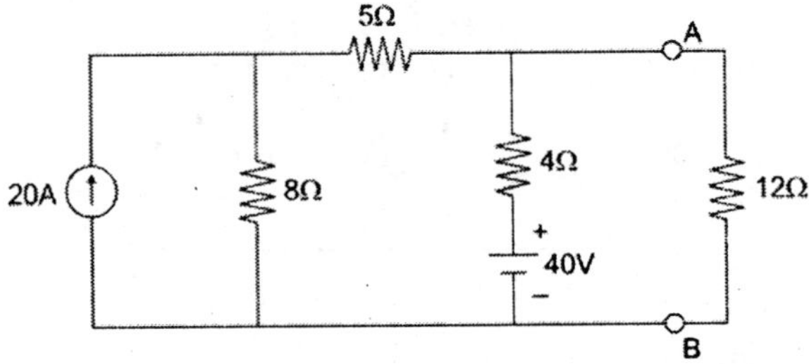

Solution: Step I: Convert the current source of 20 A into voltage source.

$$V = 20 \text{ A} \times 8\ \Omega = 160 \text{ V}$$

Above figure becomes.

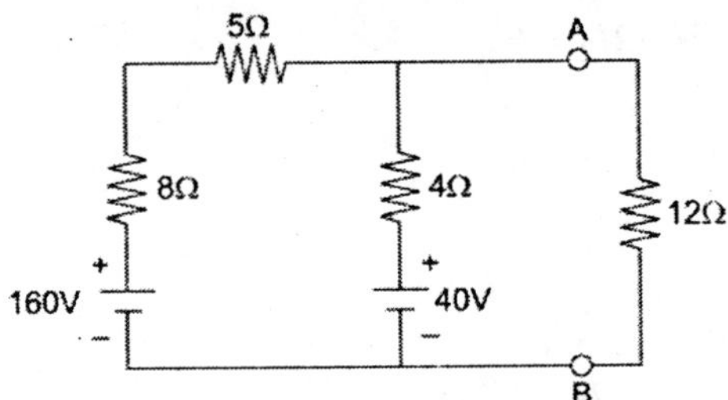

Step II: Remove the load resistance of 12 Ω and short terminal *AB*.

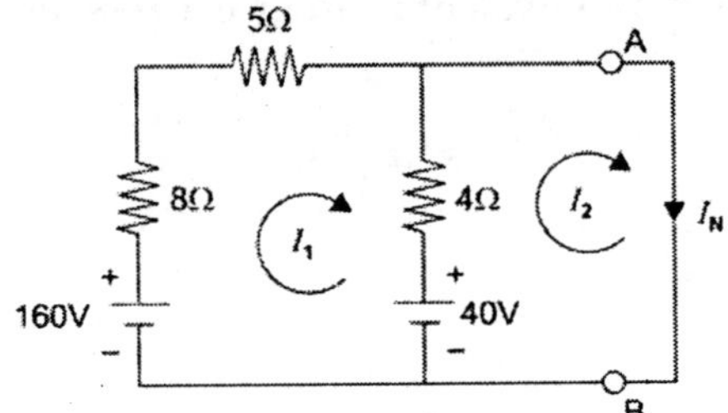

Apply KVL in loop 1.

$$160 - 8I_1 - 5I_1 - 4(I_1 - I_2) - 40 = 0 \quad ...(1)$$

Apply KVL in loop 2.

$$40 - 4(I_2 - I_1) = 0 \quad ...(2)$$

Solving Eqs (1) and (2), we get

$$I_2 = 12.3 \text{ A}$$

$$\therefore \quad I_N = I_2 = 12.3 \text{ A}$$

Step III: To find Norton's equivalent resistance R_N across terminal *AB*.
When 160 V and 40 V sources are shorted.

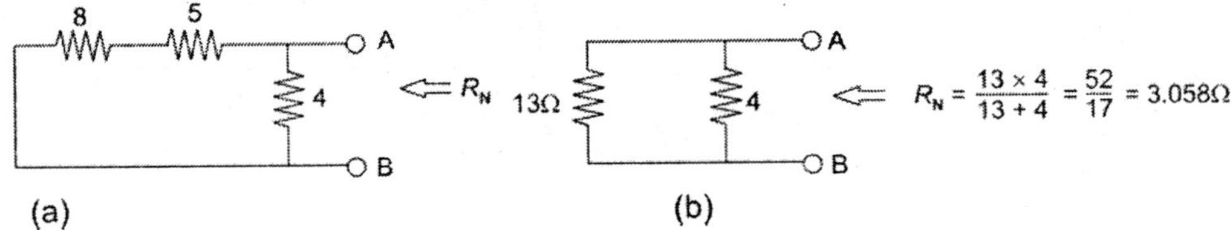

Step IV: Draw Norton's equivalent circuit.

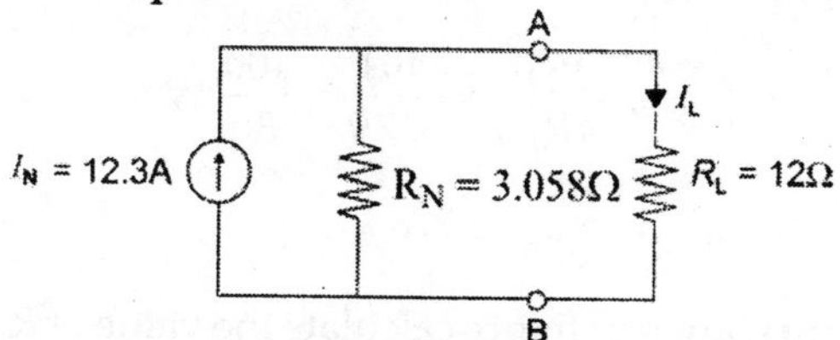

Step V: Calculate the current in 12 Ω load resistance.

$$\therefore \quad I_L = \frac{12.3 \times 3.058}{3.058 + 12} = 2.497 \text{ A} \quad \textbf{Ans.}$$

EXAMPLES BASED ON MAXIMUM POWER TRANSFER THEOREM

Example 1: In the network shown in figure below determine. **[Sem-II 02-03]**

1. The value of load resistance R_L to give maximum power transfer.
2. The power delivered to the load.

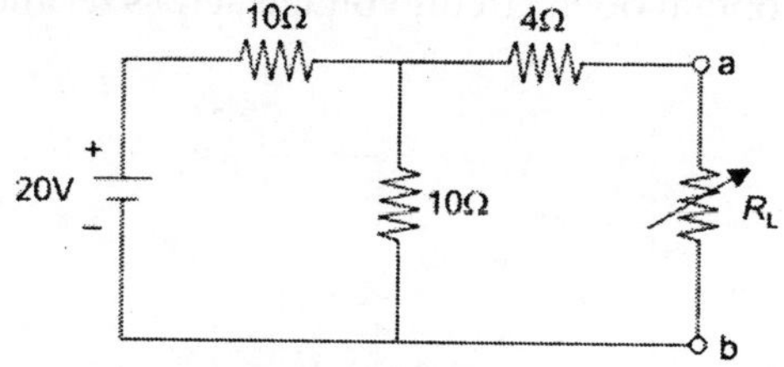

Solution: Step I: Remove the load resistance.
Find the open circuit voltage across terminal *AB*.

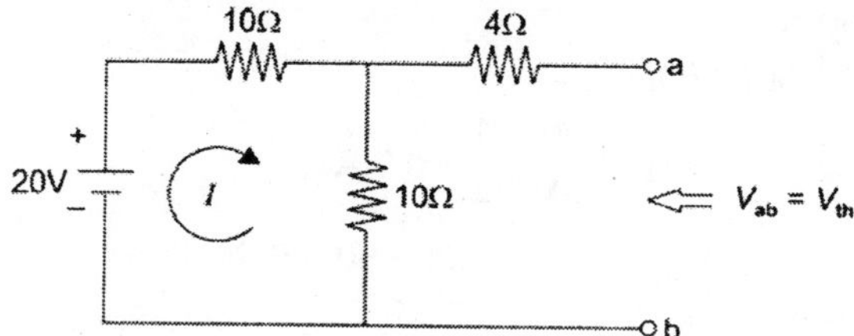

Apply KVL in loop

$$20 - 10I - 10I = 0$$

$$I = 1 \text{ A}$$

Calculate V_{ab} or V_{th}

$$\therefore \quad V_{TH} = +10I = 10 \times 1 = 10 \text{ V}$$

Step II: To find R_{TH}.

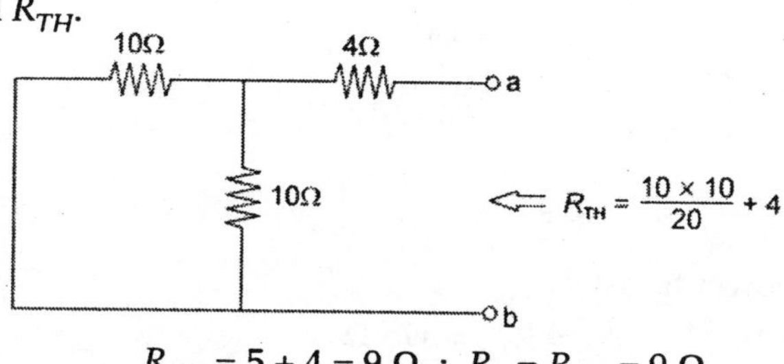

$$R_{TH} = 5 + 4 = 9\ \Omega \therefore R_L = R_{TH} = 9\ \Omega \quad \textbf{Ans.}$$

Step III: To find maximum power.

$$P_{L\max} = \frac{V_{TH}^2}{4R_{TH}} = \frac{(10)^2}{4\times 9} = \frac{100}{36}\ \text{W}$$

$$P_{L\max} = \frac{100}{36} = 2.778\ \text{W}$$ **Ans.**

Example 2: For the circuit shown in figure calculate the value of R_L to transfer maximum power to it. Also calculate the value of maximum power transfer to the load.

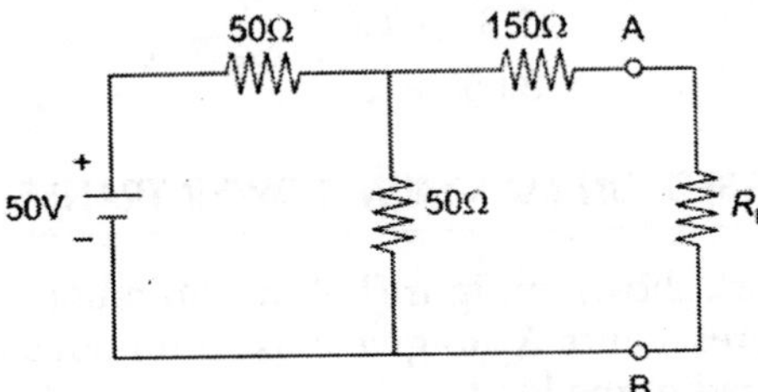

Solution: Step I: To obtain open circuit voltage across terminal *AB*.

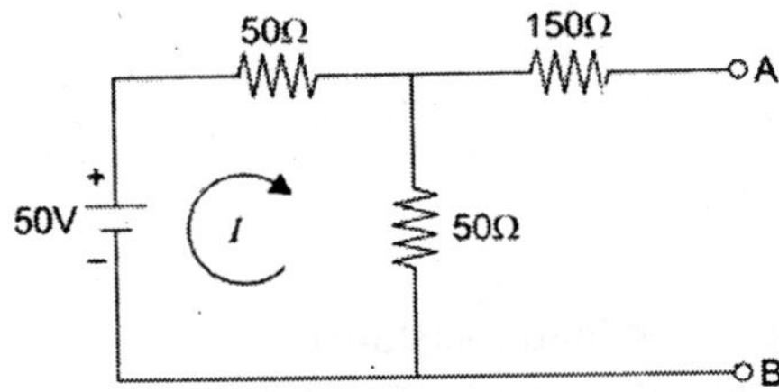

Apply KVL in loop 1

$$50 - 50I - 50I = 0$$

$$I = \frac{50}{100} = \frac{1}{2} = 0.5\ \text{A}$$

$$V_{AB} = V_{TH} = 50I = 50 \times 0.5$$

$$V_{TH} = 25\ \text{V}$$

Step II: To find R_{TH}, 50 V source are shorted.

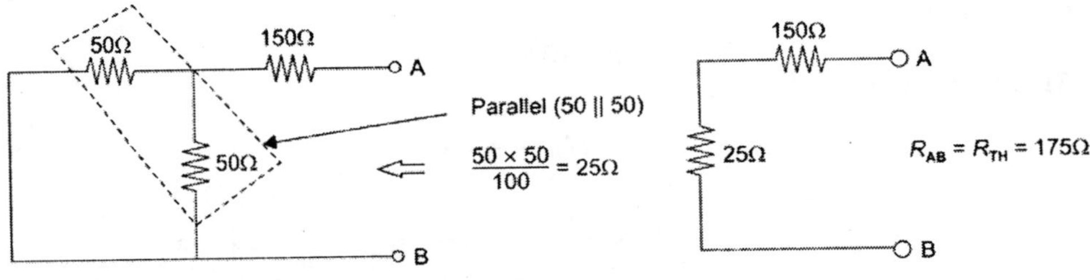

For maximum power transfer.

$$R_L = R_{TH} = 175\ \Omega$$ **Ans.**

Step III: To find the maximum power.

$$P_{L\max} = \frac{V_{TH}^2}{4R_L} = \frac{(25)^2}{4\times175}$$

$$= 0.8929\ \text{W}$$

Ans.

Example 3: Find the maximum power dissipated in the resistor R_L for the circuit shown in figure and find the value of R_L.

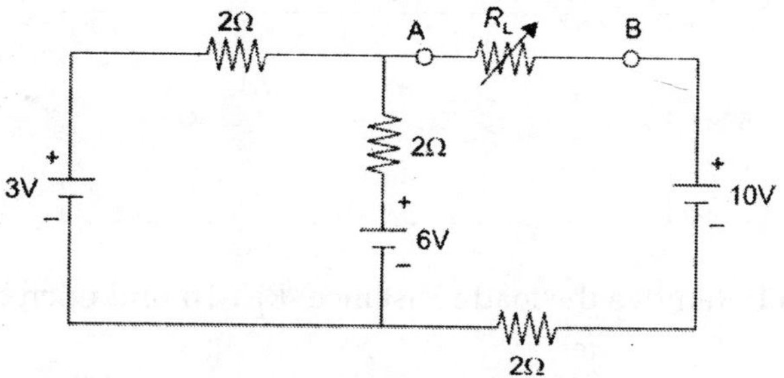

Solution: Step I: Remove the load resistance 'R_L'.

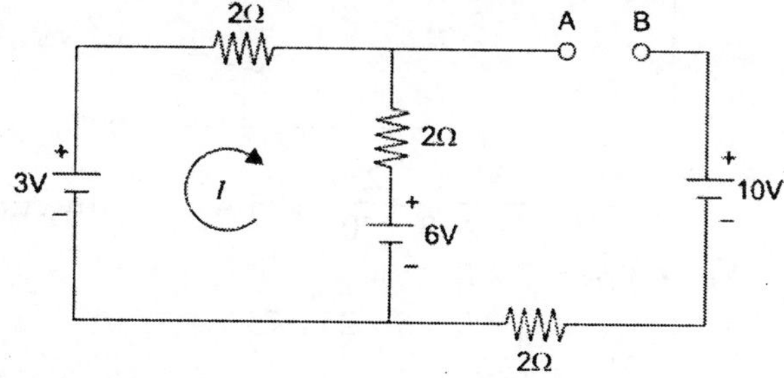

Apply KCL in above loop.

$$3 - 2I - 2I - 6 = 0$$

$$I = -\frac{3}{4}\ \text{A}$$

Calculate $V_{AB} = V_{TH}$

$$V_{TH} = 6 - 2I - 10 = -5.5\ \text{V}$$

Step II: Calculate R_{TH} across AB.

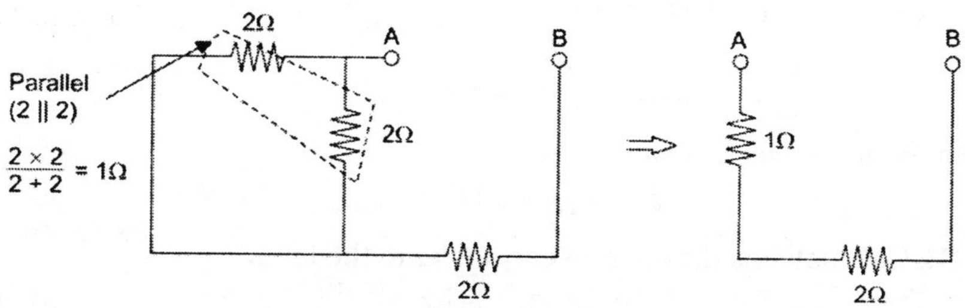

$$R_{AB} = R_{TH} = 3\ \Omega$$

For maximum power

$$R_L = R_{TH} = 3\ \Omega$$

Ans.

Step III: Calculate the maximum power

$$P_{L\max} = \frac{V_{TH}^2}{4R_L} = \frac{(5.5)^2}{4 \times 3} = 2.52 \text{ W}$$ **Ans.**

Example 4: Determine the maximum power delivered to the load in the circuit shown in figure below. **[Sem-II, 06-07]**

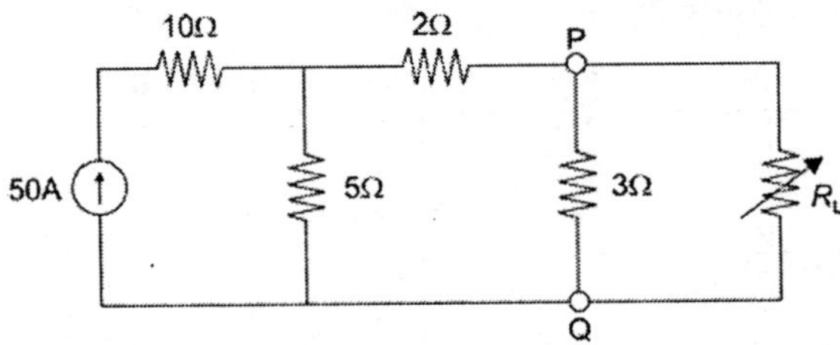

Solution: Step I: Remove the load resistance 'R_L'. To find open circuit voltage.

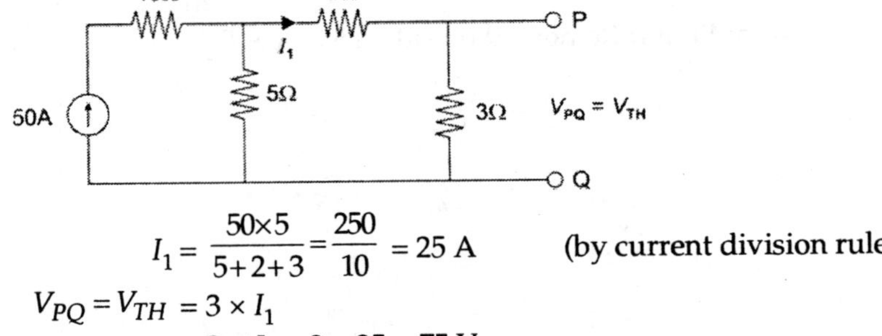

$$I_1 = \frac{50 \times 5}{5+2+3} = \frac{250}{10} = 25 \text{ A}$$ (by current division rule)

$$V_{PQ} = V_{TH} = 3 \times I_1$$

$$= 3 \times I_1 = 3 \times 25 = 75 \text{ V}$$

$$V_{TH} = 75 \text{ V}$$

Step II: To find R_{TH}

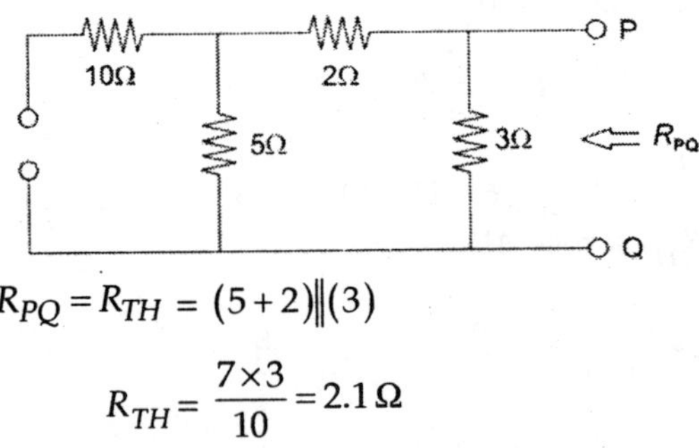

$$R_{PQ} = R_{TH} = (5+2) \| (3)$$

$$R_{TH} = \frac{7 \times 3}{10} = 2.1 \, \Omega$$

For maximum power transfer

$$R_L = R_{TH} = 2.1 \, \Omega$$ **Ans.**

Step III: Calculate maximum power transfer to the load.

$$P_{L\max} = \frac{V_{TH}^2}{4R_L} = \frac{(75)^2}{4 \times 2.1}$$

$$= 669.64 \text{ W}$$ **Ans.**

Example 5: Find the value of R to have maximum power transfer in the circuit shown in figure below. Also obtain the amount of maximum power. **[Sem-II, 03-04]**

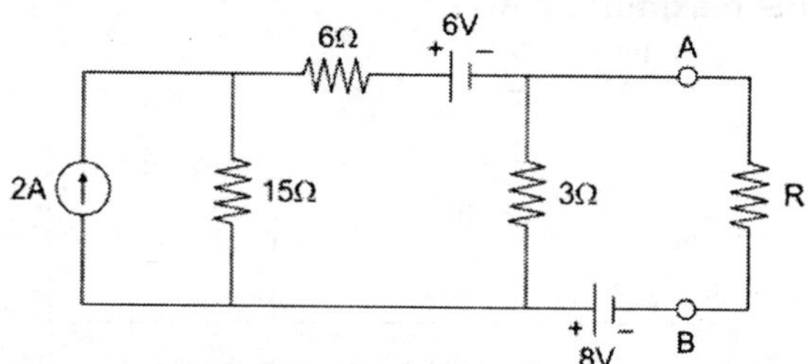

Solution: Step I: Remove the load resistance 'R'

Convert 2A current source to voltage source

$$V = IR = 2 \times 15 = 30\ V$$

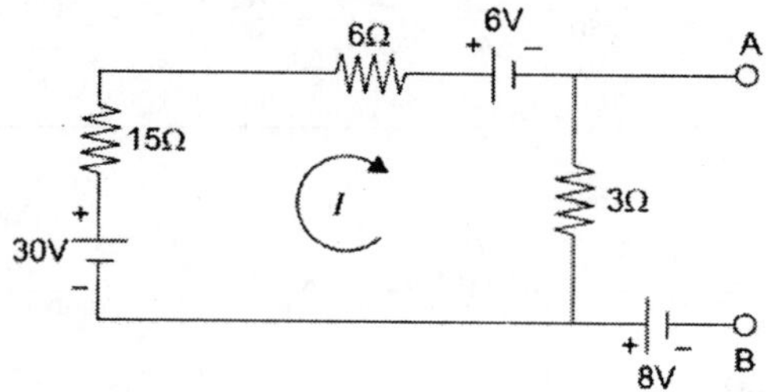

Apply KVL in loop.

$$30 - 15I - 6I - 6 - 3I = 0$$

$$I = \frac{24}{24} = 1\ A$$

Calculate voltage across AB.

i.e.
$$V_{AB} = V_{TH}$$
$$= 8 + 3I = 8 + 3 \times 1 = 1\ V$$

Step II: To find R_{TH}.

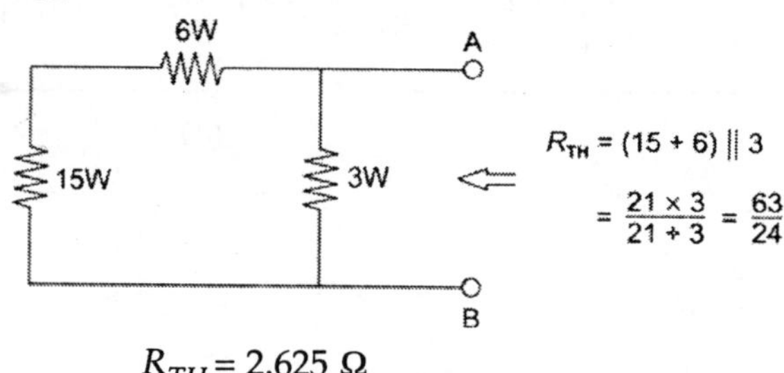

$$R_{TH} = 2.625\ \Omega$$

For maximum power transfer.

$$R_L = R_{TH} = 2.625\ \Omega$$ **Ans.**

Step III: Find maximum power

$$P_{L\max} = \frac{V_{TH}^2}{4R_L}$$

$$= \frac{(11)^2}{4 \times 2.625} = 11.52\ W$$ **Ans.**

Example 6: In the network shown in figure below find. **[Sem-I, 07-08]**

1. The value of R_L for maximum power dissipation.
2. The value of the maximum power.

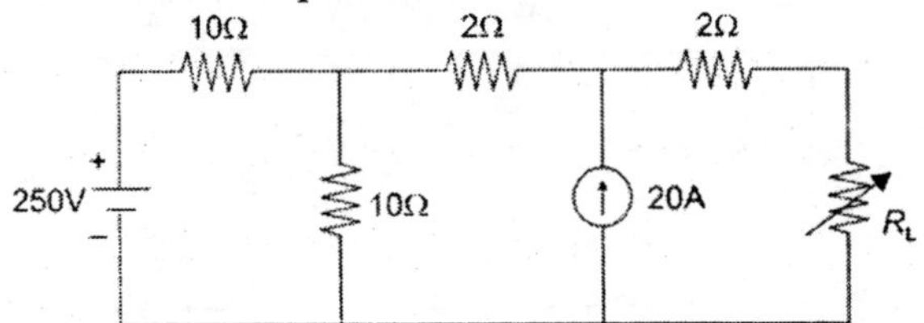

Solution: Step I: Convert 250 V source to current source.

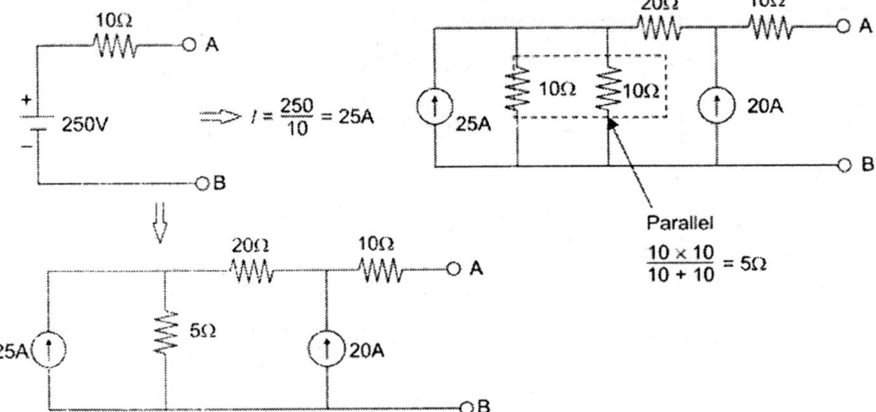

Convert the 25 A current source to voltage source.

$$V = IR = 25 \times 5 = 125 \text{ V}$$

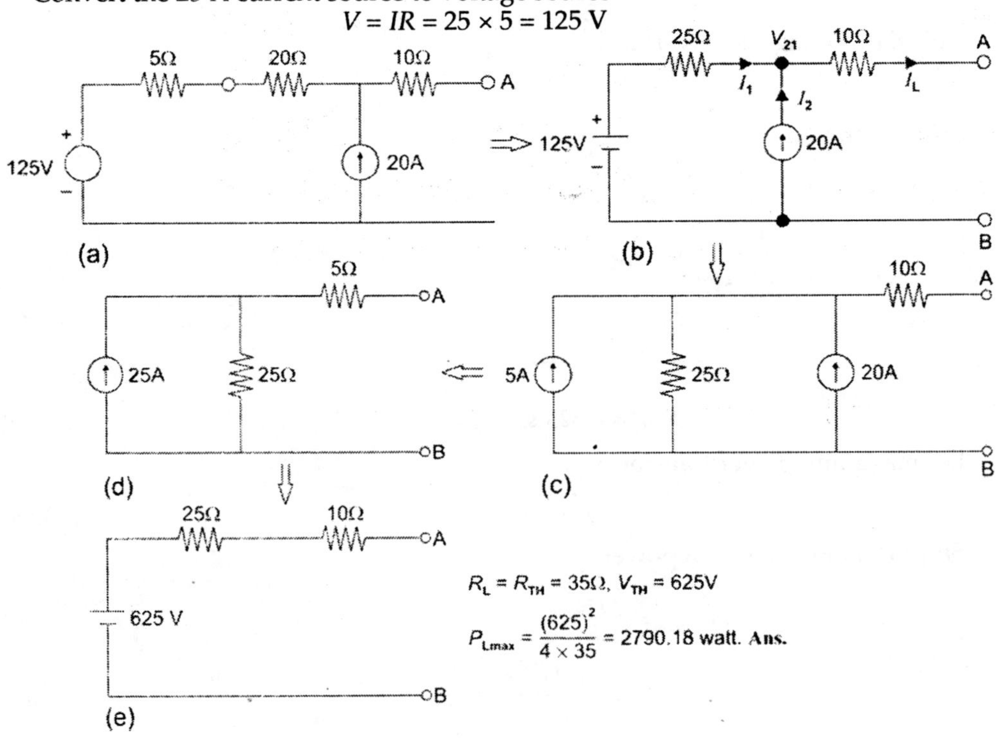

SOLVED EXAMPLES FOR PRACTICE

Example 1: In the network shown in figure below find **[UPTU 2008-09]**

1. The value of R_L for maximum power dissipation.
2. The value of the maximum power.

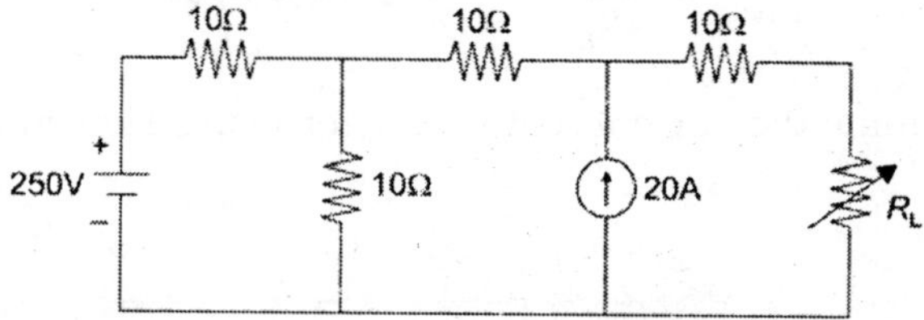

Solution: Step I: Remove the load resistance 'R_L' from the above figure.

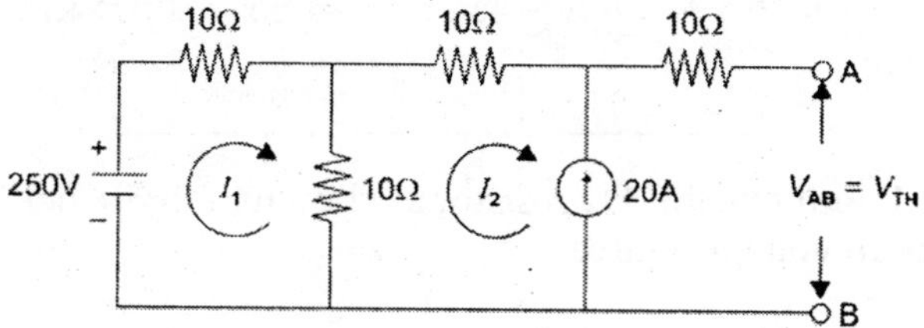

Apply KVL in loop 1

$$250 - 10I_1 - 10(I_1 - I_2) = 0$$

Apply KVL in loop 2

$$-10(I_2 - I_1) - 10I_2 = 0$$

Given $\qquad I_2 = -20$

Putting the value of I_2, we get I_1

$$-20I_1 - 10\times 20 + 250 = 0$$

$$I_1 = 2.5 \text{ A}$$

Step II: To find open circuit voltage across *AB* terminals.

Apply KVL in outer loop.

$$V_{TH} = V_{AB} = 250 - 10I_1 - 10I_2$$

$$= 250 - 10\times 2.5 + 10\times 20$$

$$= 450 - 25 = 425 \text{ volt}$$

$\therefore \qquad V_{AB} = V_{TH} = 425$ volt

Step III: Calculate the Thevenin's resistance, R_{TH}, by shorting 250 V source and opening 20 A current source as shown in the figure (a).

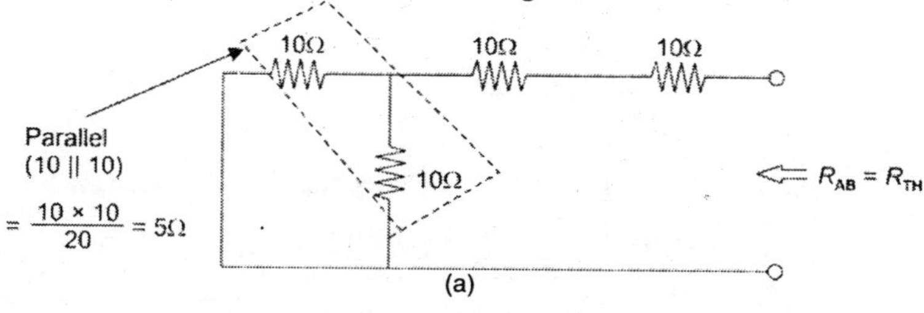

(a)

$$R_{TH} = 5 + 10 + 10 = 25\ \Omega$$

Step IV: Calculate the maximum power.
For maximum power

$$R_L = R_{TH} = 25\ \Omega$$ **Ans.**

$$P_{L\max} = \frac{V_{TH}^2}{4R_L} = \frac{(425)^2}{4 \times 25} = 1806.25\ \text{W}$$ **Ans.**

Example 2: Determine the current in 4 Ω resistor using Thevenin's theorem in the following circuit. **[UPTU 2009-10]**

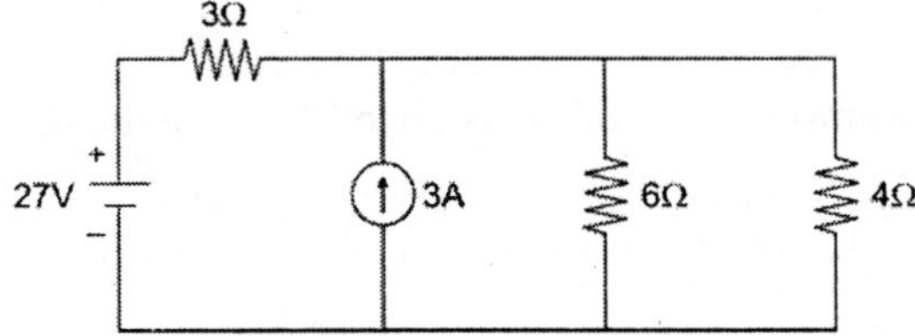

Solution: Step I: Remove the 4 Ω resistor as shown in figure below and convert the 3 A current source to voltage source.

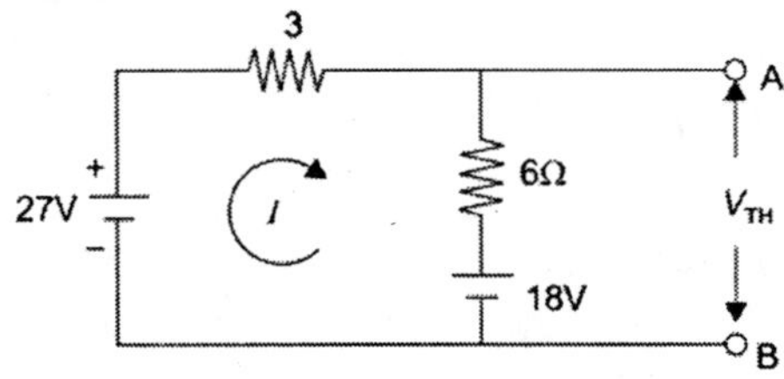

$$V = 3 \times 8 = 18\ \text{V}$$

Apply KVL in above loop.

$$27 - 3I - 6I - 18 = 0$$

$$-9I + 9 = 0$$

$$I = 1\ \text{A}$$

$$V_{TH} = 18 + 6I$$

$$= 18 + 6 \times 1$$

$$= 24\ \text{V}$$

Step II: Calculate Thevenin's equivalent resistance 'R_{TH}' by shorting voltage source and opening current source.

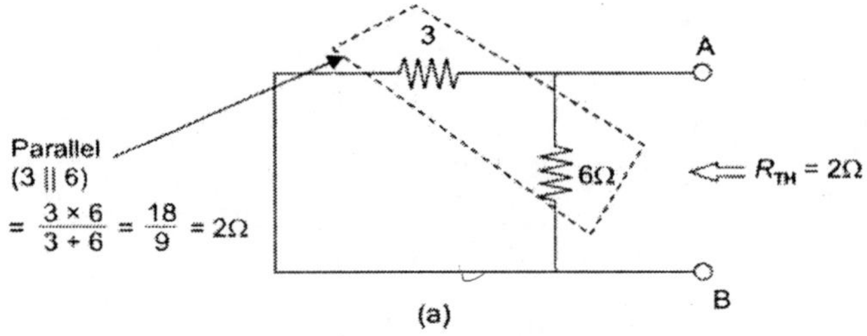

(a)

Step III: Draw Thevenin's equivalent circuit.

Step IV: Calculate the current through 4 Ω resistance.

$$I_L = \frac{V_{TH}}{R_{TH} + R_L} = \frac{24}{2+4} = 4 \text{ A}$$ **Ans.**

Example 3: Using superposition theorem, find the current in 20 Ω resistor of the circuit shown in figure below.

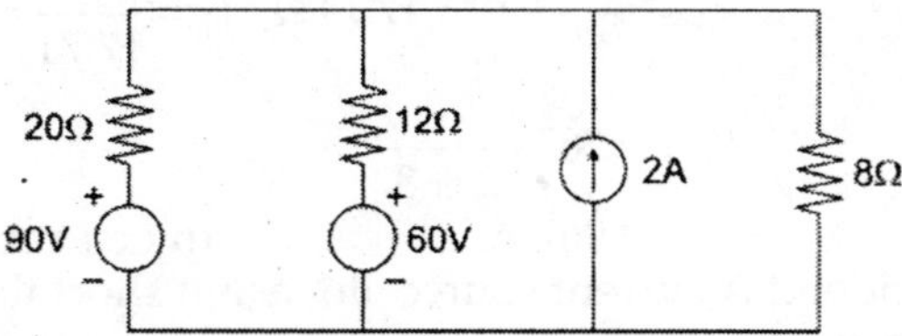

Solution: Step I: According to superposition theorem select any one source at a time keeping others deactive.

Consider 90 V source only, short 60 V source and 2 A current source is opened.

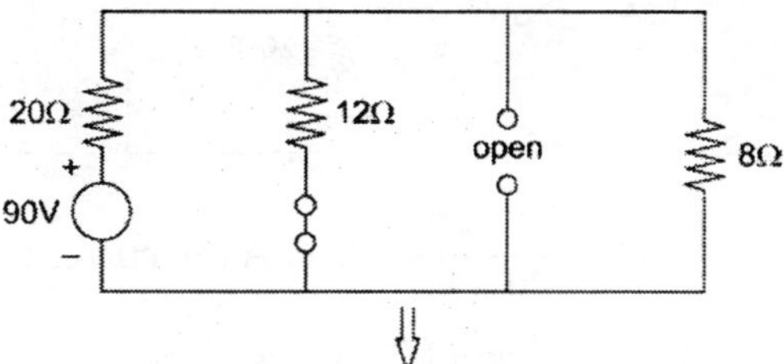

Redraw the circuit.

$$I_1' = \frac{V_1}{R_{eq1}}$$

$$R_{eq1} = (12 \| 8) + 20$$

$$= \frac{96}{20} + 20 = \frac{446}{20} = 24.8$$

$$I_1' = \frac{90}{24.8} = 3.629 \text{ A} \qquad ...(1)$$

Step II: Consider 60 V voltage source. Short 90 V voltage source and opening 2 A current source.

$$I_2 = \frac{V_2}{R_{eq2}}$$

$$R_{eq2} = (20 \| 8) + 12$$

$$= \frac{160}{28} + 12 = 17.71\,\Omega,\; I_2 = \frac{60}{17.71} = 3.387\text{ A}$$

$$I_2' = 3.387 \times \frac{8}{20+8}$$

$$= 0.967\text{ A} \qquad \text{(by current division rule)} \quad ...(2)$$

Step III: Now consider 2 A current source alone and short the two voltage sources as shown in the figure below.

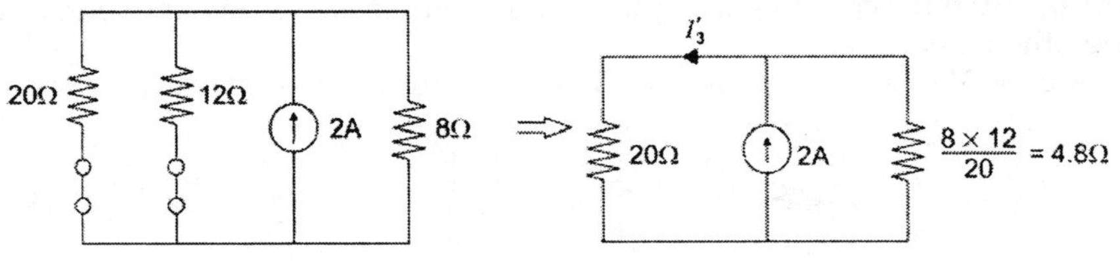

$$I_3' = \frac{2 \times 4.8}{20 + 4.8} = 0.387\text{A (by current division rule)} \quad ...(3)$$

Step IV: Calculate the current through 20 Ω resistance

From Eqs (1), (2) and (3)

$$I = I_1' - I_2' - I_3'$$

$$= 3.62 - 0.967 - 0.387$$

$$= 2.266\text{ A}$$

Ans.

Example 4: By means of superposition theorem, find the current which flows through R_2 in the circuit shown in figure. **[UPTU 2010-11, 2011-12]**

Solution: Step I: Select 120 V voltage source and short 60 V source as shown in figure below.

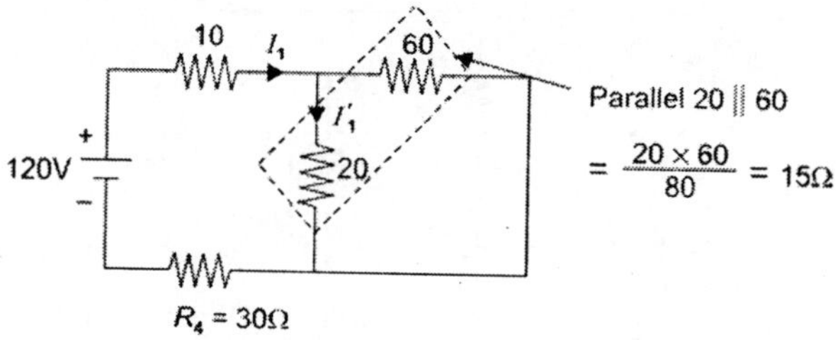

Parallel 20 || 60

$= \frac{20 \times 60}{80} = 15\Omega$

$R_4 = 30\Omega$

$$I_1 = \frac{V_1}{R_{eq1}}$$

$$R_{eq1} = (60 \| 20) + 10 + 30$$
$$= 15 + 10 + 30 = 55\ \Omega$$

$$I_1 = \frac{V_1}{R_{eq1}} = \frac{120}{55} = 2.18$$

$$I_1' = 2.18 \times \frac{60}{60+20}$$ (by current division rule)

$$= 1.63\ A$$ ...(1)

Step II: Select 60 V voltage source and short 120 V voltage source.

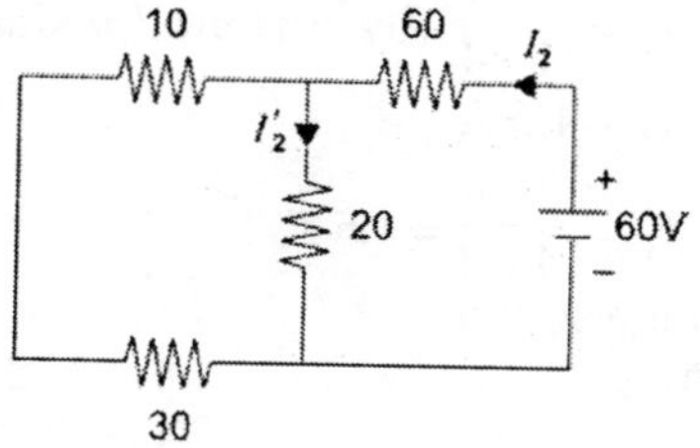

$$I_2 = \frac{V_2}{R_{eq2}}$$

$$R_{eq2} = [(10+30) \| 20] + 60$$

$$= \frac{40 \times 20}{40+20} + 60 = 73.33\ \Omega$$

$$I_2 = \frac{60}{73.33} = 0.81\ A$$

$$I_2' = 0.81 \times \frac{40}{40+20}$$

$$= 0.5454\ A$$ ...(2)

Step III: Algebraically adding Eqs (1) and (2), we get total current through 20 Ω resistance

$$I = I_1' + I_2'$$
$$= 1.63 + 0.545$$
$$= 2.175\ A$$

Ans.

Example 5: Using superposition theorem determine current in all resistance of the following network shown in figure below. **[UPTU 2011-12]**

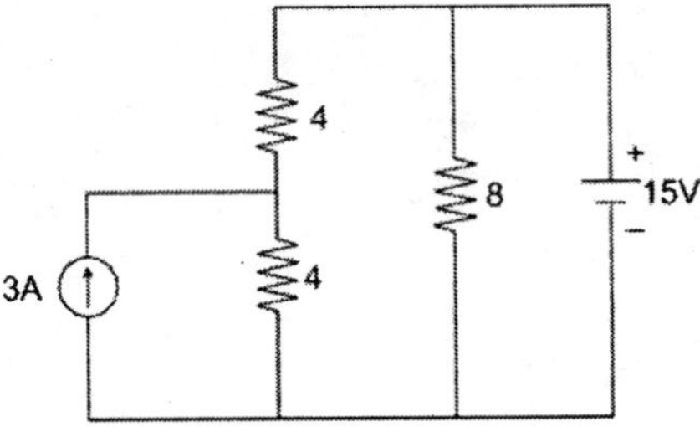

Solution: Step I: Select 3 A current source.
15 V voltage source is short.

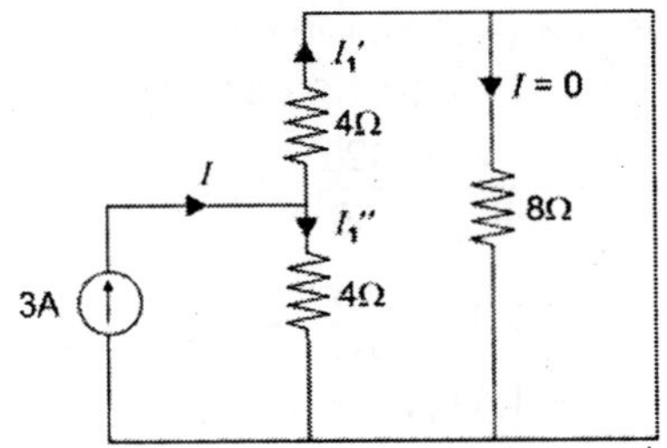

$$I_1' = \frac{3\times4}{4+4} \text{ (by current division rule)}$$

$$I_1' = 1.5 \text{ A} \qquad \text{...(1)}$$

$$I_1'' = \frac{3\times4}{4+4} = 1.5 \text{ A}$$

Step III: Select a 15 V voltage source.
3 A current source is open.

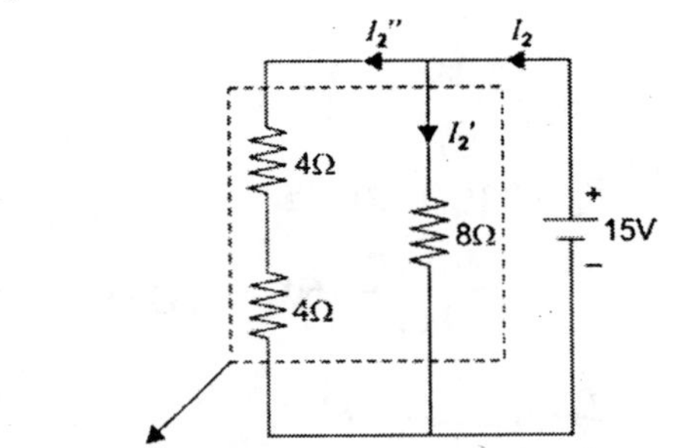

$$I_2 = \frac{V_2}{R_{eq2}}$$

$$I_2 = \frac{15}{4} = 3.75 \text{ A} \qquad \text{...(2)}$$

$$I_2' = 3.75 \times \frac{8}{8+8} = 1.875 \text{ A} \qquad \text{...(3)}$$

$$I_2'' = 3.75 \times \frac{8}{8+8} = 1.875 \text{ A} \qquad \text{...(4)}$$

Step IV: Calculate current through all resistors.
Current through upper resistor

$$4\ \Omega = 1.875 - 1.5 = 0.375\ \text{A}$$ **Ans.**

Current through lower resistor

$$4\ \Omega = 1.5 + 1.875 = 3.375\ \text{A}$$ **Ans.**

Current through all resistors

$$8\ \Omega = 0 + 1.875 = 1.875\ \text{A}$$ **Ans.**

SOLVED EXAMPLES FOR PRACTICE

Example 1: Replace the network of following figure to the left of terminals ab by its Thevenin's equivalent circuit. Hence determine I_L. **[GBTU Sem-I 2008-09]**

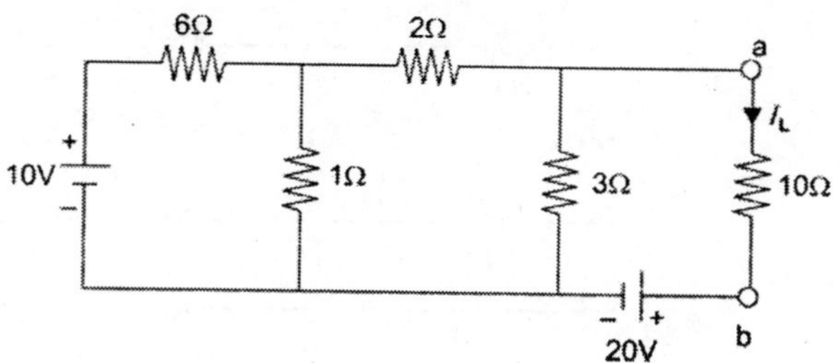

Solution: Step I: Remove the load resistance 10 Ω.
Find the open circuit voltage V_{ab} or V_{TH} across ab terminal.

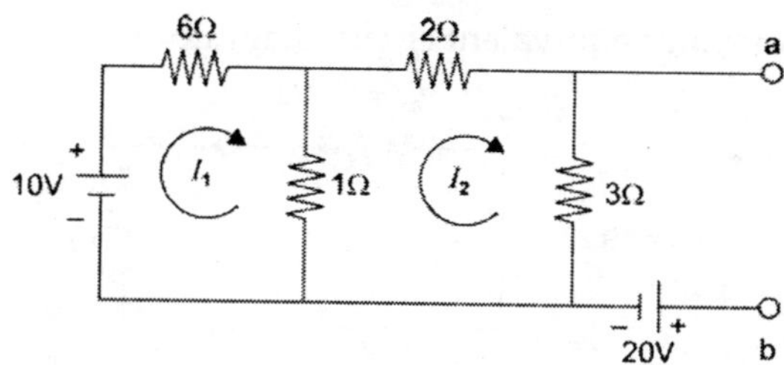

Apply KVL in loop 1.

$$10 - 6I_1 - 1(I_1 - I_2) = 0$$

$$10 - 7I_1 + I_2 = 0$$

$$7I_1 - I_2 = 10 \quad \text{...(1)}$$

Apply KVL in loop 2.

$$-1(I_2 - I_1) - 2I_2 - 3I_2 = 0$$

$$6I_2 = I_1$$

$$I_1 = 6I_2 \quad \text{...(2)}$$

From Eqs (1) and (2), we get

$$7I_1 - I_2 = 10$$

$$7 \times 6I_2 - I_2 = 10$$

$$I_2 = \frac{10}{41} = 0.24\ \text{A}$$

$$V_{ab} = V_{TH} = -20 + 3I_2$$
$$42I_2 = -20 + 3 \times 0.24$$
$$V_{TH} = -19.27 \text{ volt}$$

Step II: Calculate Thevenin's equivalent resistance across terminal '*ab*'. (when all voltage sources are shorted).

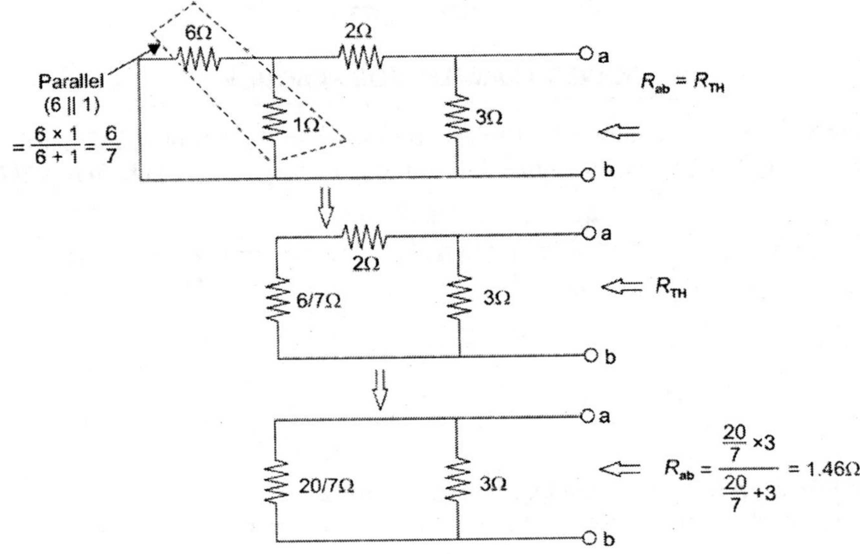

Step III: Draw Thevenin's equivalent circuit diagram.

V_{TH} = 1.46Ω

I_L

V_{TH} = 19.27V

10

$$R_{TH} = 1.46\ \Omega$$

Step IV: Calculate current through 10 Ω resistance.

$$I_L = \frac{V_{TH}}{R_{TH} + R_L} = \frac{19.24}{1.46 + 10} = 1.68 \text{ A}$$ **Ans.**

Example 2: Find the current in and voltage across the 2 Ω resistance in the figure below. **[GBTU 2008-09]**

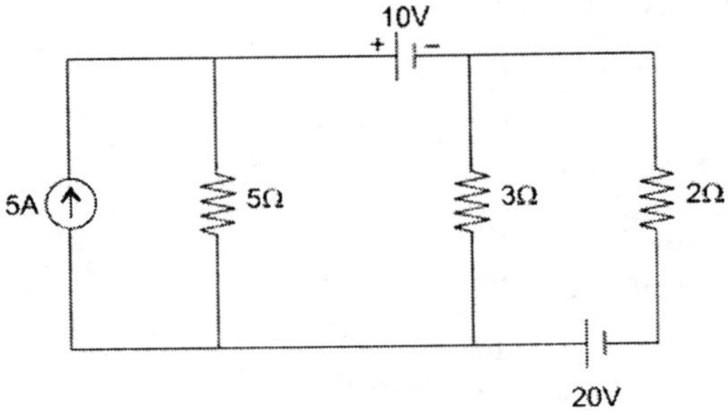

Solution: Step I: Convert 5 A current source to voltage source.

$$V = IR = 5 \times 5 = 25 \text{ V}$$

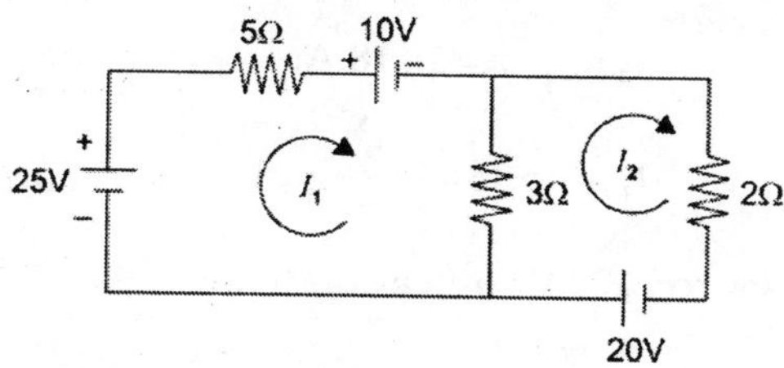

Step II: Calculate current I_2

Apply KVL in loop 1

$$25 - 5I_1 - 10 - 3(I_1 - I_2) = 0$$

$$15 - 8I_1 + 3I_2 = 0$$

$$8I_1 - 3I_2 = 15 \qquad \text{...(1)}$$

Apply KVL in loop 2.

$$-3(I_2 - I_1) - 2I_2 + 20 = 0$$

$$-5I_2 + 3I_1 + 20 = 0$$

$$3I_1 - 5I_2 = -20 \qquad \text{...(2)}$$

Solving Eqs (1) and (2), we get

$$I_2 = 5 \text{ A}$$

Net voltage in 2 Ω is

$$5 \times 2 = 10 \text{ V}$$

Ans.

Example 3: In the figure below, find the current through the 6 Ω resistor using superposition theorem. **[UPTU 2005-06]**

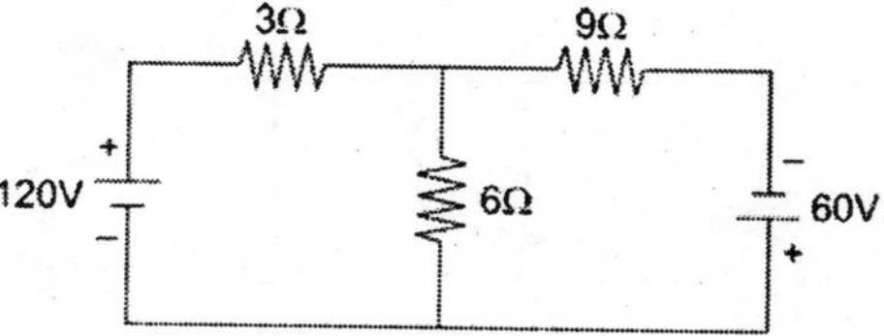

Solution: Step I: Select 120 V source. 60 V source is shorted.

$$I_1 = \frac{V_1}{R_{eq1}}$$

$$R_{eq1} = (9 \| 6) + 3$$

$$= \frac{9 \times 6}{15} + 3 = \frac{54 + 45}{15}$$

$$= \frac{99}{15} = 6.6\ \Omega$$

$$I_1 = \frac{120}{6.6} = 18.18\ \text{A}$$

$$I_1' = 18.18 \times \frac{9}{9+6} = 10.90\ \text{A (by current division rule)} \quad ...(1)$$

Step II: Select 60 V source. 120 V source shorted.

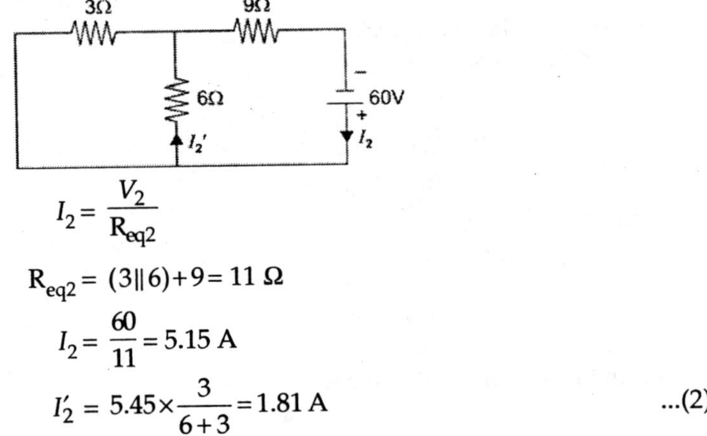

$$I_2 = \frac{V_2}{R_{eq2}}$$

$$R_{eq2} = (3 \| 6) + 9 = 11\ \Omega$$

$$I_2 = \frac{60}{11} = 5.15\ \text{A}$$

$$I_2' = 5.45 \times \frac{3}{6+3} = 1.81\ \text{A} \quad ...(2)$$

Step III: Calculate current in 6 Ω resistance.
From Eqs (1) and (2)

$$I = I_1' - I_2' = 10.91 - 1.81 = 9.09\ \text{A} \quad \textbf{Ans.}$$

Example 4: Find current I in 8 Ω resistor using superposition theorem as shown in figure below. **[UPTU 2005-06, Sem-II]**

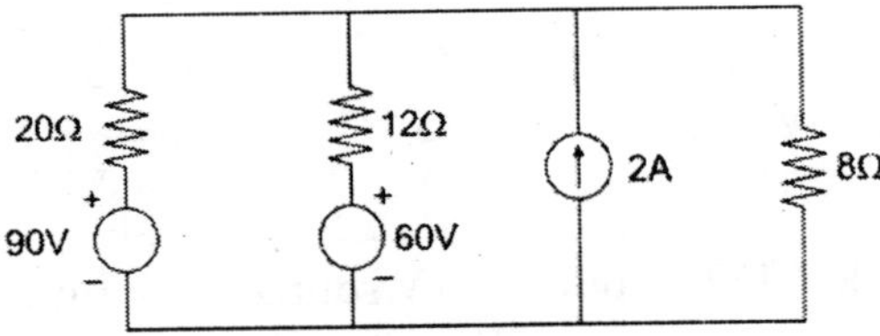

Solution: Step I: Select the voltage source 90 V.
60 V voltage source is shorted and 2 A current source is opened.

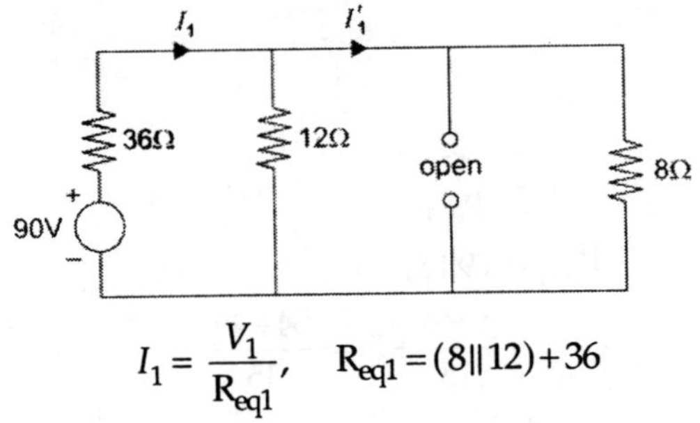

$$I_1 = \frac{V_1}{R_{eq1}}, \quad R_{eq1} = (8 \| 12) + 36$$

$$= \frac{90}{40.8} = 2.20\text{ A},\ R_{eq1} = 40.8\,\Omega$$

$$I_1' = 2.20 \times \frac{12}{12+8} = 1.32\text{ A} \qquad \text{...(1)}$$

Step II: Select 60 V source shorted the 90 V source and opened the 2 A current source.

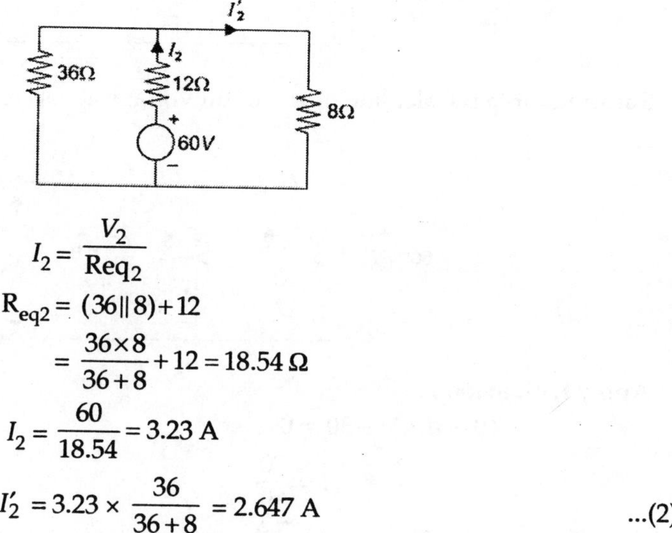

$$I_2 = \frac{V_2}{Req_2}$$

$$R_{eq2} = (36 \| 8) + 12$$

$$= \frac{36 \times 8}{36+8} + 12 = 18.54\,\Omega$$

$$I_2 = \frac{60}{18.54} = 3.23\text{ A}$$

$$I_2' = 3.23 \times \frac{36}{36+8} = 2.647\text{ A} \qquad \text{...(2)}$$

Step III: Select 2 A current source, other voltage source are deactive (shorted).

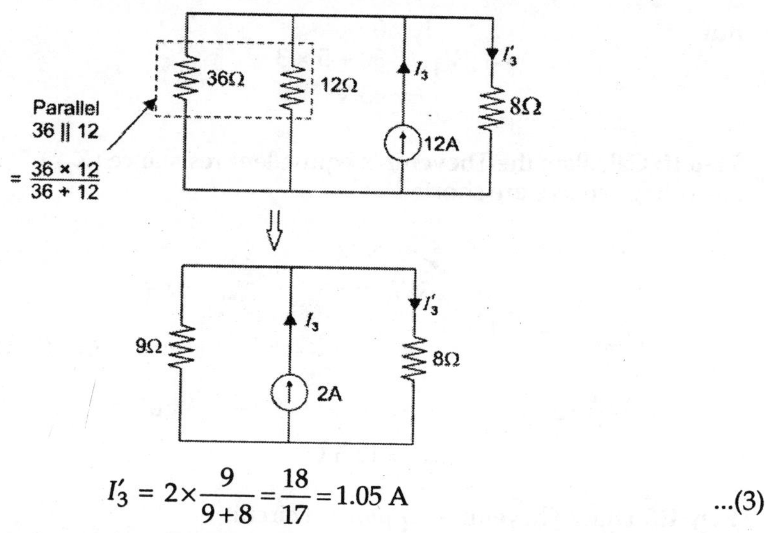

$$I_3' = 2 \times \frac{9}{9+8} = \frac{18}{17} = 1.05\text{ A} \qquad \text{...(3)}$$

Step IV: Calculate current in 8 Ω resistance.
From Eqs (1), (2) and (3), we get

$$I = I_1' + I_2' + I_3'$$
$$= 1.32 + 2.64 + 1.05$$
$$= 5.02\text{ A}$$

Ans.

Example 5: Find Thevenin's equivalent circuit. **[UPTU Sem-I, 2006-07]**

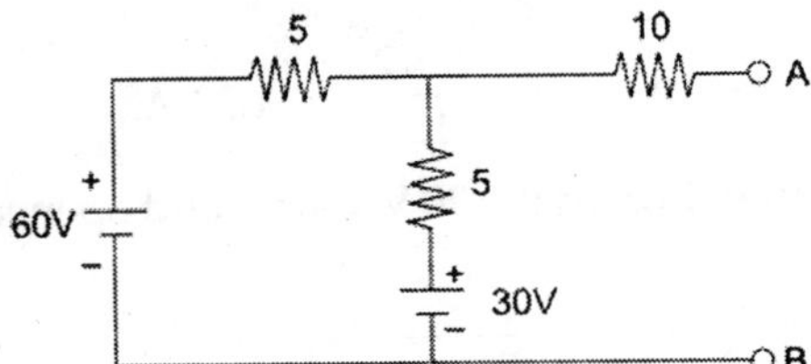

Solution: Step I: Calculate open circuit voltage across terminal AB, i.e. V_{TH}

Apply KVL in loop.

$$60 - 5I - 5I - 30 = 0$$

$$I = \frac{30}{10}$$

$$= 3\text{ A}$$

$$V_{AB} = V_{TH} = 30 - 5(I_2 - I_1) - 10I_2$$

But $$I_2 = 0$$

$$V_{TH} = 30 + 5 \times 3$$

$$= 45\text{ V}$$

Step II: Calculate the Thevenin's equivalent resistance (R_{TH}).
All voltage source are shorted.

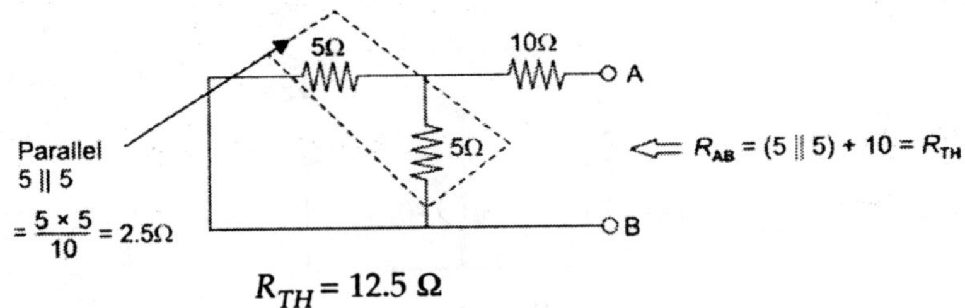

$$R_{TH} = 12.5\ \Omega$$

Step III: Draw Thevenin's equivalent circuit.

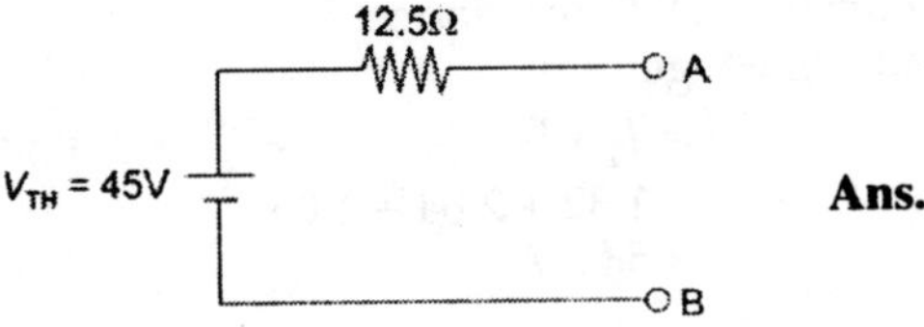

Ans.

Example 6: Determine the current flowing through 5 Ω resistor in the network shown using Thevenin's theorem. **[UPTU 2006-07]**

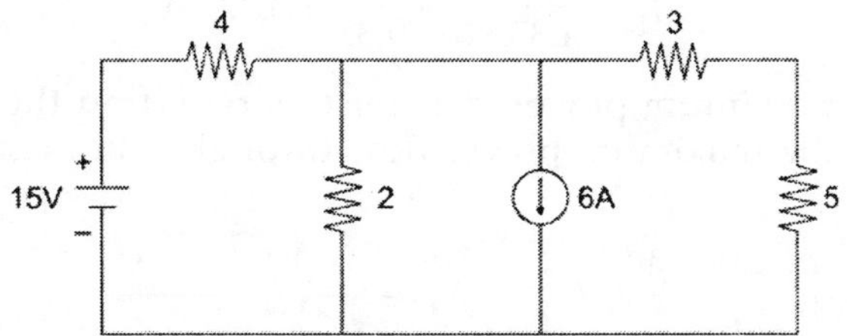

Solution: Step I: Remove the load resistance 5 Ω resistance.
Convert the 6 A current source to voltage source.

$$V = 6 \times 2 = 12 \text{ V}$$

Apply KVL in loop.

$$15 - 4I - 2I + 12 = 0$$

$$I = \frac{27}{6} = 4.5 \text{ A}$$

Voltage across *AB*

$$V_{AB} = V_{TH} = -12 + 2 \times I$$

$$= -12 + 4.5 \times 2$$

$$V_{TH} = -3 \text{ volt}$$

Step II: Calculate the Thevenin's equivalent resistance (R_{TH}).

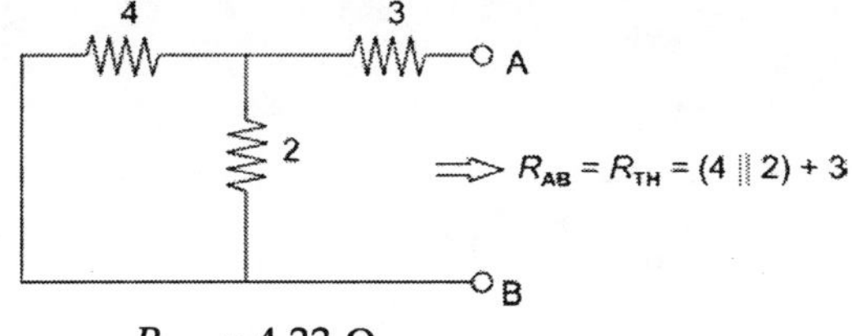

$$R_{TH} = 4.33 \ \Omega$$

Step III: Draw the Thevenin's equivalent circuit.

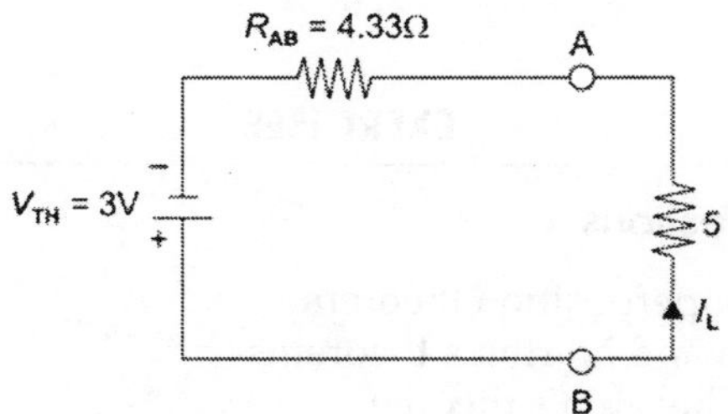

Step IV: Calculate the current in 5 Ω resistance.

$$I_L = \frac{3}{4.33+5} = \frac{3}{9.33} = 0.321 \text{ A}$$ **Ans.**

Example 7: Using maximum power transfer theorem, find the value of the load resistance 'R_L' for the maximum power flow through it in the network shown in figure below. **[UPTU 2008-09]**

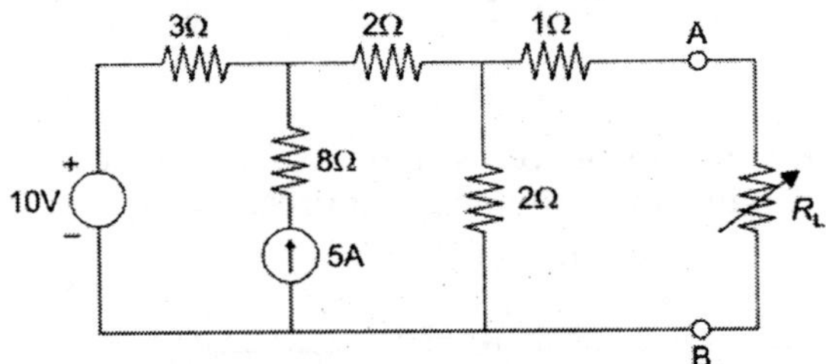

Solution: Step I: Remove the load resistance as shown in the figure below.

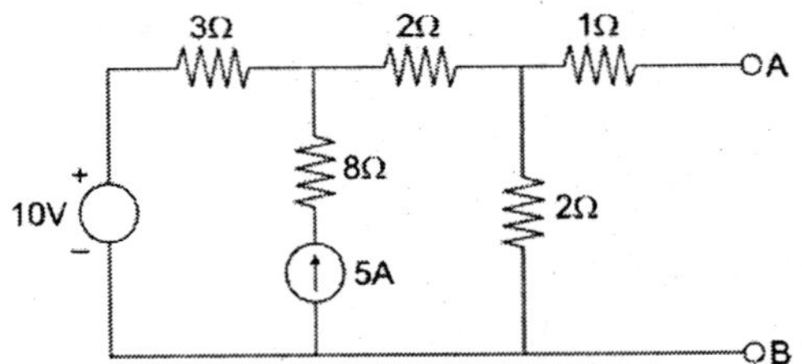

Step II: According to question, there is no need to calculate V_{TH}.

Step III: Calculate the Thevenin's equivalent resistance R_{TH} by shorting the voltage source and opening the current source as shown in figure below.

$$R_{TH} = (3+2)\|2)+1$$

$$= \frac{10}{7}+1 = \frac{17}{7} = 2.42\ \Omega$$

For maximum power $R_L = R_{TH} = 2.42\ \Omega$ **Ans.**

EXERCISES

Very Short Answer Questions

1. State and explain superposition theorem. **[Sem-I, 09-10]**
2. State superposition and Norton's theorems. **[Sem-II, 09-10]**
3. State and explain Thevenin's theorem. **[Sem-II, 09-10]**

4. Define maximum power transfer theorem and give its application in practical situation. **[Sem-I, 2012-13]**
5. In the following circuit, what will be the maximum power that can be supplied to the load. **[Sem-II, 09-10]**

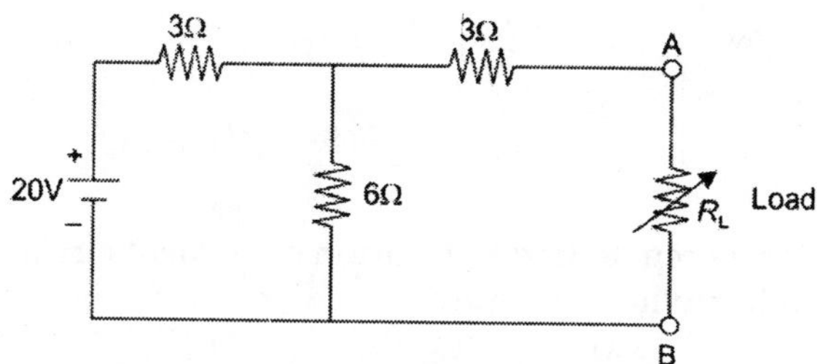

6. In the circuit of following figure, find the value of R.

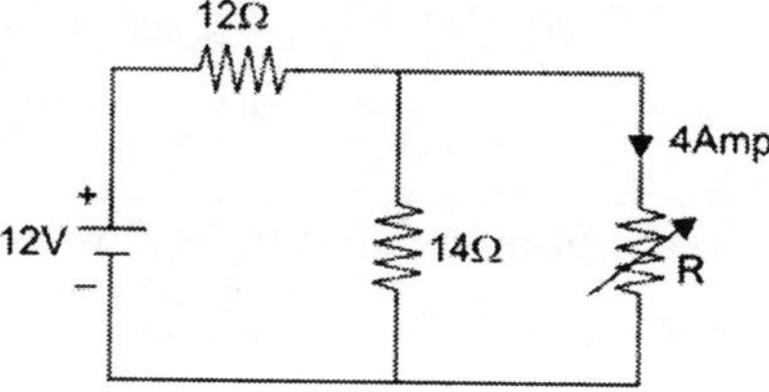

Short Answer Questions

1. Define Thevenin's theorem, give its limitations, find the current in 2 ohm resistor using this theorem. **[Sem-I, 2012-13] [Ans.** = 2.64 A**]**

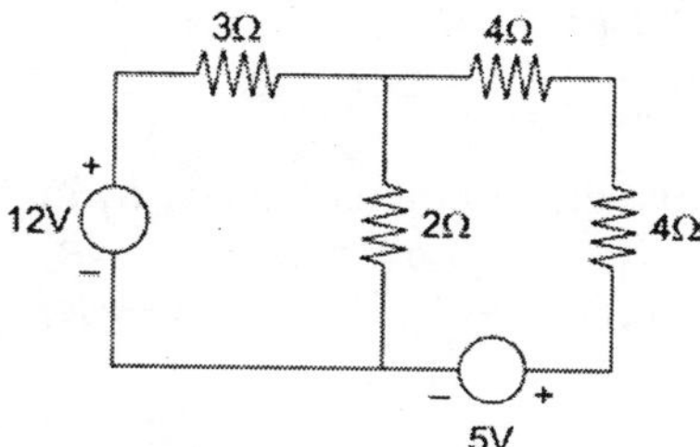

2. Determine the value of R so that the load of 20 W draws maximum power and the value of maximum power drawn by the load. **[Sem-I, 2012-13]**

   Ans. $R = 30$ W, $P_{Lmax} = 180$ W

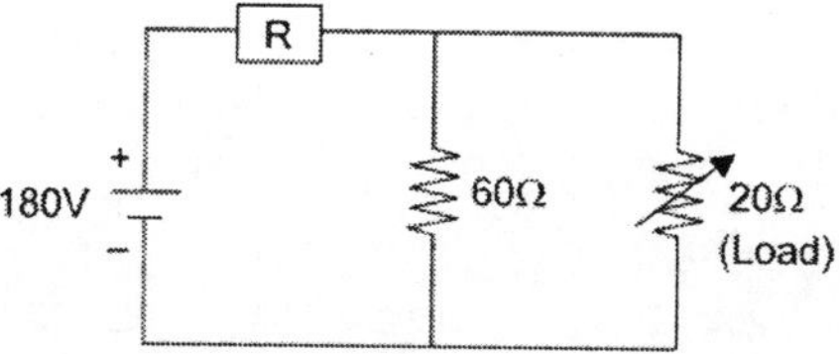

3. State and explain maximum power transfer theorem for DC circuit. **[Sem-I, 2011-12]**

4. Convert the network at terminals 'ab' by its Thevenin's equivalent circuit. Hence determine I of the circuit shown in figure below. **[Sem-II, 2010-11]**

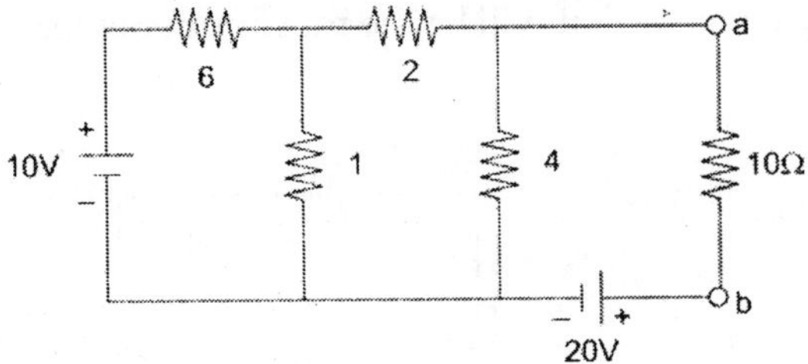

5. Apply Norton's theorem to find the Norton equivalent circuit as seen by R_L in the circuit shown in the following figure. **[Sem-II, 2008-09]**

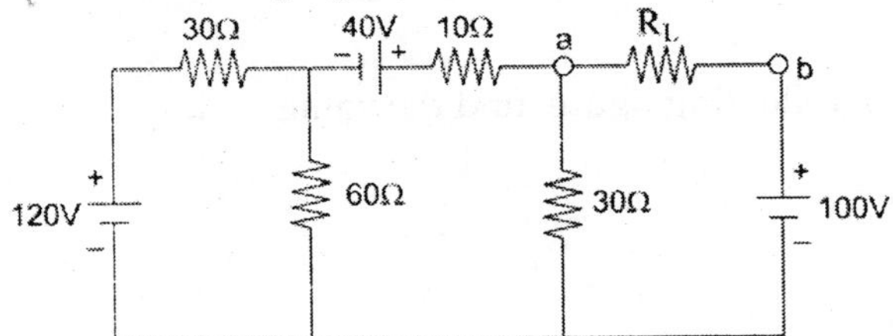

6. Using Thevenin's theorem obtain current in 13 Ω resistance in figure below.

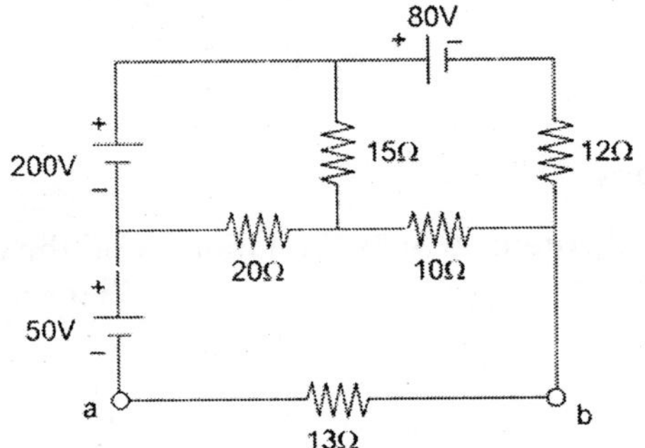

7. Find the Norton's equivalent circuit as seen by R_L in the following circuit.

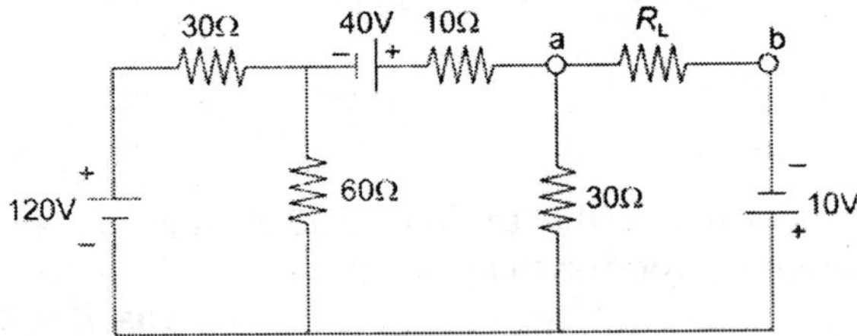

8. Use superposition theorem to find the current through the 20 Ω resistance shown in figure below. **[Sem-I, 08-09] Ans.** I = 2.226 A

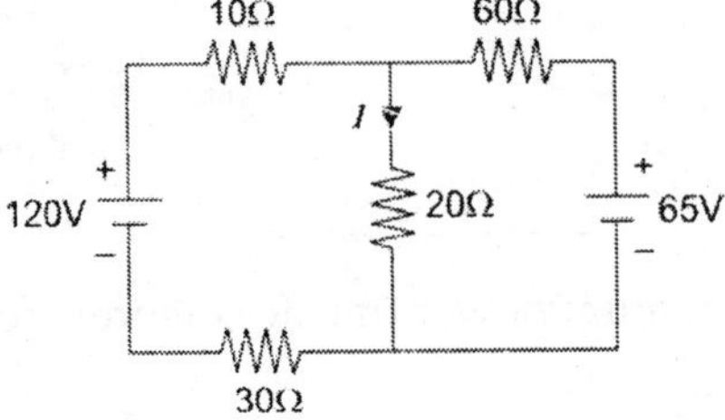

9. Calculate current through 10 Ω resistance using superposition theorem. The circuit is shown in figure below. **Ans.** I = 0.444 A, = 0.4649 A

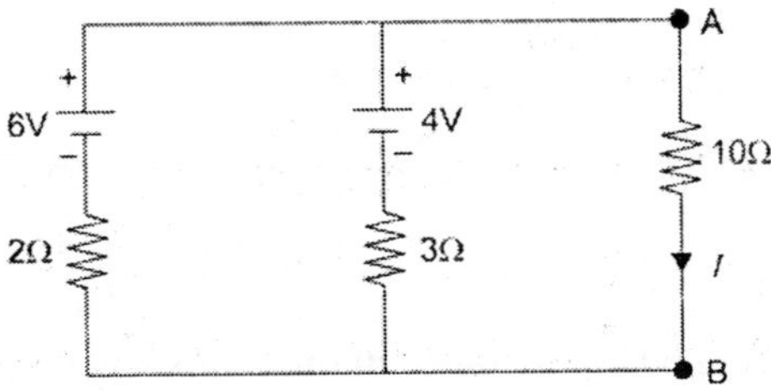

Descriptive Questions (10 Marks)

1. Define Norton's theorem. Give its limitations. Find the current in 2 ohm resistor using this theorem. **[Sem-I, 12-13]** **Ans.** I = 2.064 A

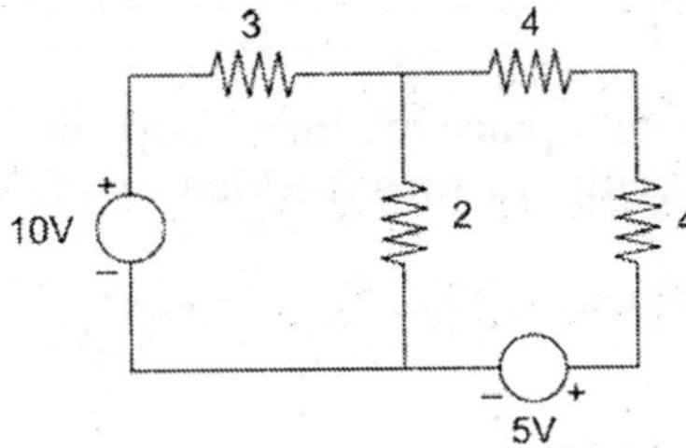

2. Using superposition theorem, find the current flowing through resistor 'R' in figure below. **[Sem-I, 2011-12] Ans.** I = 1.875 A

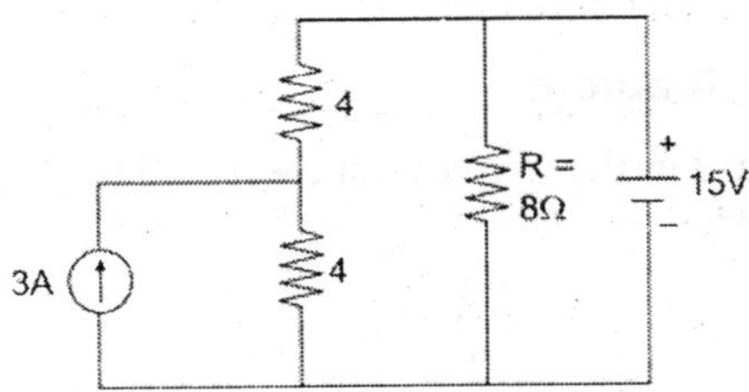

3. State superposition theorem in dc network. Determine the current i_1 and i_2 in the following network shown in figure below. **[Sem-II, 2010-11]**

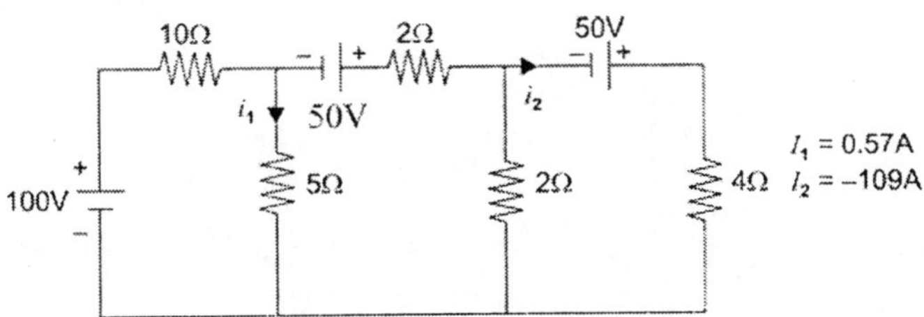

4.(i) Determine current in 4 Ω resistance using Thevenin's theorem in the following circuit **[Sem-I, 2009-10]**

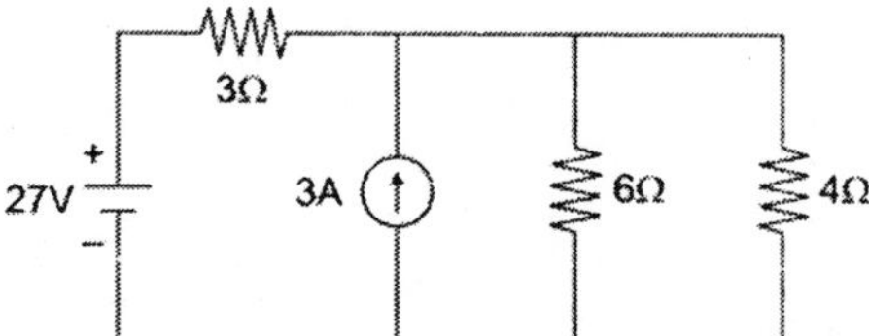

(ii) Find voltage V_1 across 60 Ω resistance in the following circuit using loop analysis method. **[Sem-I, 2009-10]** **Ans.** 12 V

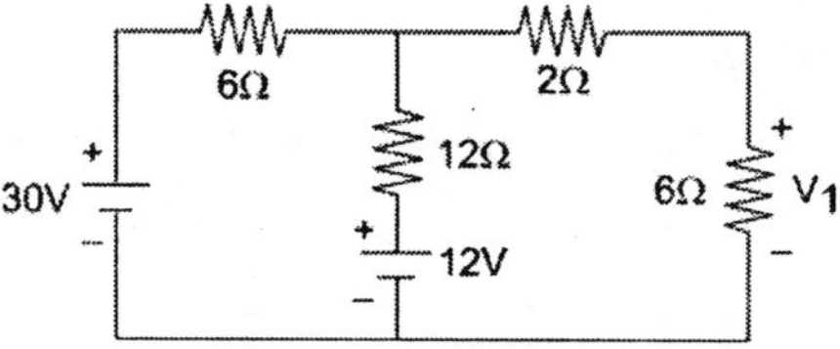

5. Use Thevenin's theorem to replace the three loop circuit of following figure by a single loop equivalent circuit in which the identify of R_L is preserved.

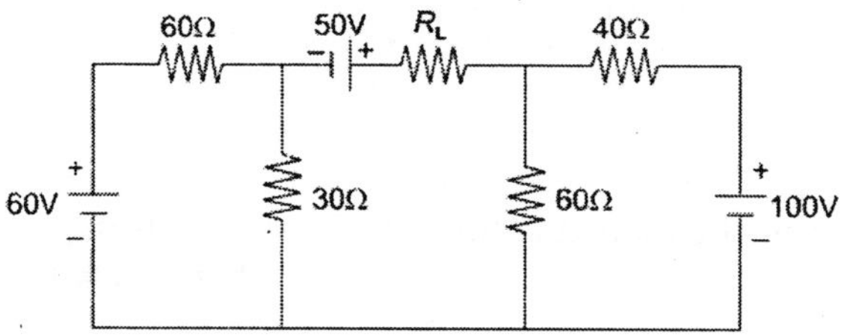

Based on Superposition Theorem

6. Determine the current I in the network shown in figure below by the principle of superposition theorem. **Ans.** $I = 4.5$ A

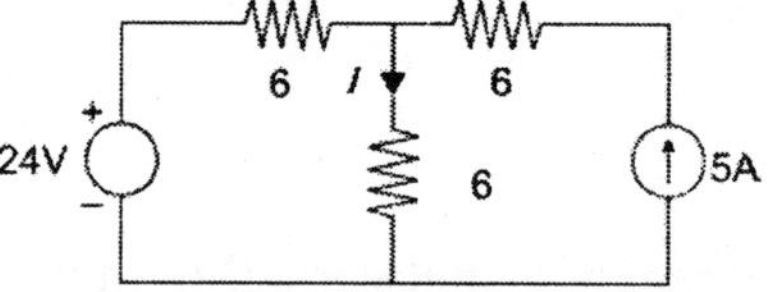

7. Determine the current I_1 in the circuit of figure below by the superposition theorem. **Ans.** $I_1 = 2$ A

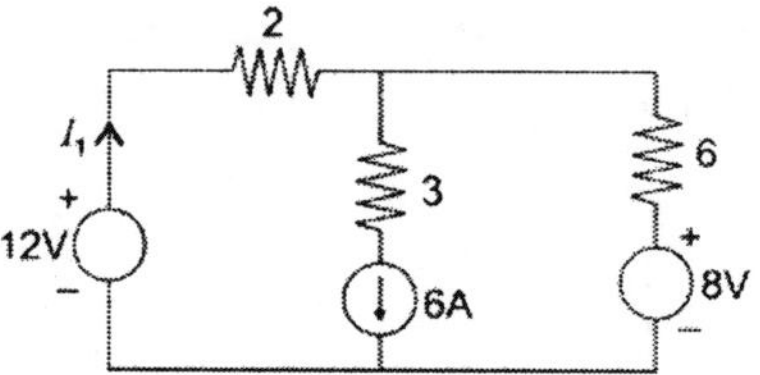

8. State superposition theorem. Use superposition theorem to determine the current through the 2 Ω resistor in the network of figure below. **Ans.** $I = \frac{2}{13}$ A

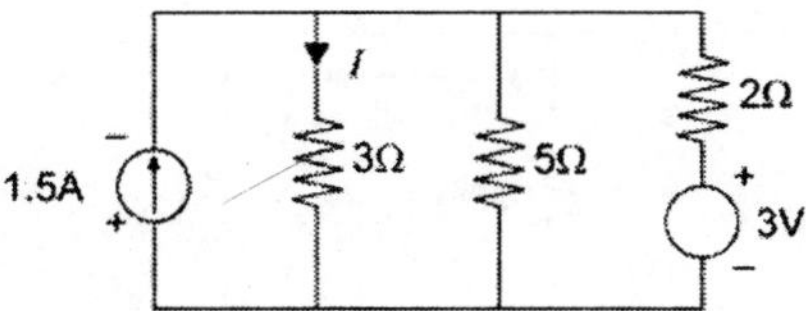

9. Use superposition theorem to determine I in the network of figure below.
Ans. $I = 7$ A

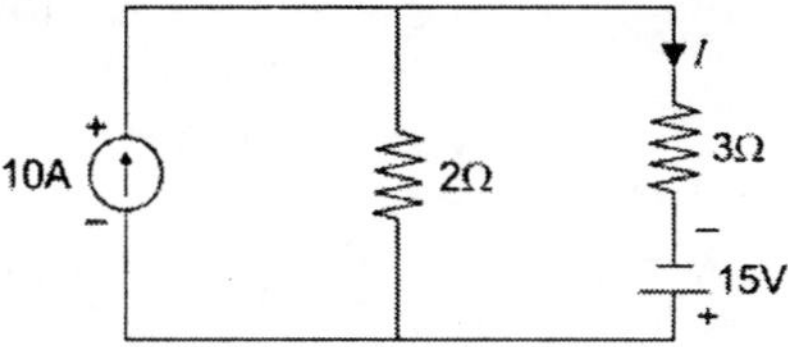

10. Determine the current I in the network of figure below by superposition theorem.

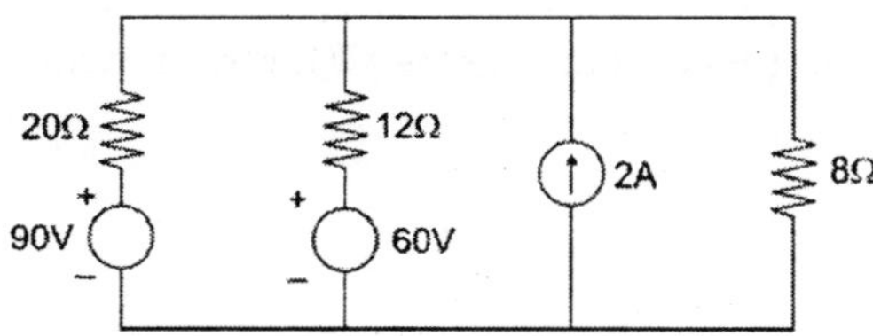

11. Using superposition theorem find the current in 20 Ω resistor of the circuit shown in figure below. **[Sem-I, 09-10]** **Ans.** $I = 2.27$ A

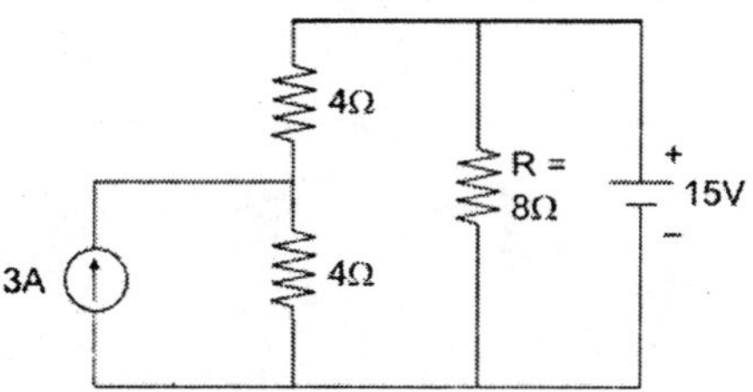

12. Using superposition theorem, find the current flowing through resistor R shown in figure below. **[MTU, 2011-12]** **Ans.** $I = 1.87$ A

13. Using superposition theorem find the current through 8 Ω for the given network. **Ans.** I = 11.75 A

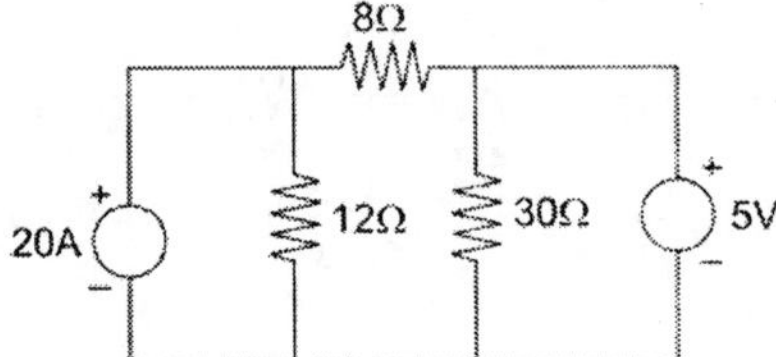

14. For the circuit of figure below, find I using superposition theorem.
[Sem-I, 2001] **Ans.** I = 1 A

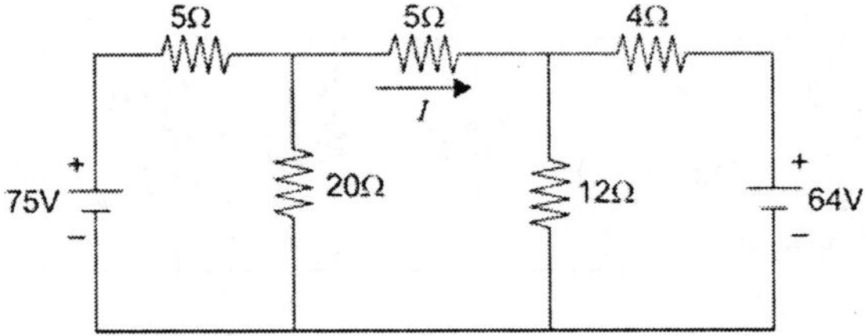

15. Determine current through 8 Ω resistor in the following network using superposition theorem. **[Sem-I, 2001]** **Ans.** I = 1.6 A

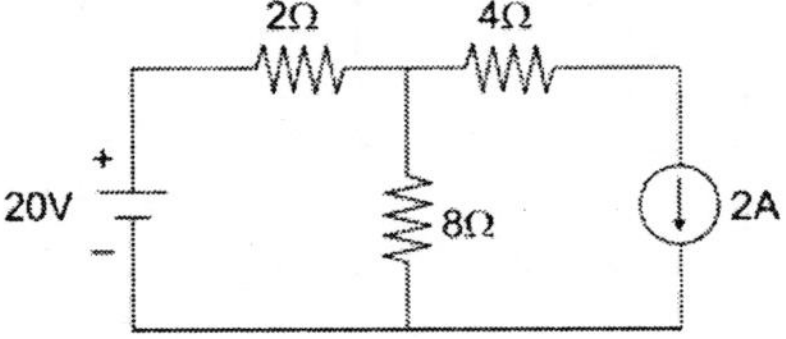

Based on Thevenin's Theorem

16. Obtain the Thevenin's equivalent across a-b for the network shown in figure below. **Ans.** 14 V, 3 W

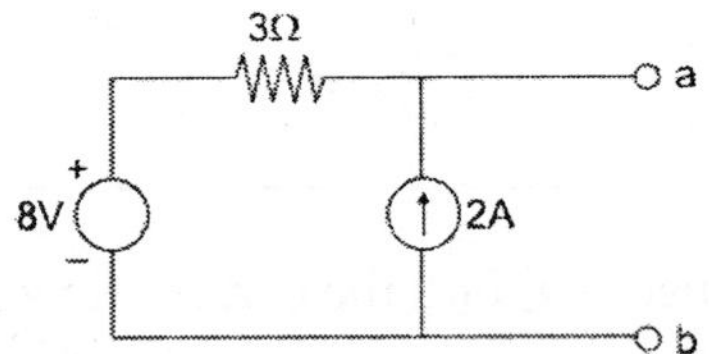

17. Find Thevenin's equivalent circuit using to the right of terminal 'ab' in figure below.

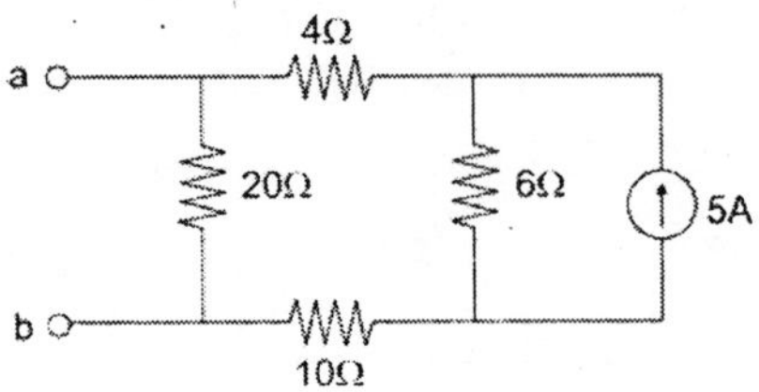

18. Determine the current through and voltage across 30 Ω resistor in figure below by applying Thevenin's theorem. **[Sem-I, 2007-08] Ans.** 0.2 A, 6 V

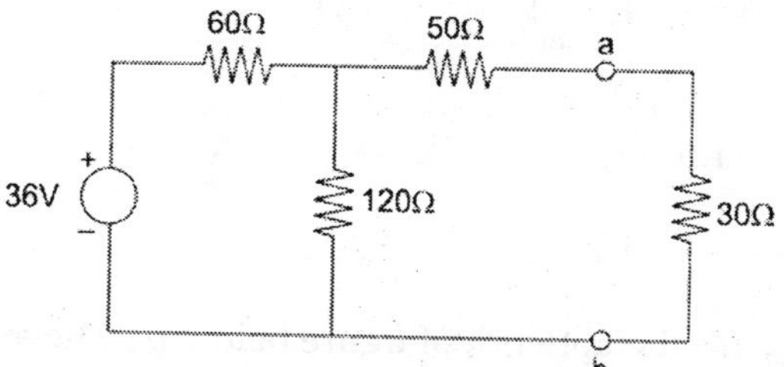

19. Determine the current I in the circuit of figure below by using Thevenin's theorem.

Ans. $I = \frac{5}{7}$ A

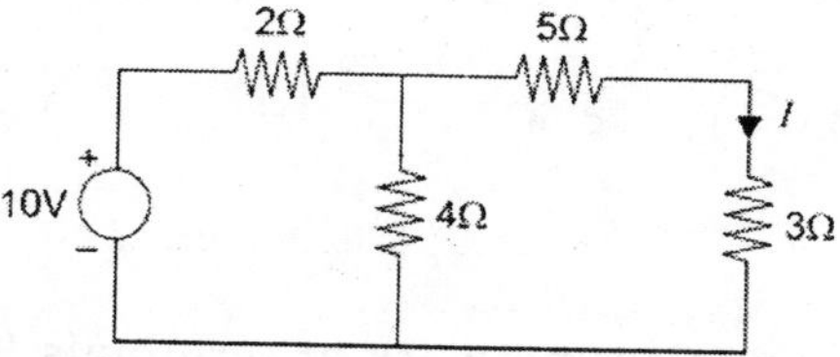

20. Determine current through 5 Ω resistor in figure below by using Thevenin's theorem.

Ans. I = 1 A

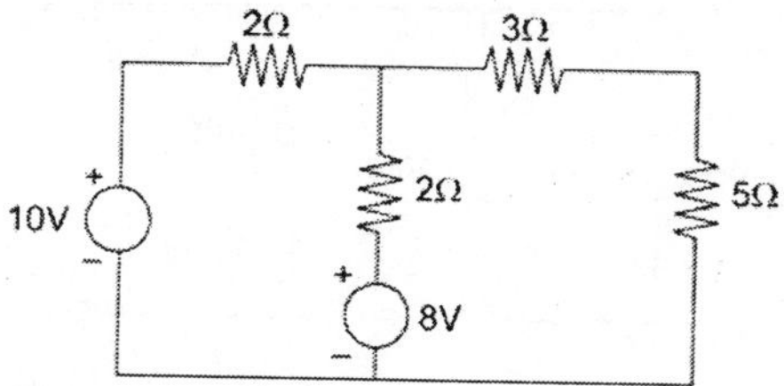

21. State Thevenin's theorem, deduce Thevenin's equivalent circuits for terminals ab in the network shown in figure below. **Ans.** I = 16 mA, V_L = 1.6 A

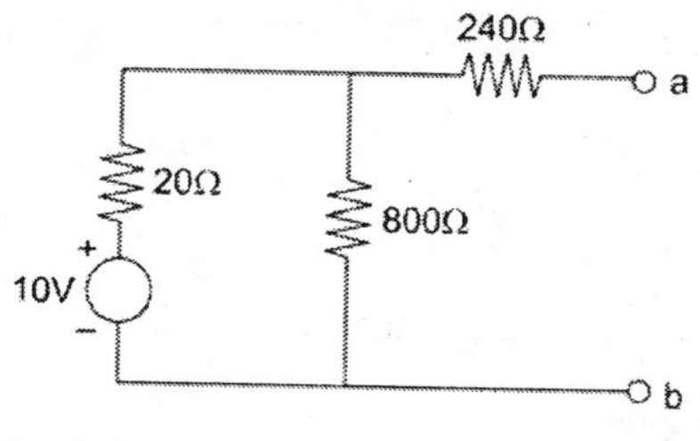

22. Obtain Thevenin's equivalent circuit at terminals ab for the network of figure below.

Ans. $V_{TH} = 5\text{ V}, R_{TH} = \frac{9}{4}\,\Omega$

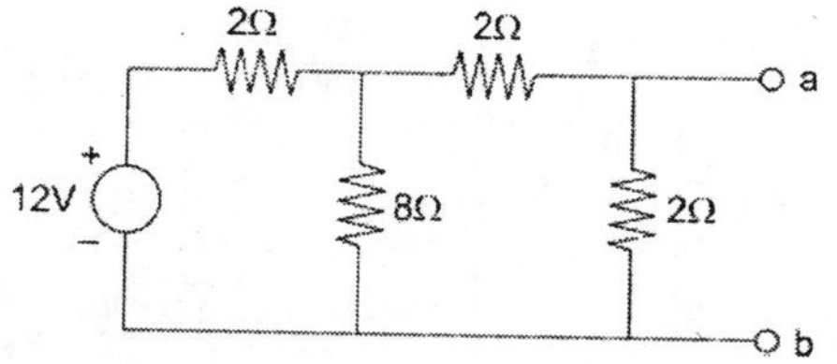

23. Find Thevenin's equivalent circuit at terminals 'ab' for the network of figure below.

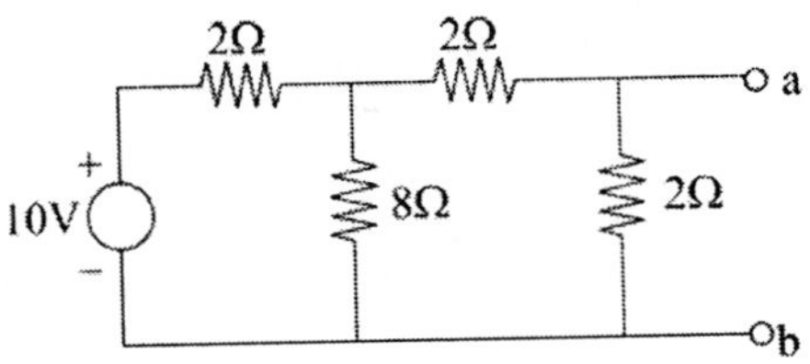

24. Find V_{ab} and R_{TH} for the network of figure below by Thevenin's theorem.

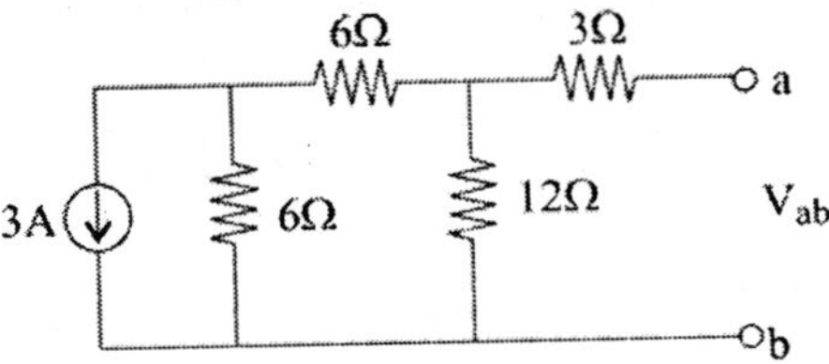

25. Find Thevenin's equivalent network at terminals 'ab' for the network of figure below. **[Sem-I, 09-10] Ans.** $V_{TH} = 5$ V, $R_{TH} = 5\ \Omega$

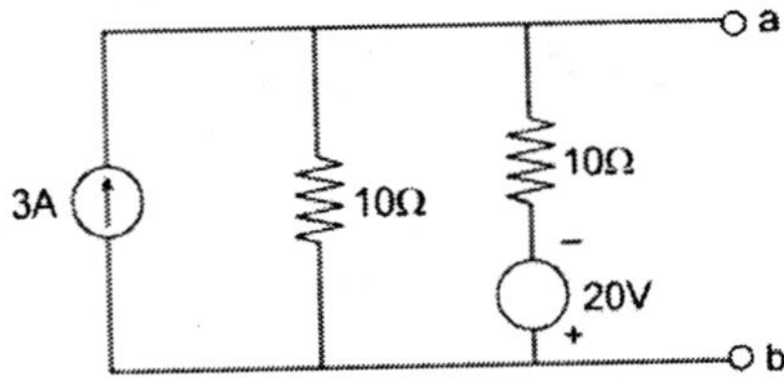

26. Determine current through 1 Ω resistance in the network of figure below by using Thevenin's' theorem. **[Sem-I, 08-09] Ans.** $I = 2$ A

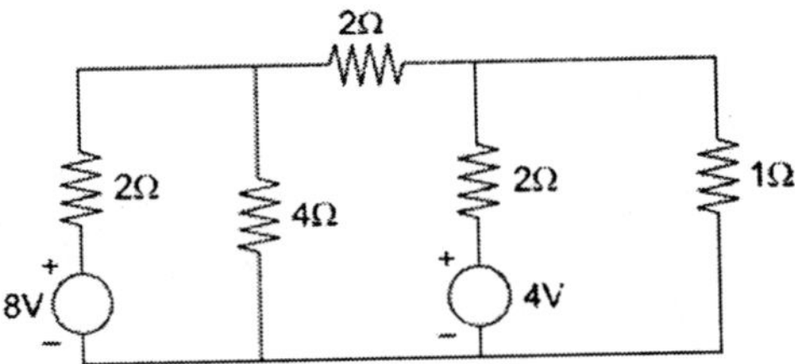

Based on Norton's Theorem

27. For the circuit shown in figure below drawn the Norton's equivalent circuit at terminal ab. **Ans.** $I_N = 3$ A, $R_N = 2.4\ \Omega$

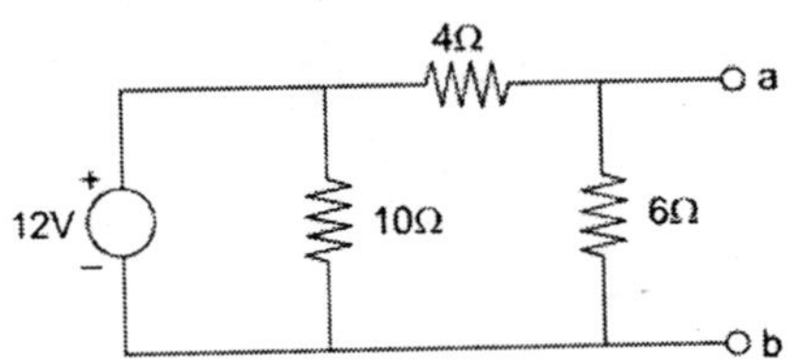

28. Determine current through 5 Ω resistor in the circuit of figure below by using Norton's theorem. **[Sem-I, 07-08] Ans.** $\frac{20}{11}$ A

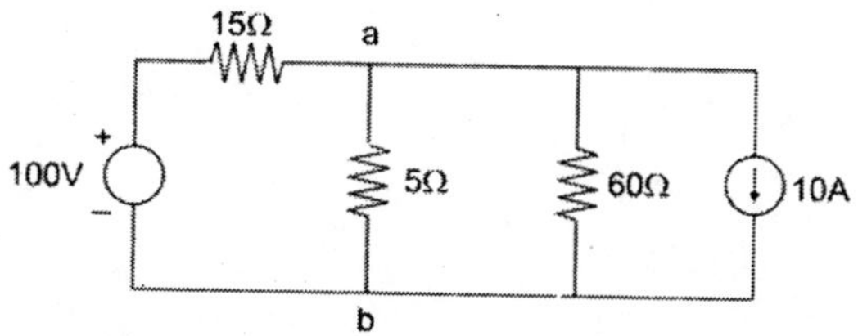

29. State Norton's theorems. Deduce Norton's equivalent circuit for terminals ab in the network shown in figure below also find the current in 100 Ω.
[Sem-II, 07-08] Ans. $I_L = 16mA$

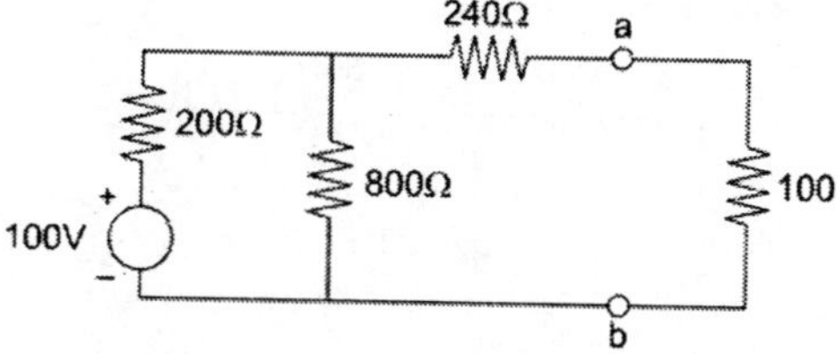

30. Determine the current through 3 Ω resistor in figure below using Norton's theorem.
Ans. $\frac{28}{13}$ A

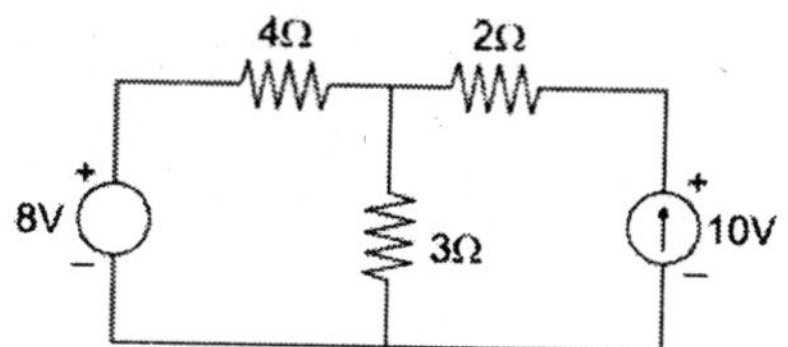

31. Find the Norton's equivalent circuits at terminals *ab* for the network of figure below. **Ans.** $R_N = \frac{7}{4}\,\Omega,\ I_N = \frac{48}{7}$ A

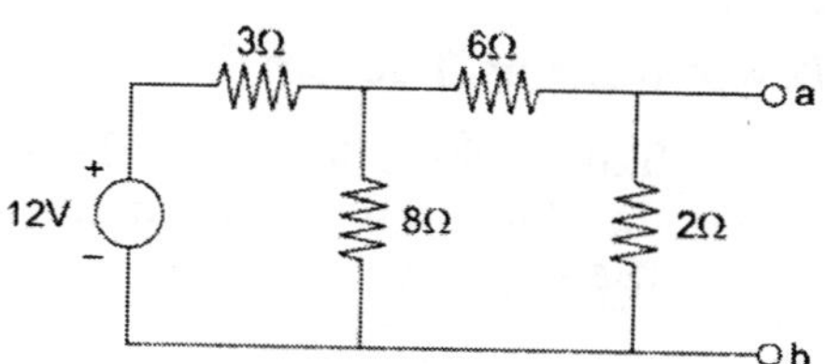

32. Determine the current through 1 Ω resistor in the network of figure below by Norton's theorem.

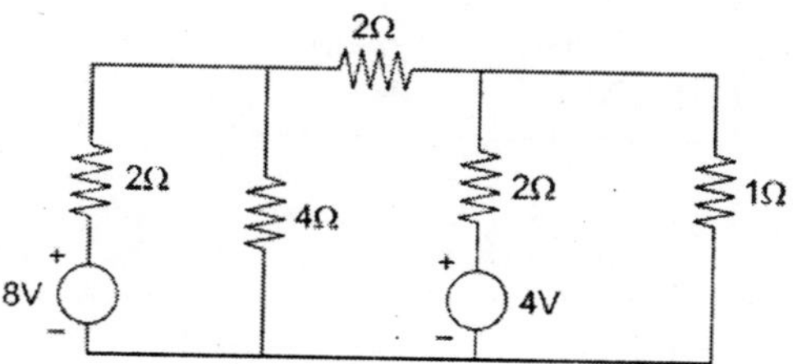

33. Find the current in 25 Ω which are connected between point *PQ* by Norton's theorem. **Ans.** $\frac{20}{7}$

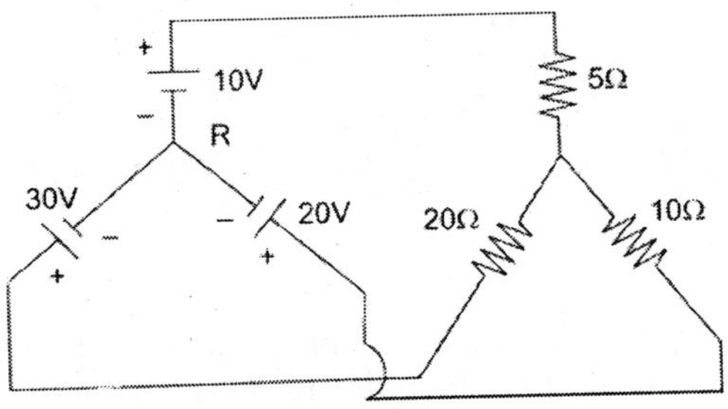

34. Determine the current through 30 Ω resistor in figure below by applying Norton's theorem. **[Sem-I, 2008-09]**

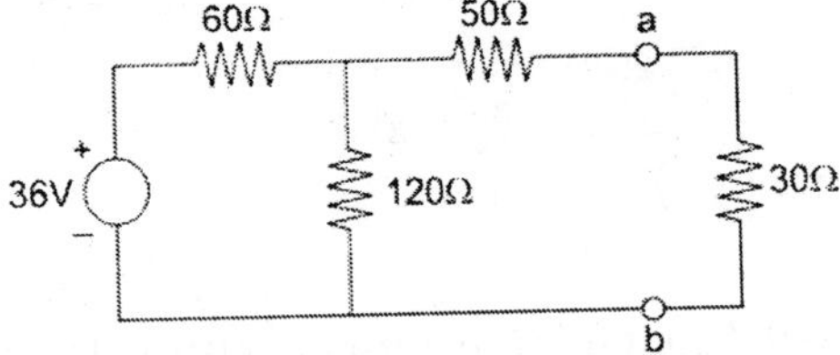

35. Find the Norton's equivalent circuit across *AB*. **[UPTU 2007-08]**

Ans. $R_N = 9$ W, $I_N = 0.66$ A

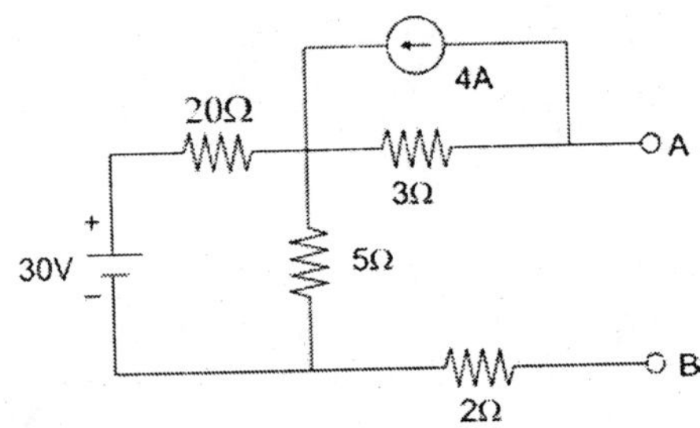

Based on Maximum Power Transfer Theorem

36. In the network shown in figure below, determine the value of the load resistance to give maximum power transfer and the power delivered to the load.

[Sem-I, 04-05] **Ans.** $R_L = 2.625\ \Omega, P_{L\max} = 11.52$ watts

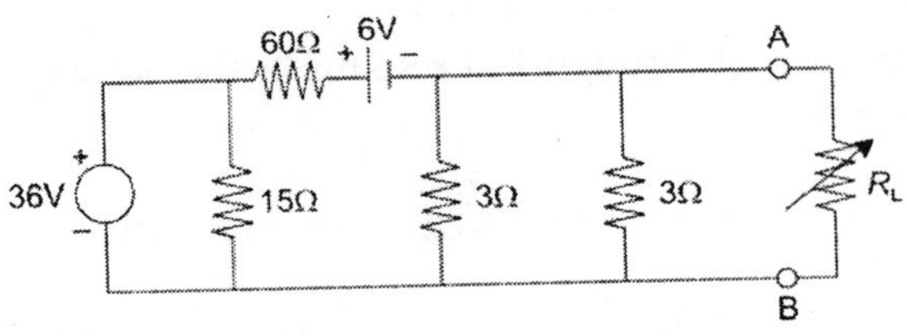

Chapter

6 AC Network Theorems

6.1 INTRODUCTION

An electric circuit or network comprises a number of interconnected single circuit elements. These networks should generally contain at least one voltage or current source. The arrangement of elements results in a new set of constraints between the current and voltages.

6.2 STAR–DELTA AND DELTA–STAR TRANSFORMATIONS

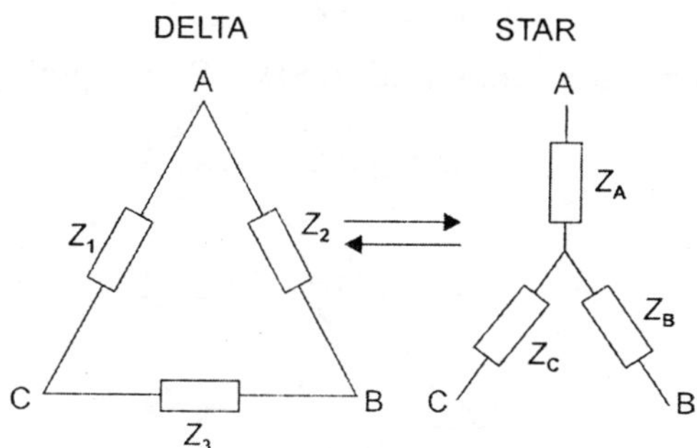

Fig. 6.1

Impedances between terminals B and C.

$$Z_{BC} = Z_B + Z_C = \frac{(Z_1 + Z_2)Z_3}{Z_1 + Z_2 + Z_3} \quad \text{...(6.1)}$$

Impedances between terminals C and A.

$$Z_{CA} = Z_C + Z_A = \frac{(Z_2 + Z_3)Z_1}{Z_1 + Z_2 + Z_3} \quad \text{...(6.2)}$$

Impedances between terminals A and B.

$$Z_{AB} = Z_A + Z_B = \frac{(Z_1 + Z_3)Z_2}{Z_1 + Z_2 + Z_3} \quad \text{...(6.3)}$$

Adding Eqs (6.1), (6.2) and (6.3), we get

$$2(Z_A + Z_B + Z_C) = \frac{2(Z_1Z_2 + Z_2Z_3 + Z_3Z_1)}{Z_1 + Z_2 + Z_3}$$

$$Z_A + Z_B + Z_C = \frac{Z_1Z_2 + Z_2Z_3 + Z_3Z_1}{Z_1 + Z_2 + Z_3} \quad ...(6.4)$$

Subtract Eqs (6.1), (6.2) and (6.3) from (6.4), we get

$$Z_A = \frac{Z_1Z_2}{Z_1 + Z_2 + Z_3} \quad ...(6.5)$$

$$Z_B = \frac{Z_2Z_3}{Z_1 + Z_2 + Z_3} \quad ...(6.6)$$

$$Z_C = \frac{Z_3Z_1}{Z_1 + Z_2 + Z_3} \quad ...(6.7)$$

Multiplying Eqs (6.5)·(6.6), (6.6)·(6.7) and (6.7)·(6.5) and adding them, we get

$$Z_AZ_B + Z_BZ_C + Z_CZ_A = \frac{Z_1Z_2^2Z_3 + Z_2Z_1Z_3^2 + Z_3Z_1^2Z_2}{(Z_1 + Z_2 + Z_3)^2}$$

$$= \frac{Z_1Z_2Z_3(Z_1 + Z_2 + Z_3)}{(Z_1 + Z_2 + Z_3)^2}$$

$$= \frac{Z_1Z_2Z_3}{(Z_1 + Z_2 + Z_3)} \quad ...(6.8)$$

Dividing Eqs (6.8)/(6.5), (6.8)/(6.6) and (6.8)/(6.7), we get

$$Z_3 = \frac{Z_AZ_B + Z_BZ_C + Z_CZ_A}{Z_A} \quad ...(6.9)$$

$$Z_1 = \frac{Z_AZ_B + Z_BZ_C + Z_CZ_A}{Z_B} \quad ...(6.10)$$

$$Z_2 = \frac{Z_AZ_B + Z_BZ_C + Z_CZ_A}{Z_C} \quad ...(6.11)$$

Equations (6.5), (6.6) and (6.7) represent the transformation from delta to star.
Equations (6.9), (6.10) and (6.11) represent the transformation from star to delta.

6.2.1 Delta to Star Conversion

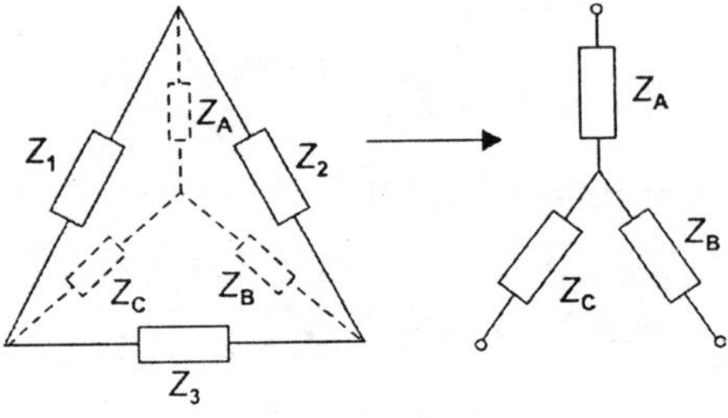

Fig. 6.2

$$Z_A = \frac{Z_1Z_2}{Z_1 + Z_2 + Z_3}$$

$$Z_B = \frac{Z_2 Z_3}{Z_1 + Z_2 + Z_3}$$

$$Z_C = \frac{Z_3 Z_1}{Z_1 + Z_2 + Z_3}$$

6.2.2 Star to Delta Conversion

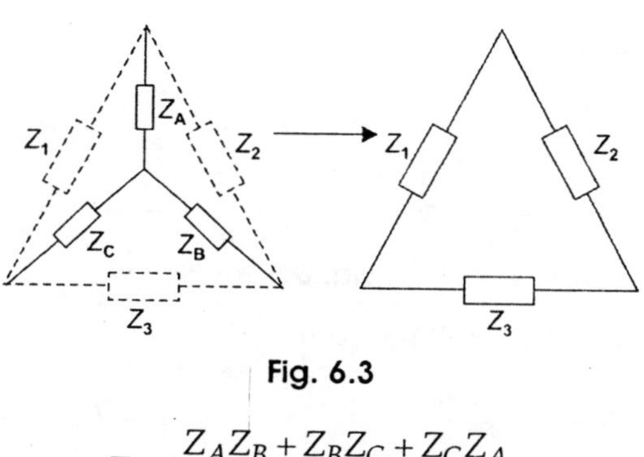

Fig. 6.3

$$Z_1 = \frac{Z_A Z_B + Z_B Z_C + Z_C Z_A}{Z_B}$$

$$Z_2 = \frac{Z_A Z_B + Z_B Z_C + Z_C Z_A}{Z_C}$$

$$Z_3 = \frac{Z_A Z_B + Z_B Z_C + Z_C Z_A}{Z_A}$$

6.3 SOURCE TRANSFORMATIONS

In the circuit analysis, a circuit with either voltage sources only or current sources only may be preferable. Because a circuit may have both, *i.e.* voltage sources and current sources, it is convenient to be able to transform voltage sources to equivalent current sources, and current sources to equivalent voltage sources. For a transformation, each voltage source should have a series internal resistance (or impedance), and each current sources have a parallel internal resistance (or impedance).

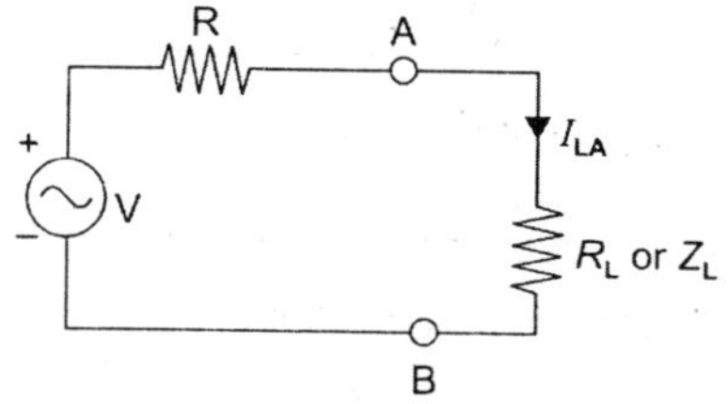

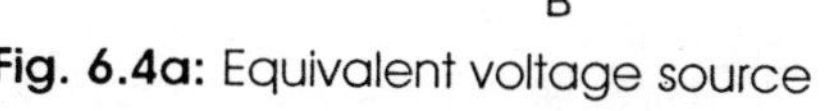

Fig. 6.4a: Equivalent voltage source

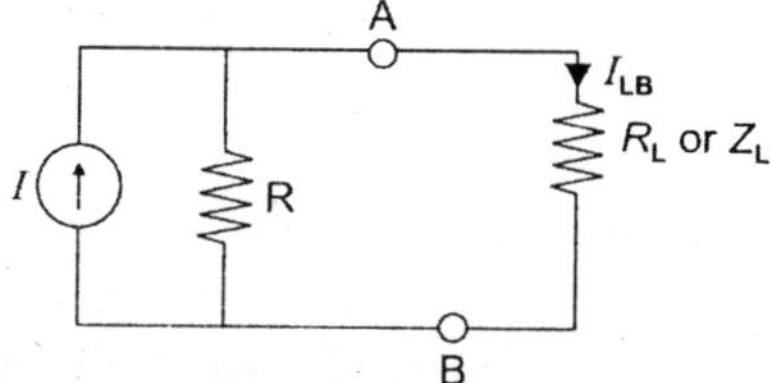

Fig. 6.4b: Equivalent current source

In both circuit current is same because load is same

i.*e.* $I_{LA} = I_{LB}$

$$I_{LA} = \frac{V}{R + R_L}, \quad I_{LB} = I \times \frac{R}{R + R_L}$$

$$I_{LA} = I_{LB}$$

$$\frac{V}{R+R_L} = I\frac{R}{R+R_L}$$

$$V = IR$$

$$I = \frac{V}{R}$$

Voltage source to equivalent current source

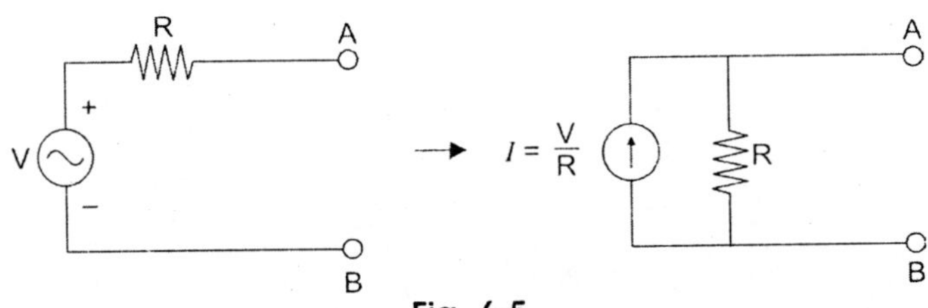

Fig. 6.5

Current source to equivalent voltage source

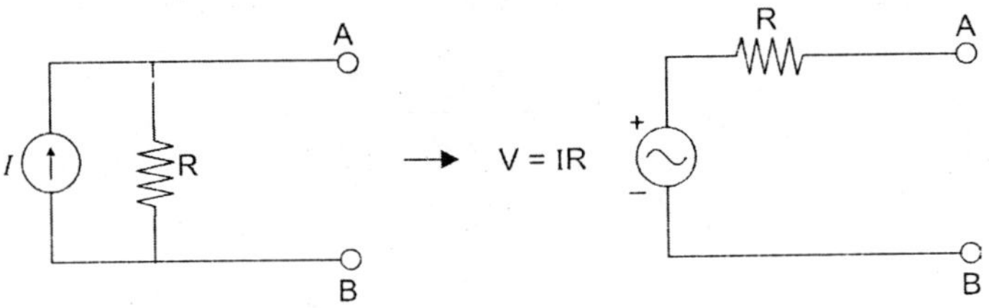

Fig. 6.6

Example: Find the voltages across the impedances in the circuit shown in figure below, then transform the voltage source 10∠30°Ω and impedance to an equivalent current source and again find the voltage, hence compare the results.

Solution: By voltage division

$$V_1 = \frac{10\angle 30° \times 50\angle 20°}{10\angle 30° + 8\angle 20°}$$

$$= \frac{500\angle 50°}{17.9\angle 25.6°} = 27.9\angle 24.4° \text{ V}$$

By Apply KVL $\quad V_2 = 50\angle 20° - 27.9\angle 24.4°$

$$= 22.3\angle 14.4° \text{ V}$$

Now transformation of the voltage source result in a current source of

$$\frac{50\angle 20°}{10\angle 30°} = 5\angle -10° \text{A}$$

$$V = I_{(Z_{eq})}$$

$$= 5\angle -10° \times \frac{10\angle 30° \times 8\angle 20°}{10\angle 30° + 8\angle 20°}$$

$$= 22.3\angle 14.4° \text{ V (verified)}$$ **Ans.**

6.4 NETWORK TERMINOLOGY

6.4.1 Loop and Mesh

A loop is any closed path of a circuit, while mesh is a loop which does not contain any other loop within it. Therefore, all the meshes are loops and a loop is not necessarily a mesh. Loop may have other loops or meshes inside it.

6.4.2 Node and Junction

A point where two or more branches meet is called a node, while a junction is a point at which three or more branches are joined together. Therefore, all the junctions are nodes and a node is not necessarily a junction.

6.4.3 Sign Convension

An electrical element having two terminals A and B known as a two-terminal element, is shown in Fig. 6.7, current i flows in the direction shown, from A to B. Voltage V drops from A to B, i.e. A is at a higher potential than B. Hence A is marked positive (+) and B negative (–).

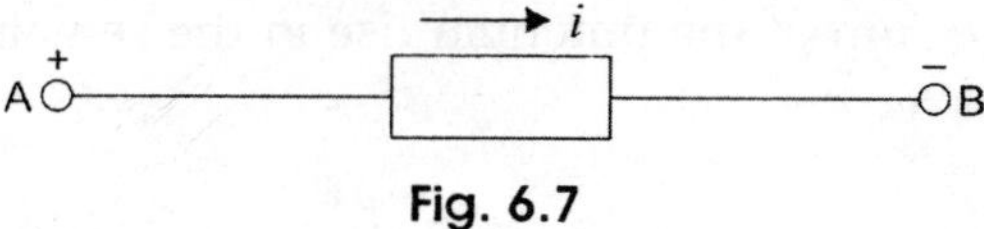

Fig. 6.7

6.5 KIRCHHOFF'S LAWS

Gustav Robert Kirchhoff derived two fundamental laws applicable to any electrical circuit. These laws concern the algebriac sum of all branch voltages around a loop and all branch currents entering or leaving a node.

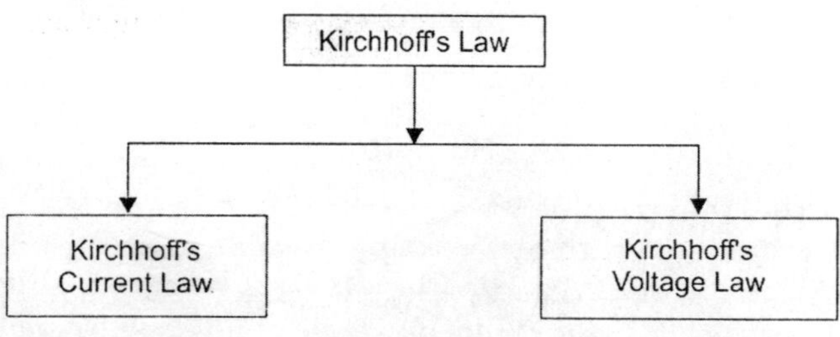

Fig. 6.8

Kirchhoff's Current Law (KCL)

It states that the algebraic sum of current meeting at a point or junction on node is equal to zero. In other words, the algebraiac sum of incoming current towards the junction or node is equal to the algebriac sum of outgoing current away from the junction or node.

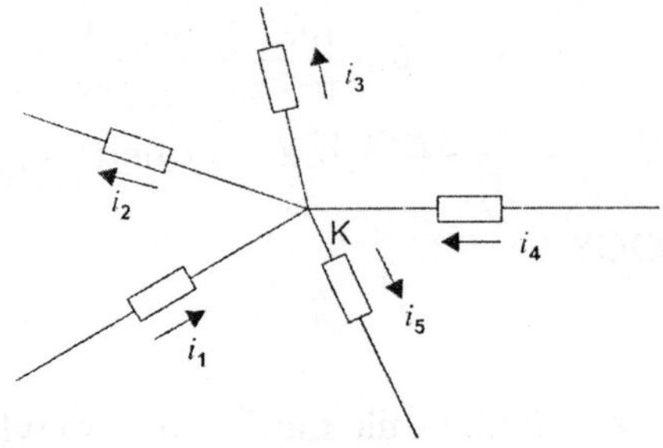

Fig. 6.9

$$i_1 - i_2 - i_3 + i_4 - i_5 = 0$$

or $$i_1 + i_4 = i_2 + i_3 + i_5$$

Kirchhoff's Voltage Law (KVL)

It states that the algebriac sum of drop (or rise) in all branch voltages in a circuit, around a loop is zero at all instant of time.

$$\sum_{i=1}^{n} v_i = 0$$

In other words, we can say, the sum of potential drops, at any instant of time, along the branches of a circuit when transversing a loop in a certain direction, clockwise is equal to the sum of the potential rise in the remaining branches forming the loop."

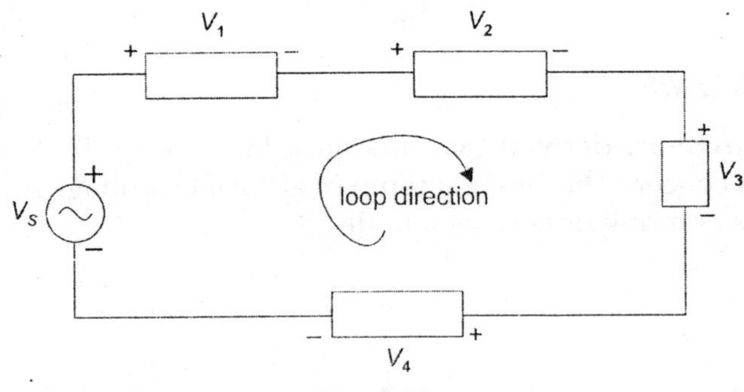

Fig. 6.10

$$V_S - V_1 - V_2 - V_3 - V_4 = 0$$

$$V_S = V_1 + V_2 + V_3 + V_4$$

6.5.1 Super-Node Analysis

Sometimes, a branch in the circuit has only a voltage source, then it is slightly difficult to apply nodal analysis (or KCL at the node at which this branch incident). In this case, we may apply supernode technique. In this technique, the adjacent nodes those are connected by a voltage source are reduced to a single node and then the KCL can be applied as usual.

Example: Calculate the current in 3 Ω resistor for the circuit shown in figure below.

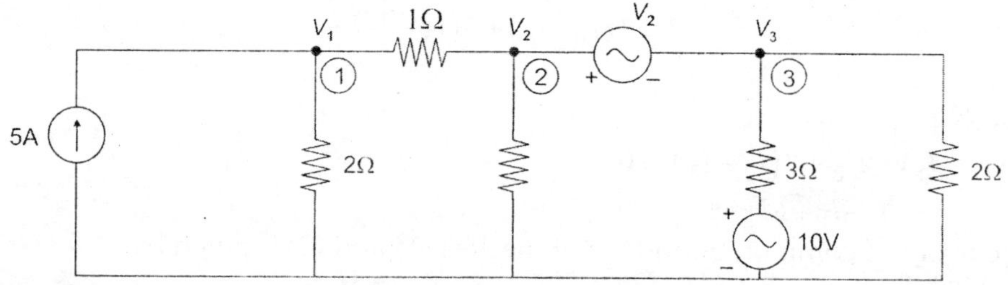

Solution: Applying KCL
At node 1:

$$5 = \frac{V_1}{2} + \frac{V_1 - V_2}{1}$$

or $$3V_1 - 2V_2 = 10 \quad ...(1)$$

At super node (*i.e.* node 2 and 3):

$$\frac{V_2 - V_1}{1} + \frac{V_2}{2} + \frac{V_3 - 10}{3} + \frac{V_3}{2} = 0$$

$$-6V_1 + 9V_3 + 5V_3 = 20 \quad ...(2)$$

The voltage between nodes 2 and 3 is given by

$$V_2 - V_3 = 20 \quad ...(3)$$

From Eqs (1) and (3)

$$3V_1 - 2V_3 = 50 \quad ...(4)$$

From Eqs (2) and (4)

$$10V_3 = 120, \text{ or } V_3 = 12 \text{ V}$$

Therefore, the current in 3 Ω resistors

$$I = \frac{V_3 - 10}{3} = \frac{2}{3} \text{ A} \quad \textbf{Ans.}$$

6.5.2 Super-Mesh Analysis

Sometimes, a branch in the circuit has a current source then it is slightly difficult to apply mesh analysis (or KVL in the loop in which this branch exist). In this case, we may apply super-mesh technique. In this techniques, a super-mesh is continued by two adjacent loops that have a common current source.

Example: Calculate the current in 3 Ω resistor for the circuit shown in figure below.

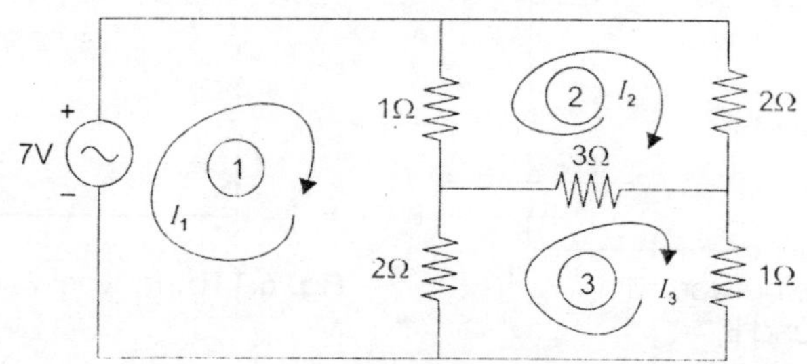

Solution: Apply *KVL*

In super-mesh (*i.e.* mesh 1 and 3);

$$7 = 1(I_1 - I_3) + 3(I_3 - I_2) + 1 \cdot I_3$$

or $$I_1 - 4I_2 + 4I_3 = 7 \quad ...(1)$$

In mesh 2:

$$1(I_2 - I_1) + 2I_2 + 3(I_2 - I_3) = 0$$

or $$-I_1 + 6I_2 - 3I_3 = 0 \quad ...(2)$$

The current of common boundary of meshes (1) and (3) is given by

$$I_1 - I_3 = 7 \quad ...(3)$$

Solving Eqs (1), (2) and (3), we get

$$I_1 = 9\text{A},\ I_2 = 2.5 \text{ A and } I_3 = 2 \text{ A}$$

Therefore, the current in 3 Ω

$$I = I_2 - I_3 = 0.5 \text{ A}$$ **Ans.**

6.6 SUPERPOSITION THEOREM

Statement: It states that: In an active linear network containing several sources (including dependent sources), the overall response (branches current or voltage) in any branch in the network equals the algebriac sum of the response (current) of each individual source considered separately with all other sources made in operative, *i.e.* replaced by their internal resistances or impedances.

To make a source operative, it is short circuited behind its internal resistance or impedance, if it is voltage source. And it is open circuited leaving behind its internal resistance or impedance, if it is a current source.

6.6.1 Applications of Superposition Theorem

The superposition theorem is applicable for any linear circuit having time-varying or time-invariant elements. It is useful in circuit analysis, when the circuit has a large number of independent sources, as it makes it possible to considered the effect of each source separately.

6.6.2 Limitations of Superposition Theorem

Not applicable to the circuit consisting of only dependent sources, circuits consisting of nonlinear elements like diode, transister etc., for calculation of power, since the power is proportional to the square (which is non-linear) of current or voltage and not useful to the circuits consisting of less than two independent sources.

6.7 THEVENIN'S AND NORTON'S THEOREMS

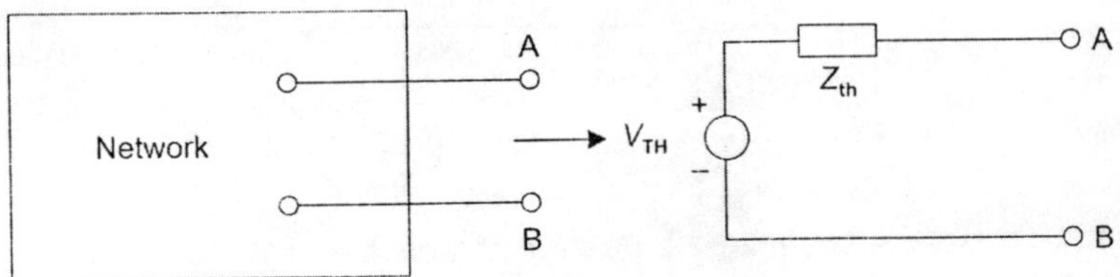

Fig. 611a: An active network with terminal A and B

Fig. 6.11b: Thevenin's equivalent

Thevenin's Theorem

Statement: It states that in any linear active network with output terminal AB may be replaced by a voltage source V_{th} in series with internal impedance Z_{th}. The voltage source V_{th} called the Thevenin's voltage, is the potential difference ($V_A - V_B$) between the terminal A and B and Zth is the internal impedance of the network as seen from the terminals A and B with all the sources set to zero, *i.e.* with all the voltage sources shorted all the current sources open circuited leaving behind their internal resistance or impedances.

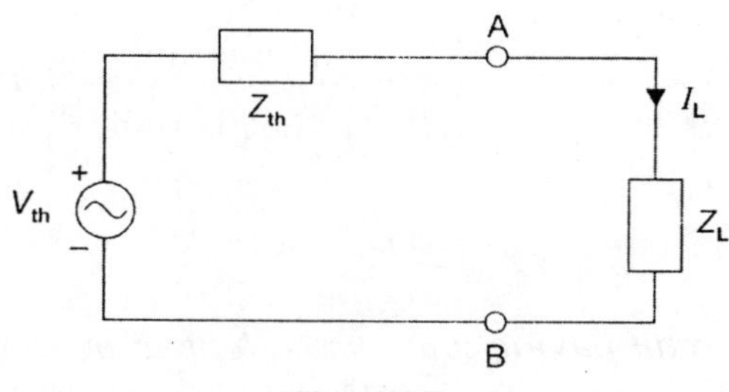

Fig. 6.12

For Thevenin's equivalent circuit

$$I_L = \frac{V_{th}}{Z_{th} + Z_L}$$

Norton's Theorem

Statement: With respect to the terminal pair AB, the network with output terminal may be replaced with a current source I_N in parallel with an internal impedance Z_n. The current source I_N called the Norton's current is the current that would flow from A to B when the terminals A and B are shorted together and Z_n is the same internal impedance as defined earlier in context to Thevenin's theorem.

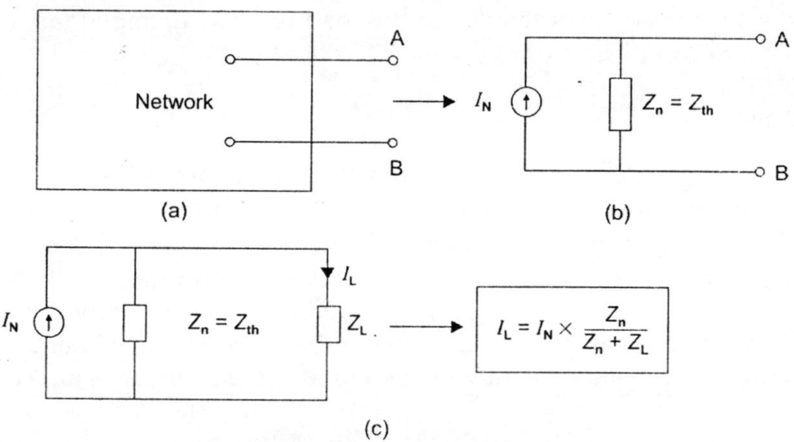

Fig. 6.13: Norton's equivalent circuit

6.7.1 Procedure to Obtain V_{th} and Z_{th} or I_N and Z_n

Step I: Remove the position of the network across which Thevenin's or Norton's equivalent circuit is to found.

Step II: Mark the terminal *AB* of the remaining 2-terminal circuit.

Step III: (*a*) Obtain the open circuit voltage at the terminal *AB*, i.e. V_{th} keeping all the sources at their normal values. (*b*) Short the terminals *AB*. Obtain the short circuit current, i.e. I_N flowing from *A* to *B* keeping all the sources of their normal values.

Step IV: Calculate $Z_{th} = Z_N$.

Case i: *If circuit having only independent sources:* In this case, set all the sources at zero values, *i.e.* with all the voltage sources shorted and all the current sources open circuited leaving behind their internal resistances or impedances.

Case ii: *If circuit having independent and dependent sources both:* In this case, we calculate V_{th} and I_N, then the internal impedance of the network N is obtained as

$$Z_{th} = Z_N = \frac{V_{th}}{I_N}$$

Case iii: *If circuit having only dependent sources:* In this case, we apply a voltage *V* at the terminal pair *AB*. A current *I* will flow due to application of *V*, then the internal impedance of the network N is obtained as:

$$Z_{th} = Z_n = \frac{V}{I}$$

Step V: Draw the equivalent circuit across *AB*: (*a*) Thevenin's voltage V_{th} in series with Z_{th} and (*b*) Norton's current I_N in parallel with Z_n.

6.7.2 Applications of Thevenin's and Norton's Theorems

One of the main applications of Thevenin's and Norton's theorems are the replacement of a large part of a network, often a complicated end uninteresting part, by a very simple equivalent. The new simpler circuit, enables one to make rapid calculations of the voltage, current and hence power which the original circuit is able to deliver to a load. It also help us to choose the best value of this load resistance/impedances required to accomplish a maximum transfer of power.

6.7.3 Limitations

Not applicable to the circuit consisting of unilateral elements like diode etc., nonlinear elements like diode transistor etc., load series or parallel with controlled or dependent sources and magnetic coupling between load and any other circuit element.

[A] As applicable to voltage sources: Consider a circuit containing *n* voltage sources $E_1, E_2, ..., E_n$ and their corresponding series impedance (internal impedance) $Z_1, Z_2, ..., Z_n$ respectively operating in parallel as shown in Fig. 6.14. Then by Millman's theorem, we can determine E_m the equivalent voltage source and Z_m the series impedance, given by

$$E_m = \frac{\sum_{i=1}^{n} E_i \cdot Y_i}{\sum_{i=1}^{n} Y_i} = \frac{E_1Y_1 + E_2Y_2 + ... + E_nY_n}{Y_1 + Y_2 + ... + Y_n}$$

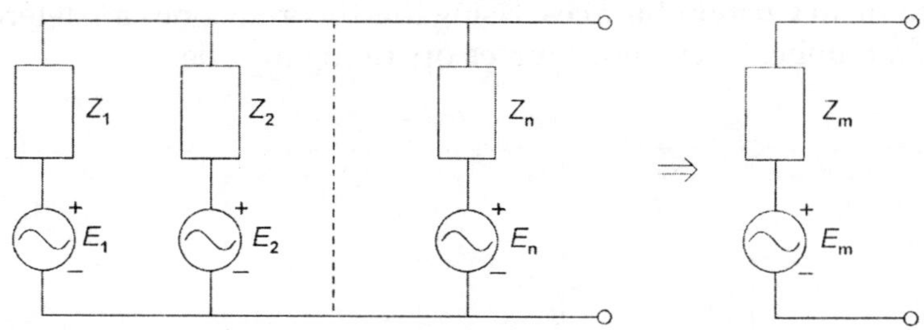

Fig. 6.14: Circuit illustrating Millman's theorem for voltage sources

$$Z_m = \frac{1}{\sum_{i=1}^{n} Y_i} = \frac{1}{Y_1 + Y_2 + ... + Y_n}$$

To prove, each Thevenin's voltage equivalent is transformed into Norton's current equivalent as shown in Fig. 6.15a, using

$$I_1 = \frac{E_i}{Z_i} = E_i Y_i;\ i = 1,2,...,n$$

and $$Y_i = \frac{1}{Z_i};\ i = 1,2,...,n$$

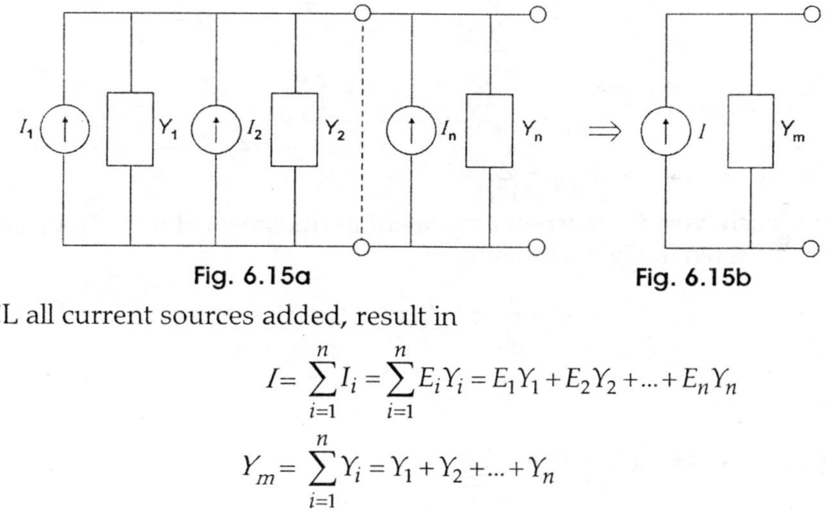

Fig. 6.15a

Fig. 6.15b

By KCL all current sources added, result in

$$I = \sum_{i=1}^{n} I_i = \sum_{i=1}^{n} E_i Y_i = E_1 Y_1 + E_2 Y_2 + ... + E_n Y_n$$

and $$Y_m = \sum_{i=1}^{n} Y_i = Y_1 + Y_2 + ... + Y_n$$

Then transforming back to voltage source E_m in series with impedance Z_m as shown in Fig. 6.15b.

$$E_m = \frac{1}{Y_m} = \frac{\sum_{i=1}^{n} E_i Y_i}{\sum_{i=1}^{n} Y_i}$$

and $$Z_m = \frac{1}{Y_m} = \frac{1}{\sum_{i=1}^{n} Y_i}$$

As Applicable to Current Sources: Using this theorem, one can determine Norton's equivalent of a number of current sources operating in series.

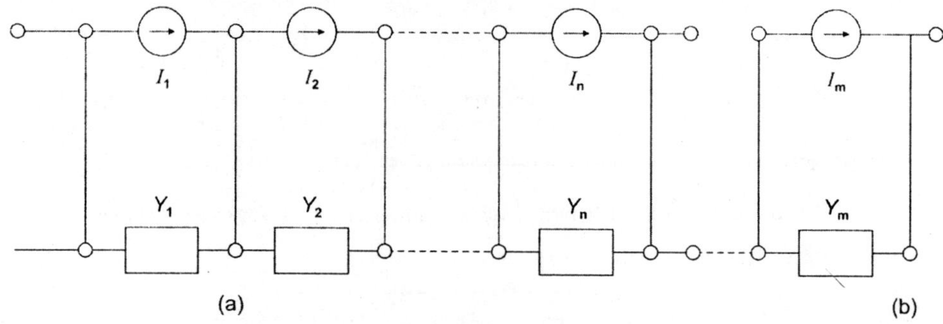

Fig. 6.16: Circuit illustrating Millman's theorem for current sources

Consider a circuit containing n current sources I_1, I_2,... I_n and their corresponding parallel admittances (Internal admittances) Y_1, Y_2,..., Y_n respectively operating in series as shown in Fig. 6.16a. Then by Millman's theorem, we can determine I_m, the equivalent current source and Y_m, the parallel admittance, given by

$$I_m = \frac{\sum_{i=1}^{n} I_i Z_i}{\sum_{i=1}^{n} Z_i} = \frac{I_1 Z_1 + I_2 Z_2 + ... + I_n Z_n}{Z_1 + Z_2 + ... + Z_n}$$

and
$$Y_m = \frac{1}{\sum_{i=1}^{n} Z_i} = \frac{1}{Z_1 + Z_2 + ... + Z_n}$$

To prove, each Norton's current equivalent in transformed into Thevenin's voltage equivalent as shown in Fig. 6.16a using

$$E_i = \frac{I_i}{Y_i} = I_i Z_i ; i = 1,2,...,n$$

and
$$Z_i = \frac{1}{Y_i} ; i = 1,2,...,n$$

All voltage sources added, result in

$$E = \sum_{i=1}^{n} E_i = \sum_{i=1}^{n} I_i Z_i = I_1 Z_1 + I_2 Z_2 + ... + I_n Z_n$$

and
$$Z_m = \sum_{i=1}^{n} Z_i = Z_1 + Z_2 + ... + Z_n$$

$$I_m = \frac{E}{Z_m} = \frac{\sum_{i=1}^{n} I_i Z_i}{\sum_{i=1}^{n} Z_i} \text{ and } Y_m = \frac{1}{Z_m} = \frac{1}{\sum_{i=1}^{n} Z_i}$$

6.7.4 Application of Millman's Theorem

Millman's theorem is an extension of Thevenin's or Norton's theorem for the circuit consisting of a number of independent voltage or current sources repsectively. In other words, we can say, this theorem provides the equivalent circuits which are either Thevenin's equivalent or Norton's equivalent circuits. It is to be noted that this theorem applies only to the independent voltage sources with their internal series impedances connected directly in parallel or independent current sources with their internal series admittance connected directly in series.

6.7.5 Limitations of Milliman's Theorem

Not applicable to the circuits consisting of impedances between the independent sources, dependent sources between the independent sources and not useful to the circuits consisting of less than two independent sources.

6.8 MAXIMUM POWER TRANSFER THEOREM

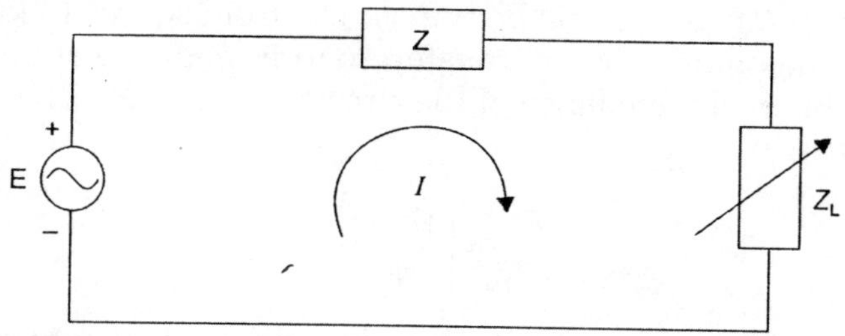

Fig. 6.17: Circuit diagram of maximum power transfer theorem

Case I: Maximum power output is obtained from an AC circuit when the load impedance is equal to the complex conjugate of the internal impedance of the circuit as seen from the terminals of the load. The maximum power transfer theorem aims at finding Z_L such that the power dissipated in it is maximum.

From Fig. 6.17

$$I = \frac{E}{Z + Z_L}$$

Power dissipated in the load

$$P = |I|^2 R_L$$

where $Z = R + JX$ and $Z_L = R_L + JX_L$

So $$P = \frac{E^2}{(R + R_L)^2 + (X + X_L)^2} R_L$$

For maximum power $\frac{\partial P}{\partial X_L}$ must be zero.

Now
$$\frac{\partial P}{\partial X_L} = \frac{0 - E^2 R_L \cdot 2(X + X_L)}{\left[(R+R_L)^2 + (X+X_L)^2\right]^2} = 0$$

or
$$E^2 \cdot R_L \cdot 2(X + X_L) = 0$$

or
$$X + X_L = 0$$
$$X_L = -X$$

i.e. the reactance of the load impedance is of opposite sign to the reactance of internal impedance of the circuit.

Putting $X_L = -X$

$$P = \frac{E^2 R_L}{(R+R_L)^2}$$

Again for maximum power $\frac{\partial P}{\partial R_L} = 0$

$$\frac{\partial P}{\partial R_L} = \frac{(R+R_L)^2 E^2 \cdot 1 - E^2 R_L (2)(R+R_L)}{(R+R_L).4} = 0$$

or
$$E^2 (R+R_L) - 2E^2 RL = 0$$

or
$$R_L = R$$

Therefore, maximum power will be transferred from source to load if $R_L = R$ and $X_L = -X$, *i.e.* for maximum power transfer, load impedance should be a complex conjugate of the internal impedance of the circuit, *i.e.* $Z_L = Z^*$. The maximum power transferred will be

$$P_{max} = \frac{E^2}{4R_L} = \left[\frac{(E/2)^2}{R_L}\right]$$

So, the overall efficiency of a circuit supplying maximum power is 50%.

Case II: Maximum power output is obtained from an AC circuit when the value of the load resistance is equal to the magnitude of the internal impedance of the circuit as seen from the terminals of the load.

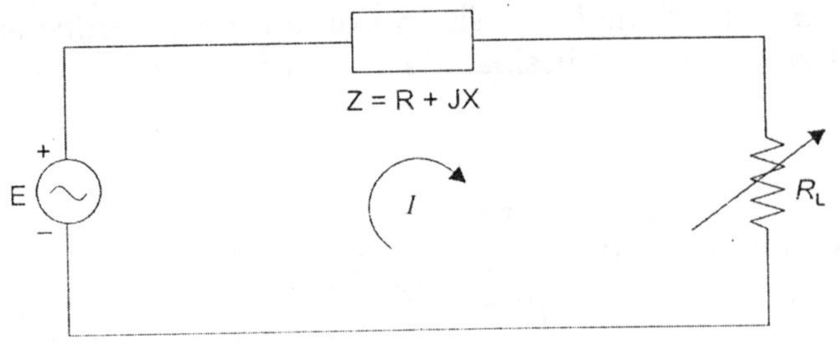

Fig. 6.18

From Fig. 6.19,
$$I = \frac{E}{R + R_L + JX}$$

Power dissipated in the load is

$$P = (I)^2 R_L = \frac{E^2}{(R+R_L)^2 + X^2} R_L$$

For maximum power, $\frac{dP}{dR_L}$ must be zero.

Now, $$\frac{dP}{dR_L} = \frac{\left[(R+R_L)^2 + X^2\right]E^2 - E^2 R_L \cdot 2(R+R_L)}{\left[(R+R_L)^2 + X^2\right]^2} = 0$$

or $$\left[(R+R_L)^2 + X^2\right]E^2 = E^2 R_L \cdot 2(R+R_L)$$

or $$R^2 + R_L^2 + 2RR_L + X^2 = 2RR_L + 2R_L{}^2$$

$$R_L^2 = R^2 + X^2$$

or $$R_L = \sqrt{R^2 + X^2} = |Z|$$

Thus, the maximum power will be transferred from source to resistive load R_L is the value of R_L is the magnitude of the internal impedance of the circuit.

Example: In the circuit shown in figure below, determine Z_L so that power absorbed by it is maximum and the value of the power absorbed.

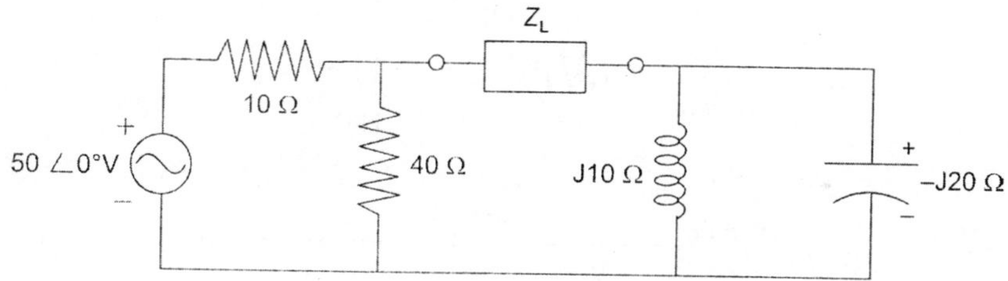

Solution: For (figure below) V_{th} is the voltage across 40 Ω, *i.e.*

$$V_{th} = 50\angle 0° \times \frac{40}{40+10} = 40\angle 0° \text{ V}$$

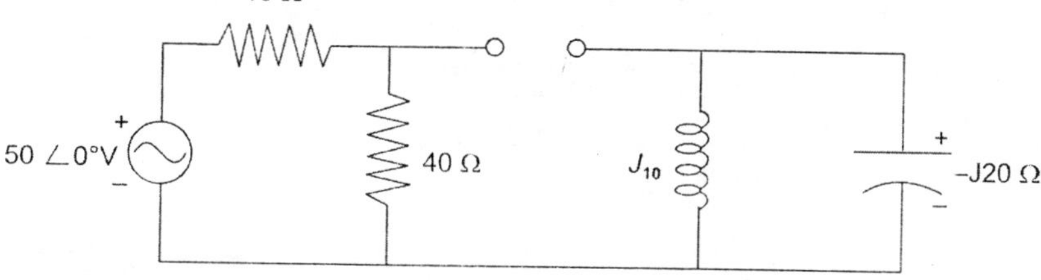

For Z_{th}: From figure below, we get

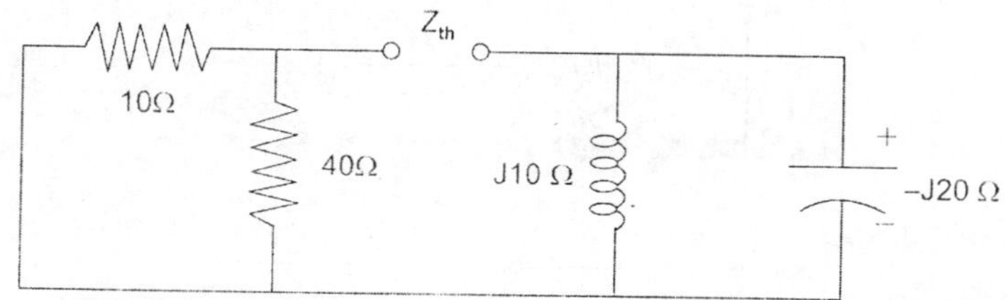

$$Z_{th} = (10 \| 40) + (-J20 \| J10)$$

$$Z_{th} = 8 + \frac{200}{-J10} = 8 + J20$$

Therefore $$Z_L = Z_{th}^{*} = (8 - J20)\,\Omega \qquad \textbf{Ans.}$$

$$P_{max} = \frac{V_{th}^2}{4R_L} = \frac{(40)^2}{4 \times 8} = 50 \text{ W} \qquad \textbf{Ans.}$$

SOLVED EXAMPLES FOR PRACTICE

Example 1: Determine the current in the capacitor branch by the superposition theorem in the circuit of figure below. **[UPTU 2003 MTU 2010]**

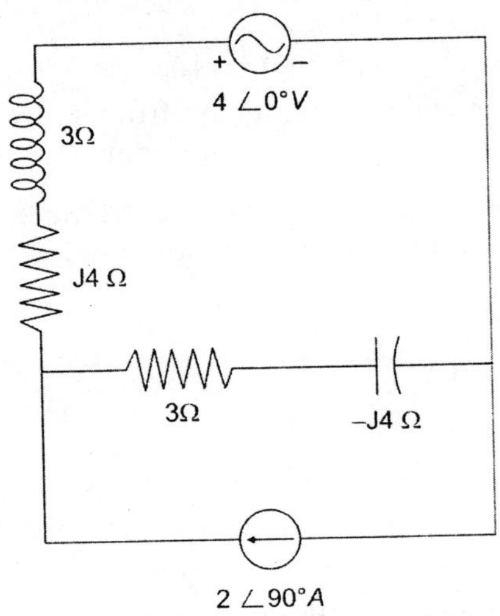

Solution: Step I: Select $4\angle 0°$ V source, current source is open circuited

$$I' = \frac{4\angle 0°}{(3 + j4) + (3 - j4)} = \frac{2}{3}\angle 0° = \frac{2}{3} \text{ A}$$

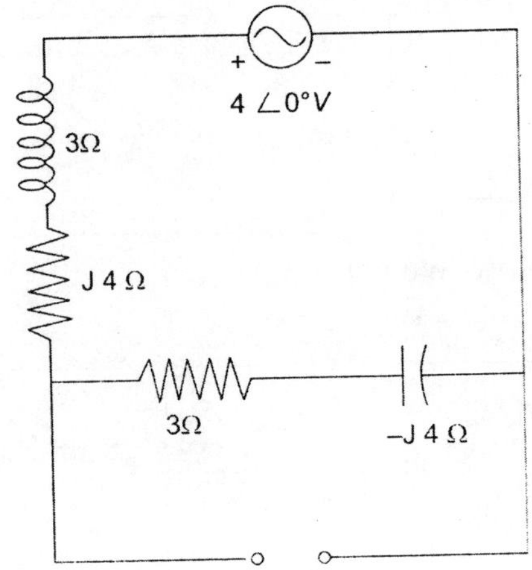

Step II: Select $2\angle 90°$ A current source, voltage source is short circuited.

$$I'' = 2\angle 90° \frac{(3+j4)}{(3+j4)+(3-j4)}$$

$$= \frac{j2(3+j4)}{6} = \frac{-4+j3}{3}$$

$$= \left(\frac{-4}{3}+j\right)\text{A}$$

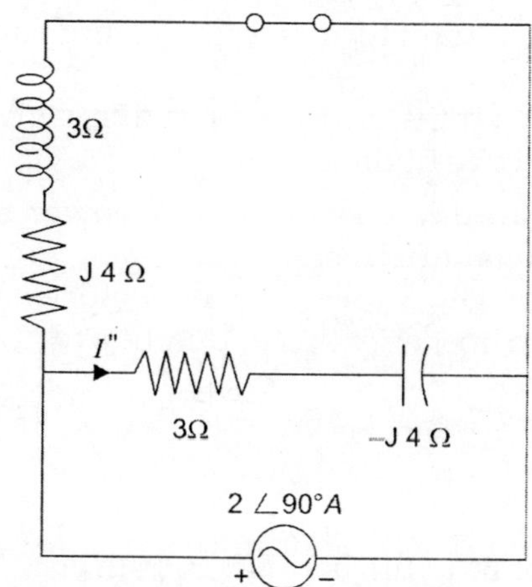

Total current in capacitor branch

$$I = I' + I''$$

$$= \frac{2}{3} - \frac{4}{3} + j = -\frac{2}{3} + j = 1.2\angle 123.7°\ \text{A}$$

Example 2: By superposition theorem, calculate current I in the circuit shown in figure below.

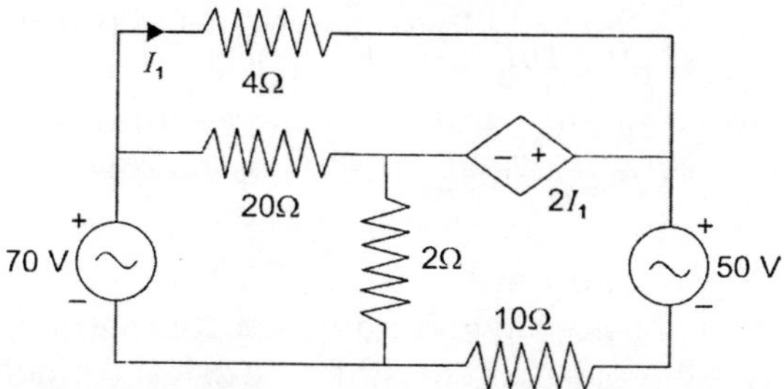

Solution: Step I: Select 70 V source

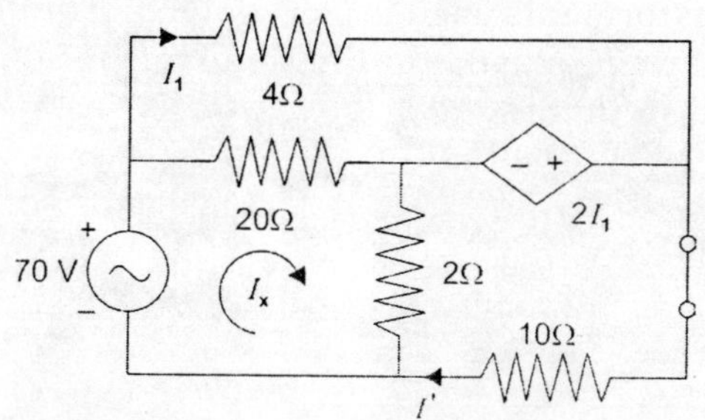

Applying *KVL*,

$$70 = 20(i_x - I_1) + 2(i_x - I') \quad ...(1)$$

$$2I_1 = 10I_1' + 2(I' - i_x) \quad ...(2)$$

$$4I_1 + 2I_1 + 20(I_1 - i_x) = 0$$

or $$I_1 = \frac{10}{13} i_x \text{ in Eq (1)}$$

Solving, we get $I' = 3.425$ A

Step II: Select 50 V source

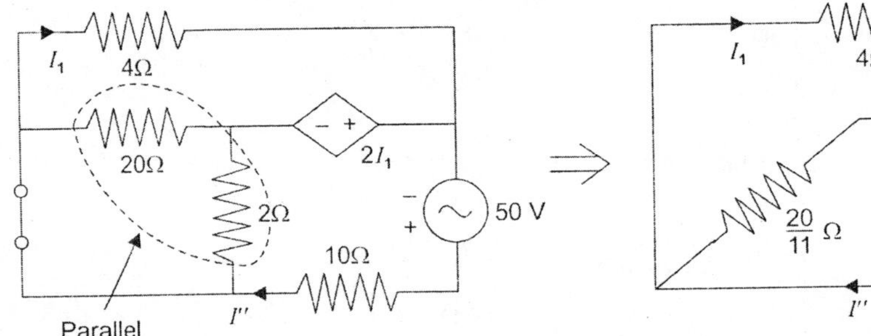

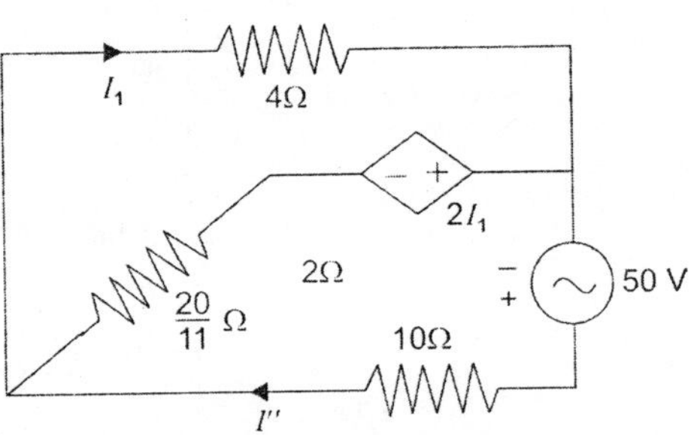

Applying *KVL*

$$50 = 10I'' + \frac{20}{11}(I'' - I_1) - 2I_1$$

and $$0 = 4I_1 + 2I_1 + \frac{20}{11}(I_1 - I'')$$

or $$I_1 = \frac{10}{43} I''$$

Putting $$I_1 = \frac{10}{43} I'' \text{ in Eq. (1), we have}$$

$$50 = 10I'' + \frac{20}{11}\left(I'' - \frac{10}{43}I''\right) - 2\left(\frac{10}{43}\right)I''$$

Solving, we get

$$I'' = 4.575 \text{ A}$$

By Superposition theorem

$$I = I' + I''$$

$$I = 3.425 + 4.575 = 8 \text{ A} \qquad \textbf{Ans.}$$

Example 3: Verify reciprocity theorem for the circuit as shown in figure below.

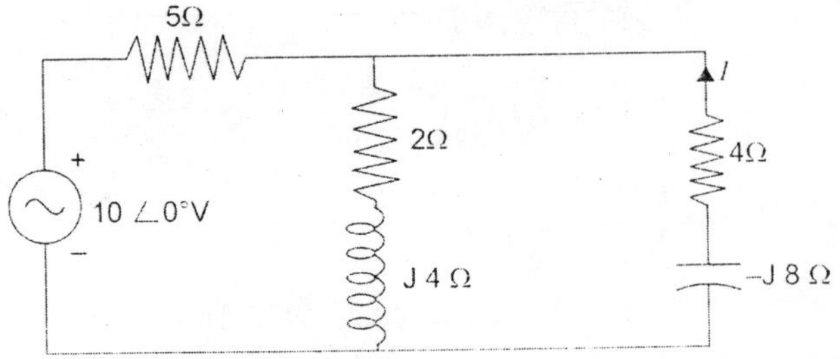

Solution: Step 1: Consider circuit 6.24

$$Z_{eq} = (4-j8) \| (2+j4)+5$$

$$= \frac{(4-j8)(2+j4)}{4-j8+2+j4}+5$$

$$= \frac{8+j16-j16+32}{6-j4}+5$$

$$= \frac{40}{6-j4}+5 = \frac{70-j20}{6-j4} = 10.1\angle 17.75° \, \Omega$$

Therefore, $$I = \frac{10\angle 0°}{10.1\angle 17.75°} \cdot \frac{(2+j4)}{(2+j4)+(4-j8)}$$

$$= 0.614 \angle 79.3° \text{ A}$$

Step II: For the circuit shown in figure below

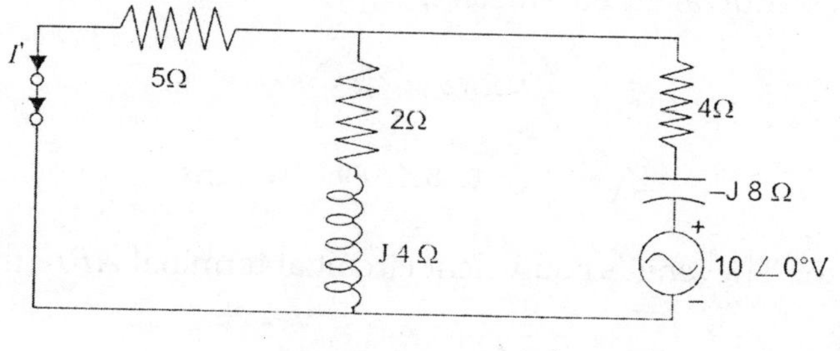

Therefore, $$I' = \frac{10\angle 0°}{9.03\angle -45.64°} \cdot \frac{(2+j4)}{(2+j4)+5}$$

$$= 0.614\angle 79.3° \text{ A}$$

Since $I = I'$

Hence reciprocity theorem is verified.

Example 4: Obtain the thevenin's theorem equivalent parameters of the circuit as shown in figure below at terminal *AB*. Then obtain Norton's equivalent parameters.

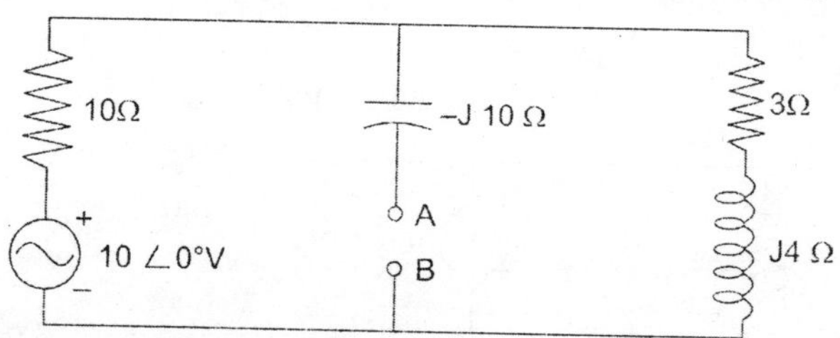

Solution: To find V_{TH}; from above figure.

V_{th} is voltage across $(3 + j4)$ *i.e.*

$$V_{th} = \frac{10}{(3+j4)+10} \times (3+j4)$$

$$V_{th} = \frac{50\angle 53.13}{13.7\angle 17.10} = 3.67\angle 36° \text{ V}$$

For Z_{th}: From figure below

$$Z_{th} = (10) || (3 + j4) + (-j10)$$

$$= \frac{30 + j40}{13 + j4} - j10$$

$$= 3.67°\angle 36° - j10 = 8.38\angle -69.13°\ \Omega$$

Therefore, Thevenin's equivalent parameters.

$$V_{th} = 3.67\angle 36°\ V,\ Z_{th} = 8.38\angle -69.13°\ \Omega \ \textbf{Ans.}$$

Hence, Norton's equivalent parameters;

$$I_N = \frac{V_{th}}{Z_{th}} = 0.438\angle 105.3°\text{A}$$

$$Z_N = Z_{th} = 8.38\angle -69.3°\ \Omega \ \textbf{Ans.}$$

Example 5: Find the Thevenin's equivalent circuit at terminal *AB* of the circuit given in figure below.

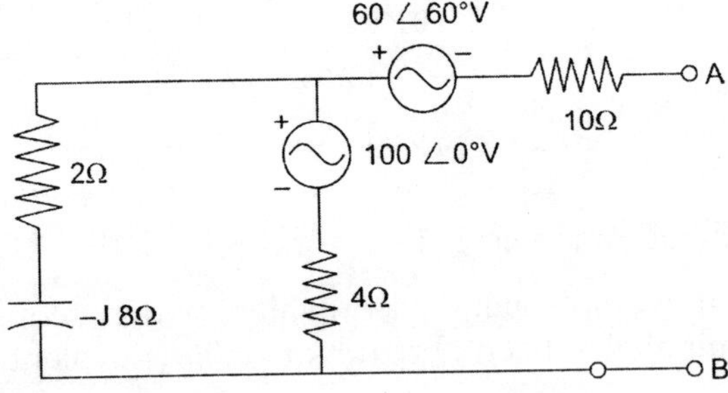

Solution: For finding $V_{th} = V_{AB}$

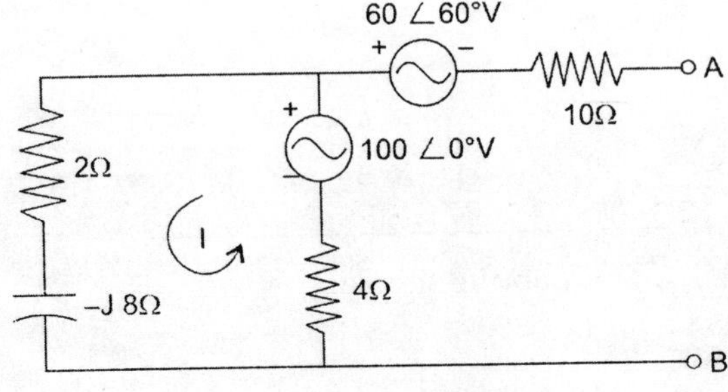

Applying *KVL*,

$$I = \frac{+100}{2 - j8 + 4} = \frac{+100\angle 0°}{6 - j8} = (6 + j8)\text{ A}$$

Voltage drop across 4 Ω is = $(6 + j8)4 = 24 + j32$

Therefore, $V_{th} = V_{AB} = -60\angle 0° + 100\angle 0° - (24 + j32)$

$V_{th} = 46 - j84 = 96\angle -61.3°$ V

For Z_{th},

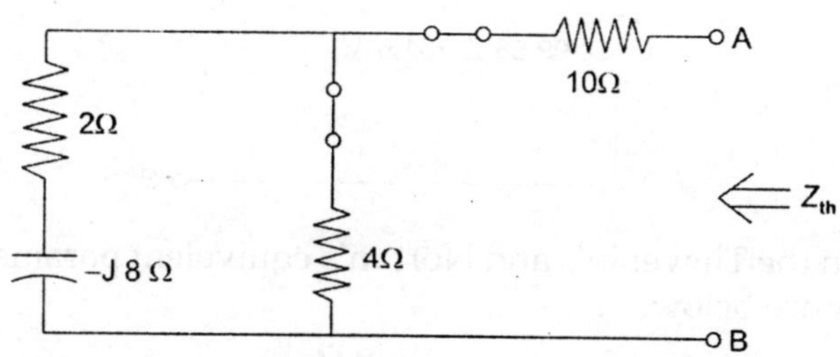

For Z_{th},

$$Z_{th} = (2 - j8) || (4) + 10 = (13 - j1.28)\,\Omega$$

The Thevenin's equivalent circuit is shown in figure below

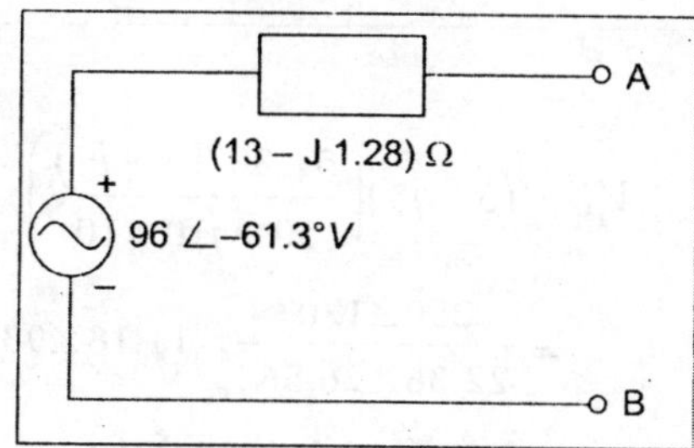

Example 6: Find the Thevenin's equivalent circuit at terminals *AB* for the circuit shown in figure below.

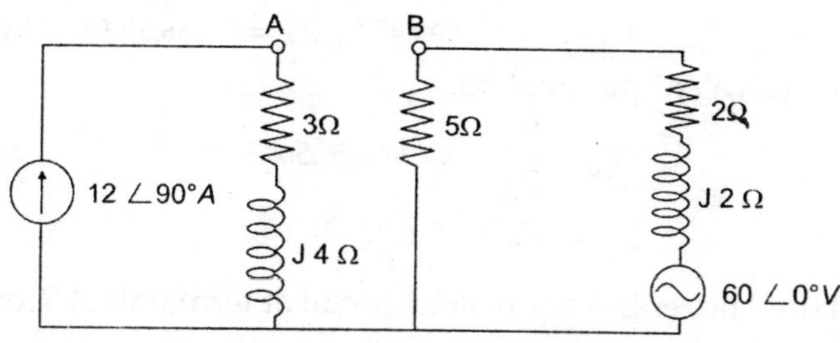

Solution: To find $V_{th} = V_{AB}$.

$$\therefore \quad V_{th} = V_A - V_B = 12\angle 90°(3 + j4) - 5\left(\frac{60\angle 0°}{2 + j2 + 5}\right)$$

$$= 99.56\angle 151.62°\ \text{V}$$

For Z_{th}

$$Z_{th} = (3 + j4) + [5 || (2 + j2)]$$

$$= 6.818\angle 46.42°\ \Omega$$

Therefore, Thevenin's equivalent circuit is shown in figure below.

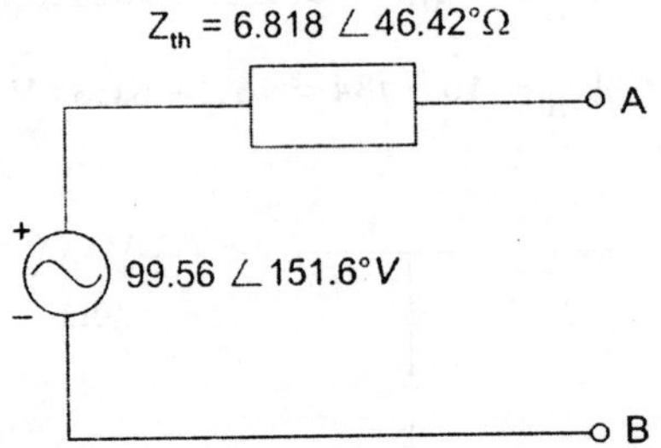

Example 7: Obtain the Thevenin's and Norton's equivalent parameters at terminals *AB* of the circuit in figure below.

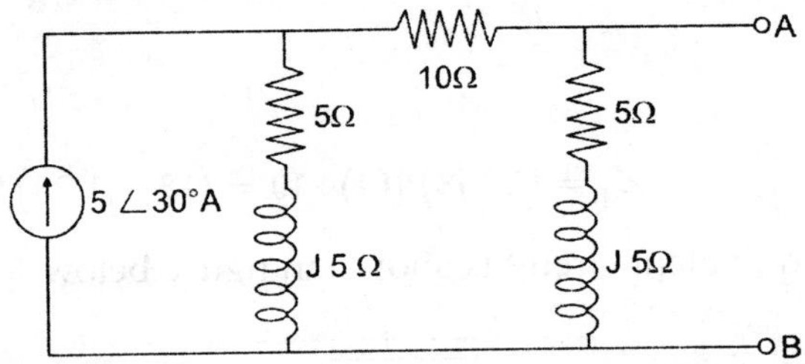

Solution: For V_{th}

$$V_{th} = (5 + j5)\left(\frac{5\angle 30°(5 + j5)}{10 + j10 + 10}\right)$$

$$= \frac{250\angle 120°}{22.36\angle 26.56°} = 11.18\angle 93.44°$$

For Z_{th}: As current source is open circuit, therefore

$$Z_{th} = \{(5 + j5) + 10\} \,||\, (5 + j5) = \frac{111.80\angle 63.43°}{22.36\angle 26.56°}$$

$$= 5\angle 36.87°\ \Omega$$

Therefore, Thevenin's equivalent parameters:

$$V_{th} = 11.18\angle 93.4°\ \text{V},\ Z_{th} = 5\angle 36.87\ \Omega$$ **Ans.**

and Norton's equivalent parameters:

$$I_N = \frac{V_{th}}{Z_{th}} = 2.236\angle 56.56°\text{A}$$

$$Z_N = Z_{th} = \angle 36.87\ \Omega$$

Example 8: Find the Thevenin's equivalent circuit at terminals *AB* for the circuit shown in figure below.

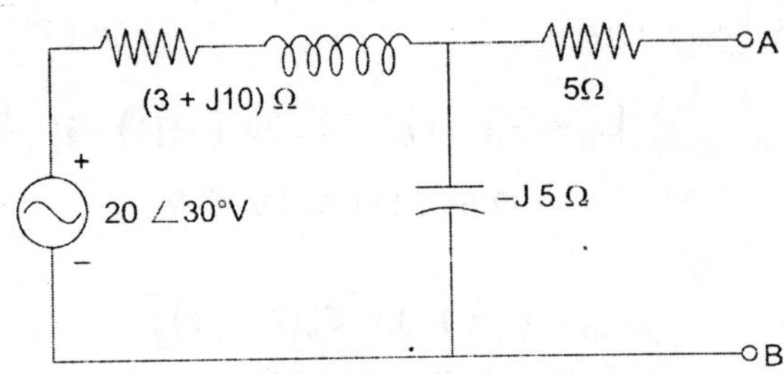

Solution: For V_{th}

$$V_{th} = \text{voltage across } (-j5)\,\Omega$$

$$= (-j5)\frac{20\angle 30^\circ}{(3+j10)+(-j5)} = 17.15\angle -11.9^\circ \text{ V}$$

For Z_{th}

$$Z_{th} = 5+(3+j10)\,||\,(-j5)$$

$$= 11.28\angle -50.3^\circ\,\Omega$$

Therefore, the Thevenin's equivalent circuit is shown in figure below.

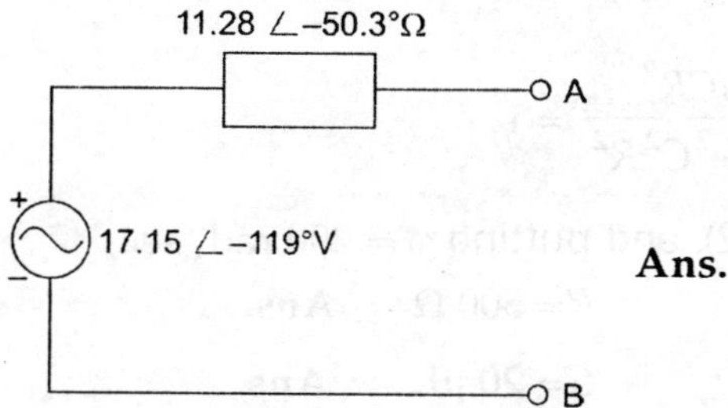

Ans.

Example 9: A loudspeaker is connected across the terminals *A* and *B* of the circuit shown in figure below. What should be the impedance of the speaker to obtain the maximum power transferred to it and what is the maximum power C.

Solution: From example (10):

For maximum power, impedance of the loudspeaker,

$$Z_L = Z_{th}^{*} = (7.21 - j7.67)^{*} = 7.21 + j7.67$$

$$= 11.28\angle 50.3^\circ\,\Omega$$

Maximum power $$P_{max} = \frac{V_{th}^2}{4R_L} = \frac{(17.15)^2}{4\times 7.21} = 10.2 \text{ W}$$ **Ans.**

Example 10: In the circuit shown in Fig. 6.30, determine the value of *R* and *C* so that maximum power is absorbed by *R*. Determine the power for these value. The signal frequency $\omega = 200$ rod/sec, $V_S = 200\angle 0^\circ$ V.

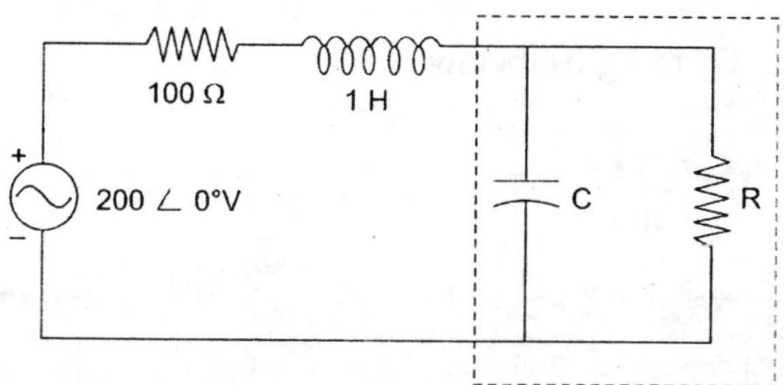

Solution: The load impedance

$$Z_L = R\,||\,\frac{1}{j\omega C} = \frac{R}{1+j\omega CR}$$

$$= \frac{R - j\omega C R^2}{1+\omega^2 C^2 R^2}$$

For maximum power transfer, Z_L should be equal to complex conjugate of the internal impedance of the circuit *i.e.*

$$Z_L = (100 + j1)^* = 100 - j1$$

or
$$\frac{R - j\omega CR^2}{1 + \omega^2 C^2 R^2} = 100 - j1$$

Equating real and imaginary parts, we get

$$\frac{R}{1 + (\omega CR)^2} = 100 \quad \text{...(1)}$$

$$\frac{\omega CR^2}{1 + \omega^2 C^2 R^2} = 1 \quad \text{...(2)}$$

Dividing Eq (1) by (2), and putting $\omega = 200$ rad/sec

$R = 500\ \Omega$ **Ans.**

$C = 20\ \mu F$ **Ans.**

Then; $R_i = R_L = 100\ \Omega$

$$P_{max} = \frac{V^2}{4R_L} = \frac{(200)^2}{4 \times 100} = 100 \text{ W} \quad \textbf{Ans.}$$

Example 11: In the circuit shown in figure below. Determine Z_L so that the power absorbed by it is maximum and the value of the power absorbed.

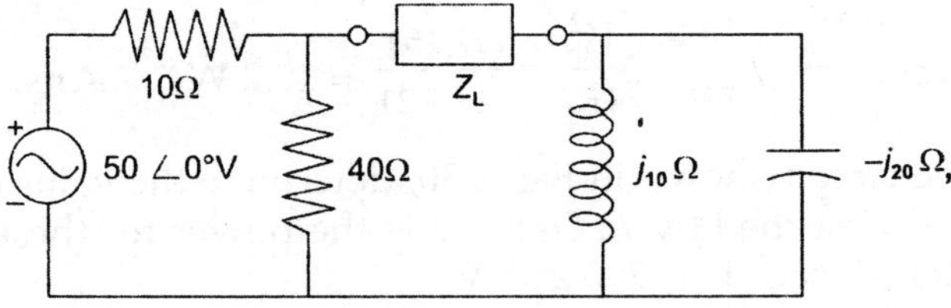

Solution: For V_{th}: From figure below.

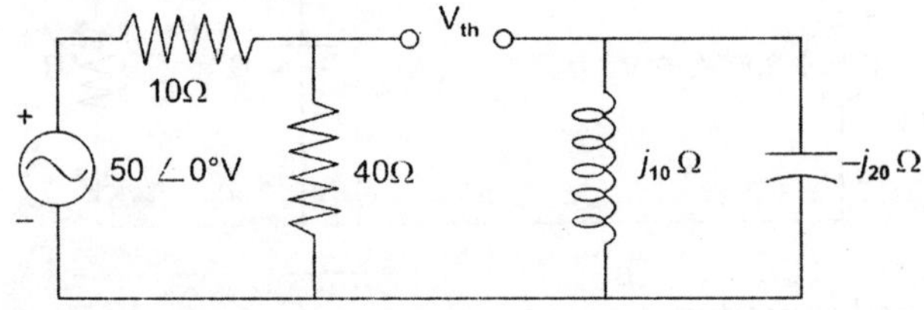

∴ V_{th} is voltage across 40 Ω is

$$V_{th} = 50\angle 0° \times \frac{40}{40 + 10} = 40\angle 0° \text{ V}$$

For Z_{th}: From figure below

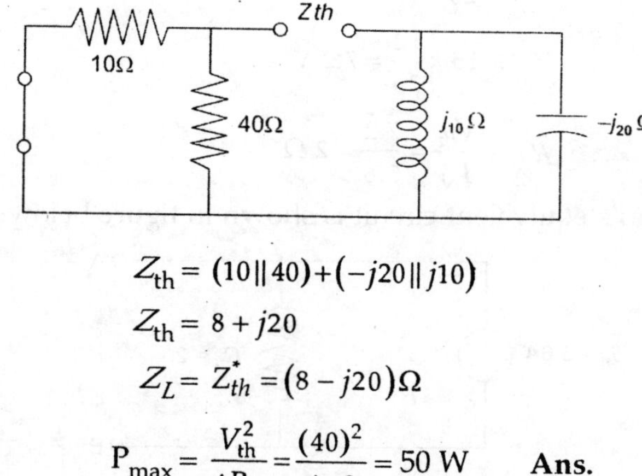

$$\therefore \quad Z_{th} = (10 \| 40) + (-j20 \| j10)$$

$$Z_{th} = 8 + j20$$

Therefore,

$$Z_L = Z_{th}^* = (8 - j20)\Omega$$

$$P_{max} = \frac{V_{th}^2}{4R_L} = \frac{(40)^2}{4 \times 8} = 50 \text{ W} \quad \textbf{Ans.}$$

Example 12: Find the Norton's equivalent circuit across terminals AB of the circuit shown in figure below.

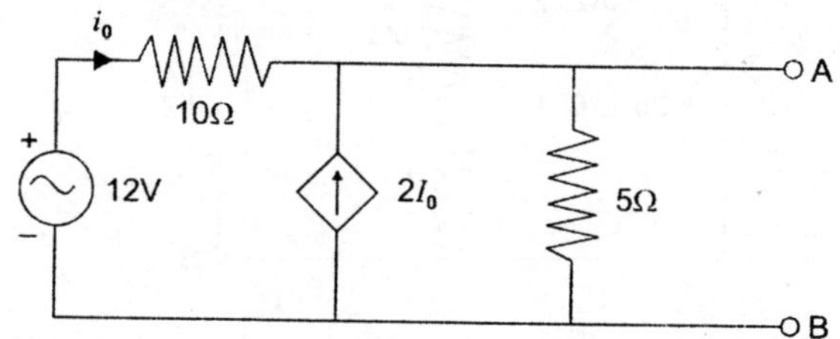

Solution: For I_N: (5 Ω resistance is short circuited) from the circuit shown in figure below.

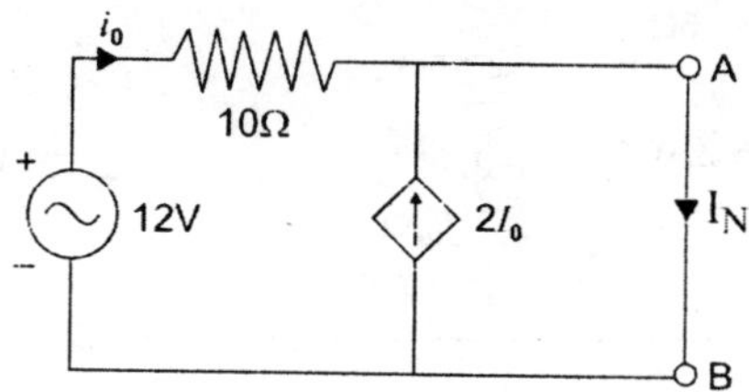

Apply *KVL* gives

$$12 = 10i_0$$

$$i_0 = 1.2 \text{ A}$$

Applying *KCL* at *A*

$$I_N = i_0 + 2i_0 = 3i_0$$

$$= 3.6 \text{ A}$$

or $\quad V_{th} = 5 \times 3i_0 =$ voltage across 5 Ω resistance

Now applying *KVL*

$$12 = 10i_0 + 5(i_0 + 2i_0)$$

$$= 25i_0$$

$$i_0 = \frac{12}{25}$$

$$V_{th} = 15 \times \frac{12}{25} = 7.2 \text{ V}$$

Therefore, $$R_N = \frac{V_{th}}{I_N} = \frac{7.2}{3.6} = 2\ \Omega$$

Hence, three Norton's equivalent circuit is shown in figure below.

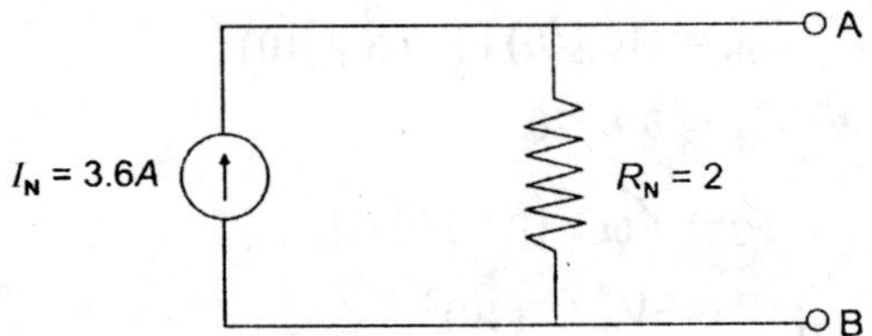

Example 13: Determine the value of Z_L to be connected across AB in figure below for maximum power transfer. Given $V_S = 25$ V, obtain the power absorbed by Z_L.

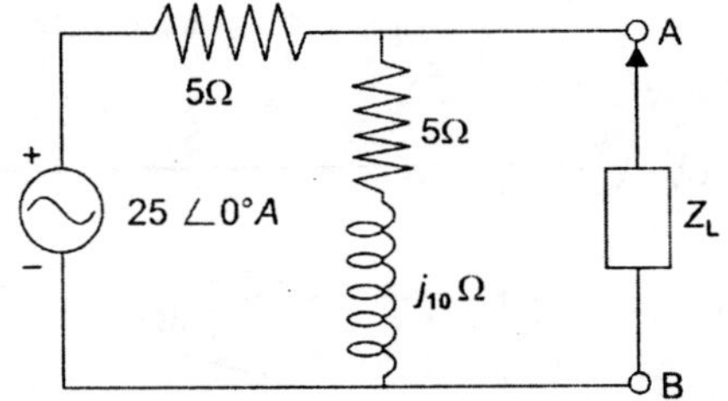

Solution: For V_{th}

V_{th} is the voltage across $(5 + j10)\Omega$, *i.e.* $25\angle 0° \times \dfrac{(5 + j10)}{5 + j10 + 5} = 19.77\angle 18.43°$ V

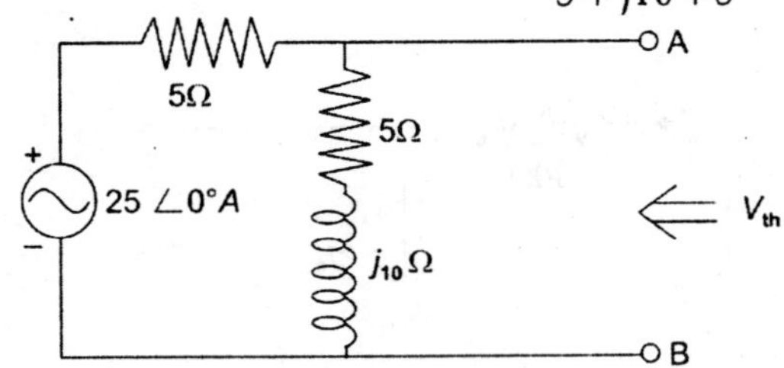

For Z_{th}:

A
5Ω
5Ω
Zth = (5) || (5 + J 10)
j10 Ω
B

$$Z_{th} = \frac{5(5 + j10)}{5 + 5 + j10} = \frac{25 + j50}{10 + j10} = (3.75 + j1.25)\ \Omega$$

$$Z_{th} = (3.75 + j1.25)\,\Omega$$

Therefore $$Z_L = Z_{th} = 3.75 - j1.25\ \Omega$$

$$P_{max} = \frac{V_{th}^2}{4R_L} = \frac{(19.77)^2}{4 \times 3.75} = 26.06\ \text{W}$$ **Ans.**

Example 14: Determine the value of R_L to be connected across AB in Fig. 6.34, for maximum power transfer. Also calculate the maximum power absorbed by R_L.

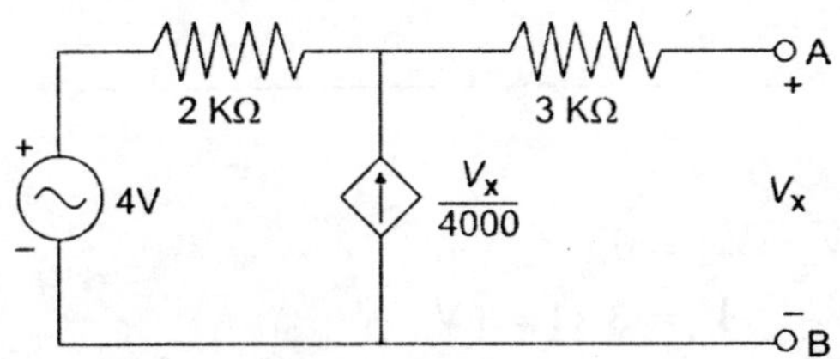

Solution: For V_{th}: From figure above

$$\frac{4 - V_{th}}{2000} = \frac{-V_x}{4000} \text{ and } V_{th} = V_x$$

$$8 - 2\,V_{th} = -V_{th} \text{ or } V_{th} = 8\ \text{V}$$

For I_{SC} or I_N:

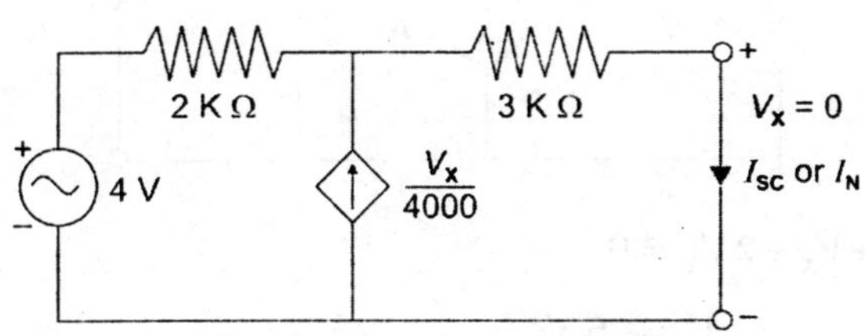

As $$V_x = 0$$

Therefore, current source is zero, *i.e.* open circuited,

then $$I_{SC} = I_N = \frac{4}{2000 + 3000} = 8 \times 10^{-4}\ \text{A}$$

Therefore, the value of R_L for maximum power

$$R_L = R_{th}$$

$$= \frac{V_{th}}{I_N} = \frac{8}{8 \times 10^{-4}}$$

$$= 10\ \text{k}\Omega$$

and maximum power

$$P_{max} = \frac{V_{th}^2}{4R_L}$$

$$= \frac{(8)^2}{8 \times 10 \times 10^3}$$

$$= 1.6\ \text{mW}$$ **Ans.**

Example 15: Calculate the current in the 6 Ω resistor of the circuit of figure below, by (i) Thevenin's theorem and (ii) Superposition theorem.

Solution: (i) Thevenin's theorem:

For V_{th}:

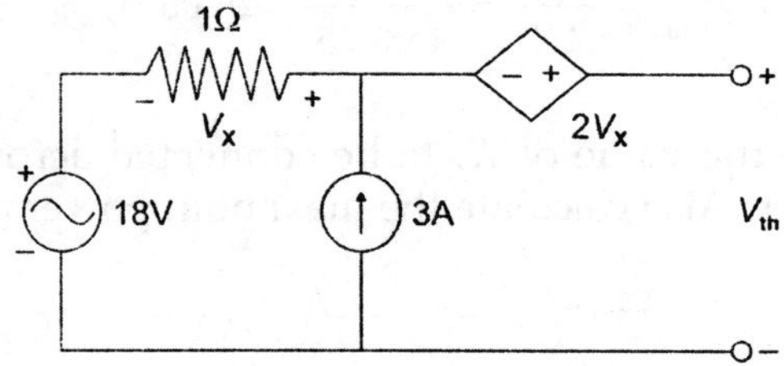

Applying *KVL* gives

$$18 + V_x + 2V_x - V_{th} = 0$$

and $$V_x = 3 \times 1 = 3 \text{ V}$$

Therefore $$V_{th} = 18 + 3V_x = 27 \text{ V}$$

For I_N

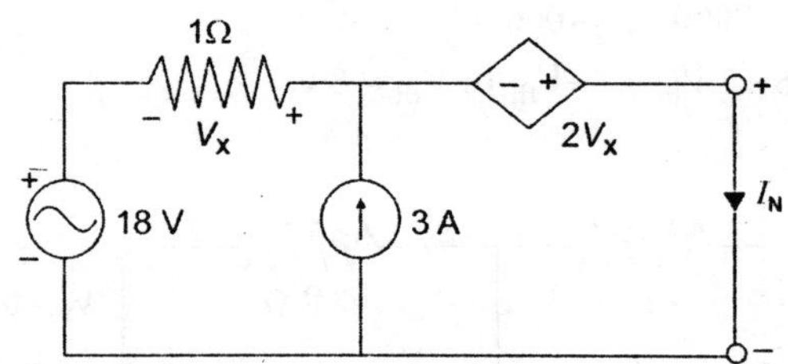

Now $$18 + V_x + 2V_x = 0$$

or $$V_x = -6 \text{ V}$$

and $$V_x = 1(3 - I_N)$$

$$-6 = 3 - I_N \text{ or } I_N = 9 \text{ A}$$

Therefore $$R_{th} = \frac{Vth}{I_N} = \frac{27}{9} = 3 \ \Omega$$

Using Thevenin's theorem equivalent circuits.

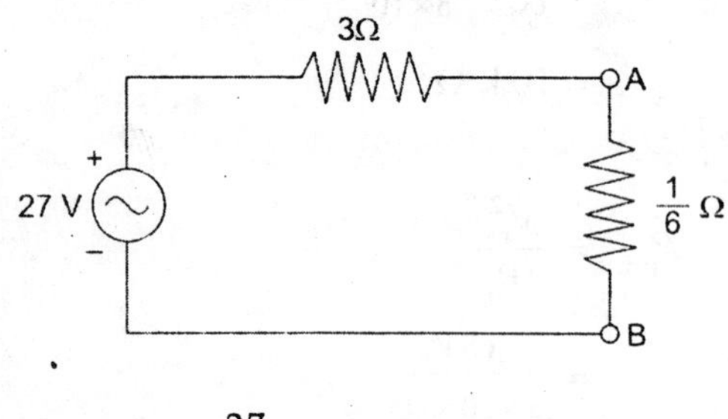

$$I = \frac{27}{3 + 6} = 3 \text{ A}$$ **Ans.**

(ii) Superposition theorem: Step I: Select 18 V source only at a time.

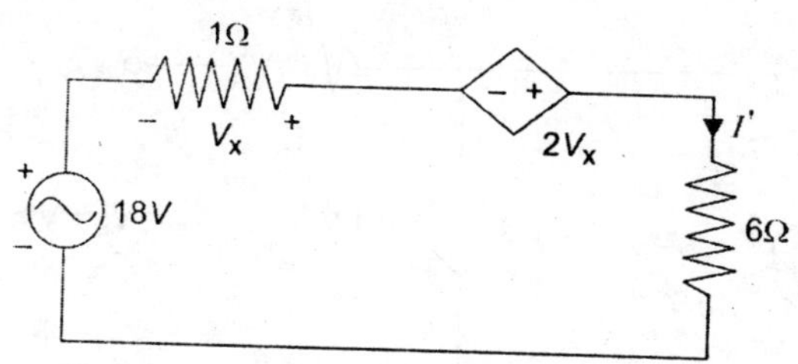

Applying *KVL*,

$$18 + V_x + 2V_x - 6I' = 0 \text{ or } 18 + 3V_x = 6I'$$

and

$$V_x = -I'$$

Therefore

$$18 - 3I' = 6I' \text{ or } I' = 2 \text{ A}$$

Step II: Select 3 A current source.

Applying *KCL* at *A*,

$$3 = \frac{V_x}{1} + \frac{V_x + 2V_x}{6}$$

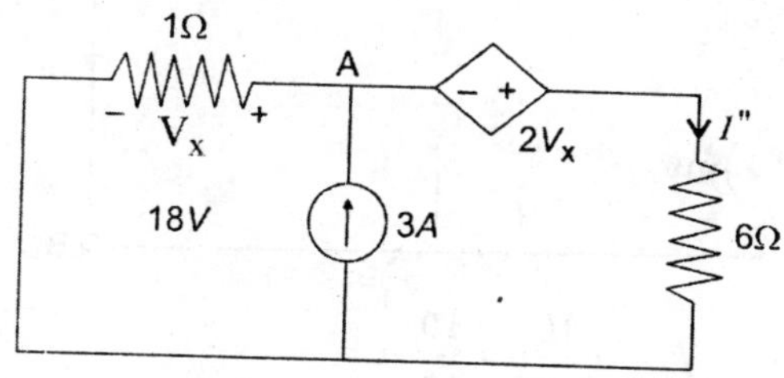

or

$$3 = \frac{V_x}{1} + \frac{V_x}{2} \text{ or } V_x = 2 \text{ V}$$

Therefore

$$I'' = \frac{V_x + 2V_x}{6} = \frac{6}{6} = 1 \text{ A}$$

Hence

$$I_{6\Omega} = I' + I'' = 2 + 1 = 3 \text{ A} \quad \text{Ans.}$$

Example 16: By Thevenin's theorem find the current in the 14 Ω resistor of the circuit of figure below.

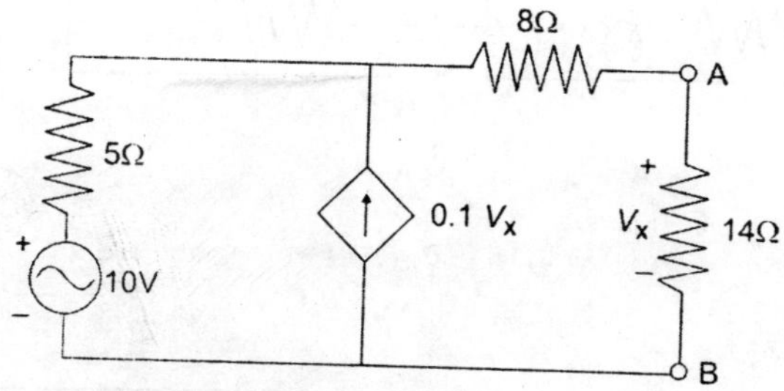

Solution: For V_{th}: We open terminal AB

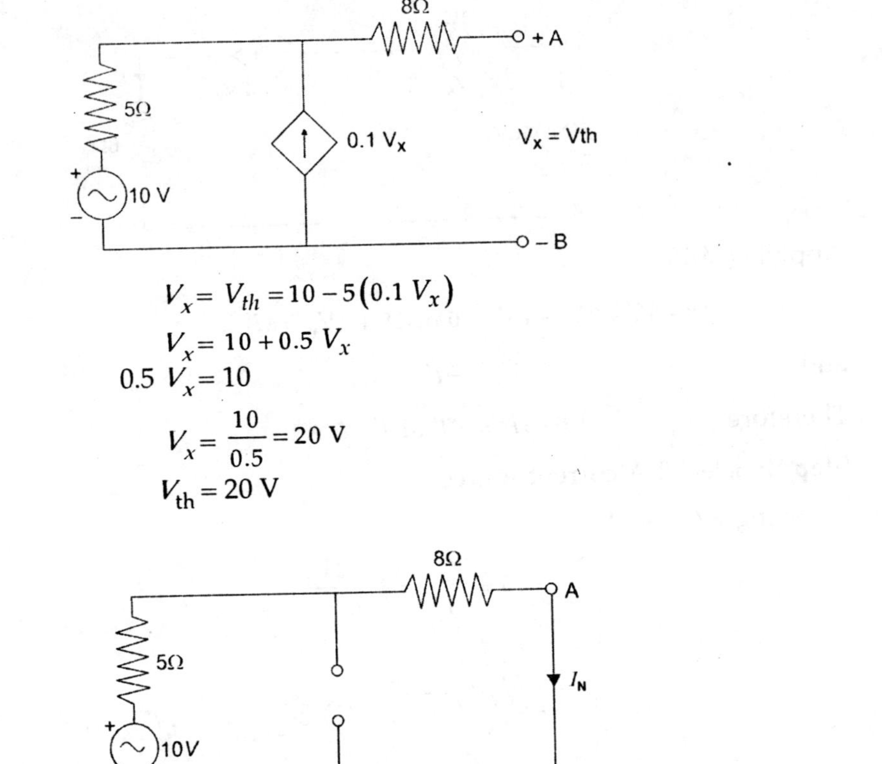

Thus
$$V_x = V_{th} = 10 - 5(0.1\ V_x)$$
$$V_x = 10 + 0.5\ V_x$$
$$0.5\ V_x = 10$$
$$V_x = \frac{10}{0.5} = 20\ \text{V}$$

$\therefore$
$$V_{th} = 20\ \text{V}$$

For I_N

$$I_N = \frac{10}{5+8} = \frac{10}{13}\ \text{A}$$

So,
$$R_{th} = \frac{V_{th}}{I_N} = \frac{20}{\frac{10}{13}} = 26\ \Omega$$

and
$$I_{14\Omega} = \frac{V_{th}}{R_{th} + R_L} = \frac{20}{26+14} = 0.5\ \text{A}$$ **Ans.**

Example 17: Using Thevenin's theorem, find the power in $(4 + j6)$ impedance connected across terminals AB in figure below.

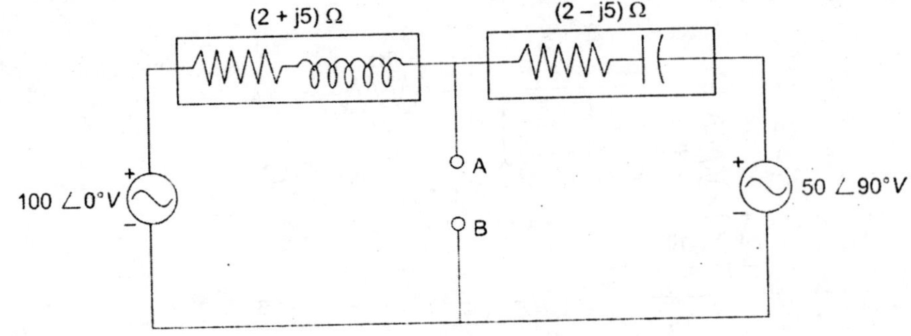

Solution: For V_{th};

$V_{th} \rightarrow$ drop across $= (2+j5)\,\Omega$

$$V_{th} = 100\angle 0° - (2+j5)\left(\frac{100\angle 0° - 50\angle 90°}{(2+j5)+(3-j5)}\right)$$

$$= 10 - j80$$

$$V_{th} = 80.62\ \angle -82.87°\ \text{V}$$

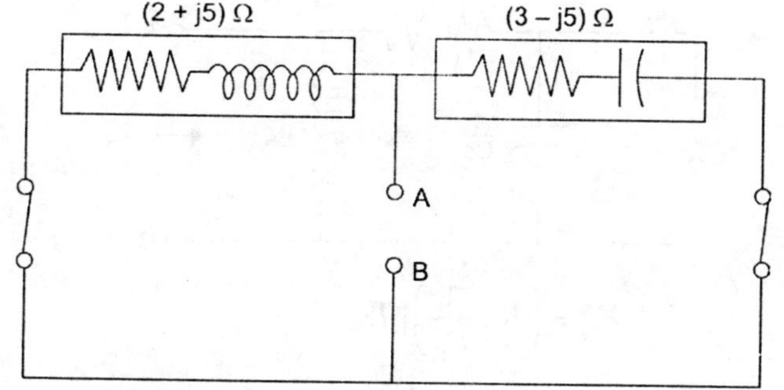

For Z_{th};

$$Z_{th} = \frac{(2+j5)(3-j5)}{2+j5+3-j5} = \frac{31+j5}{5} = (6.2+j1)\Omega$$

Then current in $Z_L = (4+j6)\Omega$ is given by

$$I_L = \frac{V_{th}}{Z_{th}+Z_L} = \frac{80.62\angle -82.87°}{(6.2+j1)+(4+j6)}$$

$$= 6.52\ \angle -117.33°\ \text{A}$$ **Ans.**

Power in $(4+j6)\Omega = I_L^2 \times R_L = (6.52)^2 \times 4$

$$P = 170.04\ \text{W}$$ **Ans.**

Example 18: Find Norton's equivalent circuit parameters across *AB* in *s*-domain figure below. Hence find Thevenin's equivalent circuit parameters.

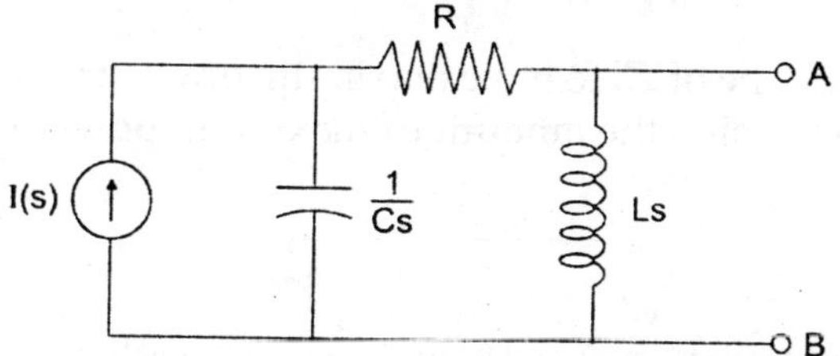

Solution: For I_N: Let us apply short circuit across *AB* as shown in figure below.

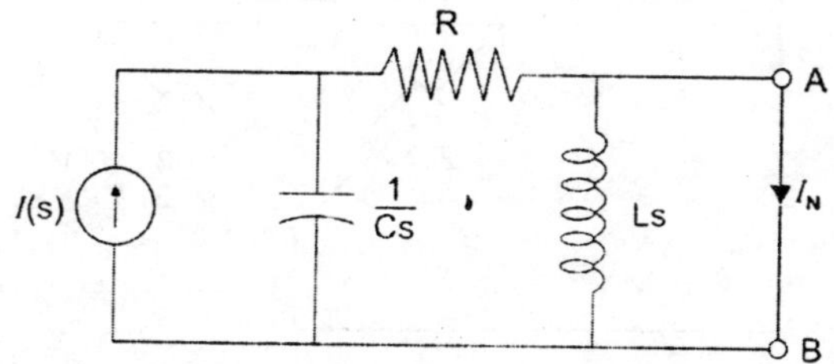

$$I_N = I(s)\cdot\frac{\frac{1}{Cs}}{\frac{1}{Cs}+R}$$

$$= I(s)\cdot\frac{1}{1+RCs}$$

For Z_N

$$Z_N = \left(R+\frac{1}{Cs}\right)\|Ls$$

$$= \frac{Ls\left(R+\frac{1}{Cs}\right)}{R+Ls+\frac{1}{Cs}}$$

$$= \frac{L_s(1+RCs)}{L\cdot C\cdot s^2+1}$$

Then, Thevenin's equivalent circuit parameters are

$$V_{th} = I_N\cdot Z_N = \frac{I(s)}{1+RCs}\left[\frac{L_s(1+RCs)}{L\cdot C\cdot s^2+R\cdot C\cdot s^2+1}\right]$$

$$= I_{es}\cdot\frac{L_s}{LCs^2+RCs^2+1}$$

and $$Z_{th} = Z_N$$

Example 19: Find the volume of Z_L to have maximum power transfer from the $10\angle 0°$ V voltage source. Also determine the amount of maximum power in figure below.

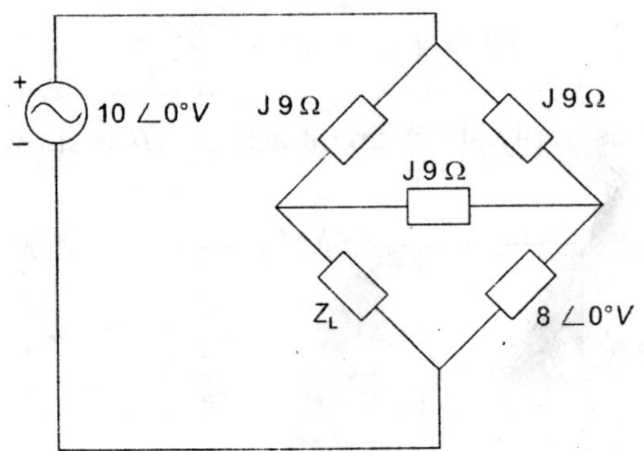

Solution: Let us first remove Z_L and apply delta-star transformation, we have

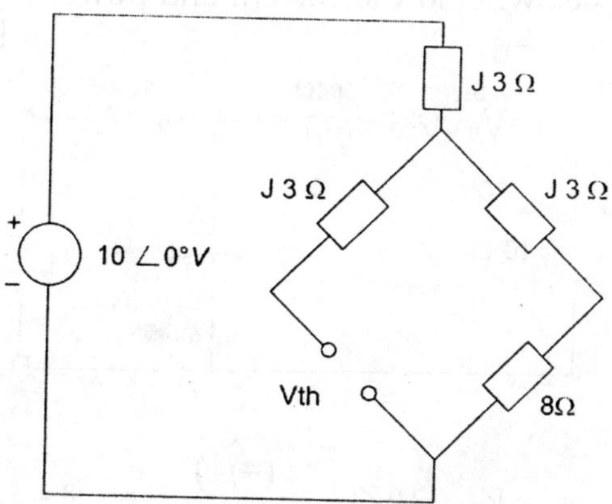

For V_{th}: V_{th} = voltage drop a across impedance $(j3+8)\Omega$

$$= (j3+8)\left[\left(\frac{10\angle 0°}{j3+j3+8}\right)\right] = \frac{10(8+j3)}{8+j6}$$

$$V_{th} = 8.854 \angle -16.31°\ \text{V}$$

For Z_{th}: From figure below

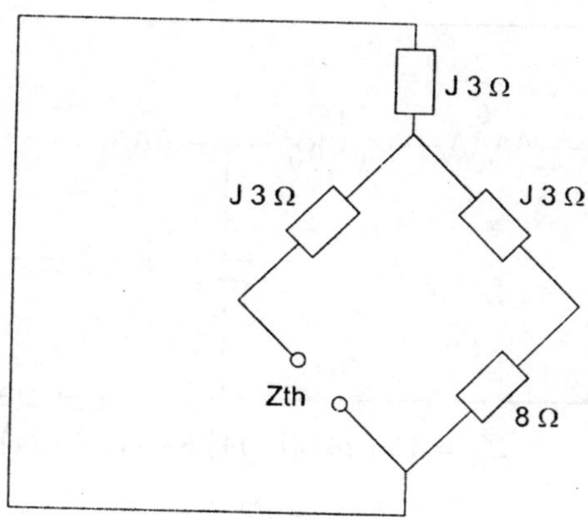

$$Z_{th} = j3 + (j3+8)\,||\,(j3)$$

$$= j3 + \left[\frac{-9+j24}{8+j6}\right]$$

$$= 5.507 \angle 82.49°$$

$$= (0.72 + j5.46)\,\Omega$$

Thus to have maximum power transfer, Z_L must be complex conjugate of Z_{th}, *i.e.*

$$Z_L = Z_{th}^{*} = (0.72 - j5.46)\Omega$$

Also, $$P_{max} = \frac{V_{th}^2}{4R_L} = \frac{(8.54)^2}{4 \times 0.72}$$

$$= 25.32\ \text{W}$$

Ans.

Example 20: By Thevenin's equivalent circuit, replace the network to the left of terminals AB in figure below. Find the current and power delivered to the load Z_L, if $Z_L = (4 + j4)\Omega$. **[UPTU 2002, MTU 2011]**

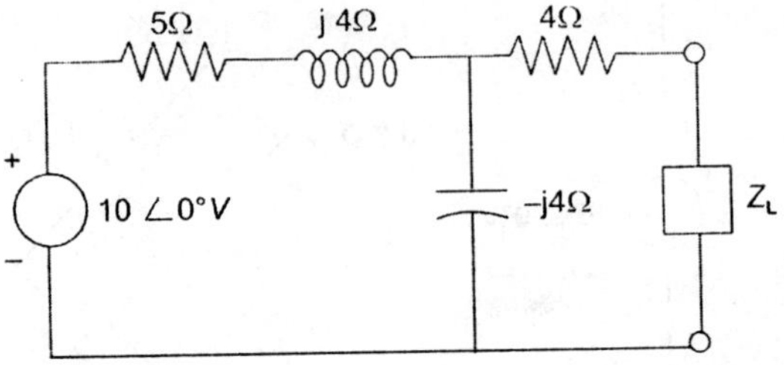

Solution: For V_{th}

$$V_{th} = 10\angle 0° \frac{(-j4)}{-j4 + 5 + j4} = -j8 = 8\angle -90° \text{ V}$$

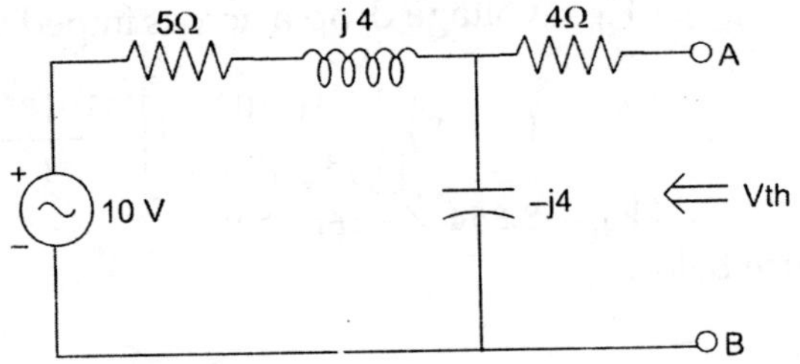

For Z_{th};

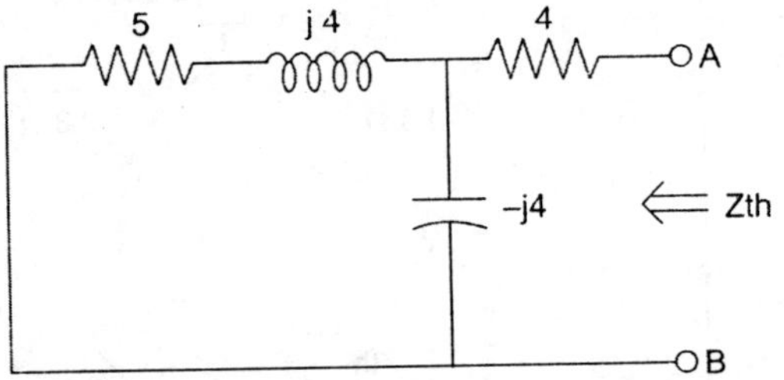

$$Z_{th} = (5 + j4) \| (-j4) + 4 = (7.2 - j4)\Omega$$

$$I_L = \frac{8\angle -90°}{7.2 - j4 + 4 + j4}$$

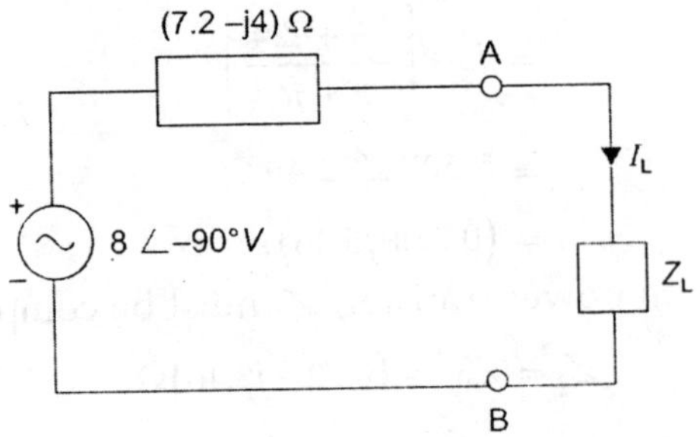

$$I_L = 0.71 \text{ A}$$ **Ans.**

Power delivered, $$P = I_L^2 \cdot R_L = (0.71)^2 = 2 \text{ W}$$ **Ans.**

Example 21: Using Thevenin's theorems determine an equivalent network for the terminals $a-b$ for zero initial conditions in figure below.

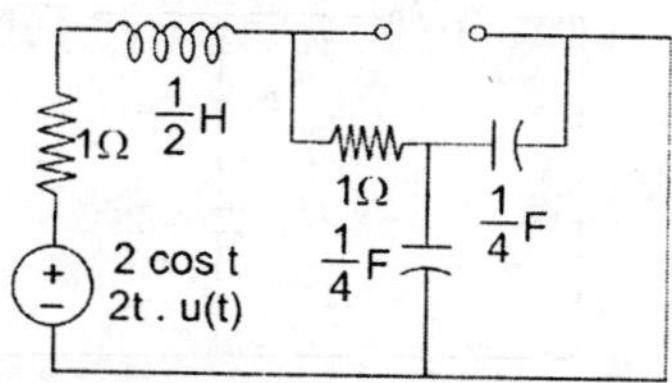

Solution: Redraw the circuit of above figure, in the transform domain as shown in figure below.

$$C_{eq} = C_1 + C_2 = \frac{1}{4} + \frac{1}{4} = \frac{1}{2}$$

For $V_{th}(s)$

Now,
$$V_{th}(s) = \frac{2s}{s^2+4} \cdot \frac{\left(1+\frac{2}{s}\right)}{\left(1+\frac{2}{s}+1+\frac{s}{2}\right)} = \frac{4s}{\left(s^2+4\right)(s+2)}$$

For
$$Z_{th}(s) = \left(1+\frac{2}{s}\right) || \left(1+\frac{s}{2}\right)$$

$$= \frac{(s+2)(s+4)}{2s+4+2s+s^2} = 1$$

Example 22: Determine current I using superposition theorem in figure below.

[UPTU 2006, MTU 2012]

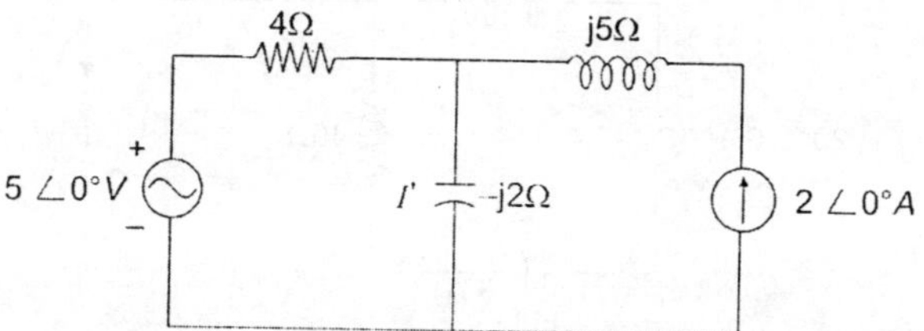

Solution: Step I: Select $5\angle 0°$ V, voltage source.

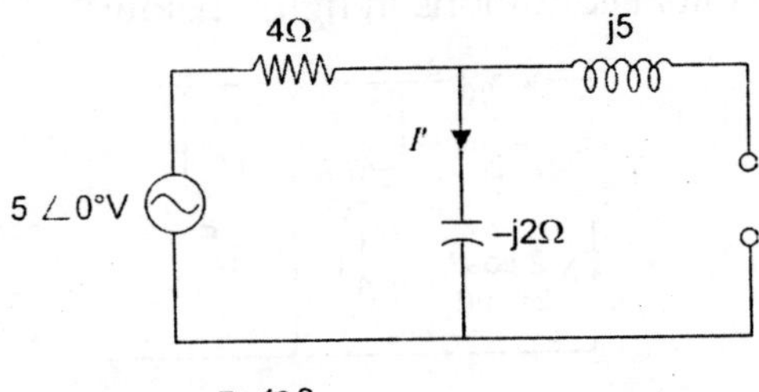

$$I' = \frac{5\angle 0°}{4 - j2} = 1 + j0.5$$

Step II: Select $2\angle 0°$ A, current source

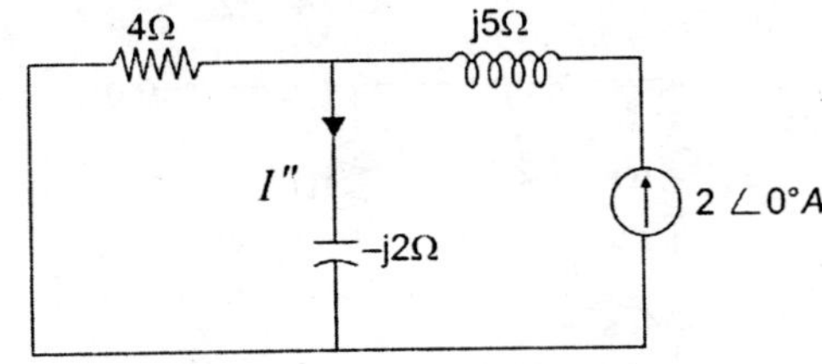

$$I'' = 2\angle 0°\left(\frac{4}{4 - j2}\right) = 1.6 + j0.8$$

Therefore, current $I = I' + I''$

$$= 2.6 + j1.3 = 2.9\angle 26.56°\text{ A}$$ **Ans.**

Example 23: Given the network of figure below, find Norton's equivalent circuit to the left side of terminals $a - b$.

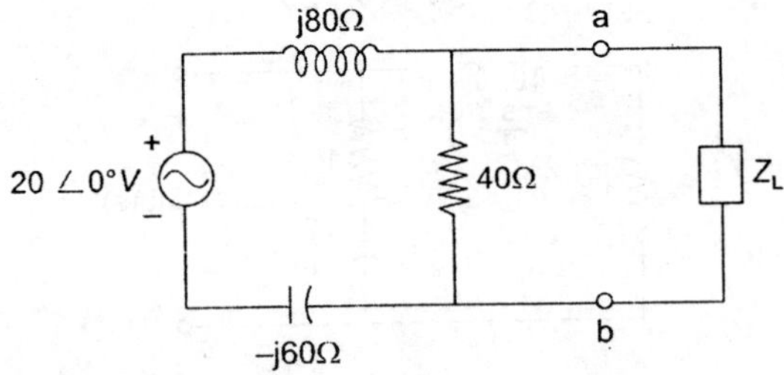

Solution: For I_N: From figure below

$$I_N = \frac{20\angle 0°}{j80 - j60} = 1\angle -90°\text{ A}$$

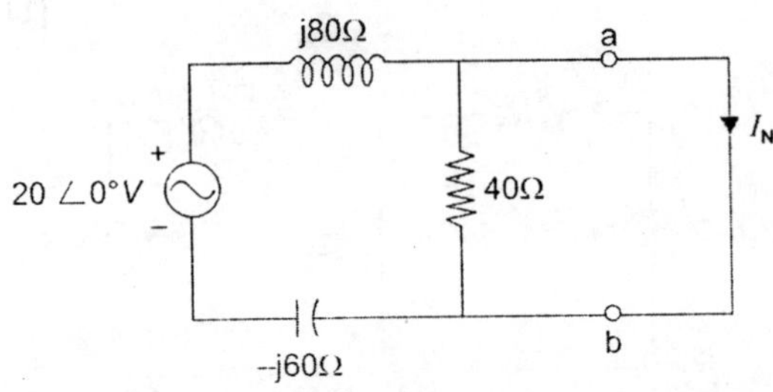

For Z_n: From figure below

$$Z_n = 40 \,||\, j20 = \frac{j800}{40 + j20} = 8 + j16 = 17.89\angle 63.43°$$

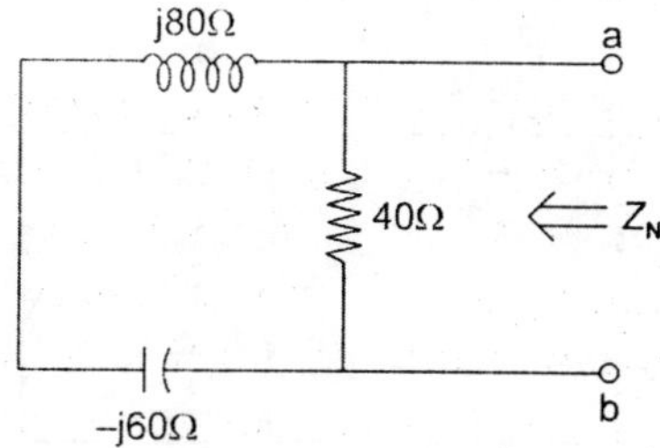

∴ Norton's equivalent circuit is shown in figure below.

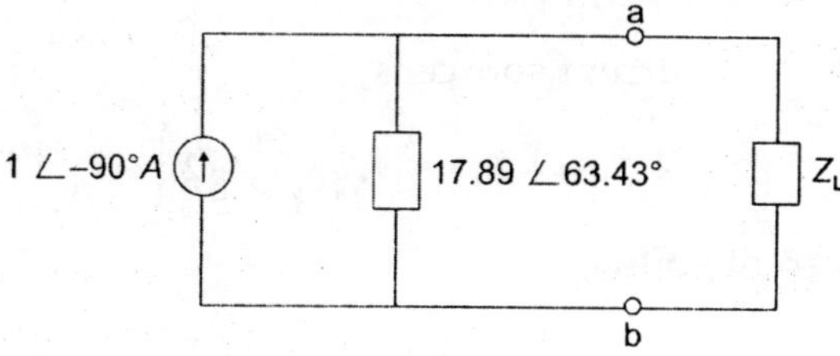

Example 24: For the circuit shown in figure below, obtain the voltage across each current source, using superposition theorem. **[UPTU 2004, GBTU 2008]**

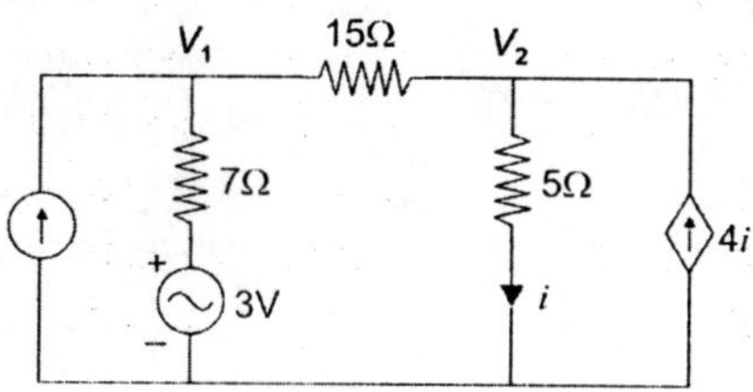

Solution: Step I: Select 2A current source

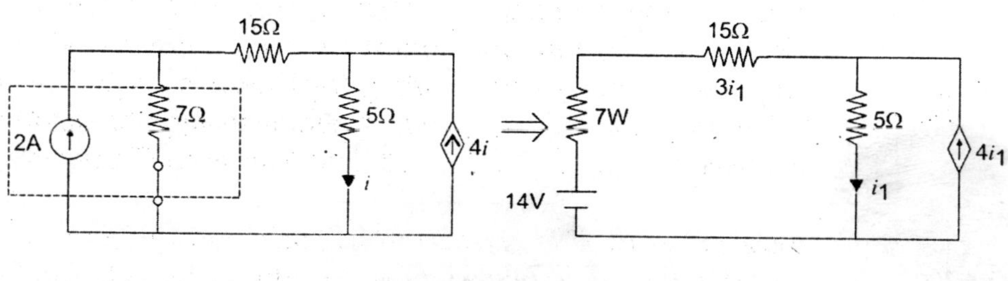

$$14 = (15 + 7)(-3i_1) + 5i_1$$

$$= -61\,i_1$$

$$i_1 = -\frac{14}{61}$$

Step II: Select 3 V, voltage source in figure below

$$3 = (15 + 7)(-3i_2) + 5i_2$$

$$i_2 = -\frac{3}{61}$$

Therefore, using superposition theorem,

$$i = i_1 + i_2 = \frac{-17}{61}$$

Hence, voltage across 2A current source is

$$= 7(3i + 2) + 3 = 7\left(\frac{-51}{61} + 2\right) + 3 = 11.15 \text{ V}$$ **Ans.**

Voltage across $4i$ current source,

$$= 5i = 5\left(\frac{-17}{61}\right) = -1.39 \text{ V}$$

Example 25: Using superposition theorem, calculate the current through $(2 + j3)\Omega$ impedance of the circuit shown in figure below. **[UPTU 2004, GBTU 2007]**

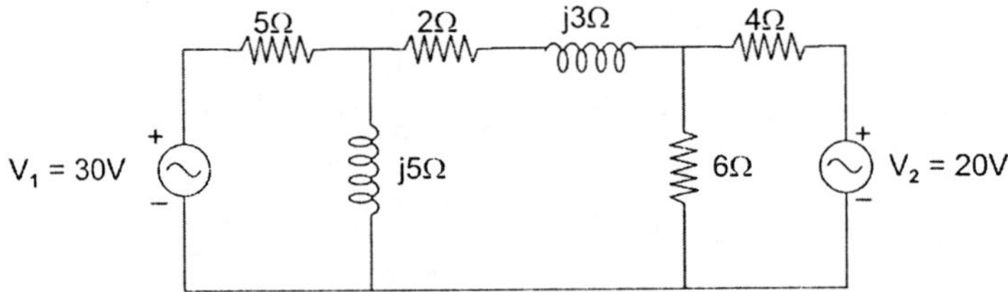

Solution: Step I: Select $V_1 = 30$ V source

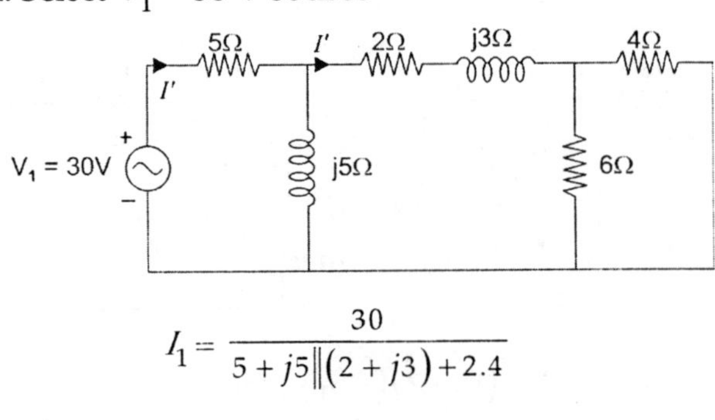

$$I_1 = \frac{30}{5 + j5 \| (2 + j3) + 2.4}$$

$$I' = \frac{I_1 \times (j5)}{j5 + 2 + j3 + 2.4} = 2.40\angle 6.4° \text{ A}$$

Step II: Select $V_2 = 20$ V source

$$I_2 = \frac{20}{4+(6\,||\,(2+j3)+5\,||\,j5)} = \frac{20(10.5+j5.5)}{69+j55}$$

$$I'' = I_2 \cdot \frac{6}{(6+4.3+j5.5)} = 1.36\angle -37.6°\text{ A}$$

Therefore, the current

$$I = I' - I'' = 1.74\angle 40°\text{ A}$$ **Ans.**

Example 26: Find the Thevenin's equivalent for the network shown in figure below at the right of terminals *ab* and hence find the source current. **[UPTU 2005, GBTU 2008]**

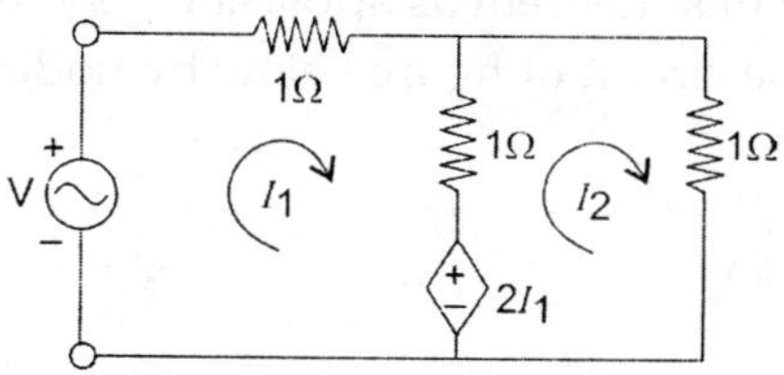

Solution: As the circuit of figure below, does not have any independent source, hence $V_{th} = 0$,

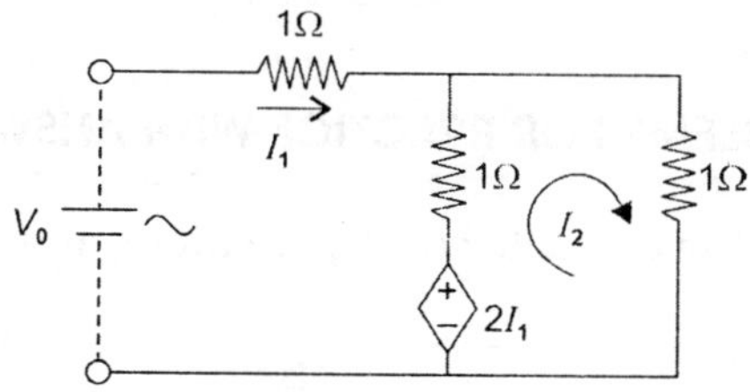

For R_{th}: In this case a voltage V_a is applied and let current I_1, which would flow due to V_0 as

$\therefore$ $$R_{th} = \frac{V_0}{I_1}$$

Applying *KVL* $$V_0 = 1\cdot I_1 + 1(I_1 - I_2) + 2I_2$$

or $$= 4I_1 - I_2 \quad ...(1)$$

and $$2I_1 = I(I_2 - I_1) + I_2$$

or $$3I_1 = 2I_2 \quad ...(2)$$

Solving Eqs (1) and (2), we get

$$V_0 = 4I_1 - \frac{3}{2}I_1 = \frac{5}{2}I_1$$

$$R_{th} = \frac{V_0}{I_1} = \frac{5}{2}\Omega$$

Therefore, Thevenin's equivalent circuit as shown in figure below

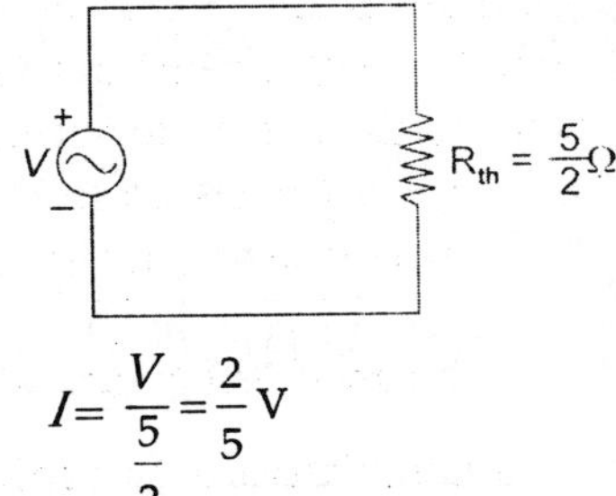

$$\therefore \qquad I = \frac{V}{\frac{5}{2}} = \frac{2}{5}\text{V} \qquad \textbf{Ans.}$$

EXERCISES

1. State superposition theorem and write its limitations.
2. State Thevenin's and Norton's theorems and write their limitations.
3. State and prove Millman's theorem as applicable to voltage sources.
4. Find the current I in the circuit of figure below by nodal analysis.

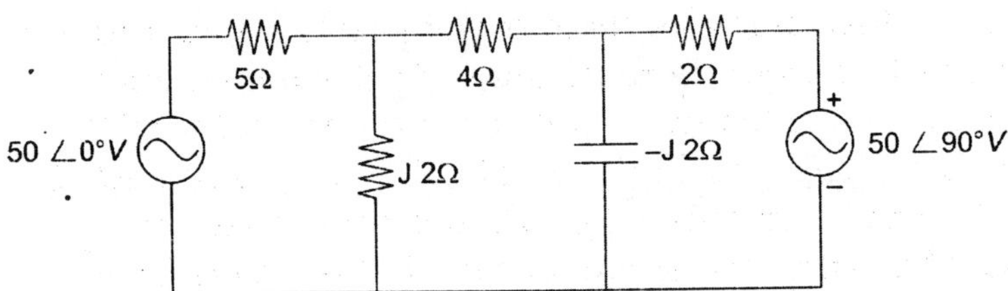

PROBLEMS FOR PRACTICE WITH ANSWERS

1. Find current through the capacitor of the circuit of figure below.

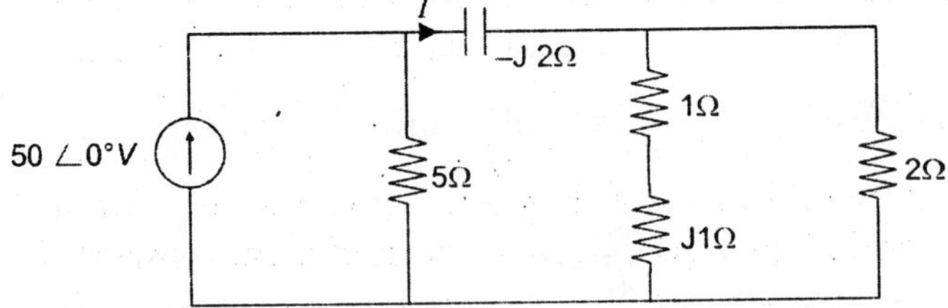

2. Determine the current I_1 in the current of figure below, by mesh analysis.

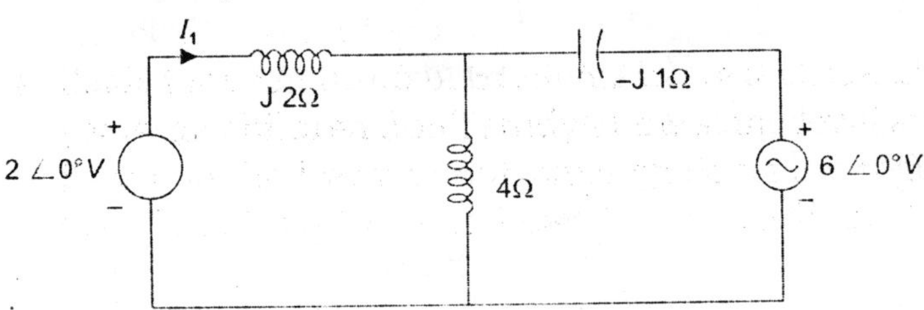

3. Determine the current I_1 in the current of above figure, by super position theorem.
4. Solve I shown in circuit of figure below, by mesh analysis.

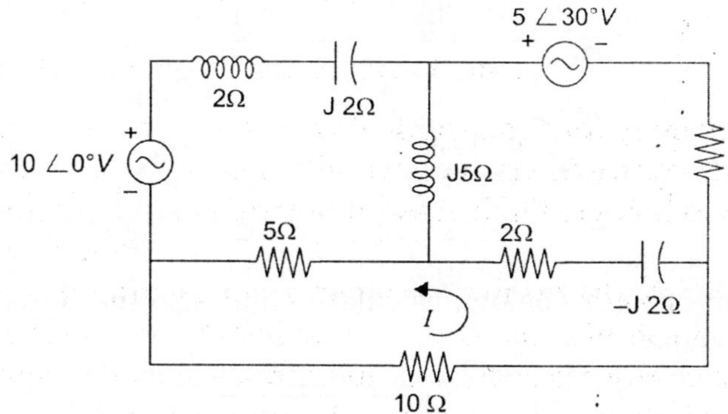

5. The circuit of figure below has a voltage source and a dependent current source. Determine the current through 25 Ω resistor.

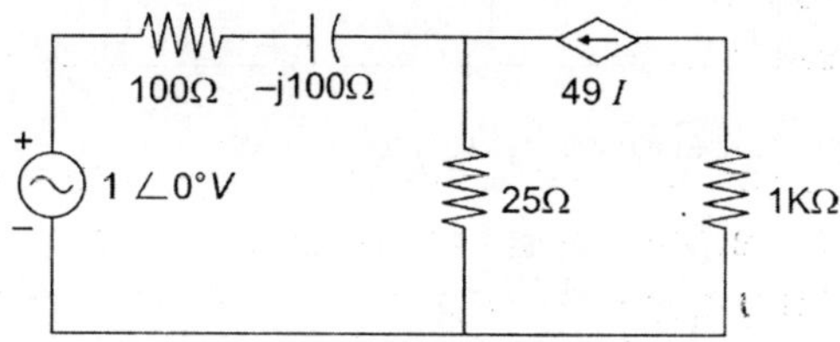

6. Determine the load that must be connected across the terminal AB of the circuit of figure below to draw the maximum power from the source. Also find the maximum power.

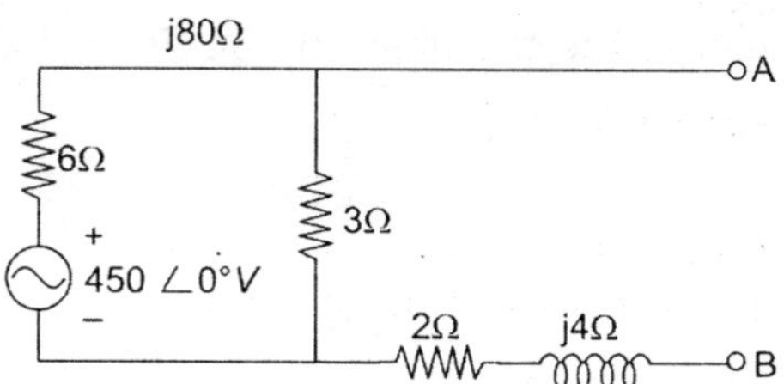

7. In the circuit shown in figure below, determine Z_L so that the power absorbed by it is maximum and also determine the power absorbed.

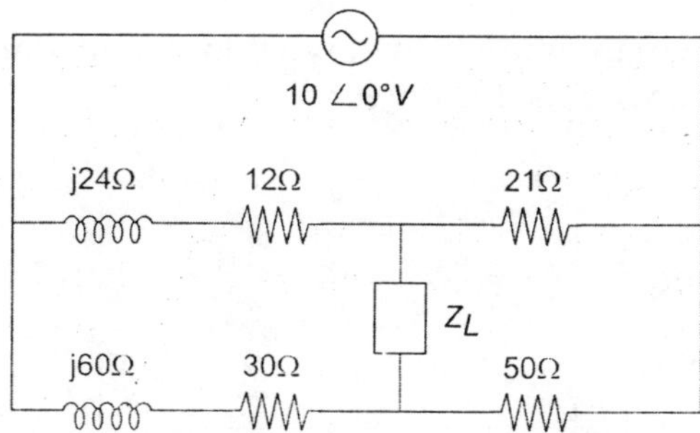

8. Obtain Thevenin's equivalent circuit across *AB* terminals for the circuit shown in figure below.

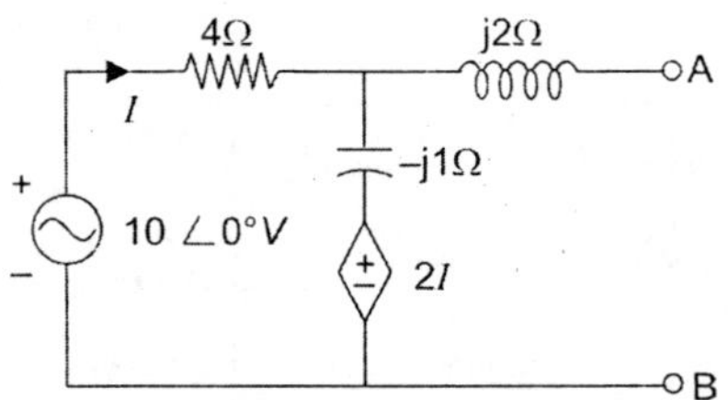

9. In the circuit of figure below, calculate *I* and also the power absorbed by the dependent source.

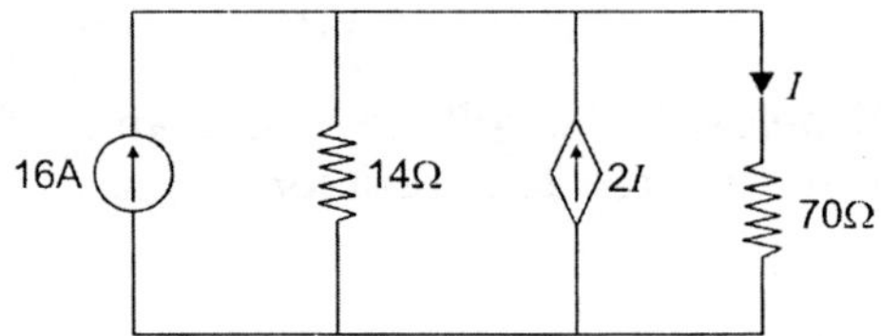

10. Solve for *I* in the circuit shown in figure below.

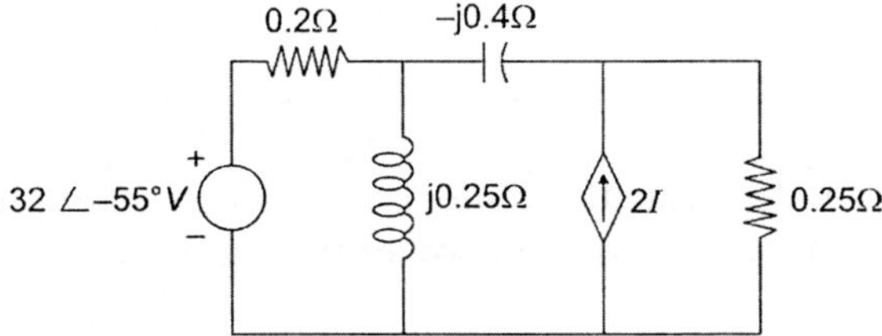

11. Find the node voltages in the circuit shown in figure below

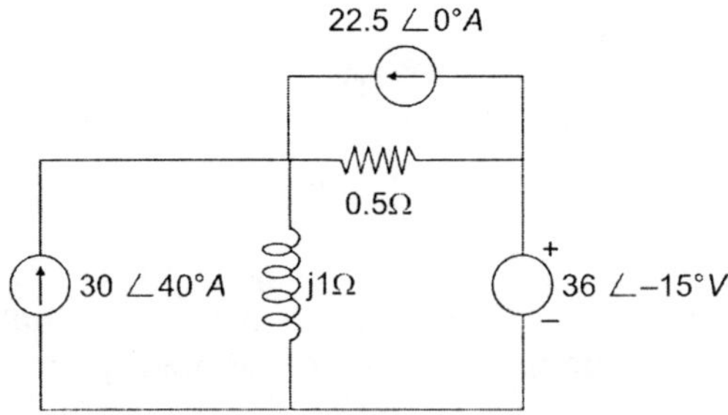

12. For the circuit shown in figure below, what load impedance ZL absorb maximum average power and what is this power.

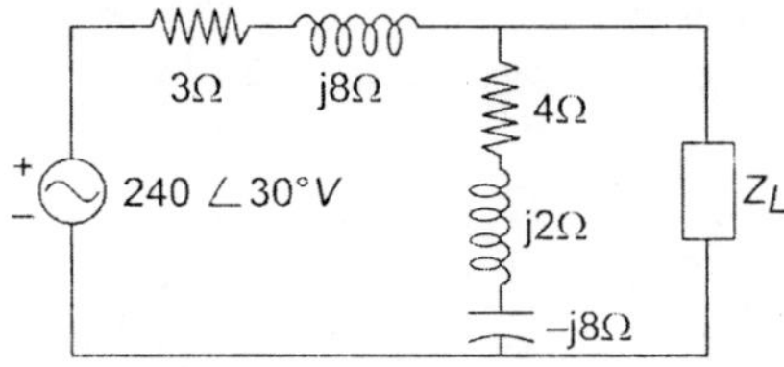

13. Find the current I for the circuit shown in figure below, using Norton's theorem.

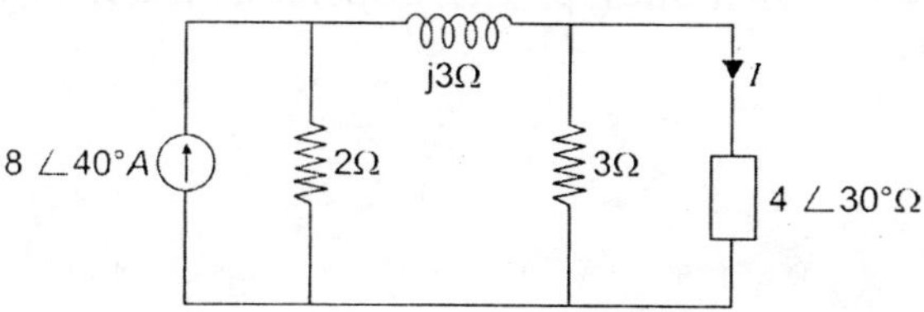

14. For the circuit shown in figure below, find the voltage source V_1 for which is the current in the voltage source $V_2 = 20\angle 0°\text{ V}$ will be zero.

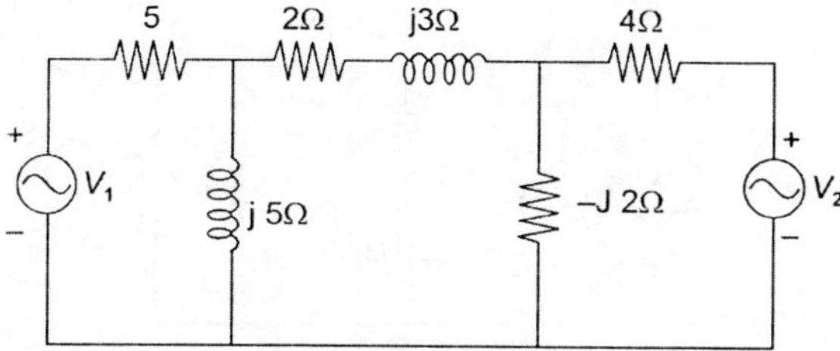

15. Calculate the current through the branch AB of the given network of figure below using (i) Thevenin's theorem (ii) Norton's theorem.

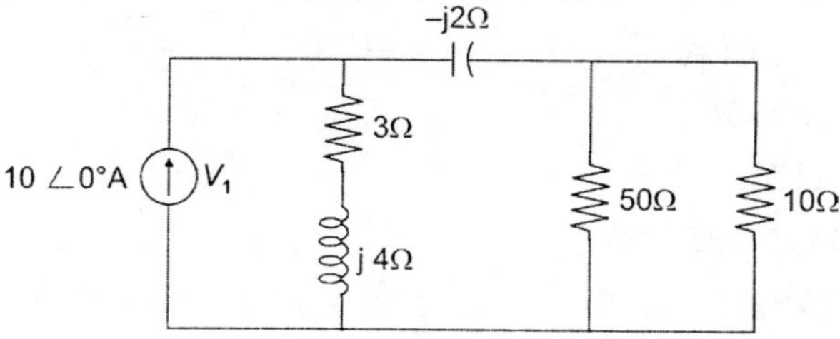

16. Determine the currents in all the branches of the circuit shown in figure below.

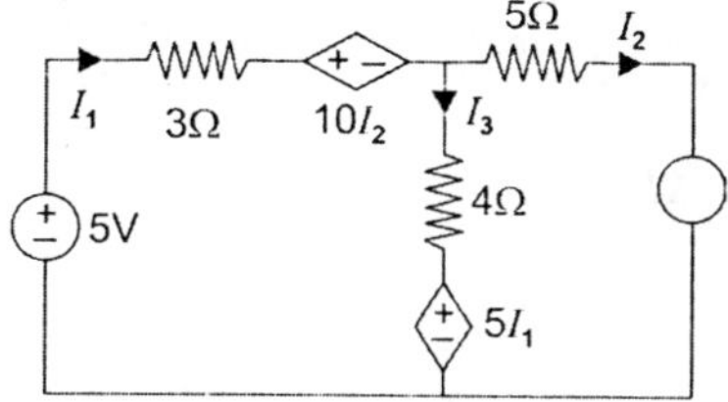

17. Determine the current through the branch AB of the circuit shown in figure below using principle of superposition theorem.

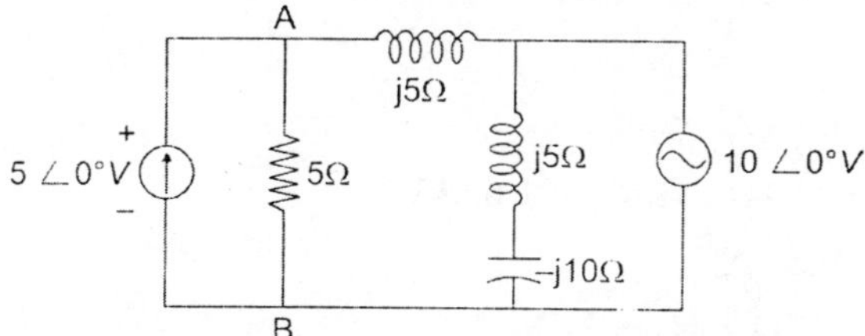

18. In the circuit shown in figure below, R_s is a variable between 2 Ω and 55 Ω. What value of R_s result in maximum power transfer to the load R_L. Also calculate the maximum power.

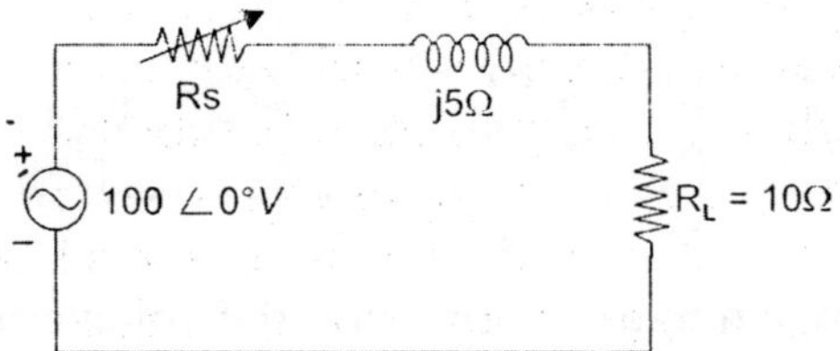

19. Use superposition theorem to find the voltage V in the circuit of figure below.

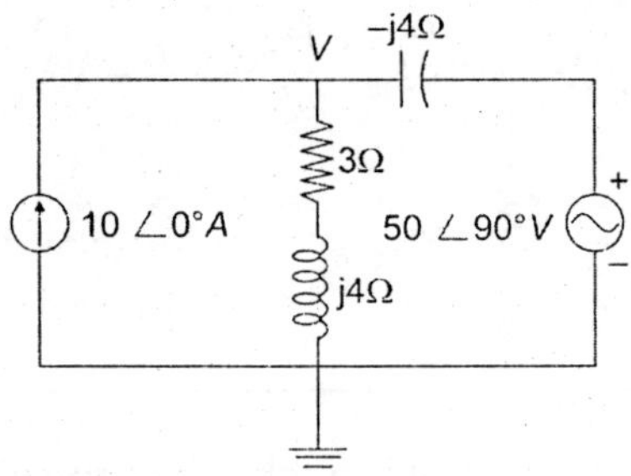

ANSWERS

1. $I = 4.16\angle 15.4$ A
2. $I_1 = 3.6\angle 123.7°$ A
4. $I_1 = 3.6\angle 123.7°$ A
5. $I = 0.435\angle -194.7°$ A
6. $Z_L = (4 - j4)\Omega$

   $P_{max} = 1406.25$ W
8. $Z_L = (42.19 - j21.49)\Omega$

   $P_{max} = 0.163$ W
9. $V_{th} = 3.67\angle -17.1°$ V

   $Z_{th} = (0.109 + j1.35)\ \Omega$
11. $V_1 = 10$ V, $V_2 = 118$ V
12. $I = 3$ A
13. $V_1 = 96$ V
14. $I = 2$ A, P = 560 W
15. $I = -253\angle 34°$ A $= 253\angle -146°$ A
16. $V_1 = 10.8\angle -155°$ V

    $V_2 = 36\angle -165°$ V
17. $Z_L = (8.45 + j0.414)\ \Omega$, $P_m = 1.67$ kW
18. $1.41\angle -19.5°$ A
19. $V_1 = 55.7\angle -17.4°$

Chapter

7 Three Phase AC Circuit

7.1 INTRODUCTION

A three phase (poly-) system has certain advantages over the single phase system, hence they are preferred. Some of these advantages are as follows:

i. **More output:** For the same size, the output of the polyphase machines is always higher than that of the single phase machine.
ii. **Smaller size:** For producing the same output, the size of three phase machine is always smaller than that of the single phase machine.
iii. **3-ϕ (phase) motor are self starting:** As the three phase ac supply is capable of producing a rotating magnetic field when applied to stationary windings. The three phase AC motors are self starting. The single phase motor needs to use an additional starting winding.
iv. **Better power factor:** The power factor of three phase machine is better than that of the single phase machines.
v. **More power is transmitted:** In the transmission system, it is possible to transmit more power using a 3-ϕ system, than the single phase system, by using two conductor of same cross-sectional area.
vi. **Smaller cross-sectional area of conductors:** If same amount of power is to be transmitted than the cross-sectional area of the conductors used for 3-ϕ system is small as compared to that for the single-phase system.

7.2 THREE PHASE ELECTRIC SYSTEM

A three-phase electrical system may be considered as three separate single-phase systems displaced from each other by 120°.

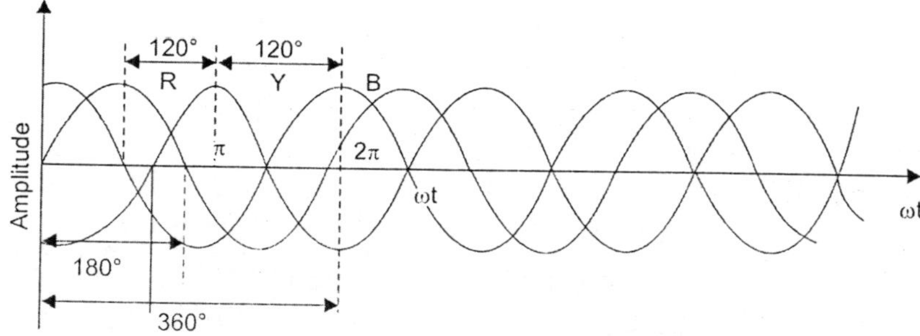

Fig. 7.1

The resultant current is given by

$$i_R + i_Y + i_B = I_m \sin\omega t + I_m \sin(\omega t - 120°) + I_m \sin(\omega t + 120°)$$

$$= I_m \sin\omega t + I_m \sin\omega t \cos 120° - I_m \cos\omega t \sin 120° + I_m \sin\omega t \cos 120°$$

$$= I_m \sin\omega t + 2I_m \sin\omega t \cos 120$$

$$= I_m \sin\omega t + (2I_m \sin\omega t)(-1/2)$$

$$= I_m \sin\omega t - I_m \sin\omega t = 0$$

The current through the neutral axis in case balance load is zero.

$$I_N = I_R + I_Y + I_B = 0$$

7.2.1 Comparison of Single Phase and Three Phase Systems

S.No.	Parameter	1-ϕ system	3-ϕ system
1.	Voltage	Low (230 V)	High (415 V)
2.	Transmission	Low	High efficiencies
3.	Size	Larger	Smaller
4.	Cross-sectional area	Larger	Smaller
5.	Use	Domestic, small power applications	Industries, large power application

7.3 BALANCED OR UNBALANCED LOAD

A star or delta type load can be further classified into two categories (i) balanced load (ii) unbalanced load.

Balanced load: A balance load is that in which magnitude of all impedance connected in the load are equal and the phase angle of them are also equal and of same type, i.e. *L*, *R* or *C*.

Unbalanced load: If a load does not satisfy the condition of being balance, then it is called as unbalanced load.

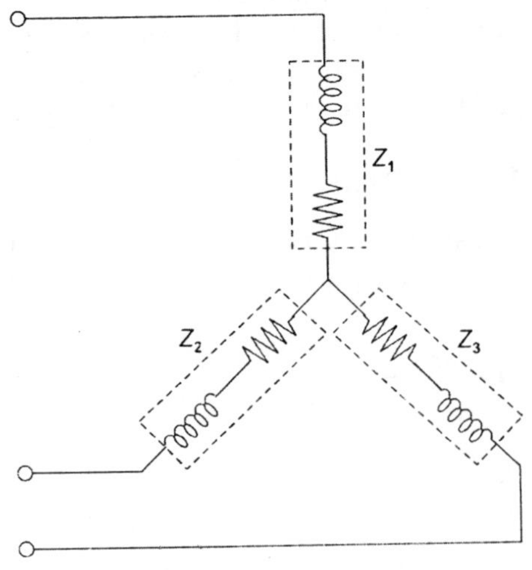

Fig. 7.2: Three phase load

$$Z_1 = Z_2 = Z_3 \qquad \text{(for balanced load)}$$

$$Z_1 \neq Z_2 \neq Z_3 \qquad \text{(for unbalanced load)}$$

7.4 GENERATION OF 3-φ EMFs

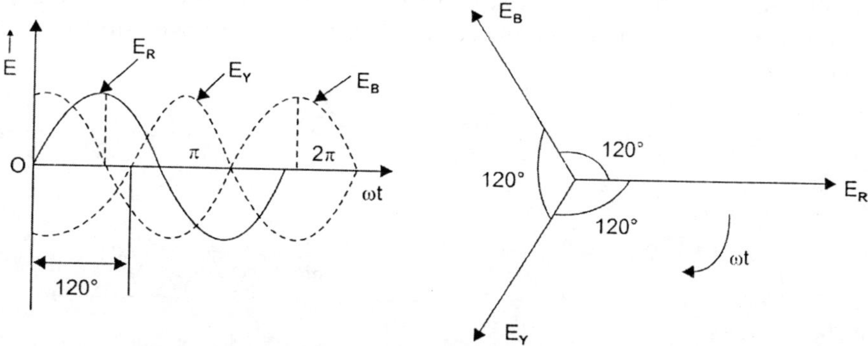

Fig. 7.3: Generation of EMF of waveform and Phasor

Instantaneous value of the emfs induced in coils *R, Y* and *B*.

$$E_R = E_m \sin \omega t$$

$$E_Y = E_m \sin(\omega t - 120°)$$

$$E_B = E_m \sin(\omega t - 240) \text{ or } E_m \sin(\omega t + 120°)$$

where $t = 0$, corresponds to the instant when the voltage (or) emf of coils *R* passes through zero and increasing in positive direction.

7.5 PHASE VOLTAGE, PHASE CURRENT, LINE VOLTAGE AND LINE CURRENT

Line and neutral voltage: The voltage between any two lines is known as line voltage. V_R, V_Y and V_B are phase voltages and V_{RY}, V_{YB} and V_{BR} are line current.

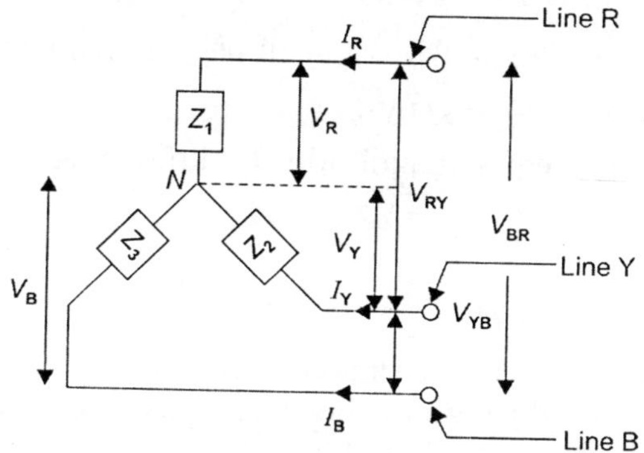

Fig. 7.4: Star connection

Similarly, the current through any phase is known as phase current (i.e. current passing through Z_1 or Z_2 or Z_3) and current through any line is line current, i.e. I_R, I_Y or I_B).

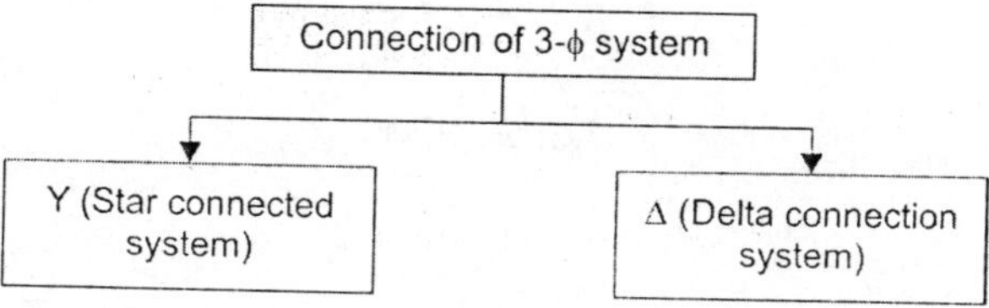

Fig. 7.5

7.6 STAR (Y) CONNECTED SYSTEM

In a star connected system similar ends of the coils are joined together (either starting or finishing) and dissimilar ends are connected to three phase supply as shown in Figs 7.6 and 7.7.

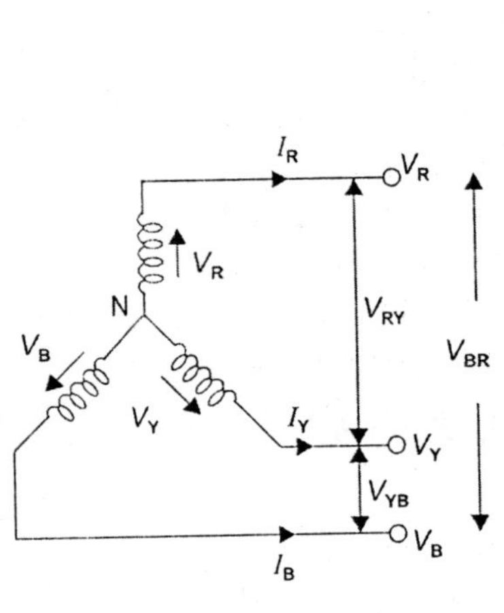

Fig. 7.6: Star connected system

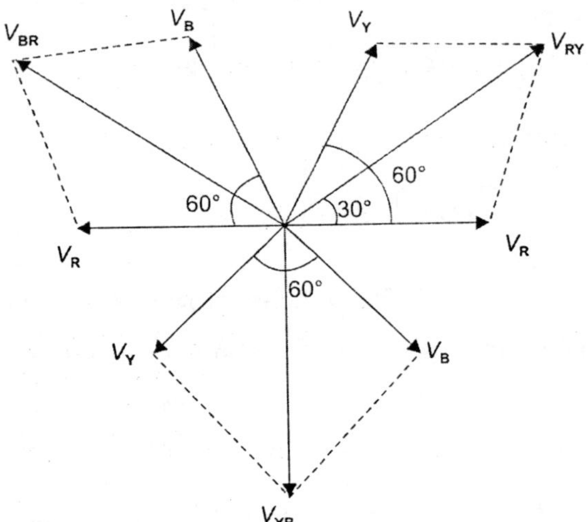

Fig. 7.7: Phase diagram

$$V_{RY} = V_R - V_Y$$

or $$V_{RY} = V_R + (-V_Y)$$

$$V_{RY} = \sqrt{(V_R)^2 + (V_Y)^2 + 2(V_R)(V_Y)\cos 60°}$$

Since $|V_R| = |V_Y| = |V_B| = |Vph|$ for balanced system

$$V_{RY} = \sqrt{3}\,V_{ph}$$

V_{RY}, V_{YB} and V_{BR} are in equal magnitude and known as line voltage (V_L).

$\therefore$ $$V_L = \sqrt{3}\,V_{ph}$$

$$V_{ph} = \frac{V_L}{\sqrt{3}} \quad \text{or} \quad E_{ph} = \frac{E_L}{\sqrt{3}}$$

Since in star-connected system each line conductor carries the current through a phase and hence current flowing through the line and phase are same.

Line current (I_L) = Phase current (I_{ph})

7.6.1 Power in 3-ϕ AC system

Active power $$P = \sqrt{3}V_{ph}I_{ph}\cos\phi \text{ W}$$

$$= 3\frac{V_L}{\sqrt{3}}I_2\cos\phi = \sqrt{3}V_L I_L \cos\phi \text{ W}$$

Reactive power $$Q = \sqrt{3}V_{ph}I_{ph}\sin\phi$$

$$= 3\cdot\frac{V_L}{\sqrt{3}}\cdot I_2 \sin\phi$$

$$= \sqrt{3}\,V_L I_L \sin\phi \text{ VAR}$$

Apparent power $S = 3V_{ph}I_{ph}$ VA

$$= \sqrt{3}\frac{V_L}{\sqrt{3}}I_L \text{ VA} = \sqrt{3}\,V_L I_L \text{ VA}$$

Note: It should be noted that in a balanced star-connected system line voltages are 120° apart, 30° ahead of the respective phase voltages, $\sqrt{3}$ times of phase voltage, equal to phase currents and at balance condition of y-connected system $V_{NR} + V_{NY} + V_{NB} = 0$

7.7 DELTA (Δ) CONNECTION SYSTEM

In delta connected system, finishing end of one coil is connected with starting end of next coil. These points are connected with the three phase supply.

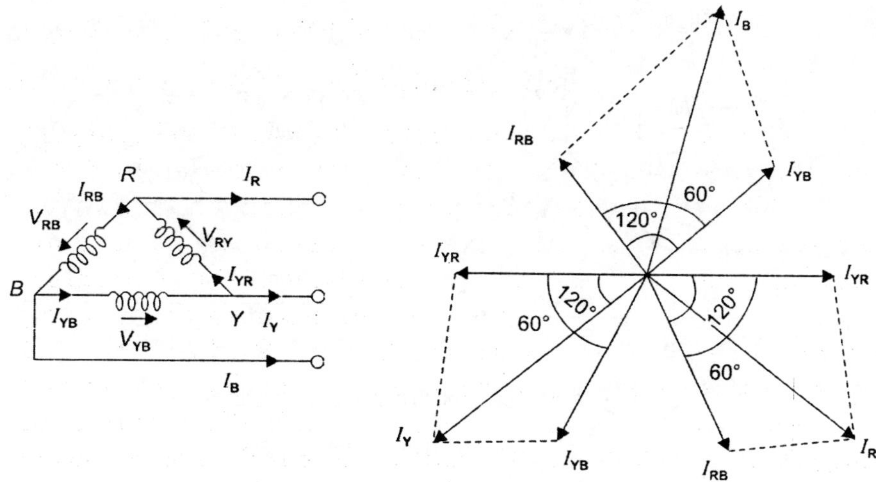

Fig. 7.8: Star connected system **Fig. 7.9:** Phasor diagram

$$I_R = I_{YR} - I_{RB}$$

$$I_Y = I_{BY} - I_{YR}$$

$$I_B = I_{RB} - I_{BY}$$

Line current

$$I_R = I_{YR} + (-I_{RB}),$$

$$= \sqrt{(I_{YR})^2 + (I_{RB})^2 + 2(I_{YR})(I_{RB})\cos 60°}$$

$$I_{YR} = I_{RB} = BY = I_{ph} \text{ and } I_R I_L = I_Y = I_B$$

$$I_R = I_L = \sqrt{(I_{ph})^2 + (I_{ph})^2 + 2\times(I_{ph})(I_{ph})\cos 60°}$$

$$I_L = \sqrt{3}I_{ph}$$

∴ $$I_{ph} = \frac{I_L}{\sqrt{3}}$$

and line voltage, V_L = Phase voltage, V_{ph}.

∴ $$V_{ph} = V_L$$

7.8 MEASUREMENT OF POWER IN 3-ϕ AC CIRCUIT

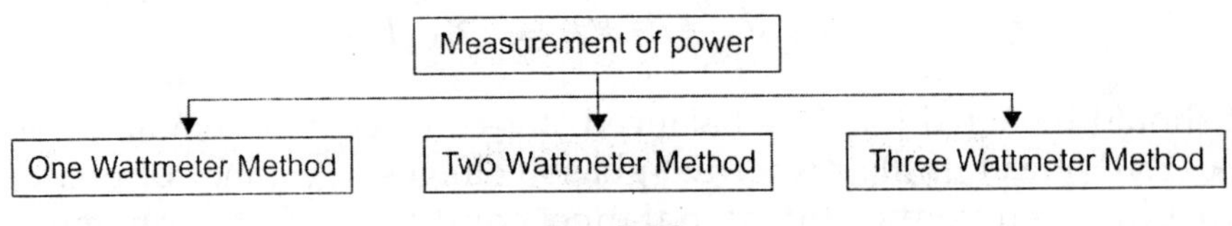

Fig. 7.10

7.8.1 One Wattmeter Method

In this method, one wattmeter is used and its reading is multiplied by 3 to get three phase power. It is suitable only if load is balanced.

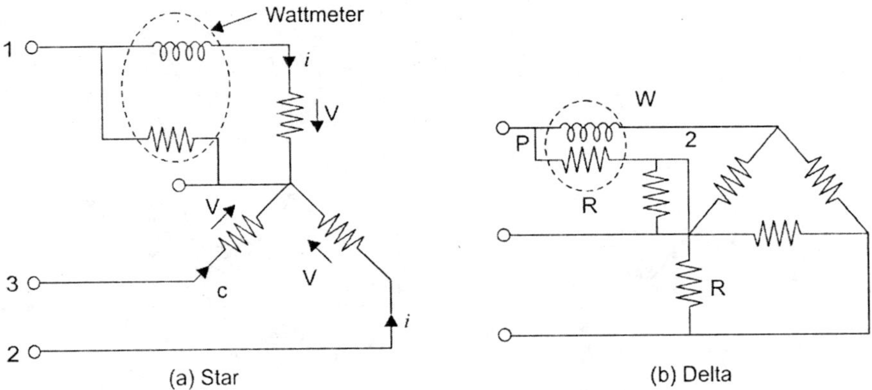

Fig. 7.11: One wattmeter connections

$$P = 3 \times \text{wattmeter reading}$$

7.8.2 Two Wattmeter Method

This is the generally used method for measurement of power in 3-ϕ, 3-wire load circuits.

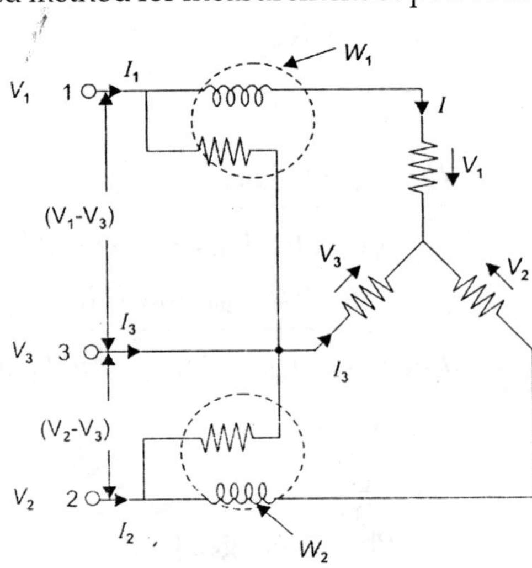

Fig. 7.12: Star connected two wattmeter connections

For Fig. 7.12 star connected system two wattmeter

$$I_1 + I_2 + I_3 = 0 \text{ (at balance)}$$

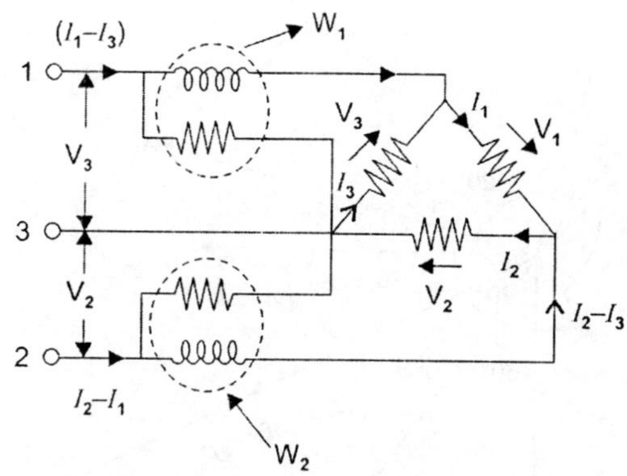

Fig. 7.13: Delta connected two wattmeter connections

Instantaneous power $= V_1I_1 + V_2I_2 + V_3I_3$ ...(7.1)

Wattmeter reading $W_1 = (V_1 - V_3)I_1$

$W_2 = (V_2 - V_3)I_2$ ...(7.2)

Total power $P = W_1 + W_2$

$$= (V_1 - V_3)I_1 + (V_2 - V_3)I_2$$

$$= V_1I_1 + V_2I_2 - V_3(I_1 + I_2)$$

$$= V_1I_1 + V_2I_2 + V_3I_3 \text{ (since } I_1 + I_2 = -I_3\text{)}$$

For Fig. 7.13 delta connected system

Wattmeter reading $W_1 = (I_1 - I_3)(-V_3)$

$W_2 = (I_2 - I_1)(V_2)$

Total power $P = W_1 + W_2$

$$= (I_1 - I_3)(-V_3) + (I_2 - I_1)(V_2)$$

$$= -V_3I_1 + V_3I_3 + I_2V_2 - I_1V_2$$

$$= V_2I_2 + V_3I_3 - I_1(V_2 + V_3)$$

We know at balance for delta connected system

$$V_1 + V_2 + V_3 = 0$$

$$V_2 + V_3 = -V_1$$

$$P = V_2I_2 + V_3I_3 - I_1(-V_1)$$

$$= V_1I_1 + V_2I_2 + V_3I_3$$

Determination of Power Factor (cos φ) from Wattmeter Readings

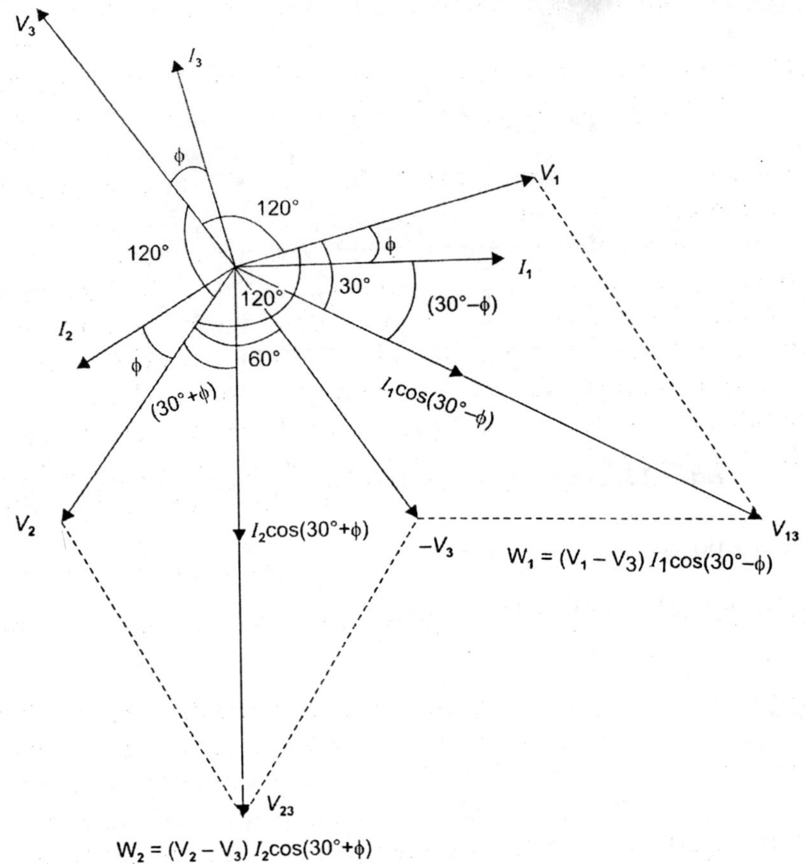

Fig. 7.14

Assume lagging PF and star-connected system (for inductive load)

$$I_1 = I_L,\ I_2 = I_L$$

$$V_{13} = V_1 - V_3 = V_L$$

$$V_{23} = V_2 - V_3 = V_L$$

$$W_1 = V_L I_L \cos(30° - \phi)$$

$$W_2 = V_L I_L \cos(30° + \phi)$$

Sum of two wattmeter readings

$$W_1 + W_2 = V_L I_L (\cos 30° - \phi) + V_L I_L \cos(30° + \phi)$$

$$= V_L I_L (\cos 30°.\cos\phi + \sin 30°.\sin\phi + \cos 30°.\cos\phi - \sin 30°.\sin\phi)$$

$$= 2V_L I_L \cos 30°.\cos\phi$$

$$= 2V_L I_L \cos\phi \times \frac{\sqrt{3}}{2} = \sqrt{3} V_L I_L \cos\phi$$

$$= \sqrt{3} V_L I_L \cos\phi \qquad \text{...(7.3)}$$

and Difference of two wattmeter reading

$$\therefore \quad W_1 - W_2 = V_L I_L \cos(30° - \phi) - V_L I_L \cos(30° + \phi)$$

$$= V_L I_L \{(\cos(30° \cos\phi + \sin 30° \sin\phi - \cos 30° \cos\phi + \sin 30° \sin\phi)\}$$

$$= 2V_L I_L \sin 30°.\sin\phi = 2 \times V_L I_L \times \frac{1}{2} \sin\phi$$

$$= V_L I_L \sin\phi \qquad ...(7.4)$$

Dividing Eq (7.4) by Eq (7.3)

$$\frac{W_1 - W_2}{W_1 + W_2} = \frac{V_L I_L \sin\phi}{\sqrt{3} V_L I_L \cos\phi}$$

$$\therefore \quad \tan\phi = \sqrt{3}\left(\frac{W_1 - W_2}{W_1 + W_2}\right)$$

$$\phi = \tan^{-1}\sqrt{3}\left(\frac{W_1 - W_2}{W_1 + W_2}\right)$$

$$\text{pf} = \cos\phi = \cos\tan^{-1}\sqrt{3}\left(\frac{W_1 - W_2}{W_1 + W_2}\right)$$

Variation in wattmeter readings:

$$W_1 = V_L I_L \cos(30° - \phi)$$
$$W_2 = V_L I_L \cos(30° + \phi)$$

Case I: When pf of load is unity $(\phi = 0°)$

$$W_1 = V_L I_L \cos 30° = \frac{\sqrt{3}}{2} V_L I_L$$

$$= \frac{1}{2} \text{ of total power}$$

$$W_2 = V_L I_L \cos 30° = \frac{1}{2} \text{ of total power}$$

$$\therefore \quad W_1 = W_2$$

Case II: When $\phi = 60°$, pf load is 0.5

$$W_1 = V_L I_L \cos(30° - 60°) = \frac{\sqrt{3}}{2} V_L I_L$$

$$W_2 = 0$$

$$\therefore \quad W_1 \neq W_2$$

Case III: When the pf load is zero (i.e. $\phi = 90°$)

$$W_1 = V_L I_L \cos(30° - 90°) = \frac{1}{2} V_L I_L$$

$$W_2 = V_L I_L \cos(30° + 90°) = -\frac{1}{2} V_L I_L$$

$$\therefore \quad W_1 = -W_2$$

Similarly wattmeter readings for capacitive loads, i.e. leading pf

$$W_1 = V_L I_L \cos(30° + \phi)$$

$$W_2 = V_L I_L \cos(30° - \phi)$$

7.8.3 Three Wattmeter Method

In this method, a wattmeter is connected in each phase and total power is calculated as sum of all the three wattmeter readings.

The disadvantages of this method is that for delta connected load current coil of wattmeter is connected by breaking the delta connected load circuit.

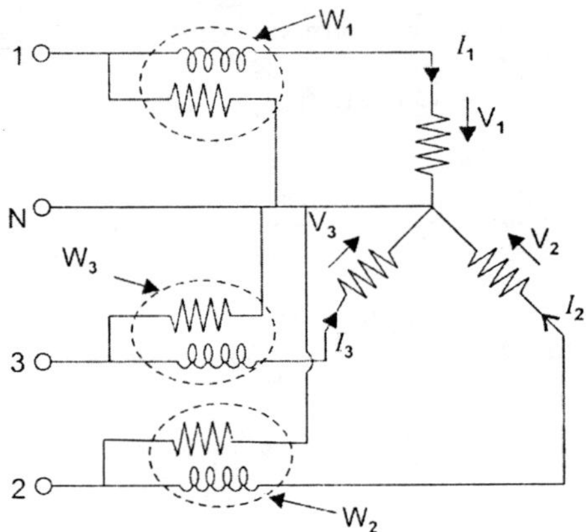

Fig. 7.15: For star connected

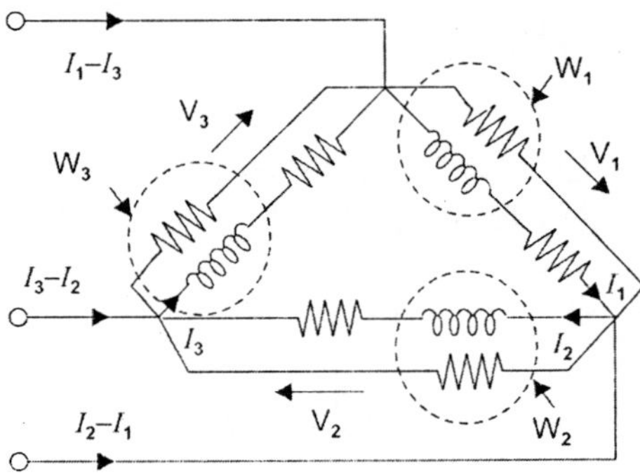

Fig. 7.16: Δ-Connected

∴ Total power $P = W_1 + W_2 + W_3$

UNIVERSITY SOLVED EXAMPLES

Example 1: A balanced star-connected load of $(8 + j6)\Omega$ per phase is connected to a balanced 3-ϕ, 400 V supply. Find the line current, pf, power in VA. **[UPTU 2005-06]**

Solution: Given data,

$$Z_{ph} = (8+j6)\Omega/\text{phase}$$

$$V_L = 400 \text{ V}$$

Y for connected system

$$\therefore \quad V_{ph} = \frac{V_L}{\sqrt{3}} = \frac{400}{\sqrt{3}} = 231 \text{ V}$$

$$I_{ph} = \frac{V_{ph}}{Z_{ph}} = \frac{231}{8+j6} = \frac{231}{\sqrt{8^2+6^2}} = \frac{231}{10} = 23.1 \text{ A}$$

∴ For *Y*-connected system

line current I_L = phase current, I_{ph} $\therefore I_{ph} = I_L$

$$I_L = I_{ph} = 23.1 \text{ A}$$

$$\cos\phi = \frac{R_{ph}}{Z_{ph}} = \frac{8}{10} = 0.8(\text{lag})$$

Total power, $P = \sqrt{3}V_L I_L \cos\phi$

$$= \sqrt{3} \times 400 \times 23.1 \times 0.8$$

$$P = 12800 \text{ W}$$ **Ans.**

or $S = \sqrt{3}V_L I_L = \sqrt{3} \times 400 \times 23.1 = 18000 \text{ VA}$ **Ans.**

Also, $P = 3I_{ph}^2 \times R_{ph} = 3 \times (23.1)^2 \times 8 = 12800 \text{ W}$ **Ans.**

Example 2: For star-connected system in a 3 – φ circuit prove that $V_L = \sqrt{3}Vph$ and $I_L = I_{ph}$ A 3-phase, 400 V supply is connected to a 3-phase star connected balanced load. The line current is 20 A and the power consumed by the load is 12 kW. Calculate the impedance of the load, phase current and power factor. **[UPTU 2006-07]**

Solution: For $V_L = \sqrt{3}V_{ph}$ and $I_L = I_{ph}$ (Refer to Section 7.6)

Given,

$$P = 12 \times 10^3 \text{ W} ;\ V_L = 400 \text{ V};\ I_L = 20 \text{ A}$$

$$V_{ph} = \frac{V_L}{\sqrt{3}} = \frac{400}{\sqrt{3}} = 231 \text{ V}$$

$$I_{ph} = I_L = 20 \text{ A}$$

Load impedance, $Z_{ph} = \frac{V_{ph}}{I_{ph}} = \frac{231}{20} = 11.547\ \Omega/\text{phase}$ **Ans.**

$$\text{pf} = \cos\phi = \frac{P}{\sqrt{3}V_L I_L} = \frac{12000}{\sqrt{3} \times 400 \times 20} = 0.866$$ **Ans.**

Example 3: A balanced 3-phase star-connected load of 18 kW taking a leading current of 60 amperes when connected across a 3-phase 440 V, 50 Hz supply. Find the values and the nature of the load. **[UPTU 2007-08]**

Solution: Given data

$$V_L = 440 \text{ V};\ f = 50 \text{ Hz};\ p = 18 \times 10^3\ W;\ I_L = 60 \text{ A}$$

$$V_{ph} = \frac{V_L}{\sqrt{3}} = \frac{440}{\sqrt{3}} = 254 \text{ V}$$

$$I_{ph} = I_L = 60 \text{ A}$$

Load impedance $Z_{ph} = \frac{V_{ph}}{I_{ph}} = \frac{254}{60} = 4.234\ \Omega$

$$\text{pf} = \cos\phi = \frac{P}{\sqrt{3}V_L I_L} = \frac{18000}{\sqrt{3} \times 440 \times 60} = 0.393\ \ (\text{lead})$$ **Ans.**

$$R_{ph} = Z_{ph} \cos\phi$$

$$= 4.234 \times 0.393 = 1.667\ \Omega/\text{phase}$$ **Ans.**

$$X = Z_{ph} \sin\phi$$

$$= 4.234\sqrt{1-(0.393)^2} = 4.234 \times 0.9193$$

$$X = 3.89\Omega/\text{phase}$$ **Ans.**

Example 4: A $3-\phi$, 3-wire, Y-connected system has 150 V between two phases. Each phase has $Z = 5\angle -30°\ \Omega$. Find (i) current in each phase (ii) total power (iii) Draw phasor diagram. **[UPTU 2001, 2007-08]**

Solution: Given data

$$V_L = 150 \text{ V}$$

$$Z_{ph} = 5\angle -30°\ \Omega.$$

$$\therefore \quad V_{ph} = \frac{150}{\sqrt{3}} = 86.6 \text{ V}$$

(i) Current in each phase

$$I_{ph} = \frac{V_{ph}}{Z_{ph}} = \frac{86.6}{5} = 17.32 \text{ A}$$ **Ans.**

$$pf = \cos 30° = 0.866 \text{ (lagging)}$$

(ii) Total power

$$P = \sqrt{3} V_L I_L \cos 30°$$

$$= \sqrt{3} \times 150 \times 17.32 \times \cos 30° = 3897 \text{ W}$$ **Ans.**

(iii) This phasor diagram is shown below.

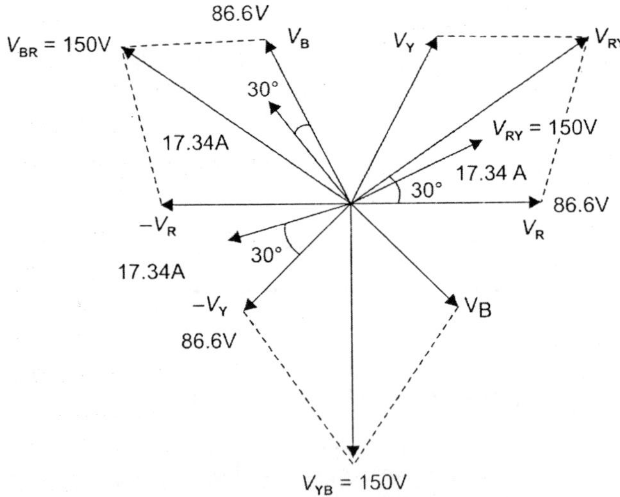

Example 5: A balanced 3-phase star-connected load of 120 kW takes a leading current of 85 A, when connected across a $3-\phi$, 1100 volts, 50 Hz supply. Obtain the values of three resistances impedances, and capacitances of the load per phase and also calculate the power factor of the load. **[UPTU 2003-04]**

Solution: Given data

$$V_L = 1100 \text{ V}$$

$$I_L = 850 \text{ A} = I_{ph}, \qquad P = 120 \times 10^3 \text{ W}$$

$$\cos\phi = \frac{P}{\sqrt{3}V_L I_L} = \frac{120\times10^3}{\sqrt{3}\times1100\times85} = 0.741 \text{ (lead)}$$ **Ans.**

$$V_{ph} = \frac{V_L}{\sqrt{3}} = \frac{1100}{\sqrt{3}}$$

$$Z_{ph} = \frac{V_{ph}}{I_{ph}} = \frac{1100/\sqrt{3}}{85} = 7.472\ \Omega$$

$$R_{ph} = Z_{ph}\cos\phi = 7.47\times0.741 = 5.536\ \Omega$$ **Ans.**

$$X_C = \sqrt{Z_{ph}^2 - R_{ph}^2} = \sqrt{(7.472)^2-(5.536)^2}$$

$$= 5.02\ \Omega$$

$$C = \frac{1}{2\pi X_C\times f} = \frac{1}{2\pi\times5.02\times50} = \mathbf{634\ \mu F}$$ **Ans.**

Example 6: Three identical coils connected in delta across 400 V, 50 Hz, 3-ϕ ac supply, take a line current of 17.32 A at power factor of 0.8 lagging. Calculate (i) The phase current (ii) The resistance and inductance of each coil (iii) The power drawn by each coil. **[UPTU 2002]**

Solution: Given data

$$V_L = 400\text{ V};\ I_L = 17.32\text{ A};\ pf = 0.8$$

∴ and $V_L = V_{th}$ for delta

(i)
$$I_{ph} = \frac{I_L}{\sqrt{3}} = \frac{17.32}{\sqrt{3}} = 10\text{ A}$$ **Ans.**

$$Z_{ph} = \frac{V_{ph}}{I_{ph}} = \frac{400}{10} = 40\ \Omega$$ **Ans.**

(ii)
$$R_{ph} = Z_{ph}\cos\phi = 40\times 0.8 = 32\ \Omega$$ **Ans.**

$$X_{ph} = \sqrt{Z_{ph}^2 - R_{ph}^2} = \sqrt{40^2-32^2} = 24\ \Omega$$ **Ans.**

$$L = \frac{X_{ph}}{2\pi\times f} = \frac{24}{2\pi\times50} = \mathbf{76.4\ mH}$$ **Ans.**

(iii) Power drawn by each coil

$$= I_{ph}^2\times R_{ph}$$

$$= (10)^2\times32 = 3200\text{ W}$$ **Ans.**

Example 7: A balanced Δ-connected load of (8 + *j*6)Ω per phase is connected to 3-phase, 230 V supply. Find the line current.

Solution: Given data

$$V_L = 230 = V_{ph}$$

$$Z_{ph} = \sqrt{8^2+6^2} = 10\ \Omega$$

$$I_{ph} = \frac{V_{ph}}{Z_{ph}} = \frac{230}{10} = 23 \text{ A}$$

$$I_L = \sqrt{3} I_{ph} = \sqrt{3} \times 23 = 39.84 \text{ A}$$ **Ans.**

Example 8: Derive the relationship between the line and phase voltage of an alternator. Three similar coils each having a resistance of 8 Ω and an inductance of 0.0191 H in series in each phase is connected across a 400 V, three phase, 50 Hz supply. Calculate the line current, power input, kVA and kVAR taken by the load.

Solution: For derivation of line and phase voltage refer to Section 6.6.

Part II: Given data

$$R_{ph} = 8\ \Omega$$
$$L_{ph} = 0.0191 \text{ H}$$
$$V_L = 400 \text{ V}$$

Calculate, I_L, kVA, kVAR and input power (kW).

$$X_{Lph} = 2\pi \times 50 \times 0.191 = 6\ \Omega$$

$$Z_{ph} = \sqrt{R_{ph}^2 + X_{Lph}^2} = \sqrt{8^2 + 6^2} = 10\ \Omega$$

$$\cos\phi = \frac{R_{ph}}{Z_{ph}} = \frac{8}{10} = 0.8 \text{ (lagging)}$$

When coil connected in star

$$V_{ph} = \frac{V_L}{\sqrt{3}} = \frac{400}{\sqrt{3}} = 23$$

$$I_{ph} = \frac{V_{ph}}{Z_{ph}} = \frac{231}{10} = 23.094 \text{ A}$$

$$I_L = I_{ph} = 23.094 \text{ A}$$

Power input

$$P = \sqrt{3}\, V_L I_L \cos\phi$$

$$= \sqrt{3} \times 400 \times 23.094 \times 0.8 = 12.8 \text{ kW}$$ **Ans.**

$$S = \sqrt{3} V_L I_L$$

$$= \sqrt{3} \times 400 \times 23.094 = 16 \text{ kV·A}$$ **Ans.**

$$Q = \sqrt{3} V_L I_L \sin\phi$$

$$= \sqrt{3} \times 400 \times 23.094 \times 0.6 = 9.6 \text{ kVAR}$$ **Ans.**

When coils are connected in Delta

$$I_{ph} = \frac{I_L}{\sqrt{3}}$$

$$I_{ph} = \frac{V_{ph}}{Z_{ph}} = \frac{400}{10} = 40 \text{ A}$$

$$I_L = \sqrt{3} \times I_{ph}$$

$$= \sqrt{3} \times 40 = 68.282 \text{ A}$$

$$P = \sqrt{3} V_L I_L \cos\phi$$

$$= \sqrt{3} \times 400 \times 68.282 \times 0.8 = 38.8 \text{ kW}$$ **Ans.**

$$S = \sqrt{3}V_L I_L$$
$$= \sqrt{3} \times 400 \times 68.282 = 48\ kVA \qquad \textbf{Ans.}$$
$$Q = \sqrt{3}V_L I_L \sin\phi$$
$$= \sqrt{3} \times 400 \times 68.28 \times 0.6 = 28.8 \text{ kVAR} \qquad \textbf{Ans.}$$

Example 9: Each phase of a delta connected load has a resistance of 25 Ω an inductance of 0.15 H and a capacitance of 120 μF in series. The load is connected across a 400 V, 50 Hz, 3-ϕ supply. Determine the line current, active power and reactive volt-ampers. **[UPTU-2002]**

Solution: Given data

$$R_{ph} = 25\ \Omega$$
$$X_{Lph} = 2\pi \times 50 \times 0.15 = 47.124\ \Omega$$
$$X_{Cph} = \frac{1}{2\pi f_C} = \frac{1}{2\pi \times 50 \times 120 \times 10^6} = 26.25\ \Omega$$
$$V_L = V_{ph} = 400\ \text{V}$$
$$X_{ph} = X_{Lph} - X_{Cph}$$
$$= 47.129 - 26.25 = 20.6\ \Omega$$
$$Z_{ph} = \sqrt{R_{ph}^2 + X_{ph}^2}$$
$$= \sqrt{25^2 + (20.6)^2} = 32.4\ \Omega$$
$$\cos\phi = \frac{R_{ph}}{Z_{ph}} = \frac{25}{32.4}$$
$$\phi = \tan^{-1}\left(\frac{X_{ph}}{R_{ph}}\right) = \tan^{-1}\left(\frac{20.6}{25}\right) = 39.50°(\text{lagg})$$
$$I_{ph} = \frac{V_{ph}}{Z_{ph}} = \frac{400}{32.4} = 12.35\ \text{A}$$
$$I_L = \sqrt{3} \times I_{ph} = \sqrt{3} \times 12.35 = 21.38\ \text{A} \qquad \textbf{Ans.}$$
$$P = \sqrt{3}V_L I_L \cos\phi = \sqrt{3} \times 400 \times 21.38 \times \cos 39.5°$$
$$= 11.43\ \text{kW} \qquad \textbf{Ans.}$$
$$Q = \sqrt{3}V_L I_L \sin\phi = \sqrt{3} \times 400 \times 21.38 \times \sin 39.5°$$
$$= 9.42\ \text{kVAR} \qquad \textbf{Ans.}$$

Example 10: Three identical resistors of 20 Ω each are connected in star to a 415 V, 50 Hz, three-phase supply. Calculate (i) The total power consumed (ii) The total power consumed if they are connected in delta (iii) The power consumed, if one of the resistor is opened.

Solution: Total power consumed from 415, 50 Hz, 3-ϕ supply when 20 Ω resistors are connected in each phase.

(i) Star

$$P_S = 3 \times \frac{\left(\frac{V_L}{\sqrt{3}}\right)^2}{R}$$

$$= \frac{V_L^2}{R} = \frac{(415)^2}{20} = 8.811 \text{ kW} \qquad \textbf{Ans.}$$

(ii) Delta $\quad P_D = 3 \times \dfrac{(V_L)^2}{R}$

$$= 3 \times \frac{(415)^2}{20} = 25.82 \text{ kW} \qquad \textbf{Ans.}$$

(iii) If one of the three resistors is open

(*a*) $\quad P_S = \dfrac{2 \times \left(\dfrac{V_L}{2}\right)^2}{R} = \dfrac{V_L^2}{2R} = 4.366 \text{ kW} \qquad$ **Ans.**

(*b*) $\quad P_D = \dfrac{2 \times V_L^2}{R} = \dfrac{2 \times 415^2}{20} = 17.225 \text{ kW} \qquad$ **Ans.**

Example 11: In two wattmeter method, power measured was 30 kW at 0.7 pf lagging. Find the reading of each wattmeter. **[UPTU 2006], V.V.V**

Solution: Given data

$$P = 30 \text{ kW}; \ \cos\phi = 0.7 \text{ (lagging)}; \ \phi = 45.57°$$

$$V_L I_L = \frac{30 \times 10^3}{\sqrt{3}\cos\phi} = \frac{30000}{\sqrt{3} \times 0.7} = 24.743 \text{ kVA}$$

$$W_1 = V_L I_L \cos(30° - \phi)$$
$$= 2474.3 \cos(30° - 45.57°) = 23.835 \text{ kW} \qquad \textbf{Ans.}$$

$$W_2 = V_L I_L \cos(30° + \phi)$$
$$= 2474.3 \cos(30° + 45.57°) = 6.165 \text{ kW} \qquad \textbf{Ans.}$$

Example 12: A 3-phase balanced load connected across a 3-ϕ, 400 V AC supply draws a line current of 10 A. Two wattmeters are used to measure input power. The ratio of two wattmeter readings is 2 : 1. Find the reading of two wattmeters.

Solution: Given data

$$\frac{W_2}{W_1} = r = \frac{1}{2} = 0.5$$

We know that, $\quad \tan\phi = \sqrt{3}\dfrac{(W_1 - W_2)}{(W_1 + W_2)}$

$$= \sqrt{3}\frac{\left(1 - \dfrac{W_2}{W_1}\right)}{\left(1 + \dfrac{W_2}{W_1}\right)} = \sqrt{3}\frac{(1-r)}{(1+r)}$$

$$= \sqrt{3}\frac{(1-0.5)}{(1+0.5)} = 30°$$

$$pf = \cos\phi = \cos 30° = 0.866$$

$$W_1 = V_L I_L \cos(30° - \phi)$$
$$= 400 \times 10 \cos(30° - 30°) = 4 \text{ kW} \qquad \textbf{Ans.}$$

$$W_2 = V_L I_L \cos(30° + \phi)$$
$$= 400 \times 10 \cos 60° = 2 \text{ kW}$$ **Ans.**

Example 13: Three equal impedances, each consisting of *R* and *L* in series are connected in star and are supplied from a 400 V, 50 Hz, 3-ϕ, 3-wire balanced supply system. The power input to the load is measured by 2-wattmeter method and the two wattmeters reads 3 kW and 1 kW. Determine the value of *R* and *L* connected in each phase.

[UPTU 2002-03]

Solution: Given data

$$W_1 = 3 \text{ kW}; W_2 = 1 \text{ kW}$$

Total power $P = W_1 + W_2 = 3 + 1 = 4 \text{ kW}$

$$\text{pf} = \cos\phi = \cos\tan^{-1}\sqrt{3}\frac{(W_1 - W_2)}{(W_1 + W_2)}$$

$$= \cos\tan^{-1}\sqrt{3}\left(\frac{3-1}{3+1}\right) = \cos 40.89°$$

$$\text{pf} = 0.755 \text{ (lagging)}$$

$$I_L = \frac{P}{\sqrt{3}V_L\cos\phi} = \frac{4000}{\sqrt{3} \times 400 \times 0.755} = 7.6316 \text{ A}$$

$$Z_{ph} = \frac{V_{ph}}{I_{ph}} = \frac{400/\sqrt{3}}{7.637} = 30.237\ \Omega$$

$$R_{ph} = Z_{ph}\cos\phi = 30.237 \times 0.7559 = 22.856\ \Omega$$ **Ans.**

$$X_{Lph} = \sqrt{Z_{ph}^2 - R_{ph}^2} = \sqrt{(30.23)^2 - (22.85)^2} = 19.796\ \Omega$$

$$L = \frac{X_{Lph}}{2\pi \times 50} = \frac{19.796}{2\pi \times 50} = 0.063 \text{ H}$$ **Ans.**

Example 14: A star-connected three-phase load has a resistance of 8 Ω and an inductive reactance of 6 Ω in each phase. It is fed from a 400 V, 3-ϕ balanced supply. Determine the line current, power factor, active and reactive powers. Draw phasor diagram showing phase and line voltages and currents. If power measurement is made using two wattmeter method, what will be the reading of both wattmeters?

[UPTU 2005-06]

Solution: Given data

$$R_{ph} = 8\ \Omega; X_{Lph} = 6\ \Omega; V_L = 400 \text{ V}$$

To find $V_{ph} = \frac{V_L}{\sqrt{3}} = \frac{400}{\sqrt{3}} = 213 \text{ V}$

$$Z_{ph} = \sqrt{R_{ph}^2 + X_{Lph}^2} = \sqrt{8^2 + 6^2} = 10\ \Omega$$

$$I_{ph} = \frac{V_{ph}}{Z_{ph}} = \frac{231}{10} = 23.1 \text{ A}$$

Line currents I_L = Phase current, $I_{ph} = 23.1$ A

$$\cos\phi = \frac{R_{ph}}{Z_{ph}} = \frac{8}{10} = 0.8$$

$$\phi = \cos^{-1}(0.8) = 36.86 \text{ (leading)}$$

$$P = \sqrt{3}V_L I_L \cos\phi$$

$$= \sqrt{3} \times 400 \times 23.1 \times 0.8 = 12.8 \text{ kW}$$ **Ans.**

$$Q = \sqrt{3}V_L I_L \sin\phi = \sqrt{3} \times 400 \times 23.1 \times 0.6 = 9.6 \text{ kVAR}$$ **Ans.**

Wattmeter readings

$$W_1 = V_L I_L \cos(30° - \phi)$$

$$W_1 = 400 \times 23.1 \cos(30° - 36.86) = 9171.3 \text{ watt}$$ **Ans.**

$$W_2 = 400 \times 23.1 \cos(30° + 36.86) = 3628.7 \text{ watt}$$ **Ans.**

Phasor diagram

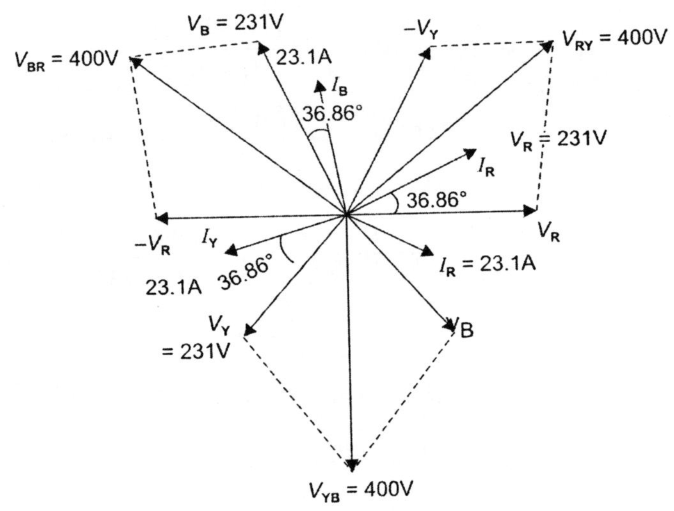

Phasor diagram of current and voltages

Example 15: A balanced star-connected load of $(8 + j6)\ \Omega$ per phase is connected to a 3–ϕ, 230 V, 50 Hz supply. Find the line current, pf, power volt-ampers and reactive power. Draw the phasor diagram for the above circuit. **[UPTU 2003-04]**

Solution:

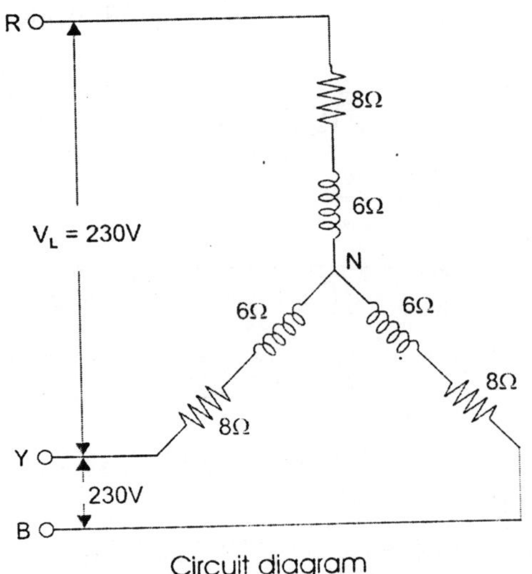

Circuit diagram

Given

$$V_L = 230 \text{ V}$$
$$Z_{ph} = 8 + j6\ \Omega$$
$$V_{ph} = \frac{V_L}{\sqrt{3}} = \frac{230}{\sqrt{3}} = 132.8 \text{ V}$$
$$Z_{ph} = \sqrt{8^2 + 6^2} = 10\ \Omega$$
$$I_{ph} = I_{ph} = \frac{V_{ph}}{Z_{ph}} = \frac{132.8}{10} = 13.28 \text{ A}$$

Line current $I_L = I_{ph} = 13.28$ A **Ans.**

$$\cos\phi = \frac{R}{Z} = \frac{8}{10} = 0.8$$

$\therefore$

$$\phi = 38.87°$$
$$P = \sqrt{3} V_L I_L \cos\phi$$
$$= \sqrt{3} \times 230 \times 13.28 \times 0.8 = 4.232 \text{ kW}$$ **Ans.**
$$Q = \sqrt{3} V_L I_L \sin\phi$$
$$= \sqrt{3} \times 230 \times 13.28 \times 0.6 = 3.179 \text{ kVAR}$$ **Ans.**
$$S = \sqrt{3} V_L I_L$$
$$= \sqrt{3} \times 230 \times 13.28 = 5.29 \text{ kVA}$$ **Ans.**

Phasor diagram

Example 16: Each phase of a star connected load consists of a resistance of 100 Ω is in parallel with a capacitance of 31.8 μ*F*. Calculate the line current, power absorbed, total kVA and power factor of the load when connected to a 416 *V*, 3-ϕ, 4 wire, 50 Hz supply. **[UPTU 2003]**

Solution: Given data

$$V_L = 416V, f = 50 \text{ Hz}$$
$$R_{ph} = 100\ \Omega \text{ and } C = 31.8\ \mu\text{F}$$

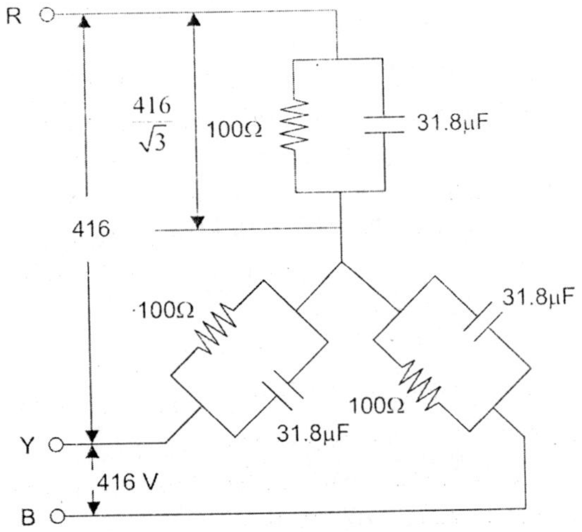

Circuit diagram

$$X_{ph} = \frac{1}{2\pi \times 50 \times 31.8 \times 10^{-6}}$$

$$= \frac{V_L}{\sqrt{3}} = \frac{416}{\sqrt{3}} = 240.2 \text{ V}$$

Admittance per phase

$$Y_{ph} = \frac{1}{R} + Jwc = \frac{1}{100} + j2\pi \times 50 \times 31.8 \times 10^{-6}$$

$$= (0.01 + j0.01)$$

$$= 0.01414\angle 45° \, S$$

$$I_L = V_{ph} \times Y_{ph}$$

$$= 240.2\angle 0° \times 0.014 \text{ A}\angle 45° = 3.397\angle 45°$$

$$I_L = I_{ph}$$

$\therefore$ $I_L = 3.397\ \angle 45°\text{A}$ **Ans.**

pf $\cos\phi = \cos 45°$ {since $\phi = 45°$}

$pf = 0.707$ (leading)

$$P = \sqrt{3}V_L I_L \cos\phi = \sqrt{3} \times 416 \times 3.397 \times 0.707$$

$= 1.73$ kW **Ans.**

$S = \sqrt{3}V_L I_L = \sqrt{3} \times 416 \times 3.397 = 2.45$ kVA **Ans.**

Example 17: A balanced star-connected load is supplied from a symmetrical 3-phase, 410 V system. The current in each phase is 30 A and lags 30° behind the phase voltage, find (i) phase voltage (ii) total power (iii) reactive power drawn by load. **[RGPV 2001]**

Solution: Given data

$$I_{ph} = I_L = 30 \text{ A}$$

$$V_L = 410, \therefore V_{ph} = \frac{V_L}{\sqrt{3}} = \frac{410}{\sqrt{3}} = 236.7 \text{ V}$$

(i) $V_{ph} = 236.7$ V

$\phi = 30°$

pf $= \cos\phi = \cos 30° = 0.866$ (lagging) **Ans.**

(ii) $P = \sqrt{3}V_L I_L \cos\phi = \sqrt{3} \times 410 \times 30 \times 0.866 = 18.45$ kW **Ans.**

(iii) Reactive power $Q = \sqrt{3}V_L I_L \sin\phi = \sqrt{3} \times 410 \times 30 \times 0.5 = 10.652$ kVA **Ans.**

Example 18: Three phase star connected load when supplied from a 400 V, 50 Hz source takes a line current of 10 A at 66.86° with respect to its line voltage. Calculate (i) impedance parameters (ii) pf and active power consumed. Draw the phasor diagram. **[NU 1998]**

Solution: From the given data, we have to draw the phasor diagram.

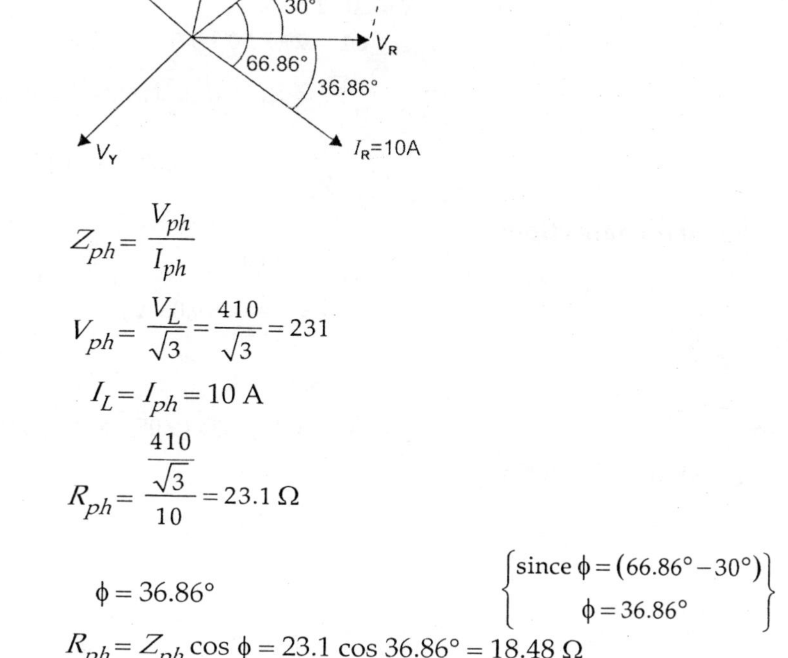

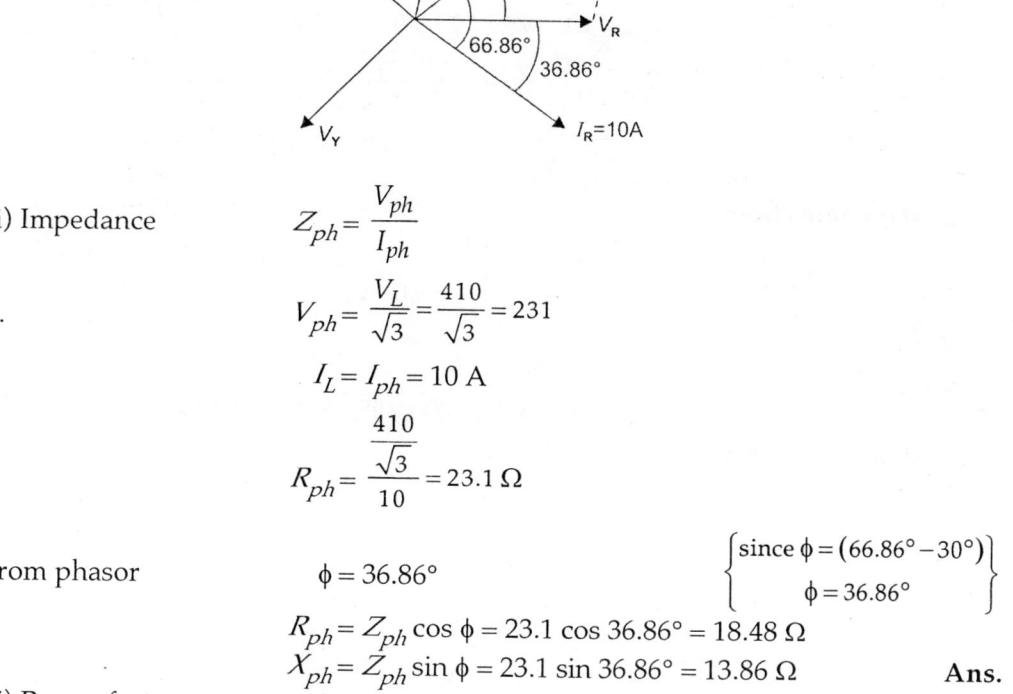

(i) Impedance $Z_{ph} = \dfrac{V_{ph}}{I_{ph}}$

$\therefore$ $V_{ph} = \dfrac{V_L}{\sqrt{3}} = \dfrac{410}{\sqrt{3}} = 231$

$I_L = I_{ph} = 10$ A

$R_{ph} = \dfrac{\dfrac{410}{\sqrt{3}}}{10} = 23.1\ \Omega$

From phasor $\phi = 36.86°$ $\left\{\begin{array}{c}\text{since } \phi = (66.86° - 30°) \\ \phi = 36.86°\end{array}\right\}$

$R_{ph} = Z_{ph}\cos\phi = 23.1 \cos 36.86° = 18.48\ \Omega$

$X_{ph} = Z_{ph}\sin\phi = 23.1 \sin 36.86° = 13.86\ \Omega$ **Ans.**

(ii) Power factor $\cos\phi = \cos 36.86 = 0.8$ (lag)

$P = \sqrt{3}V_L I_L \cos\phi$

$= \sqrt{3} \times 410 \times 23.1 \times 0.8 = 5.544$ kW **Ans.**

Example 19: A 3-phase balanced load draws 10kW power from a 400 V, 3-phase, 50 Hz, 4-wire supply at 0.8 lagging pf

(i) Determine the line current.

(ii) What would be the line current if power factor is raised to unity, power remaining the same?

(iii) How can the power factor be improved to unity?

Solution: Given

$$P = 10 \text{ kW}; \ V_L = 400 \text{ V}; \cos\phi = 0.8 \text{ (lagging)}$$

(i) Line current $I_L = \dfrac{P}{\sqrt{3}V_L \cos\phi} = \dfrac{10 \times 1000}{\sqrt{3} \times 400 \times 0.8} = 18.04 \text{ A}$ **Ans.**

(ii) Line current when power factor is raised to unity, power remaining the same

$$I_L = \frac{10 \times 1000}{\sqrt{3} \times 400 \times 1} = 14.43 \text{ A}$$

(iii) For power factor improvement to unity by using capacitors across the load.

Example 20: Three similar coils each having a resistance of 20 Ω and an inductance of 0.05 H are connected in star to a 3-phase, 50 Hz supply with 400 V between lines. Calculate power factor, total power absorbed and line current. If the same coils are connected in delta across the same supply what will be the power factor, total power absorbed and line current? **[N.U. 2003]**

Solution:

$$R = 20 \ \Omega$$

$$X_{Lph} = \omega L = 2\pi \times 50 \times 0.5 = 15.7 \ \Omega$$

$$Z_{ph} = \sqrt{R^2 + X_L^2} = \sqrt{20^2 (15.7)^2} = 25.43 \ \Omega$$

$$\cos\phi = pf = \frac{R_{ph}}{Z_{ph}} = \frac{20}{25.43} = 0.7844 \text{ (lag)}$$ **Ans.**

For star connection:

$$I_L = \frac{V_{ph}}{Z_{ph}} = \frac{\frac{400}{\sqrt{3}}}{25.43} = 9.08 \text{ A}$$

$$I_L = I_{ph} = 9.08 \text{ A}$$ **Ans.**

$$P = 3I_{ph}^2 \times R_{ph} = 3 \times (9.08)^2 \times 20 = 4.948 \text{ kW}$$ **Ans.**

For delta connections:

$$I_{ph} = \frac{V_{ph}}{Z_{ph}} = \frac{400}{25.93} = 15.73 \text{ A}$$

$$I_L = \sqrt{3} I_{ph} = \sqrt{3} \times 15.73 = 27.24 \text{ A}$$ **Ans.**

$$P = 3I_{ph}^2 \times R_{ph} = 3 \times (15.73)^2 \times 20$$

$$= 14.84 \text{ kW}$$ **Ans.**

Example 21: Three identical impedances of $30\angle 30° \ \Omega$ are connected to a 3-ϕ, 208 V, *abc* system by conductors which have impedance of (0.8 + j0.6) Ω. Find the magnitude of the voltage at the load end. **[PTU 1990]**

Solution: The equivalent star load of the delta-connected load is given as

$$Z_S = \frac{Z_D}{3} \text{ i.e., } \frac{30\angle 30°}{3} = 10\angle 30° \ \Omega$$

$$Z_{eq} = 0.8 + J0.6 + 10\angle 30° = 10.993\angle 30.62° \ \Omega$$

$$V_{ph} = \frac{208}{\sqrt{3}} = 120.1\angle 0° \text{ V}$$

$$I_{ph} = \frac{V_{ph}}{Z_{eq}} = \frac{120.1\angle 0°}{10.993\angle 30.62°}$$

$$= 10.925\angle -30.62° \text{ A}$$

$$\text{Voltage, across load} = I_{ph}Z_{ph}$$

$$= 10.925\angle -30.62 \times 10\angle 30°$$

$$V_{Lph} = 10.925\angle 0.62° \text{ V}$$ **Ans.**

Line voltage at the load $V_L = \sqrt{3} \times V_{Lph}$

$$= \sqrt{3} \times 109.25$$

$$= 189.2 \text{ V}$$ **Ans.**

Example 22: In two wattmeter method of power measurement in a 3 phase circuit, the reading of the watt meters are 1200 W and 300 W. What is the pf of the load.

[MDU 2003]

Solution: Given

$$W_1 = 1200 \text{ W}; \; W_2 = 300 \text{ W}$$

We know,

$$\text{pf} = \cos\phi = \cos\tan^{-1}\left(\frac{W_1 - W_2}{W_1 + W_2}\sqrt{3}\right)$$

$$= \cos\tan^{-1}\left(\frac{1200 - 300}{1200 + 300}\sqrt{3}\right)$$

$$\text{pf} = \cos\phi = 0.6934 \text{ (lag)}$$ **Ans.**

Example 23: Two wattmeters are connected to measure the total power in a 3-phase balanced circuit, one measures 4800 W, while the other reads backwards on reversing the latter it is found to read 400 W. What is the total power and power factor?

[RGPV 2001]

Solution:

$$W_1 = 4800 \text{ W}; \; W_2 = -400 \text{ W}$$

$$P = 4800 + (-400) = 4400 \text{ W}$$

Power factor of the circuit

$$= \cos\tan^{-1}\left(\frac{W_1 - W_2}{W_1 + W_2}\sqrt{3}\right)$$

$$= \cos\tan^{-1}\left(\sqrt{3}\,\frac{4800 - (-400)}{4800 + (-400)}\right)$$

$$= \cos\tan^{-1}(2.047)$$

$$\text{pf} = 0.438 \text{ (lead)}$$ **Ans.**

OBJECTIVE TYPE QUESTIONS

1. In a balanced 3-phase, star-connected system, the phase difference between phase voltage and their respective line voltage are:
   (*a*) 30° (*b*) 60°
   (*c*) 120° (*d*) 45°
2. In a balanced 3-phase, star-connected system, the relation between phase voltage (V_{ph}) and line voltage (V_L) is
   (*a*) $V_{ph} = \sqrt{3}V_L$ (*b*) $V_{ph} = 0.577\ V_L$
   (*c*) $V_{ph} = \sqrt{2}V_L$ (*d*) None of these
3. In a 3-phase balanced load, the power consumed is given by the relation?
   (*a*) $\sqrt{3}V_L I_L \cos\phi$ (*b*) $3V_{ph}\ I_{ph} \cos\phi$
   (*c*) both (a) and (*b*) (*d*) None of these
4. Wattmeter is an instrument which measures:
   (*a*) instantaneous power (*b*) average real power
   (*c*) apparent power (*d*) reactive power
5. In two-wattmeter method of power measurement in 3-phase balanced load, both the wattmeters give equal reading when the load pf is
   (*a*) 0.5 (*b*) zero
   (*c*) between 0.5 and one (*d*) one
6. In a 3-phase symmetrical and balanced system, the sum of instantaneous values of the currents of three phases is:
   (*a*) $i_R + i_Y + i_B$ (*b*) $i_R - i_Y - i_B$
   (*c*) $i_R - i_Y + i_B$ (*d*) always zero
7. For a 3-phase star connected balanced circuit having inductive load the angle between the line currents and the corresponding line voltages is equal to
   (*a*) 30° (*b*) 30° – ϕ
   (*c*) 30° + ϕ (*d*) ϕ
8. In a Δ-system, a phase voltage of 100 V produces a line voltage of
   (*a*) 58 V (*b*) 71 V
   (*c*) 100 V (*d*) 173 V
   (*e*) 141 V
9. In *Y*-system a line voltage of 220 V produces a phase voltage of
   (*a*) 381 V (*b*) 311 V
   (*c*) 220 V (*d*) 156 V
   (*e*) 127 V
10. The minimum no. of wattmeters to measure the power in a 3-phase unbalanced load star connected load is:
    (*a*) One (*b*) Two
    (*c*) Three (*d*) Four

ANSWERS

1. (*a*)	2. (*b*)	3. (*c*)	4. (*b*)	5. (*d*)
6. (*a*)	7. (*c*)	8. (*c*)	9. (*e*)	10. (*b*)

EXERCISES

1. A star-connected load has impedance of $(6 + j8)\Omega$ in each phase and is connected across a balanced 400 V, 3-phase supply. Obtain the line currents, total real power and real power and reactive power consumed by the load.
[RGBV 2003] [**Ans.** 23.1, 9.6 kW, 12.8 KV_{AR}]
2. Three similar coils each of impedance $Z = (6 + j8)\ \Omega$ are connected in star and supplied from 3-phase, 400 V, 50 Hz, supply. Find the line circuit, power factor, power and total volt-amperes. **[N.V. 2003]**
[**Ans.** 18.03 A, 0.624 (lag); 7.8 kW, 12.5 kVA]
3. A balanced star-connected load of $(8 + j6)\ \Omega$ is connected to a 3-phase 230 V supply. Find the line circuit a power factor, power, reactor volt-amperes and total volt-amperes. **[UTU 2003]**
[**Ans.** 13.28 A, 0.8 (lag), 4.252 kW, 3.774 VAR, 5.29 kVA]
4. A balanced three-phase, star-connected load of 100 kW takes a leading current of 80 A, when connected across a 3-phase, 1100 V, 50 Hz supply. Find the circuit constants of the load per-phase. **[NU 1996]** [**Ans.** 7.94 W, 5.21 W, 530-8μ*f*]
5. A balanced 3-phase star-connected load of 100 kW takes a leading current of 100 A when connected across a 3-phase 1100 V, 50 Hz, supply. Calculate the circuit constants of the load per phase. [**Ans.** 3.334 W, 589.5 μ*f*]
6. A delta-connected 3-phase load has a resistance of 6 Ω and an inductive reactance of 8 Ω in each branch line. Line voltage is 230 V, 50 Hz. What are the rms values of current and voltage in each branch? Calculate the total power consumed by the circuit and power factor. **[PTU 2001] Ans.** 230 V, 23 A, 0.6 (lag), 9.522 kW
7. Three coils each of impedance $20\angle 60°\ \Omega$ are connected in delta across a 400 V, 3-phase, 50 Hz ac supply. Calculate the line current and total power.
[VTU 2003] [**Ans.** 34.64 A, 12 kW]
8. In the two wattmeter method of power measurement in a three-phase, the reading of the wattmeter are 10000 W and 550 W. What is the power factor of the load?
[UPTU 2001] [**Ans.** 0.893 (lag)]
9. For a certain load, one of the wattmeter reads 20 kW and the other 5 kW after the voltage of this wattmeter has been reversed. Calculate the total power and power factor. [**Ans.** 15 kW, 0.3273 (lag), 2200 W, 0.2662 (lag)]
10. The power input to a 3-phase circuit was measured by two wattmeter method and the reading were 3400 and 1200 W respectively. Calculate the total power and power factor. **[VTU 2002]** [**Ans.** 2200 W, 0.2662 (lag)]

Chapter

8 Transients

8.1 INTRODUCTION

Transients are the surges or spikes in electric currents and voltages which are transmitted through power or data lines.

In general, transients disturbances are produced whenever

(a) an apparatus or circuit is suddenly connected to or disconnected from the supply
(b) a circuit is shorted and
(c) there is a sudden change in one applied voltage from one finite value to another.

It is important to remember that the transient currents are not driven by any part of the applied voltage but are entirely associated with the changes in the stored energy in inductors and capacitors. Since there is no stored energy in resistors, there are no transients in pure resistive circuits.

8.2 TYPES OF TRANSIENTS

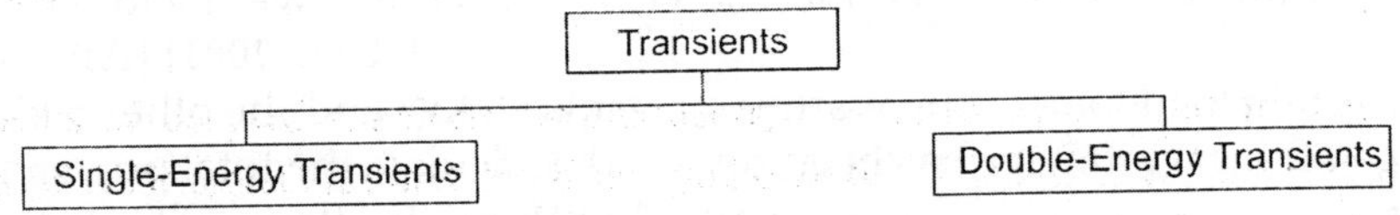

Fig 8.1: Block diagram

Single-energy transients: In which only one form of energy, either electromagnetic or electrostatic is involved as in R-L and R-C circuits.

Double-energy transients: In which both electromagnetic or electrostatic is involved as in R-L-C circuits.

In addition, transients also classified as follows:

1. **Initiation transients**: These are produced when a circuit. Which is originally dead, is energised.
2. **Subsidence transients**: These are produced when an energised circuit is rapidly deenergised and reaches an eventual steady-stage of zero current or voltage, as in the case of short-circuiting an R-L or R-C circuit suddenly.
3. **Transition transients**: These are due to sudden but energetic changes from one steady state to another.
4. **Complex transients**: These are produced in a circuit which is simultaneously subjected to two transients due to two independent disturbances or when the disturbing force producing the transients is itself variable.

5. **Relaxation transients:** In these transients, the transition occurs cyclically towards states, which when reached, become unstable themselves.

A distinction may also be made between free and forced transients which are produced due to the applied voltage being itself transient.

8.3 IMPORTANT DIFFERENTIAL EQUATIONS

For the treatment of single and double energy transient, some important differential equations, used are given below. Here both first-order and second-order differential equation will be considered.

1. First Order Equations

(i) Let $\frac{dy}{dx} + ay = 0$, where α is a constant.

Its solution is $y = ke^{-ax}$, where k is the constant of integration whose value can be found from the boundary conditions, i.e. conditions prevalent at the instant when the voltage to a circuit is applied or excluded.

(ii) If $\frac{dy}{dx} + ay = b$, where a and b are constants, then solution is $y = \frac{b}{a} + ke^{-ax}$

The value of k can again be found from boundary conditions.

(iii) If $\frac{dy}{dx} + Ay = B$ where A and B are not constants but are function of x, then the solution is given by

$$y = e^{-\int A dx} \int e^{\int A dx} B dx + ke^{-\int A dx}$$

If $A = a =$ constant, then the above equation simplifies to

$$y = e^{-ax} \int e^{ax} B dx + ke^{-ax}$$

2. Second Order Equations

(i) Suppose $\frac{d^2y}{dx^2} + a\frac{dy}{dx} + by = 0$, where a and b are constant, then the solution is

$$y = k_1 e^{\lambda_1 x} + k_2 e^{\lambda_2 x}$$

where λ_1 and λ_2 are constants of integration and whose values are

$$\lambda_1 = -\frac{a}{2} - \sqrt{\left(\frac{a^2}{4} - b\right)} \text{ and } \lambda_2 = -\frac{a}{2} + \sqrt{\left(\frac{a^2}{4} - b\right)}$$

a. If $a^2/4 > b$, the roots are real and the above solution can be applied without any difficulty.

b. If $a^2/4 < b$, the radicals contain a negative quantity, In that case, the solution is given by

$$y = e^{-\frac{1}{2}ax} (k_3 \sin \lambda_0 x + k_4 \cos \lambda_0 x)$$

where k_3 and k_4 are the new constant of integration and

$$\lambda_0 = \sqrt{\left(b - \frac{a^2}{4}\right)}$$

c. If $\frac{a^2}{4} = b$, then both roots are equal and each $= -a/2$
Hence, in this case, the solution becomes $y = k_5 e^{\lambda t} + k_6 t e^{\lambda t}$

ii. Let $\frac{d^2y}{dx^2} + a\frac{dy}{dx} + by = c$

where a, b and c are constants. In this case also, the solution will again depend on the root as discussed above.

$$y = k_1 e^{\lambda_1 x} + k_2 e^{\lambda_2 x} + \frac{c}{b}$$

iii. a. Let the differential equation be given by

$$\frac{d^2y}{dx^2} + a\frac{dy}{dx} + by = u$$

where a, b and c is constant but u is a particular function of the variable x. The solution of such an equation consists of a particular integral and a complementary function.

b. Let y be a sinusoidal function of x, then

$$\frac{d^2y}{dx^2} + a\frac{dy}{dx} + by = c \sin \omega t$$

In this case, particular integral is

$$y_1 = \frac{-c}{\sqrt{a^2\omega^2 + \left(\omega^2 - b\right)^2}} \cos\left[\omega x - \tan^{-1}\left(\frac{\omega^2 - b}{a\omega}\right)\right]$$

The complementary function is given by

$$y_2 = k_1 e^{\lambda_1 x} + k_2 e^{\lambda_2 x}$$

where $\lambda_1 = -\frac{a}{2} - \sqrt{\left(\frac{a^2}{4} - b\right)}$ and $\lambda_2 = -\frac{a}{2} + \sqrt{\left(\frac{a^2}{4} - b\right)}$

The complete solution for the above equation $y = y_1 + y_2$

Further treatment is the same as for case iii(a) above.

8.4 TRANSIENTS IN R-L CIRCUIT (DC)

If i, I_s and i_t be the resultant current, steady-state current, and transient current respectively in R-L circuit of Fig. 8.2a, then by superimposition.

The equation for the resultant current, for the duration of initiation transient.

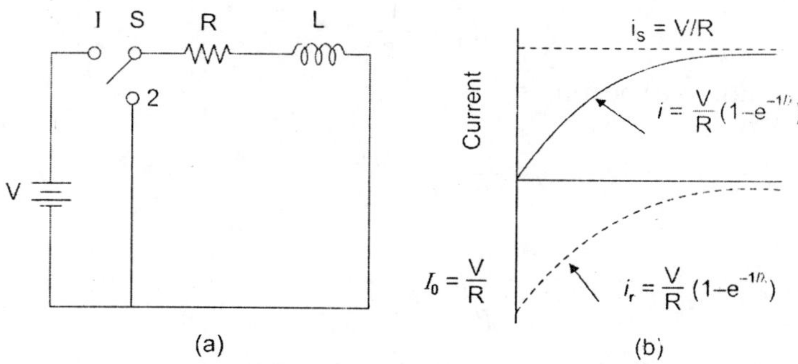

Fig. 8.2

$$i = I_s + i_t \qquad \text{...(8.1)}$$

Since the applied voltage V drives the steady-state current, hence

$$I_s = \frac{V}{R}$$

Since the transient current i_t is not associated with any voltage

$$\therefore \qquad i_t R + L\frac{di_t}{dt} = 0 \qquad \text{...(8.2)}$$

$$\text{or} \qquad \frac{di_t}{dt} = -\frac{R}{L}dt \qquad \text{...(8.3)}$$

$$\text{or} \qquad \int\frac{di_t}{dt} = -\frac{R}{L}\int dt \;\therefore\; \log hi_t = -\frac{R}{L}t + K \qquad \text{...(8.4)}$$

where K is the constant of integration whose value may be found from the initial conditions.

Now when $t = 0$, $i_t = I_0$ (say). Then from Eq. (8.4) we get, $\log_e I_0 = 0 + K$

Putting this value of K in Eq. (8.4) we have

$$\log hi_t - \log hI_0 = -\frac{R}{L}t \text{ or } \log h\frac{i_t}{I_0} = -\frac{R}{L}t = -\frac{t}{\lambda}$$

$$\therefore \qquad i_t = I_0 e^{-\frac{t}{\lambda}} \qquad \text{...(8.5)}$$

where $\lambda = \frac{L}{R}$ is called the *time-constant of the circuit.* Its reciprocal $\frac{R}{L}$ is called the damping coefficient of the circuit. The current decreases exponentially as shown in Fig. 8.2b. From Eqs (8.1) and (8.5), we have

$$i = I_s + I_0 e^{-\frac{t}{\lambda}} \qquad \text{...(8.6)}$$

If the time is reckoned when the voltage V is applied, so that when $t = 0$, $i = 0$, then from Eq (8.6), we get

$$0 = I_s + i_0 e^{-0} = I_s + I_0$$

$$\therefore \qquad I_0 = -I_S = -\frac{V}{R}$$

In that case, Eq. (8.6) becomes

$$i = \frac{V}{R} - \frac{V}{R}e^{-t/\lambda} \qquad ...(8.7)$$

$$= \frac{V}{R}\left(1 - e^{-t/\lambda}\right) \qquad ...(8.8)$$

Curves for I_s and i_t have been plotted in Fig. 8.2b. The curve for resultant current has been obtained by the superposition of steady-state current $I_s = (V/R)$ and transient current

$$i_t = \frac{V}{R}e^{-t/\lambda}$$

Theoretically, the transient current i_t takes infinite time to die off but, in practice, it disappears in a very short time.

The values of resultant, steady-state and transient voltages across the resistor can be found by multiplying Eq. (8.7) by R and shown in Fig. 8.3. The emf of self-induction $-\frac{L di_t}{dt}$ is only transient in nature and equals $i_t R$ as seen from Eq. (8.2) above.

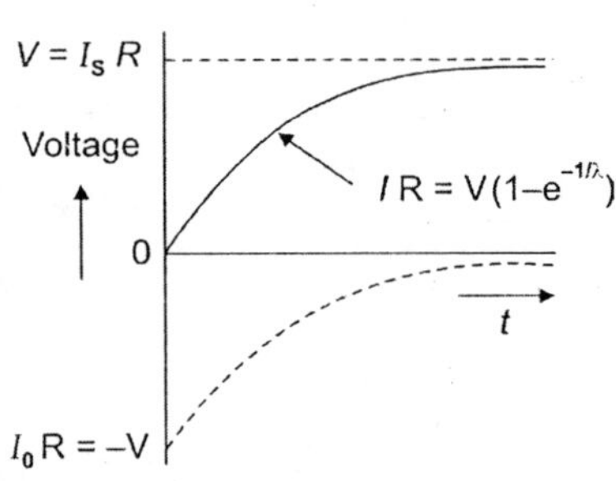

Fig. 8.3

8.5 SHORT CIRCUIT CURRENT

After some time, the transient current would disappear and the only current flowing in the circuit would be the steady-state current $I_S = \frac{V}{R}$.

Let the R-L circuit can be closed upon itself, i.e. be short-circuited by shifting the switch [Fig. 8.2a] to position 2. Since the voltage V has been excluded from the circuit, the trapped current I_s will immediately cease to be a steady-state current, but on the other hand, will become the initial value I_0 of a new subsidence transient current i_t. If time is measured at the instant of short-circuit, so that when $t = 0$, the current is $I_S = V/R$, then Eq. (8.5) becomes

$$i_t = \frac{V}{R}e^{-t/\lambda}$$

This Eq. (8.9) has been plotted in Fig. 8.4. The only voltage acting in the circuit is that due to self-induction, i.e $-\frac{L di_t}{dt}$ which equals $i_t R$.

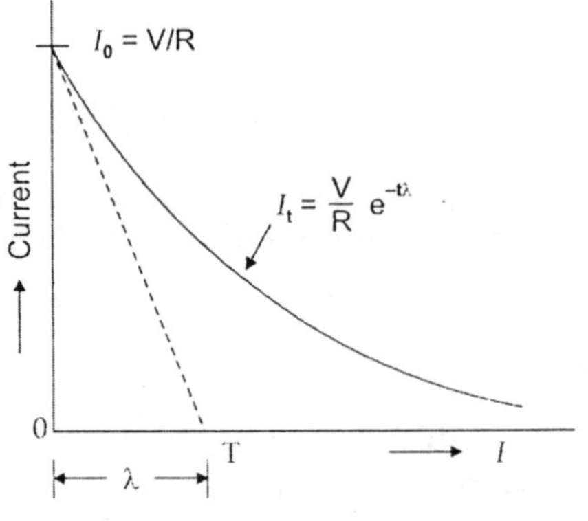

Fig. 8.4

8.6 TIME CONSTANT

The time constant of a circuit is defined as the time it would take for the transient current to decrease to zero, if the decrease were linear instead of being exponential. In other words, it is the time during which the transient current would have decreased to zero, it had maintained its initial rate of decrease. The initial rate of decrease can be found by differentiating Eq. (8.6) and putting $t = 0$

$$\therefore \quad \frac{di_t}{dt} = \frac{I_0}{\lambda} e^{-t/\lambda}$$

$$\therefore \quad \left(\frac{di_t}{dt}\right)_{t=0} = -\frac{I_0}{\lambda}$$

If the rate of decrease were constant throughout and equal to $-I_0 / \lambda$, then the straight line showing the relation between i_t and t would be given by

$$i_t = -\frac{I_0}{\lambda} t$$

The time-period would be equal to the subtangent OT drawn to the exponential curve of Fig. 8.4 at $i_t = I_0$ i.e. at the beginning of the curve.

If we put $t = \lambda$ in Eq. (8.5), then

$$i_t = I_0 e^{-1} = I_0 / e = I_0 / 2.718 = 0.37\ I_0$$

Hence, time period of a circuit is the time during which the transient current decreases to 0.37 of its initial value.

8.7 TRANSIENTS IN R-L CIRCUITS (AC)

Let a voltage given by $v = V_m \sin(\omega t + \Psi)$ be suddenly applied across an R-L circuit (Fig. 8.5a) at a time when $t = 0$. It means that voltage is applied when it is passing through the value $V_m \sin \Psi$. Since the contact may be closed at any point of the cycle, angle Ψ may have any value lying between zero and 2π radians. The resultant current, as before, is given by

$$i = i_s + i_t$$

$$I_m = \frac{V_m}{\sqrt{R^2 + X_L^2}} = \frac{V_m}{Z}$$

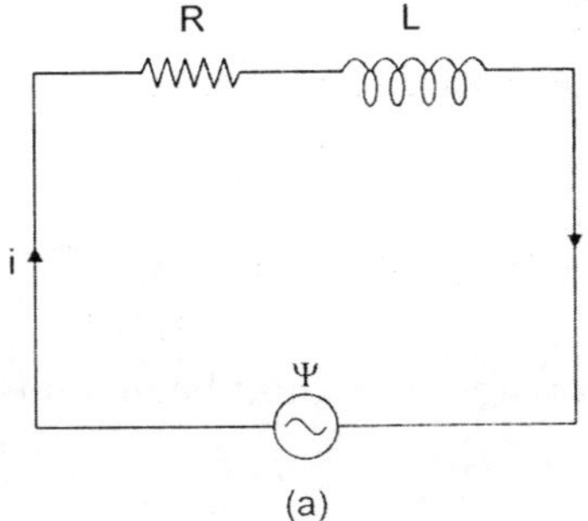

(a)

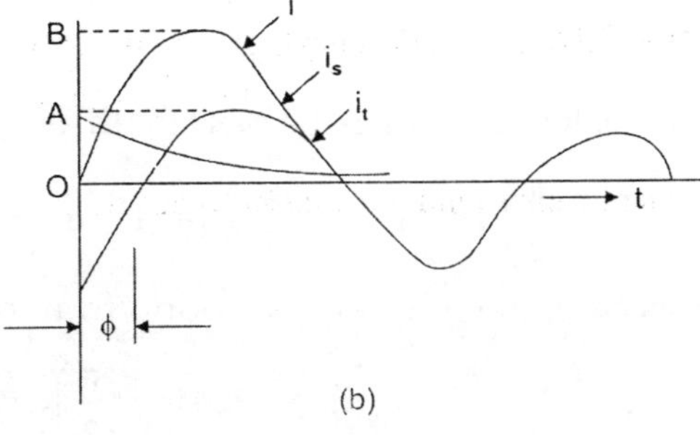

(b)

Fig. 8.5

The value of steady-state current is found by the normal circuit theory. The peak steady-state current is given by

$$I_m = \frac{V_m}{\sqrt{R^2 + X_L^2}} = \frac{V_m}{Z}$$

where $\sqrt{R^2 + X_L^2}$ is the impedance of the circuit. This current lags behind the applied voltage by an angle ϕ such that $\tan\phi = \frac{X_L}{R}$ or $\phi = \tan^{-1}\left(\frac{X_L}{R}\right)$

Hence, the equation for the instantaneous value of the steady-state current becomes

$$i_s = I_m \sin(\omega t + \Psi - \phi)$$

As before, the transient current is given by

$$i_t = I_0 e^{-t/\lambda} \quad \therefore \quad i = I_m \sin(\omega t + \Psi - \phi) + I_0 e^{-t/\lambda} \qquad \text{...(8.9)}$$

Now, when $t = 0$, $i = 0$, hence putting these values in Eq. (8.9), we get

$0 = I_m \sin 0 = I_m \sin(\Psi - \phi) + I_0 \quad \therefore I_0 = -I_m \sin(\Psi - \phi)$

Hence Eq. (8.9) can be written as

$$i = I_m \sin(\omega t + \Psi - \phi) - I_m \sin(\Psi - \phi) e^{-t/\lambda} \qquad \text{...(8.10)}$$

From Eq. (8.10), it is seen that the value of and hence the size of the transient current depends on angle, i.e. it depends on the instant in the cycle at which the circuit is closed. We will consider the following three cases:

Case 1

When $t = 0$, let the voltage pass through its zero value and become positive, i.e. let $\Psi = 0$. In that case, putting this value of Ψ in Eq. (8.10), we get

$$i = I_m \sin(\omega t - \phi) - I_m \sin(-\phi) e^{-t/\lambda} = I_m \left[\sin(\omega t - \phi) + \sin\phi e^{-t/\lambda}\right]$$

This is shown in Fig. 8.5b. It is seen that maximum instantaneous peak current OB is larger than the normal peak current OA.

Case 2

Let $t = 0$, when voltage is passing through its value $V_m \sin(\phi)$ so that $\Psi = \phi$

In that, $I_0 = 0$ there is no transient current at the time of switching on (i.e. $i_t = 0$). It corresponds to the contacts closing at the instant when the steady state current itself is zero.

Case3

When $t = 0$, let the voltage be passing through

$$V_m \sin\left(\phi \pm \frac{\pi}{2}\right) \text{ i.e. } \Psi = \phi \pm \frac{\pi}{2} \text{ and } \Psi - \phi = \pm\frac{\pi}{2}$$

In this case, the transient [as found from relation above] would be given by

$$i_t = -I_m \sin\left(\pm\frac{\pi}{2}\right) e^{-t/\lambda} = \mp I_m e^{-t/\lambda}$$

Under these conditions, the transient would have its maximum possible initial value.

8.8 TRANSIENTS IN R-C SERIES CIRCUITS (DC)

When a DC voltage V is suddenly applied to an R-C series circuit (Fig. 8.6), the voltage across the capacitor rises from zero value to the steadystate value v. If v_c is the voltage across capacitor, v_{ct} the transient voltage, then

$$v_c = V + v_{ct} \quad ...(8.11)$$

The charging current is maximum at the beginning but then is reduced to zero so that there is no steady-state current but a transient one.

Since the transient current is not associated with any applied voltage, hence

$$i_t R + v_{ct} = 0 \quad ...(8.12)$$

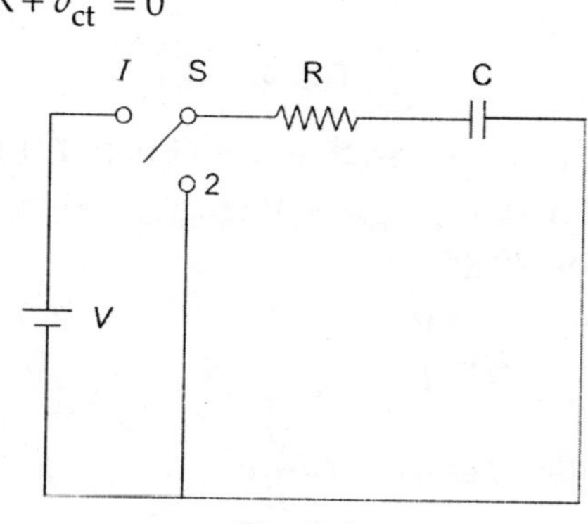

Fig. 8.6

Now, capacitor voltage $v_{ct} = \frac{q_t}{C}$

Hence, Eq. (8.12) becomes

$$i_t R + \frac{q_t}{C} = 0$$

or $$R\frac{di_t}{dt} + \frac{1}{C}\frac{dq_t}{dt} = 0$$

or $$\frac{di_t}{dt} = -\frac{1}{CR}\frac{dq_t}{dt} = -\frac{1}{CR}i_t \qquad \left(\because \frac{dq_t}{dt} = i_t\right)$$

$$\frac{di_t}{i_t} = -\frac{d_t}{CR}; \text{ As before } i_t = I_0 e^{-t/CR} = I_0 e^{-t/\lambda}$$

where $CR = \lambda$ = time constant. The reciprocal $\frac{I}{CR}$ is known as *damping coefficient.*

(i) Charging Current

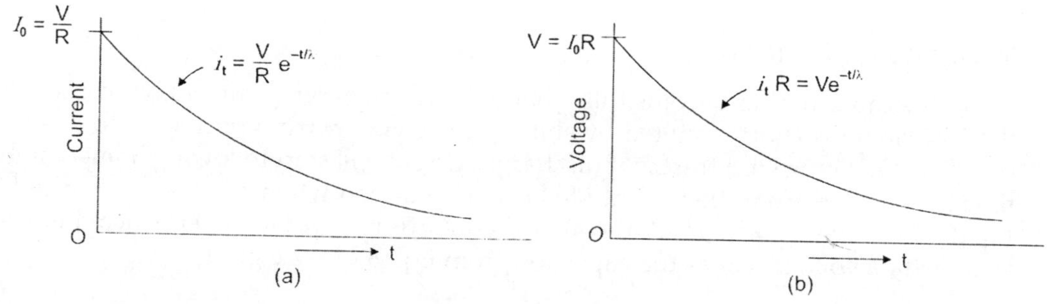

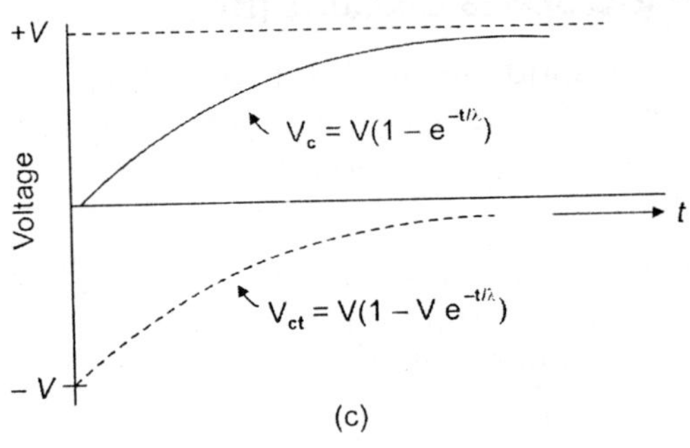

Fig. 8.7

When $t = 0$, transient current $i_t = i_0$, so that from Eq. (8.12) $v_{ct} = -I_0 R$, moreover, when $t = 0$, $v_C = 0$, Hence from Eq. (8.11), $v_{ct} = -V$

Combining these results, we get

$$I_0 = \frac{V}{R}$$

$$\therefore \quad i_t = I_0 e^{-t/\lambda} = \frac{V}{R} e^{-t/\lambda}$$

This is plotted in Fig. 8.7a. The transient voltage across the resistor R is given by

$$i_t R = \frac{V}{R} e^{-t/\lambda} \times R$$

$$= V e^{-t/\lambda} \text{ (Fig. 8.7 b)}$$

From Eq. (8.12) the value of transient voltage across the capacitor is

$$v_{ct} = -i_t R$$

Hence Eq. (8.11) becomes

$$v_c = V - i_t R = V - V e^{-t/\lambda}$$

or

$$v_c = V\left(1 - e^{-t/\lambda}\right) \qquad ...(8.13)$$

The voltage across the capacitor v_c which is the sum of transient voltage v_{ct} and steady-state V has been plotted in Fig. 8.7c.

The charge across the capacitor is given by

$$q = v_c = CV\left(1 - e^{-t/\lambda}\right) \text{ or } q = Q\left(1 - e^{-t/\lambda}\right)(\therefore Q = CV)$$

(ii) Discharge Current

When the capacitor has become fully charged so that charging current has ceased, then the R-C circuit is short-circuited by shifting the switch S from position 1 to position 2 (Fig. 8.6). On doing so, a transient discharge current will start following immediately. If time is reckoned from the instant of short-circuit, then when $t = 0$. $i_t = I_0$ hence from Eq. (8.12) above $v_{ct} = -I_0 R$. Moreover, when $t = 0$, $v_c = V$. However, since there is no steady-state voltage across the capacitor, from Eq. (8.11), we get $v_c = v_{ct}$.

Combining this result, we get

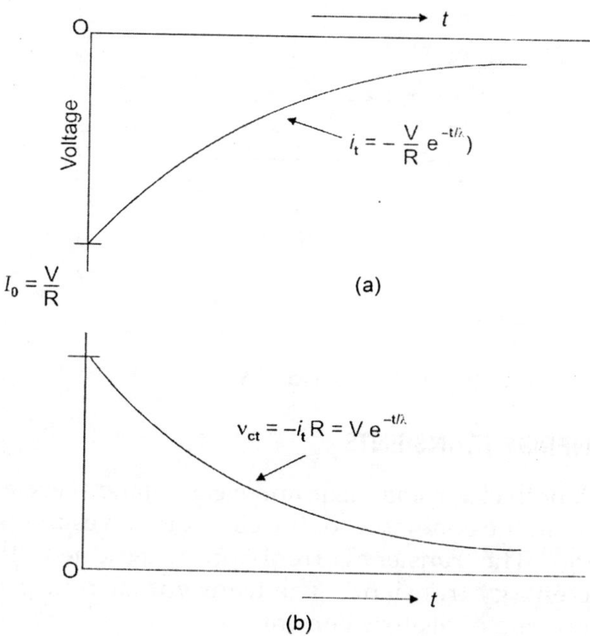

Fig. 8.8

$$I_0 = -\frac{V}{R}$$

$$i_t = -\frac{V}{R}e^{-t/\lambda}$$

It is plotted in Fig. 8.8a. Negative sign shows that discharge current follows in a direction opposite to that in which the charging current follows. That is why the curve has been below the X-axis, it may be noted that the only voltage in the circuit is v_{ct} which equals $-i_t R$.

8.9 TRANSIENTS IN R-C SERIES CIRCUITS (AC)

In this case, the resultant currents can be determined in the same way as for an R-L circuit (Section 8.7). It is given by

$$i = i_s + i_t = I_m \sin(\omega t + \psi + \phi) + I_0 e^{-t/\lambda}$$

where
$$I_m = \frac{V_m}{\sqrt{R^2 + X_c^2}}$$

and
$$v = V_m \sin(\omega t + \psi)$$

The value of I_0 as found from initial known conditions $(t = 0, i = 0)$ is given by $I_0 = -I_m \sin(\psi + \phi)$

Hence, the resultant current becomes

$$i = I_{m,} \sin(\omega t + \psi + \phi) - I_m \sin(\psi + \phi) e^{-t/\lambda}$$

As shown in Fig. 8.9, the resultant current at the moment of switch closing is OA and is made up of steady-state current OC and transient current OB.

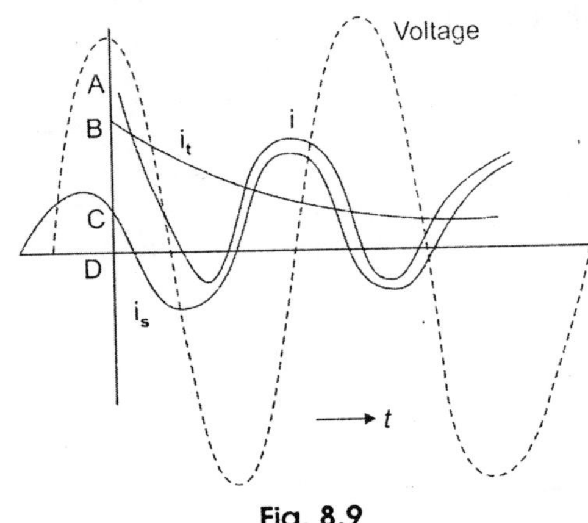

Fig. 8.9

8.10 DOUBLE ENERGY TRANSIENTS

In an R-L-C circuit, both electromagnetic and electrostatic energies are involved, hence any sudden change in the conditions of the circuit involves the redistribution of these two forms of energy. The transient currents produced due to this redistribution are known as double-energy transients. The transient current produced may be unidirectional or a decaying oscillatory current.

In an R-L-C circuit, the transient voltages across the three circuit parameters are i_t, R, $(L di_t/dt)$ and q_i/C. Hence, the equation of the transient voltage is

$$i_t R + L\frac{di_t}{dt} + \frac{q_t}{C} = 0 \qquad ...(8.14)$$

Differentiating the above Eq. (8.14) and putting i_t for dq_1/dt, we get

$$\frac{d^2 i_t}{dt^2} + \frac{R}{L}\frac{di_t}{dt} + \frac{1}{LC} i_t = 0 \qquad ...(8.15)$$

This is a linear differential equation of the second order with constant coefficient (like in case 2; Section 8.3.) Its solution is given by

$$i_t = k_1 e^{\lambda_1 t} + k_2 e^{\lambda_2 t} \qquad ...(8.16)$$

where k_1 and k_2 are constants whose values are found from the boundary conditions. The values of λ_1 and λ_2 are given by

$$\lambda_1 = -\frac{R}{2L} - \sqrt{\frac{R^2}{4L^2} - \frac{1}{LC}} \text{ and } \lambda_2 = -\frac{R}{2L} + \sqrt{\frac{R^2}{4L^2} - \frac{1}{LC}}$$

Depending on the value of λ_1 and λ_2, four different conditions of the circuit are distinguishable. We will now examine these four conditions in the case of an R-L-C circuit.

CASE 1. Loss-free Circuit, R=0, i.e. Undamped

In this case, $\lambda_1 = \sqrt{-\frac{1}{LC}} = j-1\sqrt{LC} = -j\omega$ and $\lambda_2 = -\sqrt{-\frac{1}{LC}} = -j-1\sqrt{LC} = -j\omega$

Hence, Eq. (8.16) given above becomes

$$\begin{aligned} i_t &= k_1 e^{j\omega t} + k_2 e^{-j\omega t} \\ &= k_1(\cos\omega t + j\sin\omega t) + k_2(\cos\omega t - j\sin\omega t) \end{aligned}$$

$$= (k_1 + k_2)\cos \omega t + j(k_1 - k_2)\sin \omega t$$

or $$i_t = A \cos \omega t + B \sin \omega t \qquad ...(8.17)$$

where $$A = k_1 \text{ and } k_2 \text{ and } B = j(k_1 - k_2)$$

Eq. (8.17) can be still further simplified to

$$i_t = I_m \sin(\omega t + \phi) \qquad ...(8.18)$$

where $$I_m = \sqrt{A^2 + B^2} \text{ and } \phi = \tan^{-1}(A/B)$$

As seen from Eq. (8.18), the transient current in this case is sinusoidal wave of constant peak value and frequency $f = 1/2\pi\sqrt{LC}$ as shown in Fig. 8.10a. The values of two constant terms I_m and ϕ can be determined from any two known initial circuit conditions which are (i) the initial current in the inductance and (ii) the initial voltage across the capacitor.

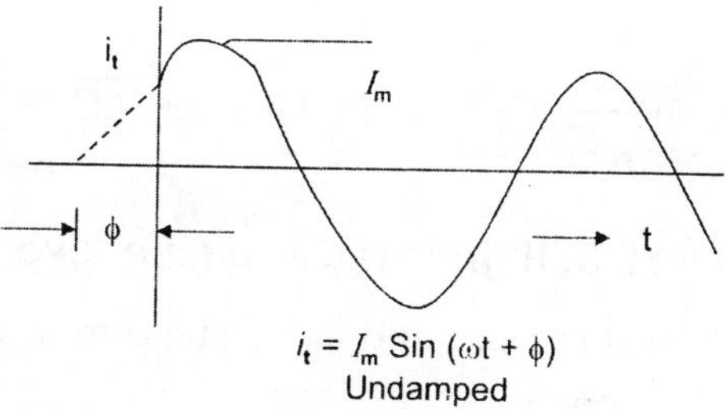

Fig. 8.10a

CASE 2. Low-loss Circuit: $\frac{R^2}{4L^2} < \frac{1}{LC}$ i.e. Underdamped

In this case, λ_1 and λ_2 would be conjugate complex numbers because the term under the square root sign in each case would be negative.

$$\therefore \qquad \lambda_1 = \frac{R}{2L} + j\sqrt{\frac{1}{LC} - \frac{R^2}{4L^2}}$$

If $a = \frac{R}{2L}$ and $\omega = \sqrt{\frac{1}{LC} - \frac{R^2}{4L^2}}$ then $\lambda_1 = -a + j\omega$ and $\lambda_2 = -a - j\omega$

Putting these values in equation (v). we get

$$i_1 = k_1 e^{(-a+j\omega)t} + k_2 e^{(-a-j\omega)t}$$

$$= a$$

This above equation can be reduced, as before, to the form

$$i_t = I_m e^{-at} \sin(\omega t + \phi) \qquad (8.19)$$

where I_m and ϕ are constants as before. Equation (vi) represents damped transient oscillatory current as shown in Fig. 8.10b.

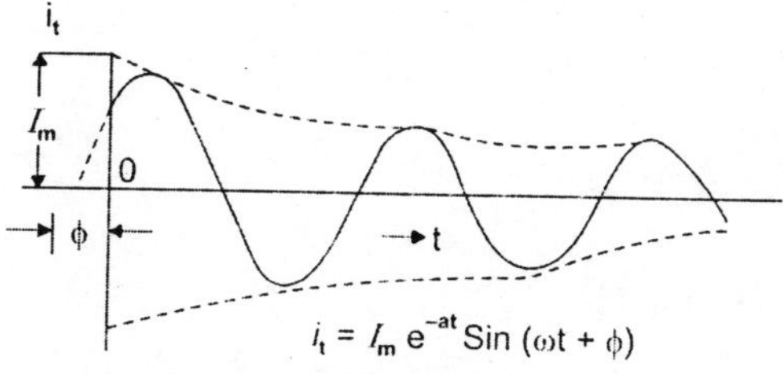

Fig. 8.10b

The exponential term e^{-at} which accounts for the delay of oscillations is called the *decay* or *damping factor* or merely decrement. It makes each current peak a definite fraction less than that preceding it. The logarithm to the Naperian base '*e*' of the ratio of peaks one cycle apart in time is $a/f = R/s\ fL$ and is referred to as logarithmic decrement. The frequency of damped oscillation is given by

$f = \sqrt{\frac{1}{LC} - \frac{R^2}{4L^2}}$ and is called the natural frequency of the circuit.

If $\frac{R^2}{4L^2} < \frac{1}{LC}$, then $f = 1/2\pi\sqrt{LC}$

CASE 3. High-loss Circuit, i.e. overdamped

In this case, λ_1 and λ_2 will be pure numbers.

$$\lambda_1 = \frac{R}{2L} + \sqrt{\frac{R^2}{4L^2} - \frac{1}{LC}} = -a + \gamma \text{ and } \lambda_2 = -a - \gamma$$

$$\therefore \qquad i_t = k_1 e^{(-a+\gamma)t} + k_2 e^{(-a-\gamma)t} = e^{-at}\left(k_1 e^{\gamma t} + k_2 e^{-\gamma t}\right)$$

Now $\qquad e^{at} = \sinh \gamma t + \cosh \gamma t$

and $\qquad e^{-\gamma t} = e^{-at}(A\cosh \gamma t + B\sinh \gamma t)$

A typical curve of the above equation is shown in Fig. 8.10c.

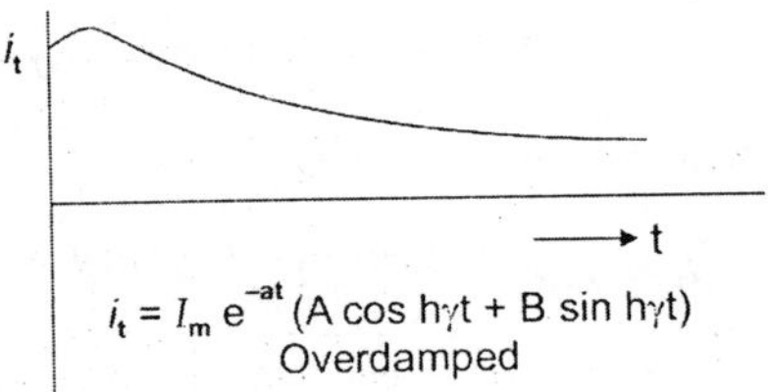

Fig. 8.10c

CASE 4. $\frac{R^2}{4L^2} = \frac{1}{LC}$, i.e. Critical Damping

In this case, $\lambda_1 = \lambda_2 = -\frac{R}{2L}$

Hence, Eq. (8.16) is reduced to

$(k_1 + k_2 t)e^{-\frac{R}{2L}t}$ or $i_t = (k_1 + k_2 t)e^{-at}$

It is a case of critical damping because current is reduced to almost zero in the shortest possible time. Eq. (8.19a) has been plotted in Fig. 8.10d.

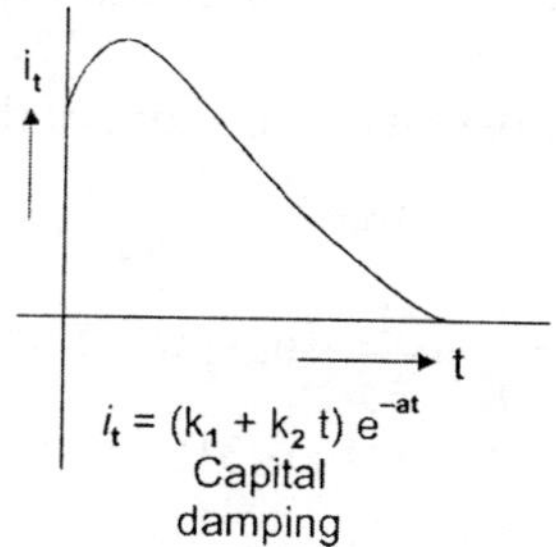

Fig. 8.10d

Hence, we can summarize as follows:

1. Transient current is an undamped sine wave if $R = 0$
2. Transient current is non-oscillatory if $R < 2\sqrt{\frac{L}{C}}$
3. Transient current is non-oscillatory if $R \geq 2\sqrt{\frac{L}{C}}$
4. Critical damping occurs if $R = 2\sqrt{\frac{L}{C}}$

SOLVED EXAMPLES

Example 1. A circuit of resistance 10 W and inductance 0.1 H in series has a direct voltage of 200 V suddenly applied to it. Find the voltage drop across the inductance at the instant of switching on and at 0.01 second. Find also the flux-linkages at these instants.

[Bombay Univ; Basic Electricity]

Solution. (i) Switching instant

At the instant of switching on, $i = 0$, so that i$R = 0$, hence all applied voltage must drop across the inductance only. Therefore, voltage drop across inductance = 200 V.

Since at this instant $i = 0$, there are no flux linkages of the coil.

(ii) When $t = 0.01$ second

As time passes, current grows so that the applied voltage is partly dropped across the resistance and partly across the coil. Let us first find iR drop for which purpose we need the value of i at $t = 0.01$ second.

Now, time period of the circuit is $\lambda = \frac{L}{R} = \frac{0.1}{10} = 0.01$ second. Since the given time happens to be equal to time constant.

$$\therefore\ i = \left(\frac{200}{10}\right) \times 0.632 = 12.64 \text{ A}\ ;\ iR = 12.64 \times 10 = 126.4 \text{ V}$$

$$\text{Drop across inductance} = \sqrt{200^2 - 126.4^2} = 155 \text{ V}$$

$$\text{Now, } L = \frac{N\phi}{i} \qquad \text{or } N\phi = Li$$

$\therefore$ Flux-linkages $Li = 0.1 \times 12.64 = 1.264$ Wb-turns. **Ans.**

Example 2. A 1.0 H choke has a resistance of 50 Ω. This choke is supplied with AC voltage given by $e = 141 \sin 314\, t$. Find the expression for the transient component of the current flowing through the choke after the voltage is suddenly switched on.

[Jadavpur University]

Solution. The equation of the transient component of the current is (Section 8.7) Case 1)

$$i_t = I_m \sin\phi e^{-t/\lambda}$$

Here,
$$\lambda = \frac{L}{R} = \frac{1}{50} = 0.02 \text{ S}$$

$$Z = 50 + j314 = 318\angle 80.95°$$

$$I_m = \frac{V_m}{Z} = \frac{141}{318} = 0.443 \text{ A}$$

$$\sin 80.95° = 0.9875$$

$\therefore$
$$i = 0.443 \times 0.9875 e^{-t/0.02} = 0.4376 e^{-t/0.02}$$ **Ans.**

Example 3. A 50 Hz sinusoidal voltage of maximum value of 400 V is applied to a series circuit of resistance 10 Ω and inductance 0.1 H. Find the expression for the value of the current at any instant after the voltage is applied, assuming that voltage is zero at the instant of application. Calculate its value 0.02 second after switching on.

[Punjab Univ. 1990]

Solution. In such cases, as seen from Section 8.7 (Case 1), the current consists of a steady state component and a transient component. The equation of the resultant current is

$$\underbrace{I_m \sin(\omega t - \phi)}_{\text{steady-state current}} + \underbrace{I_m \sin\phi e^{t/\lambda}}_{\text{transient current}}$$

where
$$I_m = V_m / Z;\ \phi = \tan^{-1}(X_L/R);\ \lambda = L/R \text{ S}$$

$$R = 10 \text{ W};\ XL = 314 \times 0.1 = 31.4 \text{ W}$$

$$Z = 10 + j31.4 = 33\angle 72.3°$$

$$I_m = 400/33 = 12.1 \text{ A};\ \phi = 72.3° = 1.26 \text{ rad}$$

$$\sin\phi = \sin 72.3 = 0.9527;\ \lambda = 0.1/10 = 1/100 \text{ S}$$

$$i = 12.1\left\{\sin(314t - 1.262) + 0.9527 e^{100t}\right\}$$

Substituting $t = 0.02$ S, we get

$$i = 12.1\left\{\sin(314 \times 0.02 - 1.262) + 0.9527 e^{-2}\right\}$$

$$= 12.1\left(\sin 5.02 + 0.9527 e^{-2}\right)$$

$$= 12.1\left(\sin 288° + 0.9527 e^{-2}\right)$$

$$= 12.1(-\sin 72° + 0.9527 \times 0.1353)$$

$$= 12.1(-0.9511 + 0.1289) = -9.95 \text{ A}$$ **Ans.**

Example 4. In a simple saw-tooth generator circuit with thyratron switches on at 150 V and switches off at 10 V. If this circuit is supplied with 250 V DC source; find the time period of saw-tooth wave. The resistance and capacitance have the values of 10 kΩ and 1 μF respectively.

[Jadavpur University]

Solution. With reference to Fig. 8.11, let
V = applied voltage
V_{c1} = switching–off voltage of the thyratron = 10 V
V_{c2} = switching-on voltage of the thyratron = 150 V

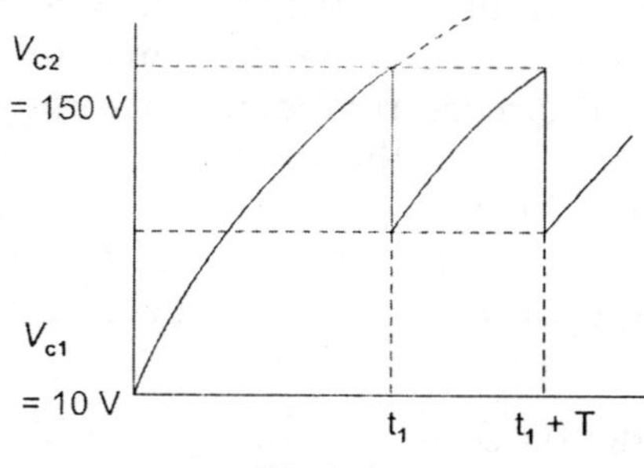

Fig. 8.11

Now, $v = V\left(1-e^{-t/\lambda}\right)$

$$V_{c1} = V\left(1-e^{-t_1/\lambda}\right) \quad \text{... (1)}$$

$$V_{c2} = V\left(1-e^{-t_1/\lambda}\right) \quad \text{...(2)}$$

where T is the time-period of the saw-tooth wave. From Eqs (i) and (ii) we get

$$T = \lambda \log_e (V - v_{c1})/(V - v_{c2})$$

Now, $\lambda = CR = 10^4 \times 10^{-6} = 10^{-2}$ S

$V = v_{cl} = 250 - 10 = 240$ V; $V - v_{c2} = 250 - 150 = 100$ V

$\therefore \dfrac{(V - v_{c1})}{(V - v_{c2})} = \dfrac{240}{100} = 2.4 \quad \therefore\ T = 10–2$ loge $2.4 = 0.00875$ S. **Ans.**

Example 5. A coil is having an inductance of 5 H and a resistance of 2 Ω is connected in parallel with a 30 Ω resistor across a 120 V DC supply. The DC supply is suddenly disconnected. Evaluate:

(a) initial rate of change of current after switching operation.
(b) voltage across the 30 Ω resistor initially and after time $t = 0.2$ s.
(c) voltage across the contacts of the switch at the instant of separation and
(d) rate at which the coil is losing its stored energy 0.2 second after switching.

Solution. (a) Since the steady-state current is zero, $i = I_0 e^{-t/\lambda}$

Now, at time, $t = 0$, current is $= 120/2 = 60$ A. It means the current flowing through the coil immediately before the opening of the switch is 60 A.

$$\therefore \qquad I_0 = 60 \text{ A}$$

Hence, the above equation becomes $i = 60e^{-t/\lambda}$

Now $$\lambda = \frac{L}{R} = \frac{5}{32} = 0.156 \qquad \therefore\ i = 60e^{-6.4t}$$

$$\left(\frac{di}{dt}\right)_{t=0} = \left(-60 \times 6.4e^{-6.4t}\right)_{t=0} = -384 \text{ A/S}$$

The significance of negative sign as it shows that the current is decreasing.

(b) After the supply has been disconnected, the current through the 30 Ω resistor is i since it is in series with the coil.

Initial pd across the 30 Ω resistor = (current at $t = 0$) × 30 = 60 × 30 = 1800 V

Current through the resistor after 0.2 second = $60e^{-6.4\times 0.2} = 16.68$ A

∴ Voltage across the resistor after 0.2 second

= (current at $t = 0.2$ second) × 30 = 16.68 × 30 = 500.46 V

(c) The emf induced in the coil at break tends to maintain the current through it in the original position. Hence, the direction of the current through 30 Ω resistor is upwards so that the potential difference across the switch contacts will be the sum of supply voltage and the voltage across 30 Ω resistor.

∴ Initial voltage across switch contacts = 1800 + 120 = 1920 V

(d) The rate of loss of energy = power = induced emf in coil current (after 0.2 sec)

$$L\left(\frac{di}{dt}\right)_{t=0.2} \times \text{current (after 0.2 See)}$$

Now, after 0.2 second, $i = 16.68$ A

value of $\frac{di}{dt}$ after 0.2 second = $-60 \times 6.4 \times e^{-1.28} = -106.76$ A/See

∴ Rate of loss of energy = –5 × 106.76 × 16.68 = –8903.784 J/See. **Ans.**

Example 6. A damped oscillation has the equation $i = 60e^{-10t}\sin 530t$. Find the number of oscillations which occurs before the amplitude of the oscillations decays to $\frac{1}{10}$th of its undamped value.

Solution. Undamped amplitude = 60 A.

$\frac{1}{10}$th amplitude = $\left(\frac{1}{10}\right) \times 60 = 6$ A

Let the time required for this decay be t. Now, the decay of the peak of the oscillations is given by the term $60e^{-10t}$

∴ $6 = 60e_1^{-10t}$ ∴ $e_1^{10t_1} = 10$ or $10\,t_1 = \log 10 = 2.3 \log_{10} 10 = 2.3$

∴ $t_1 = 0.23$ S

Frequency of oscillations = 530/2π = 84.35 Hz.

Hence, the number of oscillations which occur before the amplitude falls to $\frac{1}{10}$th of its undamped value = 0.23 × 84.35 = 19.401. **Ans.**

EXERCISES

1. Explain the term time constant for an inductive circuit.
2. An uncharged capacitor in series with a resistor is connected to a constant supply voltage. Why does the voltage across the capacitor rise slowly? Write down an expression for the voltage across the capacitor after time (t) seconds. Sketch a curve of voltage against time.
3. When a capacitor in series with a resistor is connected to a constant voltage source the pd across the capacitor rises slowly. Explain the reason for this. Give expressions for:

   (a) The time constant of the circuit (b) The pd across the capacitor (c) The charging current, in relation to the circuit constants and time from switching on the voltage.

Chapter

9 Measuring Instruments

9.1 INTRODUCTION

Electrical quantities like voltage, current and power are not visible by eyes. The instrument which are used to measure these quantities are called electrical measuring instruments and instrument which measures voltage, current and power are known as voltmeter, ammeter and wattmeter respectively. The measuring instrument can be broadly divided into two category.

(a) absolute or primary instruments (b) secondary instruments

Absolute instruments do not provide direct reading of quantity under measurement. They provide the reading terms of meter constant and angle of deflection. These instruments are used in standard laboratories for calibration. Secondary instruments provide direct reading of quantity under measurement, they may be analog or digital type.

A. **Analog instruments:** An analog instrument is one in which measured quantity as indicated by the movement of a pointer across the face of a scale.

B. **Digital instruments:** An digital instrument is one in which measured quantity is indicated in the form of digits or a series of number displayed on a screen.

9.2 CLASSIFICATION

Secondary instruments are further classified as below.

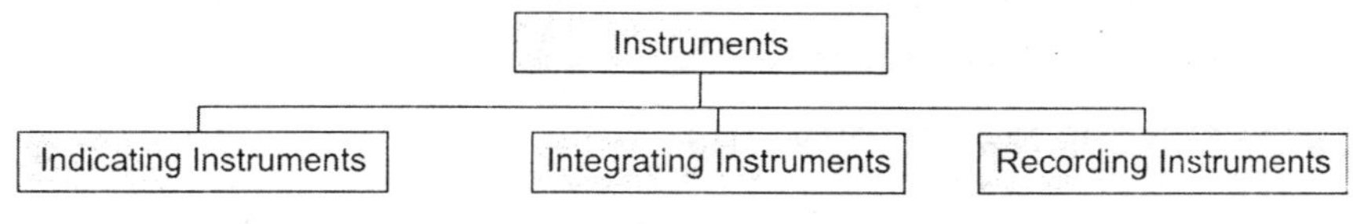

Fig. 9.1

(i) Indicating instrument: Indicating instruments are those instruments which directly indicate the value of electrical quantity with the help of pointer. **Example:** Ammeter, voltmeter and wattmeter.

(ii) Integrating instruments: Integrating instruments are those instruments which measures the total quantity of electrical energy over a specified period of time. These instrument give the summation of electrical quantity being supplied for the given time only. **Example:** Household energy meter, ampere hour meter.

(iii) **Recording instruments**: Recording instrument are those instruments which give a constinous record of the variations of the electrical quantity to be measured. **Example:** Recording voltmeters which is used in power stations to record the generated voltage.

9.3 OPERATION OF INDICATING INSTRUMENTS

For satisfactory operation of any indicating instrument, following three torques must act together appropriately.

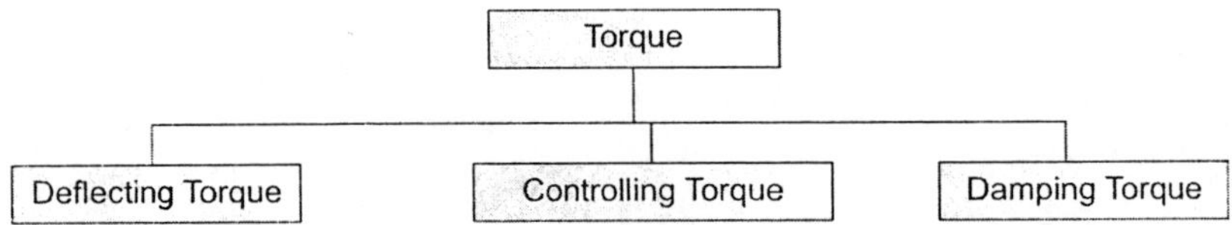

Fig. 9.2

(a) **Deflecting torque:** It causes the moving system of the instrument to move from its position of rest (indicated by zero on a dial by a pointer) and it is produced by using any one of the following effects of electric current, for example, magnetic effect, electromagnetic induction effect, heating effect, electrostatic effect.

(b) **Controlling torque:** It limits the movement of moving systems. It also ensures that magnitude of deflection is always the same for the given value of input quantity under measurement. It acts in the opposite direction to the deflecting torque. At steady state

Deflecting torque = Controlling torque

i.e. $T_d = T_c$

In practice, controlling torque is produced by two ways: (a) using spring action and (b) using gravity action.

(c) **Damping torque:** Due to deflecting torque, pointer moves in one direction while due to controlling torque pointer moves in opposite direction. Due to these opposing torques, the pointer may oscillate in the forward and backward direction if the damping torque is not present. It brings the moving system to rest quickly in its final position and acts only when the moving system is actually moving. If moving system is at rest, damping torque is zero. Thus final deflection of the instrument is not affected due to damping torque. Different methods of producing damping torque are: (a) air friction damping (b) fluid friction damping and (c) eddy current damping.

9.4 TYPES OF MEASURING INSTRUMENTS

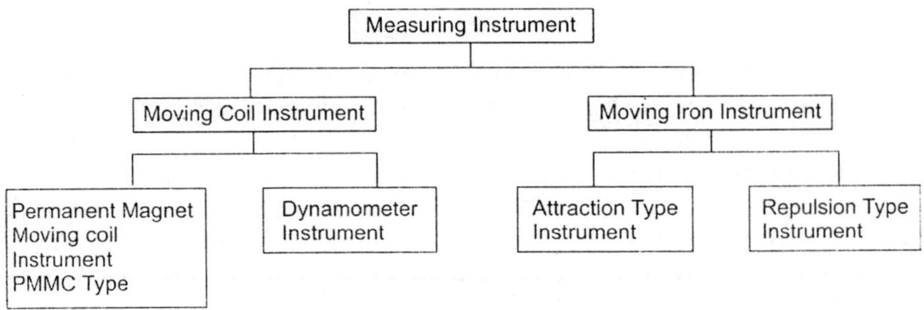

Fig. 9.3

9.4.1 Permanent Magnet Moving Coil Instrument (PMMC)

PMMC instrument are used either as ammeter or voltmeter and suitable for DC measurement only. They are not suitable for AC measurement.

Operating Principle

When the current carrying coil is placed in a magnetic field, the coil experience a mechanical force which provides necessary deflecting torque. This deflecting torque is responsible for the deflection of the pointer. The amount of force experienced by the coil is proportional to the current passing through the coil.

Construction

As the name suggest, it consist of permanent magnet and a moving coil which is mounted on a light aluminium frame. The permanent magnet is of 'U' shape and is made up of 'alnic' which is the alloy of aluminium, nickel and cobalt. The coil is mounted on the spindle and a pointer is attached to the spindle which moves over a calibrated scale as shown in Fig. 9.4.

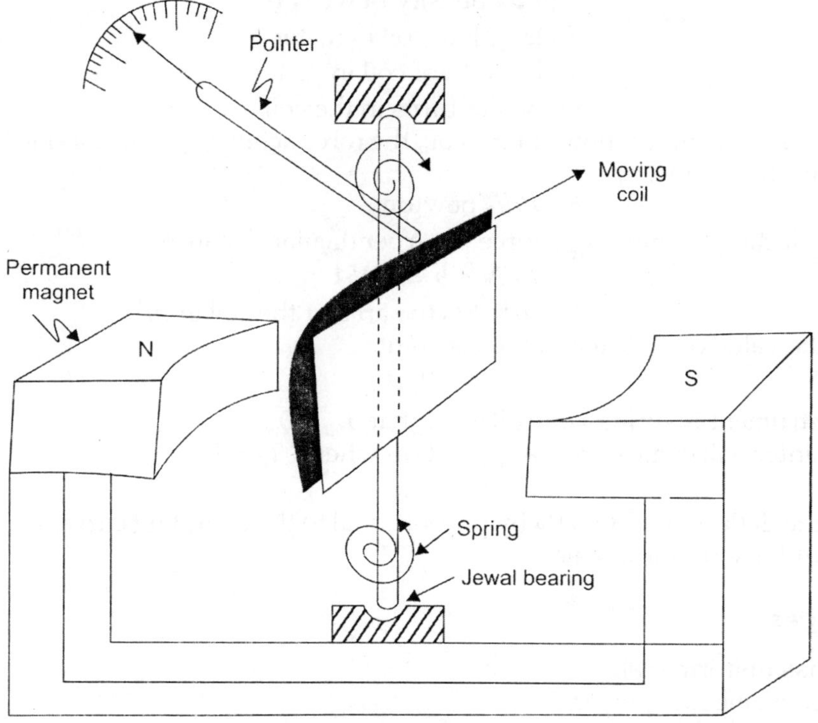

Fig. 9.4

Working

When an instrument is connected in the circuit the current flows through the coil-since the coil is carrying current and is placed in the magnetic field of the permanent magnet, a mechanical force acts on it. As a result, the pointer moves over the calibrated scale to indicate the value of current and voltage being measured.

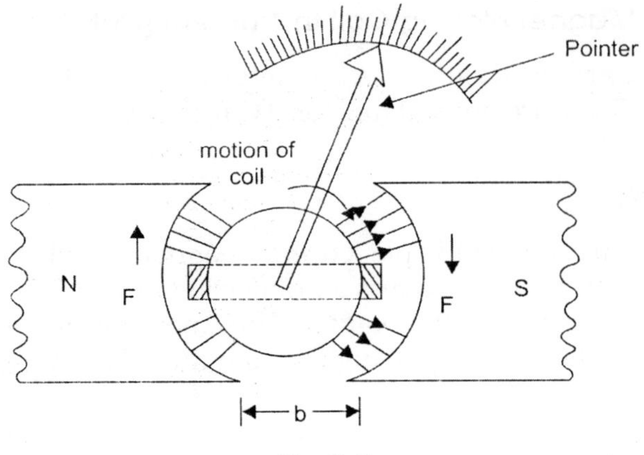

Fig. 9.5

Deflecting Torque

When current is passed through the coil, force acts on its both sides which producing the deflecting torque. Referring to Fig. 9.5.

Let, B = flux density in wb/m^2

l = length of coil in meter

b = breadth of coil in meter

N = No. of turns in the coil

If a current of I ampers flows in the coil, the force acting on each coil side is given by,

Force on each coil side,

$$F = BIlN \text{ newton}$$

and Deflecting torque, T_d = force × perpendicular distance

$$= BIlN \times b = BINA$$

where $A = (b \times l)$ is the area of the coil in m^2

Since the value of B, N and A are constant.

$$T_d \propto I$$

The instrument is spring-controlled so that $T_C \propto \theta$.

The pointer will come to rest at a position where, $T_d = T_C$.

$$\therefore \quad \theta \propto I$$

Thus, the deflection is directly by proportional to the operating current. Hence, such instrument have uniform scale.

Advantages

(1) It has uniform scale.
(2) It consume low power.
(3) It has high accuracy.
(4) The sensitivity is high.
(5) They have no hysteresis loss.

Disadvantages

(1) These instrument can not be used for ac. measurment.
(2) Effect of temperature and friction introduce error.

9.4.2 Dynamometer Type Instrument

It is also known as electrodynamic type instrument. These instruments are the modified form of permanent magnet type instrument. Here magnetic field is produced by two fixed coils placed on either sides of the moving coil. Such instrument can be used as ammeter or as voltmeter but are generally used as wattmeter. They are suitable for DC as well as AC measurment Fig. 9.6.

Principles: It works on the same principles AC that of PMMC that whenever a current carrying moving coil is placed in a magnetic field, force is exerted on the moving coil and deflection takes place.

Torque Equation

If i_f and i_m are the current flowing through the fixed and moving coil respectively. Then deflecting torque

$$T_d \propto i_f i_m$$

If T_C is controlling torque, then

$$T_C \propto \theta$$

But in equilibrium, $T_C = T_d$

$\therefore$ $\theta = i_f i_m$

If $i_m = i_f = i$

Then $q = i^2$

So the scale is not uniform.

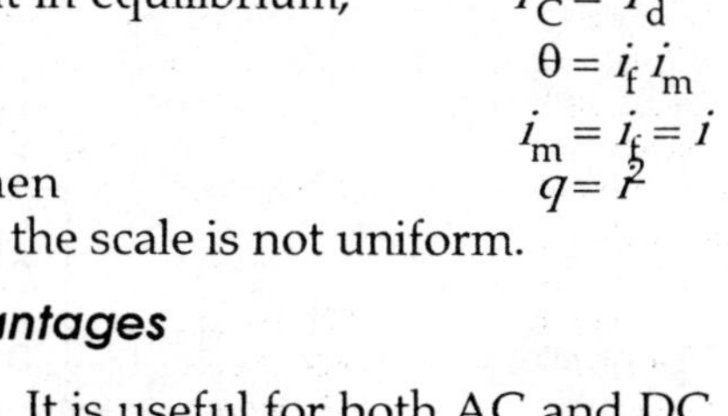

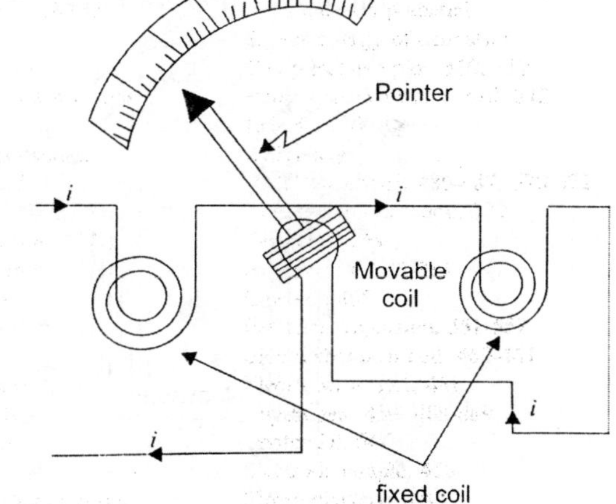

Fig. 9.6

Advantages

(1) It is useful for both AC and DC measurement.
(2) High degree of accuracy.
(3) Low power consumption and light in weight.
(4) It can be used for calibrating purpose.
(5) These instrument are free from hysteresis and eddy current loss.

Disadvantages

Scale is non-linear. It is an expensive instrument and the sensitivity of the instrument is very low.

9.4.3 DYNAMOMETER TYPE WATTMETER

Wattmeter: It is a device which is used to measure power. It consists of two coils named currents coil and pressure coil (voltage coil). The symbol of wattmeter is shown in Fig. 9.7. The most commonly used wattmeter is dynamometer type wattmeter which can measure of DC as well as AC power.

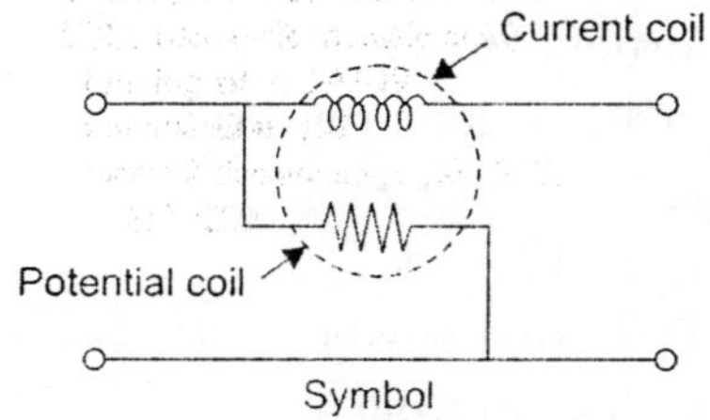

Fig. 9.7: Symbol of wattmeter

Construction

The dynamometer wattmeter is consist of two-coils, fixed coil and moving coil. The two fixed coils are placed parallel to one another to produce a uniform magnetic field. They are connected in series with the load and called current coil as shown in Fig. 9.7. The moving coil is connected across the load through a series resistance. The moving coil is known as voltage coil. The voltage coil carries current proportional to the voltage in the circuit.

Working

When the wattmeter is connected in the circuit to measure power (Fig. 9.8). The current coil carries the load current and potential coils carries current proportional to the load voltage. Due to current in the coils mechanical force exist between them. The result is that movable coil moves the pointer over the scale.

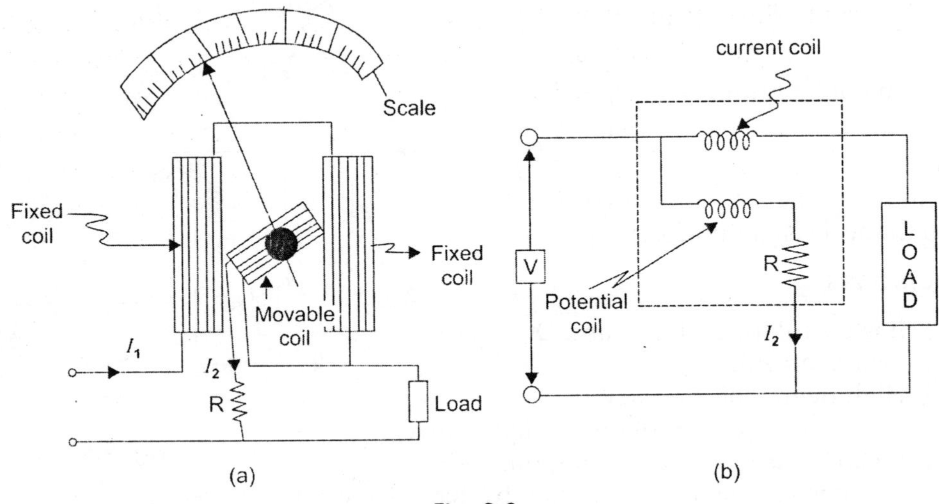

Fig. 9.8

Deflecting Torque

We shall now prove that deflection torque is proportional to load power in DC as well as AC circuit.

For DC. Circuit

Consider that the wattmeter is connected in a DC circuit to measure power as shown in Fig. 9.8. The power taken by the load is VI_1

$\therefore$ Deflecting torque $T_d \propto I_1 I_2$

Since I_2 is directly proportional to V.

$\therefore$ Deflecting torque, $T_d \propto VI_1 \propto$ load power.

Similarly for AC circuits

$$T_d \propto VI \cos \phi$$

$$T_d \propto \text{load power}$$

Since the instrument is spring controlled

$$T_c \propto \theta$$

In the steady-state position of deflection

$$T_d = T_c$$

$$\therefore \quad \theta \propto \text{load power}$$

Hence such instruments have uniform scale.

Advantages

(i) It can be used for AC as well as DC power measurement.
(ii) It consumes less power.
(iii) Uniform scale.
(iv) Instrument is free from hysterisis loss.
(v) Light weight.

Disadvantages

These instruments are expensive, produce large error at low pf.

9.5 EXTENSION OF RANGE OF MOVING COIL INSTRUMENT

If we have to measure large currents and voltages, in such situation, some means are adopted to increase the range of the instruments.

(a) Extension of Ammeter Range: The range of permanent magnet moving coil instrument (PMMC) ammeter can be extended by connecting a low resistance in parallel with the instrument as shown in Fig. 9.9.

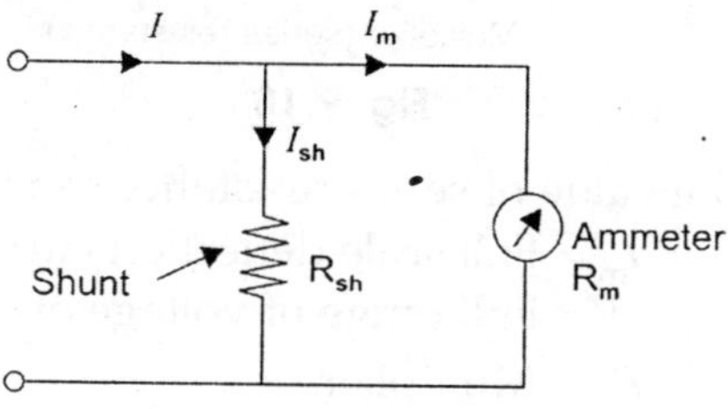

Fig. 9.9

This parallel connected resistance is called the shunt. In order to measure the high current most of the current is passed through shunt and it allows flowing small current through the meter.

Let,

R_m = Internal resistance of meter
R_{sh} = Shunt resistance
I_m = Full scale deflection current
I_{sh} = Shunt current
I = Full current to be measured

From Fig. 9.9 voltage drops across the shunt and meter must be same

$$\therefore \quad I_m R_m = I_{sh} R_{sh}$$

$$\therefore \quad R_{sh} = \frac{I_m R_m}{I_{sh}}$$

where $\quad I = I_{sh} + I_m, \; I_{sh} = I - I_m$

$$\therefore \quad R_{sh} = \frac{I_m}{I - I_m} R_m$$

If 'N' is the multiplying power, then $N = \frac{I}{I_m}$

$$\therefore \quad N = \frac{\text{Current to be measured}}{\text{Current in meter}}$$

$$\therefore \quad N = \frac{I}{I_m} = 1 + \frac{R_m}{R_{sh}}$$

Hence the value of shunt resistance

$$R_{sh} = \frac{R_m}{N-1}$$

(b) Extension of Voltmeter Range: The range of the permanent magnet moving coil voltmeter can be extended connecting a high resistance in series with the instrument as shown in Fig. 9.10. This series connected resistance is called multiplier.

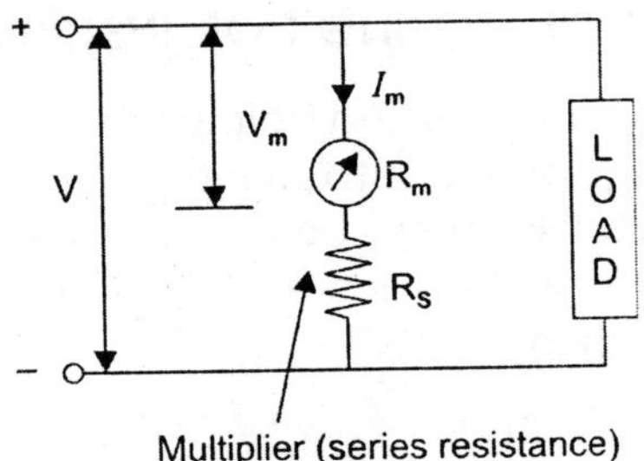

Fig. 9.10

From above Fig. 9.10, the value of series resistance can be calculated as follows:

I_m = Full scale deflection current

V = Full range of voltage of voltmeter or source voltage

R_S = Multiplier

R_m = Internal resistance of meter

V_m = Voltage across the meter

⇒ From Fig 9.10, $V_m = I_m R_m$

$$V = I_m (R_m + R_S)$$

$$R_S = \left(\frac{V - I_m R_m}{I_m}\right)$$

or,

$$R_S = \left(\frac{V}{I_m} - R_m\right)$$

The multiplying factor $N = \frac{\text{Voltage to be measured}}{\text{Voltage across meter}} = \frac{V}{V_m}$

$$\therefore \quad = \frac{V}{V_m} = \frac{I_m (R_m + R_S)}{I_m R_m}$$

$$= \left(1 + \frac{R_S}{R_m}\right)$$

Therefore the value of multipliers is given by

$$R_S = (N-1)R_m$$

9.6 MOVING IRON INSTRUMENT

Moving iron instrument are commonly used in measurement of voltage and current. These instrument can be used in AC and DC, so they are universally employed in laboratory, test labs and industries, are cheap, simple in construction and accurate. These are classified into two categories:

9.6.1 Attraction Type Moving Iron Instrument

This type of instrument is shown in Fig. 9.11. The basic principle of operation is that, a soft iron piece if brought near a magnet gets attracted by the magnet. Figure 9.11 shows a fixed coil C and an oval shaped soft iron piece centrally mounted on the spindle. The spindle is supported between jewel bearings and it carries the pointer. The instrument may be spring controlled or gravity controlled. Damping is provided by a piston moving in an air chamber. This piston is attached to the main spindle. For such instruments, eddy current damping is not used because the presence of a permanent magnet required for damping purpose would affect the operating field of the instrument.

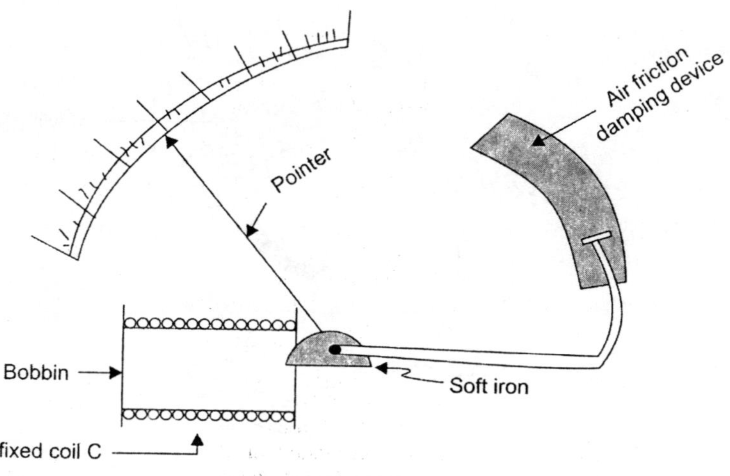

Fig. 9.11

When current to be measured is passed through the fixed coil C, it produces a magnetic field. Due to this field the soft iron piece gets attracted inside and the pointer deflects over a calibrated scale. The torque developed in this instrument is proportional to the square of the current through the coil and therefore the scale is non uniform. The scale is cramped at the beginning and open of the upper end of the scale. The shape of the soft iron piece is so adjusted that as far as possible a uniform scale is obtained. The soft iron piece is always attracted irrespective of the direction of the magnitude field of the coil. Therefore the instrument can be used for both AC as well as DC measurement.

The damping is provided by the piston attached to the spindle. The deflecting torque T_d is proportional to the square of current passing through the coil.

$$\therefore \quad T_d \propto I_2^2$$

So the deflection of the pointer is also proportional to square of the current.

$$\therefore \quad \theta \propto I^2$$

Due to this reason, the scale of this instrument is nonlinear.

Application

This type of instrument can be used for the measurement of AC as well as DC quantities. This is because irrespective of the direction of current, the deflection q will always be in the same direction.

9.6.2 Repulsion Type Moving Instrument

Figure 9.11 shows the construction of a moving iron instrument. The basic principle on which this instrument works is that if two soft iron pieces, mangetised in the same direction (north poles of both on one side and south poles on the other side) are placed very near to each other they repel. The two soft iron strips A and B are shown in Fig. 9.12. The strip A is attached to be bobbin over which the coil C is wound. The other strip B is attach to the spindle and therefore it is movable.

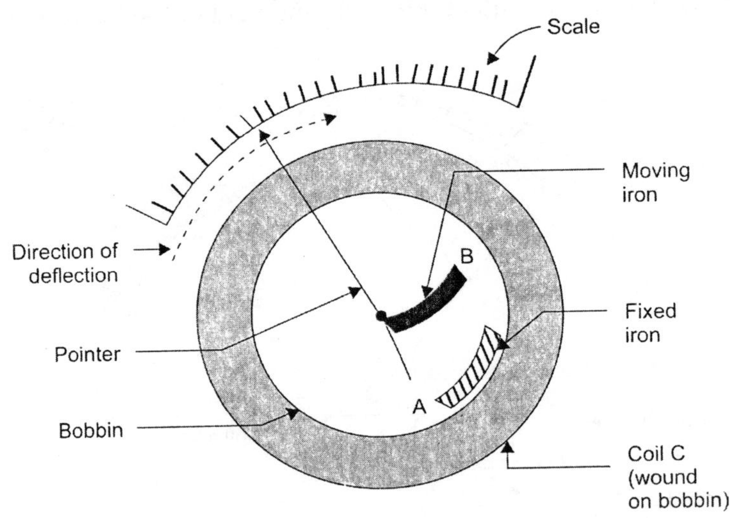

Fig. 9.12: Construction of moving iron instrument

When the current to be measured flows through coil C, A and B are magnetised in the same direction and thus repel each other. Due to this force of repulsion strip B moves away from strip A and therefore the pointer attached to the spindle deflects. The type of damping is usually the air friction type. It is provided by the piston moving in the air chamber. The force of repulsion between the two strips depends on their relative field strength. As the field strength is proportional to the current in the coil, the deflecting torque is proportional to the square of the current. Due to this, the instruments has non-uniform scale. In practice, attempt is made to make the scale move uniform by using soft iron pieces of suitable shapes. Similar to the attraction type instrument, this instrument can be used for AC as well as DC measurement.

Advantages

(1) Suitable for AC as well DC measurements.
(2) Simple and robust in construction as the moving system (soft iron piece) is free from current leads.
(3) Good accuracy.
(4) Cheaper is cost as compared to permanent magnet moving coil instrument.
(5) The instrument has high torque to weight-ratio.

Disadvantages

(1) The scale is nonuniform.
(2) Power consumed by the instrument is high as compared to that of the permanent magnet moving coil instrument.
(3) Due to the presence of iron part in the operating system, error due to the hysteresis effect is introduced. To reduce this effect nickel iron alloys are used.

Applications: Moving iron instruments are rarely used for DC measurements except for very inexpensive applications. They are used extensively on AC where 5 to 10% errors is acceptable.

SOLVED EXAMPLES BASED ON SHUNT MULTIPLIER CIRCUIT

Example 1: A moving coil ammeter has a full scale deflection of 50 μA and a coil resistance of 100 Ω. The value of the shunt resistance required for the instrument to be converted to read a full-scale reading of 1 A will be............mΩ. **[UPTU 2008-09]**

Solution: Given data

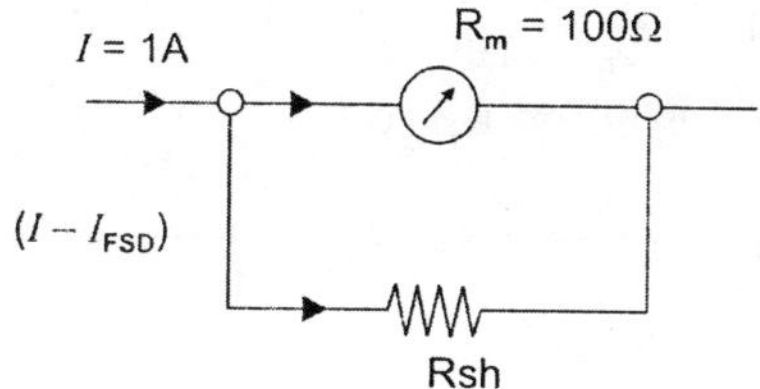

Voltage across the shunt is

$$V_{sh} = R_m \times I_{FSD}$$

$$= 100 \times 50 \times 10^{-6} = 5 \text{ mV}$$

$$= \frac{V_{sh}}{I - I_{FSD}} = \frac{5 \times 10^{-3}}{\left(1 \times 10^{-6} - 50 / 10^{-6}\right)}$$

$$= \frac{5 \times 10^{-3}}{0.9995} = 5 \text{ m}\Omega$$ **Ans.**

Example 2: The full-scale deflection current of a meter is 1 mA and its internal resistance is 100 Ω. If this meter is to have full scale deflection when 100 V is measured, the value of series resistor should be ....Ω. **[UPTU 2008-90, 2010-11]**

Solution: Given data:

$I_{FSD} = 1 \text{ mA}, R_m = 100\ \Omega,\ V = 100 \text{ V}$

$$V_{FS} = I_{FSD} \times R_m = 1 \text{ mA} \times 100 = 100 \text{ mV}$$

$$R_S = \frac{V - V_{FS}}{1 \text{ mA}} = \frac{100 - 01}{1 \times 10^{-3}} = 99.9 \text{ k}\Omega$$ **Ans.**

Example 3: A moving coil multi-ammeter having a resistance of 8 Ω gives full scale deflection when a current of 5 mA is passed through it. Explain these instrument can be used for measurement of (1) current up to 2 A. (2) voltage up to 8 V.

[Sem-II, UPTU 2009-10]

Solution: Given data, $R_m = 8\ \Omega, I_{FSD} = 5 \text{ mA}$

(1) Modification to measure current upto 2 A:

$I_{sh} = I - I_{FSD}$

$= 2000 \text{ mA} - 5 \text{ mA}$

$= 1995 \text{ mA}$

Voltage across the meter $= V_{\text{across}}\ R_{sh}$

$= I_{FSD} \times R_{sh}$

$= 5 \times 10^{-3} \times 8 = 40 \text{ mV}$

$$R_{sh} = \frac{V_{sh}}{I_{sh}} = \frac{40 \times 10^{-3}}{1995 \times 10^{-4}} = 0.02\ \Omega$$ **Ans.**

(2) Modification to measure voltage up to 8 V:

$$R_s = \frac{8}{I_{FSD}} - R_m = \frac{8}{5 \times 10^{-3}} - 8 = 1592\ \Omega$$ **Ans.**

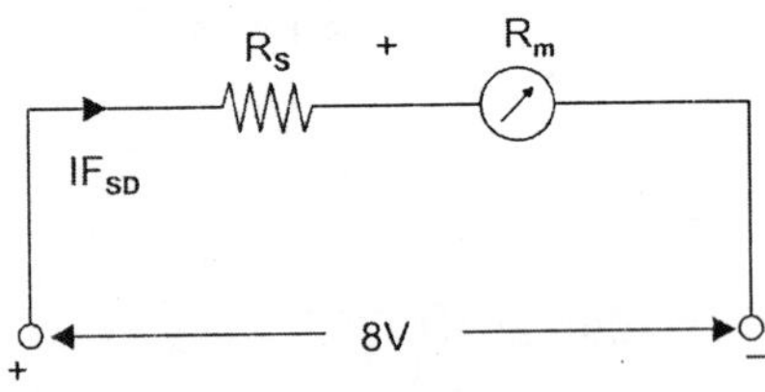

Example 4: A moving coil instrument gives a full-scale deflection of 20 mA when a potential difference of 50 mV is applied. Calculate the series resistance to measure 500 V on full scale. **[Sem-I, UPTU 2004-05]**

Solution: Given data

$$I_m = 20 \text{ mA},\ V_m = 50 \text{ mV},\ V = 500$$

We know, $$R_m = \frac{V_m}{I_m} = \frac{50 \times 10^{-3}}{20 \times 10^{-3}} = 2.5\ \Omega$$

And $$R_S = \frac{V_m}{I_m} - R_m = \frac{500}{20 \times 10^{-3}} - 2.5 = 24997.5\ \Omega$$ **Ans.**

EXERCISES

1. Describe the following measuring instruments.
   (*a*) Deflecting torque (*b*) Controlling torque
   (*c*) Damping torque
2. Write a short note on
   (*a*) Indicating instrument (*b*) Integrating instrument
   (*c*) Recording instrument
3. Enlist the advantages and disadvantages of permanent magnet moving coil (PMMC) type instruments.
4. Explain attraction type and repulsion type moving iron instruments with neat and clean diagram.
5. Explain the operation of dynamometer type wattmeter instrument.

REVIEW QUESTIONS

Very Short Answer Questions

1. What are analog and digital instrument?
2. Define the following terms.
   (*a*) Shunt (*b*) Multiplier
3. Write the name of different types of torque acting on measuring instrument.
4. Compare PMMC and MI instrument.
5. Give the classification of instruments.

Short Answer Questions

1. List various types of torques required for the operation of an indicating instrument and explain their significance.
2. Enlist the advantages and disadvantages of PMMC type instruments.
3. Explain the principle of operation of attraction type of moving iron type of instruments.
4. Explain the principle of operation of repulsion type of moving iron instruments.
5. Explain the principle of operation of electro-dynamometer wattmeter.
6. Explain the construction and working principle of PMMC type instruments.

Descriptive Questions

1. Explain the construction, working principle, advantages, disadvantages and application of PMMC types instruments.
2. Explain attraction and repulsion type moving iron instrument with neat and clean diagram.

Chapter

10 Magnetic Circuits

10.1 INTRODUCTION

All of us are familiar with a magnet, it is a piece of solid body which possesses a property of attracting iron pieces and metal pieces. This is called a magnet. Every magnet has two poles called the north pole and the south pole. There are two types of magnet (Fig. 10.1).

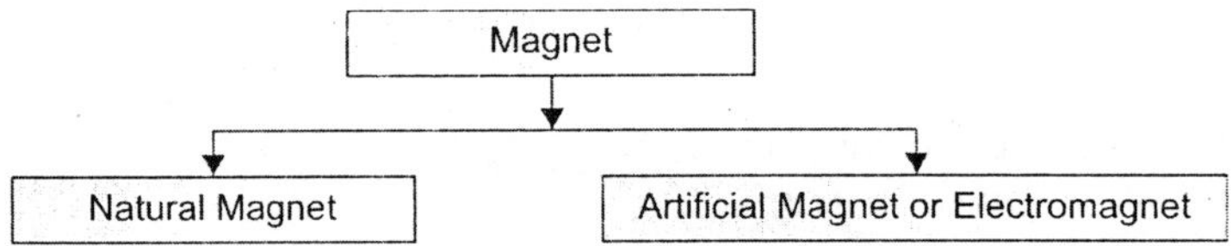

Fig. 10.1: Block diagram

Our interest is confined to artificial magnets only. Artificial magnets are formed by flow of electric current and are called electromagnets. According to Orested, every current carrying conductor is always surrounded by a magnetic field. The property of such current is called *magnetic effect of electric current.*

Note: Electromagnet was discovered by Oersted.

10.2 MAGNETIC CIRCUIT CONCEPT

(i) **Magnetic field:** The region near a magnet where a force is experienced is called the magnetic field. Magnetic field is strongest near the pole and goes on decreasing in strength as we move away from the magnet.

(ii) **Magnetic lines of force:** The magnetic field of magnet is represented by imaginary lines around it which are called magnetic lines of force. Note that these lines have no physical existence, these are purely imaginary and were introduced by Michael Faraday to get the visualization of distribution of such lines of force.

(iii) **Magnetic flux (ϕ):** The total number of lines of force existing in a particular magnetic field is called magnetic flux. The unit of flux is weber and flux is denoted by ϕ.

$\therefore$ 1 weber= 10^8 lines of force

(iv) **Magnetic flux density (B):** It is the ratio of the magnetic flux to the cross-sectional area or it can be defined as the flux per unit area in a plane at right angles to the flux is known as flux.

Mathematically

$$B = \frac{\phi}{A} \text{ wb/m}^2 \text{ or Tesla}$$

(iv) **Magnetic field strength (*H*):** This gives quantitative measure of strongness or weakness of the magnetic field. This can be defined as the force experienced by a unit N-pole when placed at any point in a magnetic field. It is denoted by ***H*** and its unit is newton per weber or ampere-turns per meter.

∴ Mathematical

$$H = \frac{\text{Ampere turn}}{\text{Length}}$$

or $$H = \frac{NI}{l} \text{ AT/m}$$

(vi) **Permeability:** The flow of flux produced by the magnet not only depends on the magnetic field strength but also on one important property of the magnetic material called permeability. It is related to the medium in which magnet is placed. The force exerted by one magnetic pole on other depends on the medium in which magnets are placed (Fig. 10.2).

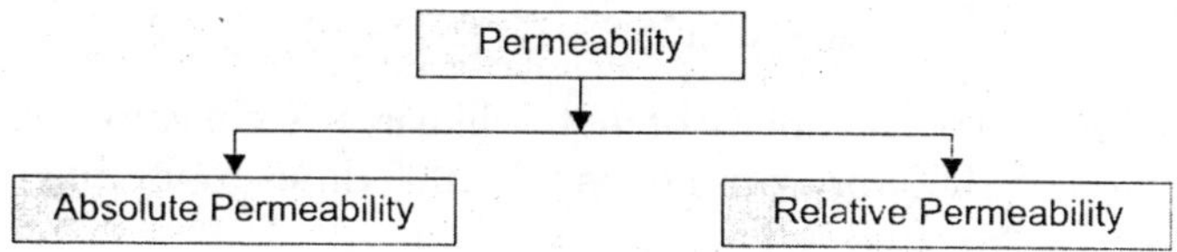

Fig. 10.2: Block diagram

(*a*) ***Absolute permeability*** **(μ):** The magnetic field strength (***H***) decides the flux density (***B***) to be produced by the magnet around it in a given medium. The ratio of magnetic flux density *B* in a particular medium (other than vaccum or air) to the magnetic field strength *H* producing that flux density is called absolute permeability of that medium. It is denoted by μ and its unit is H/m.

∴ Mathematically

$$\mu = \frac{B}{H}$$

i.e., $$B = \mu H$$

Permeability of free space or vaccum (μ_0): If the magnet is placed in a free space (or) vaccum or in air then the ratio of flux density ***B*** and magnetic field strength ***H*** is called permeability of free space or vaccum or air. It is denoted by m_0 and measured in H/m. It is experimentally found that this μ_0, i.e. ratio of ***B*** and ***H*** in vaccum remains constant every where in the vacuum and its value is $4\pi \times 10^{-7}$ H/m.

∴ $$\mu_0 = 4\pi \times 10^{-7} \text{ H/m.}$$

The ratio of *B* to *H* is constant only for free space, vaccum or air which is $\mu_0 = 4\pi \times 10^{-7}$ H/m.

(*b*) ***Relative Permeability*** **(μ_r):** The relative permeability is defined as the ratio of flux density produced in a medium (other than free space) to the flux density produced in free space, under the influence of same magnetic field strength and under identical conditions. If the magnetic field strength is ***H*** which is producing flux density ***B*** in the medium while flux density B_0 in free space then the relàtive permeability is defined as

$$\mu_r = \frac{B}{B_0} \text{ (where } H \text{ is same)}$$

For free space vaccum or air $\mu_r = 1$.
According to definition of absolute permeability we can write for given **H**

$$\mu = \frac{B}{H} \text{ (in medium)} \quad ...(10.1)$$

$$\mu_0 = \frac{B_0}{H} \text{ (in free space)} \quad ...(10.2)$$

Dividing (10.1) and (10.2), we get,

$$\frac{\mu}{\mu_0} = \frac{B}{B_0}$$

$\Rightarrow$ but

$$\frac{\mathbf{B}}{\mathbf{B_0}} = \mu_r$$

$$\frac{\mu}{\mu_0} = \mu_r$$

$$\therefore \quad \mu = \mu_0 \mu_r$$

Note: The relative permeability of metals like iron, steel varies from 100 to 100,000.
Example: If $\mu_r = 1000$ for iron means it is 1000 times more magnetic than the free space a air.

(vii) **Magnetomotive force (MMF):** We know that the flow of electrons is known as current which is basically due to electromotive force (emf).
Similarly, magnetomotive force (mmf) is defined as the amount of force which is used to drive the net amount of flux all through inside a magnetic circuit.
Let us consider a magnetic circuit in the form of toroidal ring as shown in Fig 10.4(a). Let us assume, l = the mean length of the magnetic path, A = cross-sectional area, N = number of turns of magnetising coil and I = current through coil. Then the magnetic field intensity at any point on mean path of the solenoid is

$$H = \frac{NI}{l} \text{AT/m} \quad ...(10.3)$$

But magnetic flux density in the solenoid

$$B = \mu_0 \mu_r H \quad ...(10.4)$$

where μ_0 is the relative permeability of the magnetic material of the solenoid.

$$\therefore \quad \text{Total flux produced } \phi = B \times A \quad ...(10.5)$$

or, $$\phi = \mu_0 \mu_r HA$$

$$= \frac{\mu_0 \mu_r NIA}{l} wb \quad ...(10.6)$$

or, $$\phi = \frac{NI}{l/\mu_0 \mu_r A} \quad ...(10.7)$$

or, $$\phi = F/S \quad ...(10.8)$$

or, $$F = \phi \times S \quad ...(10.9)$$

where, $F = NI$ and $S = \dfrac{l}{\mu_0 \mu_r A}$

F is called magneto-motive force (mmf) and S is called reluctance. Equation (10.9) is sometimes called ohm's law of magnetic circuit.

(viii) **Reluctance (S):** In electric circuit, current flow is opposed by the resistance of the material. Similarly there is opposition by the material to the flow of flux which is called reluctance. It is defined as the resistance offered by the material to the flow of magnetic flux through it and is denoted by 'S'. It is directly proportional to the length of the magnetic circuit while inversely proportional to the area of cross-section. Mathematically

$$S \propto \frac{l}{A} \qquad \text{(where '}l\text{' in m and '}A\text{' in m}^2\text{)}$$

$$\therefore \quad S = \frac{kl}{A}$$

where k = constant of proportionality
= reciprocal of absolute permeability of material

$$k = \frac{1}{\mu}$$

$$\therefore \quad S = \frac{l}{\mu A} = \frac{l}{\mu_0 \mu_r A} \text{ AT/Wb}$$

It is measured in ampere-turn per weber. The reluctance can be also expressed as the ratio of magnetomotive force to the flux produced.

$$\text{Reluctance} = \frac{\text{mmf}}{\text{flux}}$$

$$\therefore \quad S = \frac{NI}{\phi} \text{ AT/Wb}$$

(ix) **Permeance:** The permeance of the magnetic circuit is defined as the reciprocal of the reluctance. It can also be defined as the property of the magnetic circuit due to which it allows flow of the magnetic flux through it.

$$\therefore \quad \text{Permeance} = \frac{1}{\text{Reluctance}}$$

It is measured in weber per ampere-turn (Wb/AT)

10.3 MAGNETIC CIRCUIT WITH DC EXCITATIONS

Magnetic circuit: The closed path followed by magnetic flux is called a magnetic circuit.

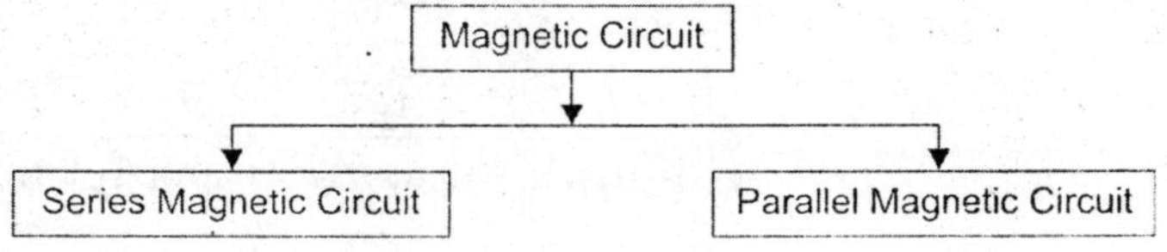

Fig. 10.3: Block diagram

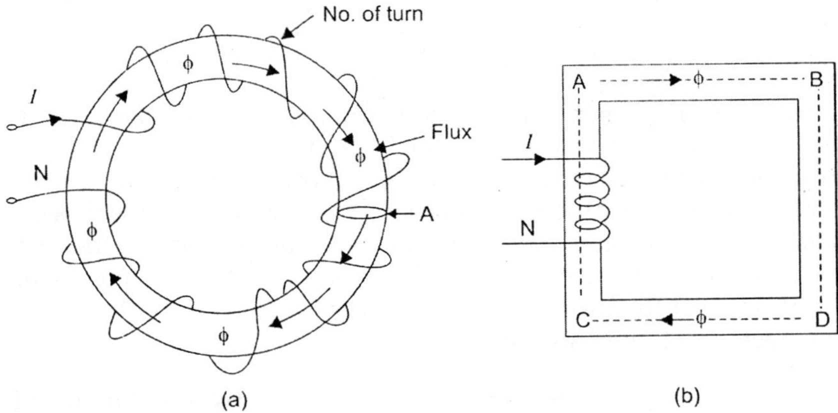

Fig. 10.4: Simple magnetic circuit

Series Magnetic Circuit

In series magnetic circuit, the same flux ϕ flows through the circuit. It can just be compared to a series electric circuit which carries the same current through out.

Analysis of Series Magnetic Circuits with Air Gap

Consider a circular ring made from different materials of length l_1, l_2 and l_3 (in Fig. 10.5) cross-sectional area A_1, A_2 and A_3 and relative permeability μ_{r_1}, μ_{r_2} and μ_{r_3} respectively with a cut of length l_g known as air gap.

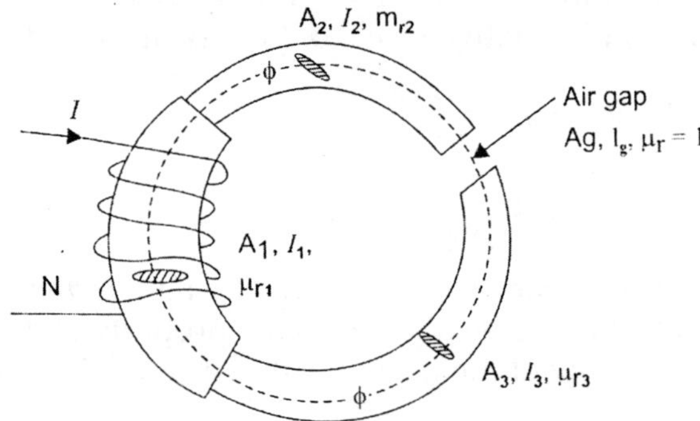

Fig. 10.5: Series magnetic circuit with air gap

∴ Total reluctance of the series magnetic circuit with air gap is

$$S = S_1 + S_2 + S_3 + S_g$$

$$S = \frac{l_1}{\mu_0 \mu_{r1} A_1} + \frac{l_2}{\mu_0 \mu_{r2} A_2} + \frac{l_3}{\mu_0 \mu_{r3} A_3} + \frac{l_g}{\mu_0 \mu_{r3} A_g}$$

[since $\mu_{r3} = 1$ for air)

$$\text{Total mmf} = \phi \times S$$

$$= \phi \left(\frac{l_1}{\mu_0 \mu_{r1} A_1} + \frac{l_2}{\mu_0 \mu_{r2} A_2} + \frac{l_3}{\mu_0 \mu_{r3} A_3} + \frac{l_g}{\mu_0 A_g} \right)$$

$$= \frac{B_1 l_1}{\mu_0 \mu_{r1}} + \frac{B_2 l_2}{\mu_0 \mu_{r2}} + \frac{B_3 l_3}{\mu_0 \mu_{r3}} + \frac{B_g l_g}{\mu_0}$$

$$= H_1l_1 + H_2l_2 + H_3l_3 + H_gl_g$$

or

Total ampere turns required = Sum of ampere turn required for individual parts of the magnetic circuit

Parallel Magnetic Circuit

A magnetic circuit which has more than one path for flux is called a parallel magnetic circuit. It can just be compared to a parallel electric circuit which has more than one path for electric circuit.

Analysis of Parallel Magnetic Circuits with Air Gap

For the circuit shown in Fig. 10.6, path ABCD and AFED are in parallel, so, ampere turns required to create flux ϕ_1 in path ABCD is equal to ampere-turns required to create flux ϕ_2 in path AFED and also equal to the ampere turns required for both of the paths. Hence total ampere-turns required for magnetic circuit.

$$\text{Total } AT = AT \text{ for path } DA + AT \text{ for path ABCD}$$
$$= AT \text{ for path } DA + AT \text{ for path AFED}$$

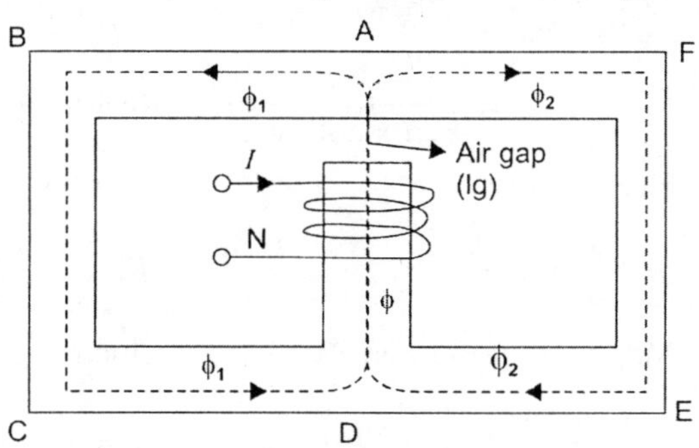

Fig. 10.6: Parallel magnetic circuit

10.4 ANALOGY BETWEEN ELECTRIC AND MAGNETIC CIRCUITS

[UPTU; 2002-03, 2004-05, 2006-07, MTU 2008-09, 2009-10]

The analogy or similarities between electric and magnetic circuits are listed below:

Table 10.1: Similarities

	Magnetic circuit	*Electric circuit*
Circuit	A B I N D C	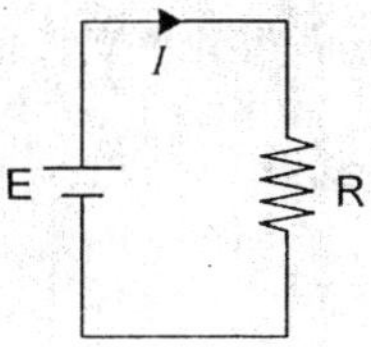
1. Definition	The closed path followed by magnetic flux is called a magnetic circuit.	The closed path followed by an electric current is called an electric circuit.

Contd.

Table 10.1: Similarities (*Contd.*)

	Magnetic circuit	*Electric circuit*
2. Driving Force	mmf	emf
3. Response	Flux $\phi = \frac{\text{mmf}}{S}$ Wb	Current $I = \frac{E}{R}$
4. Impedance	Reluctance, $S = \frac{l}{\mu_0 \mu_r A}$ **Series** $S = S_1 + S_2 + \ldots + S_n$ **Parallel** $S = \frac{1}{\frac{1}{S_1} + \frac{1}{S_2} + \ldots + \frac{1}{S_n}}$	Resistance $R = \frac{\rho l}{A}$ **Series** $R = R_1 + R_2 + \ldots + R_n$ **Parallel** $R = \frac{1}{\frac{1}{R_1} + \frac{1}{R_2} + \ldots + \frac{1}{R_n}}$
5. Admittance	Permeance $= \frac{1}{\text{Reluctance}}$ Wb/AT	Conductance $= \frac{1}{R}$ Siemen
6. Proportionality	Reluctivity $= \frac{1}{\text{Permeability}} = \frac{1}{\mu}$	Resistivity $\rho = \frac{1}{\text{Conducitivity}}\ \Omega/\text{m}$
7. Density	Flux density $B = \frac{\phi}{A}$ Wb/m^2	Current density $J = \frac{I}{A}$ A/m^2
8. Field intensity	Magnetic field intensity $H = \frac{\text{mmf}}{L} = \frac{NI}{L}$. AT/m	Electric field intensity $E = \frac{V}{x}$ Volt/m
9. Drop	mmf drop $= \phi \times S$	Voltage drop $= IR$

Table 10.2: Dissimilarities

Magnetic circuit	*Electric circuit*
1. Flux does not actually flow in a magnetic circuit.	Current does flow in an electric circuit.
2. Permeability does not largely vary from material to material and there is hardly any material which can act as an insulator to the magnetic flux.	Conductivity varies largely from material to material and that some materials are insulators to electric current and some are very good conductors.
3. For a particular temperature the permeability depends up on the flux density (or total flux).	For a particular temperature, conductivity (or resistivity) is constant and independent of current strength.
4. Flux can pass through air.	Current would not flow through the air until an arc is struck.
5. Residual flux persists after removal of mmf.	The current is reduced to zero after removal of source of emf.
6. Flux can pass through air.	Current cannot pass through air.

10.5 MAGNETIC CIRCUIT CALCULATION

There are two basic types of problems occur in magnetic circuit calculations.

1. In the first type, the value of flux ϕ or flux density B is given and mmf is to be determined. This type of calculation is straight forward.
2. In the second type, the applied mmf is known and the flux or flux density is to be determined. There is no direct analytical solution to this problem because of the nonlinear characteristics of the magnetic material usually numerical techniques or graphical methods are used to some such problems.

10.6 ELECTROMAGNETISM

We have discussed the concept of magnetism, basic properties and magnetic circuits, but we have not seen the generation of emf with the help of magnetism. Emf can be generated by different ways but the most popular and extensively used method of generating an emf is based on electromagnetism. In 1831, an English Physicist, Michael Faraday succeeded in getting emf from magnetic flux. The phenomenon by which emf is of obtained from flux is called *electromagnetic induction*. Let us discuss in brief, what is electromagnetic induction and its effects on electrical engineering.

Faraday's Experiments

Let us study first the two experiments conducted by Faraday to get understanding of electromagnetic induction.

Experiment 1

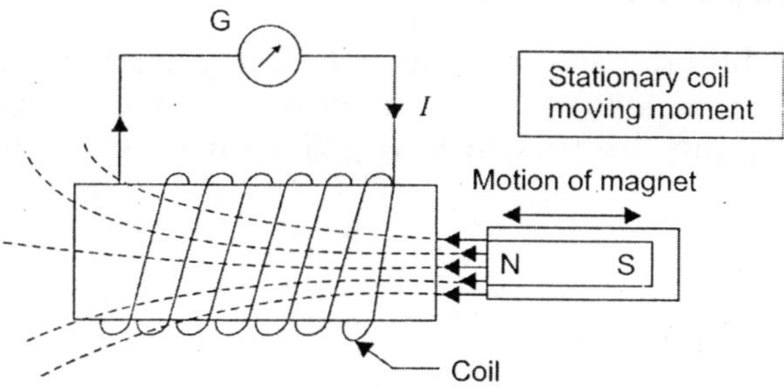

Fig. 10.7: Faraday's experiment 1

Explanation: Consider a coil having N turns connected to a galvanometer as shown in Fig. 10.7. Galvanometer indicate flow of current in the circuit. A permanent magnet is moved relative to coil, such that magnetic lines of force associated with coil get changed whenever, there is motion of permanent magnet, galvanometer deflects indicating flow of current through the circuit. The galvanometer deflects in one direction, when magnet is moved towards a coil. If deflect in other direction, when moved away from the coil. The deflection continuous as long as motion of magnet exists. Now deflection of galvanometer indicates flow of current. But to exist flow of current there must be presence of emf. Hence such movement of flux lines with respect to coil generates an emf which drives current through the coil. This is the situation where coil is fixed and magnet is moved to create relative motion of flux with respect to coil.

Experiment 2

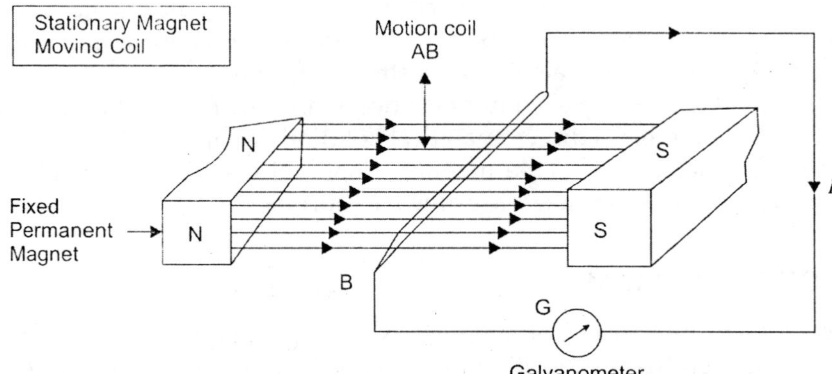

Fig. 10.8: Faraday's experiment 2

Explanation: The similar observation can be made by moving a coil in the magnetic field of fixed permanent magnet, creating relative motion between flux and coil. This arrangement is shown in Fig. 10.8. The coil AB is connected to the galvanometer and moved by some external means in the magnetic field of fixed permanent magnet. Whenever coil AB is moved in the direction shown in the Fig. 10.8, the galvanometer deflects indicating flow of current through coil AB. In both cases, basically there is change of flux lines with respect to conductor, i.e. there is cutting of flux lines and the conductor in which emf is induced with this experiments Faraday stated two laws called Faraday's law of electromagnetic Induction.

10.7 NATURE OF INDUCED EMF

We know that according to Faraday's laws of electromagnetic induction, whenever conductor cuts the magnetic flux, an emf is induced in the conductor. Such emf can be induced by changing the flux in two different ways as shown in the block diagram (Fig. 10.7).

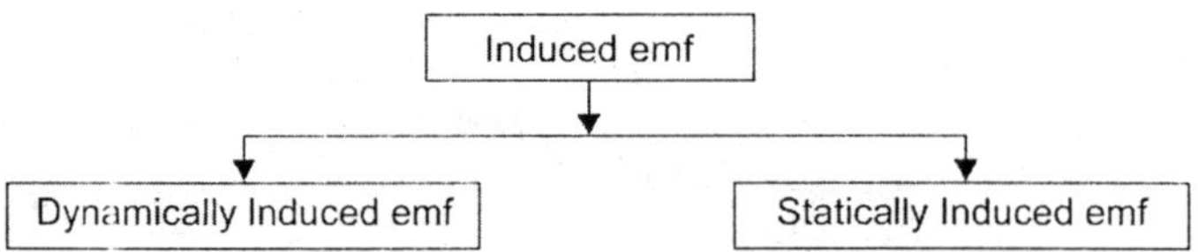

Fig. 10.9: Block diagram

(a) Dynamically induced emf: In induced emf which is due to the physical movement of conductor with respect to stationary magnetic field is called dynamically induced emf. In DC generator, we come across this type of induced emf. The direction of dynamically induced emf can be found using Fleming's right hand rule.

(b) Statically induced emf: When the conductor is stationary and magnetic field is moving or changing, the emf is induced in the conductor which is stationary. The direction of statically induced emf is found by lenz's law (Fig. 10.10).

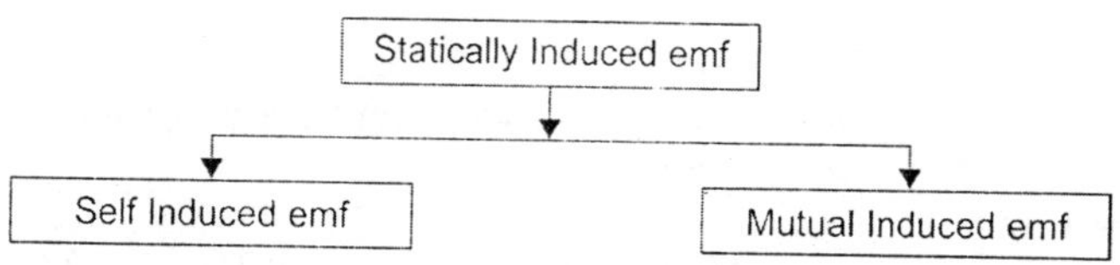

Fig. 10.10: Block diagram

(i) *Self induced emf:* If the emf is induced in the coil due to the change of its own flux, it is known as self induced emf. According to Lenz's law the direction of this induced emf will be so as to oppose the current producing it. The cause is the current hence the self induced emf will try to set up a current which is in opposite direction to that of current. This property of coil which opposes any change in the current passing through it is called self inductance or only inductance.

(ii) *Mutually induced emf:* If the emf is induced in the coil due to change of current in any other coil, this is known as mutually induced emf.

10.7.1 Magnetic Leakage and Fringing

Leakage flux is the flux which follows a leakage path as shown in Fig. 10.11. Flux in the air gap is known as *useful flux* which is utilized for various useful purposes for the purpose of calculations the iron is supposed to carry whole of the flux throughout its entire length.

The ratio of total flux (flux in the iron path) to the useful flux (flux in the air) is known as *leakage factor.*

i.e.
$$\text{Leakage factor} = \frac{\text{Total flux}}{\text{Useful flux}}$$

or
$$\text{Leakage factor} = \frac{\text{Flux in the iron path}}{\text{Flux in the air gap}}$$

It is also seen from Fig. 10.11 that the useful flux passing across the gap tends of bulge outwards, thereby increasing the effective area of gap and reducing the flux density in the gap. This effect is referred to as *fringing,* and the longer the air gap, the greater is the fringing.

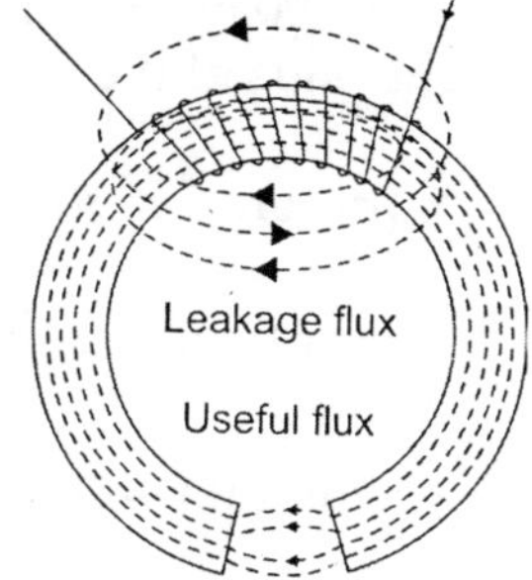

Fig. 10.11

In electrical machines (such as in generators and motors), magnetic leakage is undesirable as it causes increase in weight (not decrease in the power efficiency) and cost of manufacture. Though magnetic leakage cannot be avoided completely but can be reduced to the minimum by placing the magnetizing or exciting coils as close as possible to the air gap or to the points in the magnetic circuit where the flux is to be utilized for useful purpose.

UNIVERSITY SOLVED EXAMPLES

Example 1: An electromagnet has an gap of 4 mm and flux density in the gap is 1.3 wb/m^2. Determine the ampere-turns for the gap.

[UP Technical Univ; Electrical Engineering, Second Semester 2006-07; Mahamaya Technical Engineering, Jan/Feb. 2006]

Solution:

Magnetising force, $H_g = \frac{B}{\mu_0 \mu_r} = \frac{1.3}{4\pi \times 10^{-7} \times 1} = 1.035 \times 10^6$ AT/m

$\therefore \mu_r$ for air = 1

Ampere-turns for the gap = $H_g l_g = 1.035 \times 10^6 \times 4 \times 10^{-3} = 4.140$ **Ans.**

Example 2: A rectangular shaped core is made of mild steel plate 15 mm × 20 mm cross section. The mean length of the magnetic path is 18 cm. The exciting coil has 300 turns and current 0.7 A. Calculate: (i) magnetising force (ii) flux density (iii) reluctance (iv) flux of magnetic circuit. Assume relative permeability of mild steel as 940.

[RGPV; Basic Electrical Engineering, Jan/Feb: 2006]

Solution: Mean length of magnetic path

$$l = 18 \text{ cm} = 0.18 \text{ m}$$

Cross-sectional area of mild steel plate

$$a = 15 \text{ mm} \times 20 \text{ mm} = 300 \text{ mm}^2 = 3 \times 10^{-4} \text{ m}^2$$

(i) Magnetising force $\quad H = \frac{NI}{l} = \frac{300 \times 0.7}{0.18} = 1{,}166.6667$ AT/m **Ans.**

(ii) Flux density $\quad B = \mu_0 \mu_r H = 4\pi \times 10^{-7} \times 940 \times 1{,}166.6667 = 1.378$ T **Ans.**

(iii) Reluctance $\quad S = \frac{1}{\mu_0 \mu_r a} = \frac{0.18}{4\pi \times 10^{-7} \times 940 \times 3 \times 10^{-4}}$

$= 50.794 \times 10^4$ AT/Wb **Ans.**

(iv) Flux $\quad \phi = B \times a = 1.378 \times 3 \times 10^{-4} = 4.134 \times 10^{-4}$ Wb **Ans.**

Example 3: A coil of insulated wire of 500 turns and of resistance 4 Ω is closely wound on an iron ring. The ring has a mean diameter of 0.25 m and a uniform cross-sectional area of 700 mm². Calculate the total flux in the ring when a dc supply of 6 V is applied to the ends of the winding. Assume a relative permeability of 550.

[UP Technical Univ; Electrical Engineering, July 2002]

Solution: Length of iron ring

$$l = \pi D = \pi \times 0.25 = 0.25\,\pi \text{ m}$$

Area of cross-section of iron path

$$a = 700 \text{ mm}^2 = 0.7 \times 10^{-3} \text{ m}^2$$

Current flowing through the winding

$$I = \frac{\text{Voltage applied across coil}}{\text{Resistance of coil}} = \frac{6}{4} = 1.5 \text{ A}$$

Total flux in the ring $\quad \phi = \frac{NI \times \mu_r \mu_0 a}{l}$

$$= \frac{500 \times 1.5 \times 550 \times 4\pi \times 10^{-7} \times 0.7 \times 10^{-3}}{0.25\pi} = 0.462 \text{ mWb}$$

Example 4: A wrought iron bar 30 cm long and 2 cm in diameter is bent into a circular shape as given in figure below. It is then wound with 500 turns of wire. Calculate the current required to produce a flux of 0.5 mWb in magnetic circuit with an air gap of 1 mm, μ_r (iron) = 4,000 (assume constant).

[UP Technical Univ; Electrical Engineering, Second Semester 2004–05]

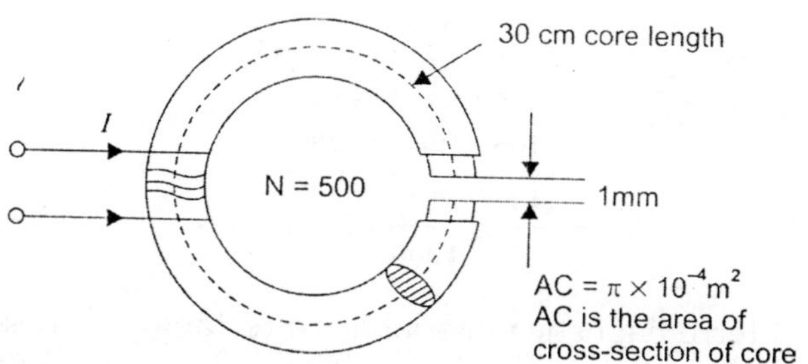

Solution:

Flux to be produced $\phi = 0.5\text{ mWb} = 0.5 \times 10^{-3}\text{ Wb}$

Area of cross-section of core

$$a = \pi \times 10^{-4}\text{ m}^2$$

Flux density required $B = \frac{\phi}{a}$

$$= \frac{0.5 \times 10^{-3}}{\pi \times 10^{-4}} = \frac{5}{\pi} = 1.5915\text{ T}$$

Airgap length $l_g = 1\text{ mm} = 0.001\text{ m}$

Core length $l_i = 30\text{ cm} = 0.3\text{ m}$

Total ampere-turns required

$$AT = \frac{B}{\mu_0} l_g + \frac{B}{\mu_0 \mu_r} l_i = \frac{1.5915}{4\pi \times 10^{-7}} \times 0.001 + \frac{1.5915}{4\pi \times 10^{-7} \times 4000} \times 0.3$$

$$= 1266 + 95 = 1,361$$

Current required $I = \frac{AT}{N} = \frac{1361}{500} = 2.72\text{ A}$ **Ans.**

Example 5: A circular ring 20 cm in diameter has an air gap 1 mm wide cut in it. The area of cross section the ring is 3.6 cm^2. Calculate the value of the direct current needed in a coil of 1000 turns uniformly wound round the ring to create a flux of 0.5 mWb in the air gap. Neglect fringing and assume relative permeability for the iron as 650.

[UP Technical Univ; Electrical Engineering, First Semester 2006-07]

Solution:

Flux to be produced $\phi = 0.5\text{ mWb} = 0.5 \times 10^{-3}\text{ Wb}$

Area of *x*-section $a = 3.6\text{ cm}^2 = 3.6 \times 10^{-4}\text{ m}^2$

Flux density required $B = \frac{\phi}{a} = \frac{0.5 \times 10^{-5}}{3.6 \times 10^{-4}} = 1.389\text{ T}$

Air gap length $l_g = 1\text{ mm} = 1 \times 10^{-3}\text{ m}$

Length of iron path $l_i = \pi d - l_g = \pi \times 0.20 - 1 \times 10^{-3} = 0.62732$

Total ampere-turns required

$$AT = \frac{B}{\mu_0} l_g + \frac{B}{\mu_0 \mu_r} l_i = \frac{1.389}{4\pi \times 10^{-7}} \times 1 \times 10^{-3}$$

$$= \frac{1.389}{4\pi\times10^{-7}\times650}\times0.62732$$

$$= 1105+1067=2172$$

Current required $I = \frac{AT}{N} = \frac{2172}{1000} = 2.172 \text{ A}$ **Ans.**

Example 6: A ring of ferromagnetic material has a rectangular cross-section The inner diameter is 7.4 in, the outer diameter is 9 in., and the thickness is 0.8 in. There is a coil of 600 turns wound on the ring. When the coil carries a current of 2.5 A, the flux produced in the ring is 1.2×10^{-3} Wb. Find: (i) magnetic field intensity (ii) reluctance (iii) permeability. **[UP Technical Univ; Electrical Engineering, Second Semester 2007-08]**

Solution: Number of turns in the coil

$$N = 600$$

Current carried by coil $I = 2.5$ A

Mean length of magnetic flux path is that of a circle midway between the inside and outside diameter, i.e.

$$l = \frac{\pi(7.4+9)}{2} = 25.45 \text{ in} = 25.45\times0.0254$$

$$= 0.64635 \text{ m}$$

Cross-sectional area of the toroidal core

$$a = (9-7.4)\times0.8 = 1.28 \text{ in}^2 = 8.26\times10^{-4} \text{ m}^2$$

(i) Magnetic flux density $\mathbf{B} = \frac{\phi}{a} = \frac{1.2\times10^{-3}}{8.26\times10^{-4}} = 14.5 \text{ Wb/m}^2$ **Ans.**

(ii) Reluctance $S = \frac{\text{MMF}}{\phi} = \frac{NI}{\phi} = \frac{600\times2.5}{1.2\times10^{-3}} = 1250\times10^3 \text{ AT/Wb}$ **Ans.**

(iii) Permeability $\mu = \frac{1}{S_a} = \frac{0.64635}{1.250\times10^3\times8.26\times10^{-4}}$

$$= 0.000623 \text{ H/m}$$

Relative permeability $\mu_r = \frac{\mu}{\mu_0} = \frac{0.000623}{4\pi\times10^{-7}} = 496$ **Ans.**

Example 7: A cast steel electromagnet has an air gap length of 3 mm and an iron path of length 40 cm. Find the number of ampere-turns necessary to produce a flux density of 0.7 Wb/m² in the gap. Neglect leakage and fringing. Assume ampere-turns required for air gap to be 70% of the total ampere-turns.

[RGPV; Basic Electrical Engineering 2001]

Solution:

Air-gap length $l_g = 3 \text{ mm} = 3\times10^{-3} \text{ m}$

Flux density required in the air gap

$$\mathbf{B}_g = 0.7 \text{ Wb/m}^2$$

Magnetising force, $\mathbf{H}_g = \frac{\mathbf{B}}{\mu_0,\mu_r} = \frac{0.7}{4\pi\times10^{-7}\times1} = 5.57\times10^5 \text{ AT/m}$ $\quad\therefore \mu_r$ for air $= 1$

Ampere-turns required for the air gap

$$AT_g = H_g l_g = 5.57\times10^5 \times 3\times10^{-3} = 1671$$

Since ampere-turns required for the air gap are 70% of the total ampere-turns i.e. $AT_g = 0.7$ AT (total ampere-turns required)

So total ampere-turns required

$$AT = \frac{AT_g}{0.7} = \frac{1671}{0.7} = 2387$$ **Ans.**

Example 8: A steel ring of 25 cm diameter and of circular section 3 cm in diameter has an air gap of 1.5 mm length. It is wound uniformly with 750 turns of wire carrying a current of 2.1 A. Calculate (i) magnetomotive force (ii) flux density in air gap (iii) magnetic flux (iv) relative permeability of steel ring. Assume that iron path takes about 35% of the total magnetomotive force. **[RGPV; Basic Electrical Engineering, February 2005]**

Solution:

Area of a section $a = \frac{\pi}{4}(d)^2 = \frac{\pi}{4}\left(3\times10^{-2}\right)^2 = 0.0007\ \text{m}^2$

(i) Magnetomotive force

$$AT = N\times I = 750\times2.1 = 1575$$ **Ans.**

Ampere-turns provided for iron path

$$AT_i = 35\%\ \text{of total}\ AT = 0.35\times1575 = 551$$

Ampere-turns provided for air gap

$$AT_g = AT - AT_i = 1575 - 551 = 1024$$

(ii) Flux density in the air gap

$$B_g = \frac{AT_g \times \mu_0}{l_g} = \frac{1024\times4\pi\times10^{-7}}{1.5\times10^{-3}} = 0.858\ \text{T}$$ **Ans.**

(iii) Magnetic flux $\phi = B_g \times a = 0.858\times0.0007 = 0.6\ \text{mWb}$ **Ans.**

Assuming negligible leakage, we have

flux density in iron path $B_i = B_g = 0.858$ T

length of iron path $l_i = \pi\times D - l_g = \pi\times0.25 - 0.0015 = 0.784$ m

(iv) Relative permeability of steel

$$\mu_r = \frac{B_i l_i}{\mu_0 AT_i} = \frac{0.858\times0.784}{4\pi\times10^{-7}\times551} = 970$$ **Ans.**

Example 9: An iron ring of mean length 50 cm and relative permeability 300 has an air gap of 1 mm. If the ring is provided with a winding of 200 turns and a current of 1 A is allowed to flow through, find the flux density across the air gap. **[UP Univ; Elec Engineering, June 2001]**

Solution: Let the flux density through iron as well as air gap be B Wb/m^2

Total ampere turns provided

$$AT = N\times1 = 200\times1 = 200$$

Total ampere-turns required

$= AT$ required for air gap + AT required for iron ring

or Total ampere-turns provided

$$= \frac{B}{\mu_0} l_g + \frac{B}{\mu_0 \mu_r} l_i$$

$$\text{or } 200 = \frac{B}{\mu_0}\left(l_g + \frac{l_i}{\mu_r}\right) = \frac{B}{\mu_0}\left(0.001 + \frac{0.5}{300}\right)$$

$$\text{or flux density, } B = \frac{200 \times \mu_0}{0.001 + \frac{0.5}{300}} = \frac{200 \times 4\pi \times 10^{-7}}{0.001 + \frac{0.5}{300}} = 0.0942 \text{ T}$$ **Ans.**

Example 10: An iron ring is made up of three parts: $l_1 = 10$ cm, $A_1 = 8$ cm^2, $A_2 = 3$ cm^2, $l_3 = 6$ cm, $A_3 = 2.5$ cm^2. It is wound with a coil of 250 turns. Calculate current required to produce flux of 0.4 mWb. $\mu_1 = 2{,}670$, $\mu_2 = 1{,}050$, $\mu_3 = 600$.

[UP Technical Univ; Electrical Engineering, Second Semester 2007-08]

Solution:

Total reluctance, $S = \frac{l_1}{\mu_0 \mu_{r_1} a_1} + \frac{l_2}{\mu_0 \mu_{r_2} a_2} + \frac{l_3}{\mu_0 \mu_{r_3} a_3}$

$$= \frac{0.1}{4\pi \times 10^{-7} \times 2{,}670 \times 8 \times 10^{-4}} + \frac{0.08}{4\pi \times 10^{-7} \times 1{,}050 \times 3 \times 10^{-4}}$$

$$+ \frac{0.06}{4\pi \times 10^{-7} \times 600 \times 2.5 \times 10^{-4}}$$

$= 0.37225 \times 10^5 + 2.021 \times 10^5 + 3.183 \times 10^5$

$= 5.57655 \times 10^5$ AT/Wb

mmf $=$ Flux $\phi \times$ Reluctance S

$= 0.4 \times 10^{-3} \times 5.57655 \times 10^{-5} = 223$ ampere-turn

Current required $I = \frac{\text{mmf}}{N} = \frac{223}{250} = 0.892$ A **Ans.**

Example 11: A rectangular magnetic core shown in figure below has square crosssection area 16 cm^2. An air gap of 2 mm is cut across one of its limbs. Find the exciting current needed in the coil having 1000 turns wound on the core to create an air-gap flux of 4 mWb. The relative permeability of the core is 2000.

[UP Technical Univ; Electrical Engineering, Feb. 2002]

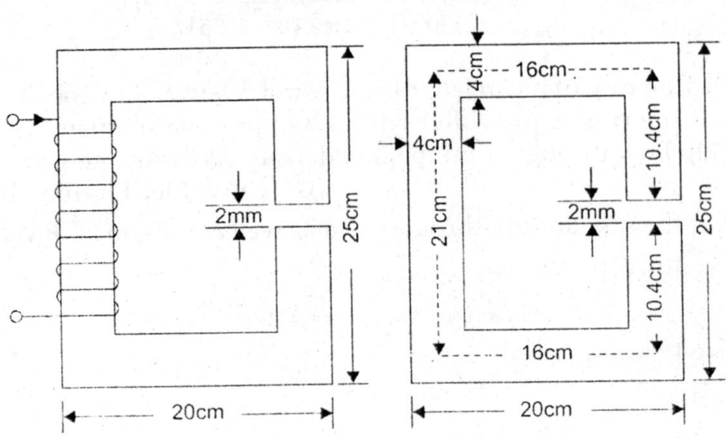

Solution: Flux to be created

$$\phi = 4 \text{ mWb} = 0.004 \text{ Wb}$$

Area of cross-section $a = 16 \text{ cm}^2 = 16 \times 10^{-4} \text{ m}^2$

Fluse density required $B = \dfrac{\phi}{a}$

$$= \frac{4 \times 10^{-3}}{16 \times 10^{-4}} = 2.5 \text{ T}$$

Length of air gap $l_g = 2 \text{ mm} = 2 \times 10^{-3} \text{ m}$

Each side of cross-section $= \sqrt{16} = 4 \text{ cm}$

Length of iron path $l_i = \left(25 - 2 \times \dfrac{4}{2} + 20 - 2 \times \dfrac{4}{2}\right) \times 2 - 0.2$

$$= 73.8 \text{ cm} = 0.738 \text{ m}$$

Total ampere-turns required

$$AT = \frac{B}{\mu_0} l_g + \frac{B}{\mu_0 \mu_r} l_i = \frac{2.5 \times 2 \times 10^{-3}}{4\pi \times 10^{-7}} + \frac{2.5 \times 0.738}{2{,}000 \times 4\pi \times 10^{-7}}$$

$$= 3979 + 734 = 4713$$

Number of turns on the coil $= 1{,}000$

Exciting current required, $I = \dfrac{AT}{N} = \dfrac{4713}{1000} = 4.713 \text{ A}$ **Ans.**

Example 12: The magnetic circuit frame shown in figure is built of iron of square cross-section of 3 cm. Each air gap is 2 mm wide and each of the coil is wound with 1,000 turns. The relative permeability of part A and B may be taken as 1,000 and 1,200 respectively. Calculate (a) reluctance of part A (b) reluctance of two air gaps (c) total reluctance of complete magnetic path (d) total *mmf* (e) total flux and (f) flux density.

Solution: Cross-sectional area

$$a = (0.03)^2 = 0.009 \text{ m}^2$$

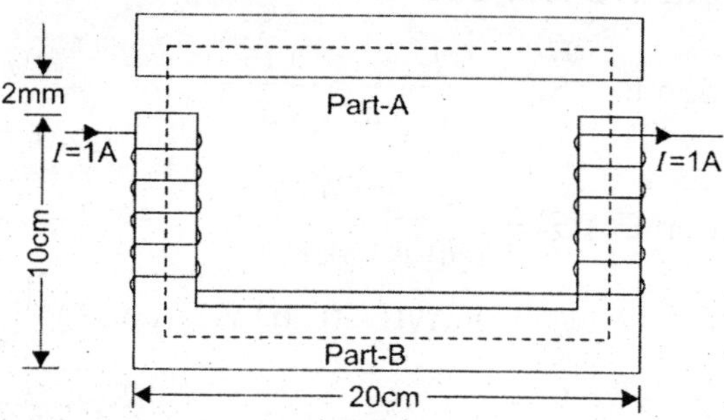

Mean length flux path in part *A*

$$l_A = 20 - (1.5 + 1.5) = 17 \text{ cm or } 0.17 \text{ m}$$

Mean length flux path in part *B*

$$l_B = (20 - 1.5 - 1.5) + (10 - 1.5) + (10 - 1.5)$$
$$= 34 \text{ cm or } 0.34 \text{ m}$$

Relative permeability of part A

$$\mu_{r_A} = 1000$$

Relative permeability of part *B*

$\mu_{r_B} = 1200$

Length of two air-gaps, $l_g = 2 \times 2 = 4$ mm $= 0.004$ m

(a) Reluctance of Part A $S_A = \dfrac{0.17}{4\pi \times 10^{-7} \times 1000 \times 0.0009} = 150313$ AT/Wb **Ans.**

Reluctance of Part B $S_B = \dfrac{l_B}{\mu_0 \mu_{r_B} \times a} = \dfrac{0.34}{4\pi \times 10^{-7} \times 1200 \times 0.0009}$

$= 250521$ AT/Wb

(b) Reluctance of two air-gaps

$$S_g = \frac{l_g}{\mu_0 a} = \frac{0.004}{4\pi \times 10^{-7} \times 0.0009} = 35.36776 \text{ AT/Wb}$$ **Ans.**

(c) Total reluctance $S = S_A + S_B + S_g = 150313 + 250521 + 3536776$

$= 3937610$ AT/Wb **Ans.**

(d) Total mmf $= 2 \times 1000 \times 1 = 2000$ AT **Ans.**

because mmf is produced by two coils on part *B* each having 1,000 turns and carrying a current of 1 A.

(e) Total flux $= \dfrac{\text{mmf}}{\text{Reluctance}} = \dfrac{2000}{3937610} = 5.08 \times 10^{-4}$ Wb

(f) Flux density $B = \dfrac{\phi}{a} = \dfrac{5.08 \times 10^{-4}}{0.0009} = 0.564 \text{ Wb/m}^2$ (or Tesla) **Ans.**

Example 13: A case steel magnetic structure made of a bar of section 2 cm × 2 cm is shown in figure. Determine the current that the 500 turn magnetizing coil on the left limb should carry so that a flux of 2 m Wb is produced in the right limb. Taken $\mu_r = 600$ and neglect leakage.

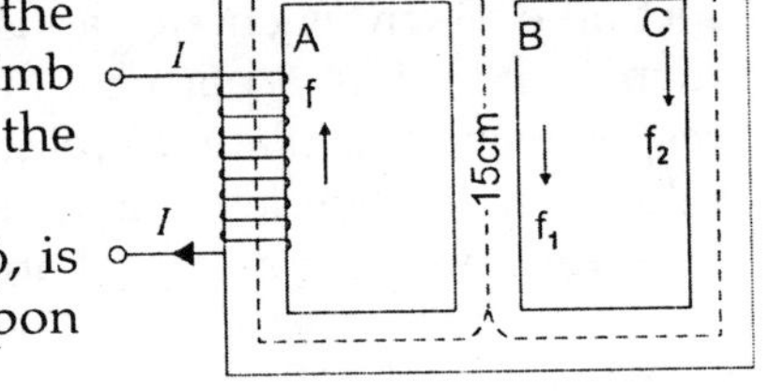

Solution: Flux created by magnetizing coil, say ϕ, is divided at junction point into two paths depending upon the reluctances of portions B and C respectively.

Reluctance of portion B $S_B = \dfrac{l_B}{\mu_0 \mu_r \times a} = \dfrac{0.15}{\mu_0 \mu_r a}$

Reluctance of portion C $S_C = \dfrac{l_C}{\mu_0 \mu_r a} = \dfrac{0.25}{\mu_0 \mu_r a}$

Flux in portion C $\phi_C = 2\text{mWb} = 0.002$ Wb (given)

Flux in portion B $\phi_B = \phi_C \times \dfrac{S_C}{S_B} = 2 \times 10^{-3} \times \dfrac{0.25/\mu_0 \mu_r a}{0.15/\mu_0 \mu_r a}$

$= 3.33 \times 10^{-3}$ Wb

Total flux in portion A, $\phi = \phi_B + \phi_C$

$= 3.33 \times 10^{-3} + 2 \times 10^{-3} = 5.33 \times 10^{-3}$ Wb

Flux density in portion A

$$B_A = \frac{\phi}{A} = \frac{5.33 \times 10^{-3}}{4 \times 10^{-4}} = 13.33 \text{ Wb/m}^2$$

AT required for portion A

$$AT_A = \frac{BA \times l_A}{\mu_0\mu_r} = \frac{13.33 \times 0.25}{4\pi \times 10^{-7} \times 600} = 4416$$

Flux density in path B $\quad B_B = \frac{3.33 \times 10^{-3}}{4 \times 10^{-4}}$

$$= 8.33 \text{ Wb/m}^2$$

At required for portion B

$$AT_B = \frac{B_B l_B}{\mu_0\mu_r} = \frac{8.33 \times 0.15}{4\pi \times 10^{-7} \times 600} = 1658$$

Total ampere-turns required

$$AT = AT_A + AT_B = 4416 + 1658 = 6074$$ **Ans.**

Example 14: A coil of 1000 turns is wound on a laminated core of steel having a cross-section of 5 cm^2, the core has an air gap of 2 mm cut at right angle. What value of current is required to have an air gap flux density 0.5 *T*. Permeability of steel may be taken as infinity. Determine the coil inductance.

[UP Technical Univ; Electrical Engineering; First Semester 2003-4]

Solution: Total ampere-turns required

$$AT = \frac{B}{\mu_0\mu_r} l_i + \frac{B}{\mu_0} l_g$$

$$= 0 + \frac{0.5}{4\pi \times 10^{-7}} \times 2 \times 10^{-3} = 796 \qquad [\because \mu_r = \infty]$$

Current required $\quad i = \frac{AT}{N} = \frac{796}{1000} = 0.796 \text{ A}$

Inductance of coil $\quad L = \frac{N\phi}{i} = \frac{1000 \times 0.5 \times 5 \times 10^{-4}}{0.796}$

$$= 0.314 \text{ H}$$

Example 15: A toroid has a core of square cross-section 2500 m^2 in area and a mean diameter of 250 mm. The core material has a relative permeability 1000. Calculate the number of turns wound on the core to obtain an inductance of 1 H.

Solution: Length of core

$$l = \pi \times D = \pi \times 0.25 = 0.25\pi \text{ meters}$$

Area of cross-section of core

$$a = 2500 \text{ mm}^2 = 0.0025 \text{ m}^2$$

Relative permeability of core material

$$\mu_r = 1000$$

$$\mu_0 = 4\pi \times 10^{-7} \text{ H/m}$$

Self inductance of coil $\quad L = 1 \text{ H}$

$$\therefore \quad L = \frac{N^2 a\mu_0\mu_r}{l}$$

Number of turns on the coil

$$N = \sqrt{\frac{L \times l}{\mu_0\mu_r a}} = \sqrt{\frac{1 \times 0.25\pi}{4\pi \times 10^{-7} \times 1000 \times 0.0025}} = 500$$ **Ans.**

Example 16: The core of a magnetic circuit is of mean length 40 cm and uniform cross-sectional area 4 cm^2. The relative permeability of the core material is 1000. An air gap of 1 mm is cut in the core, and 1000 turns are wound on the core. Determine the inductance of the coil if fringing is negligible.

[UP Technical Univ, Electrical Engineering; First Semester 2008-09)

Solution: Mean length of core

$$l_i = 40 - 0.1 = 39.9 \text{ cm} = 0.399 \text{ m}$$

cross-sectional area of core, $a = 4 \text{ cm}^2 = 0.0004 \text{ m}^2$

Relative permeability of core material

$$\mu_r = 1000$$

Air gap length $l_g = 1 \text{ mm} = 0.001 \text{ m}$

Number of turns wound on the core

$$N = 1000$$

Assuming flux density in the core to be B Wb/m^2

Total ampere-turns required

$$AT = \frac{B}{\mu_0 \mu_r} l_i + \frac{B}{\mu_0} l_g$$

$$= \frac{B}{4\pi \times 10^{-7} \times 1{,}000} \times 0.399 + \frac{B}{4\pi \times 10^{-7}} \times 0.001$$

$$= 317.5 \text{ B} + 795.8 \text{ B} = 1113 \text{ B}$$

Current required $I = \frac{AT}{N} = \frac{1.113}{1000} \text{B} = 1.113 \text{ B}$

Flux $\phi = B \times a = B \times 0.0004 = 0.0004 \text{ B}$

Inductance of coil $L = \frac{N\phi}{I} = \frac{1000 \times 0.0004\text{B}}{1.113\text{B}} = 0.359 \text{ H}$ **Ans.**

EXERCISES

1. Define terms: mmf, flux and reluctance and give their relationship.
   [Mahamaya Technical Univ Electrical Engineering, Second Semester 2011-12]
2. Describe the analogies that can be made between electric and magnetic circuit regarding the following items: driving force, field intensity, impedance drops, equivalent circuits. **[UP Technical Univ; Electrical Engineering; First Semester, 2008-09]**
3. Explain magnetic and electric circuits. Give analogy between them.
   [UP Technical Univ; Electrical Engineering; Second Semester 2006-07]
4. Give analogous characteristics of electrical and magnetic circuits.
   [UP Technical Univ; Electrical Engineering; First Semester 2007-08]
5. Establish the analogy between electric and magnetic circuits.
   [UP Technical Univ; Electrical Engineering; Second Semester 2007-08]
6. Draw and explain *B-H* curve. What is meant by saturation, coercive force, residual magnetism? Show them in diagram.
   [GB Technical Univ; Electrical Engineering; Second Semester 2011-12]
7. How is *B-H* curve of a ferromagnetic material different from that of a non-magnetic material? Name all the salient regions of ***B-H*** curve of magnetic material.
   [UP Technical Univ; Electrical Engineering; First Semester 2003-04]

8. Draw and explain hysteresis loop. What is its significance?
[GB Technical Univ; Electrical Engineering; Second Semester 2009-10]
9. State and explain Faraday's laws of electromagnetic induction, Lenz's law, Fleming's right hand rule and Fleming's left hand rule.
[VTU Belgaum; Karnataka Univ; Summer 2003]
10. State the following:
    (i) Magnetic flux and its properties
    (ii) Flux density
    (iii) Fleming's right hand rule
    (iv) Fleming's left hand rule
    (v) Lenz'slaw
[GB Technical Univ Electrical Engineering, Second Semester, 2009-10]
11. What do you understand by self-inductance? Derive its expression.
[Mahamaya Technical Univ; Electrical Engineering; First semester 2011-12]
12. Explain the concept of mutual inductance. Define coefficient of coupling and derive the expression between self-inductances of two coils, mutual inductance between them and the coefficient of coupling.
13. Define mutual inductance (M) and show that

$$K = \frac{M}{\sqrt{L_1 L_2}}, K \leq 1$$

where L_1 and L_2 are inductances of coil 1 and 2 respectively and K is coupling coefficient. **[Punjab Technical Univ; First Semester 2005-06]**

PROBLEMS FOR PRACTICE

1. A magnetic circuit has a uniform cross-sectional area of 5 cm^2 and a length of 25 cm. A coil of 120 turns is wound uniformly over the magnetic circuit. When the current in the coil is 1.5 A, the total flux is 0.3 mWb; when the current in the coil is 5 A, the total flux is 0.6 mWb. For each value of current, calculate (i) the magnetising force (ii) the relative permeability of iron as 1500. [**Ans.** 2546 AT]
2. Calculate the relative permeability of iron when the exciting current taken by the 600 turn coil is 1.2 A, and the total flux produced is 1 mWb. The mean circumference of the ring is 0.5 m and the area of cross-section is 10 cm^2. [**Ans.** 552]
3. A cast iron ring with a mean diameter of 10 cm and a cross-sectional area of 3 cm^2 has a radial gap of 0.15 cm. Calculate the current required through the winding of 1000 turns wound uniformly over the ring to produce a flux 2×10^{-4} Wb in the air gap. Take relative permeability of cast iron as 250. [**Ans.** 1.462 A]
4. A cast steel ring has a circular cross-section 3 cm diameter and a mean circumference of 80 cm. The ring is uniformly wound with a coil of 600 turns.
   (i) Estimate the current required to produce a flux of 0.5 mWb in the ring.
   (ii) If a saw cut of 2 mm wide is made in the ring, find approximately the flux produced by the current found in (i).
   Take ampere-turns per metre at the above flux density 670.
   [**Ans.** (i) 0.893 A (ii) 0.1614 mWb]
5. An iron ring of mean diameter 22 cm and cross-section 10 cm^2 has an air gap 1mm wide. The ring is wound uniformly with 200 turns of wire. The permeability of ring material is 1000. A flux of 0.16 mwb is required in the gap. What current should be passed through the wire? **[Punjab Univ; Elec. Engineering 1; April 1982]**
[**Ans.** 1075 A]

6. A flux density of 1 Wb/m^2 is required in a 2 mm air gap of an electromagnet with an iron path of 100 cm. Calculate the ampere-turns required for the same. Assume m for iron = 1900 and fringing around the air gap is neglected. **[Ans.** 2,110]
[Punjab Univ; Elec Circuits and System Nov; 1983]
7. An iron ring has a mean circumferential length of 60 cm with an air gap of 1 mm and a uniform winding of 300 turns. When a current of 1 A flows through the coil, find the flux density. The relative permeability of iron is 300. Assume $\mu = 4\pi \times 10^{-7}$ H/m **[Delhi Univ; Electrical Engg. I; 1970]** **[Ans.** 0.1256 *T*]
8. A magnetic ring has a mean circumference of 1.5 m and is of 0.01 m^2 in cross-section and is wound with 175 turns. A saw cut of 4 mm width is made in the ring. Calculate the magnetising current required to produce a flux of 0.8 mWb in the air-gap. Assume permeability of iron as 400 and leakage factor of 1.25.
[Punjab Univ; Applied Electricity Nov. 1974] **[Ans.** 3.16 A]
9. An iron ring of mean circumference 80 cm is made from round iron of area 8 cm^2. It has a saw cut of 2 mm wide and is wound with 500 turns. Find the current required to produce a flux of 0.8 mWb across the air-gap. Assume a relative permeability for iron as 625 and leakage factor of 1.25. **[Ans.** 5.73 A]
10. The magnetic circuit shown in figure below is built-up of iron of square cross-section, 2 cm wide. Each air gap is 2 mm wide, m for part A may be taken as 900 and for B as 1250. Each of the exciting coils is wound with 1200 turns and the exciting coil is carrying current 0.8 ampere. Find:
    (i) Reluctance of A (*iv*) Total reluctance
    (ii) Reluctance of B (*v*) Total flux
    (iii) Reluctance of two air gap (*vi*) Flux density (neglecting leakage)
[RGPV Bhopal; Basic Electrical Engineering June, 2007]

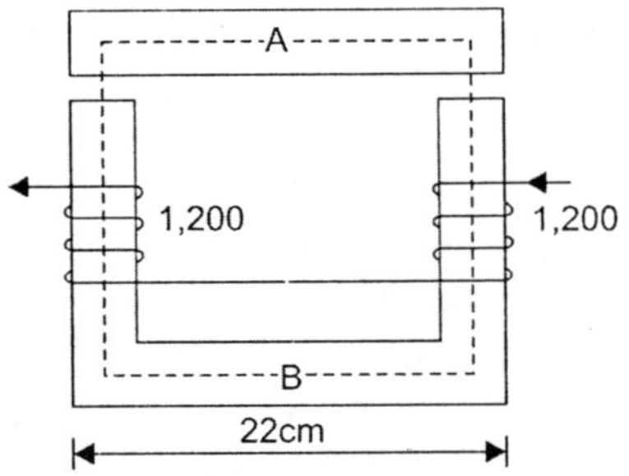

[Ans. (i) 442,100 AT/Wb, (ii) 626,620 AT/Wb, (iii) 7,957,750 AT/Wb, (iv) 9,036,470 AT/Wb, (v) 0.2125 mWb (vi) 0.53 Wb/m^2 or Tesla]

Chapter

11 Single Phase Transformer

11.1 INTRODUCTION

The transformer is probably one of the most useful electrical device. It is an static device which is used to transfer electric power from one circuit to another without changing its frequency. The main function of transformer is to raise as lower, the voltage in a circuit with corresponding decrease or increase in current at the same frequency. It works on the principle of Faraday's law of electromagnetic induction. Tranformer have no moving parts, rugged and durable in construction. The efficiency of transformer is very high and lie between 92% and 95%.

11.2 TRANSFORMER AS A DEVICE

Transformer is a static device (there is no rotating part). It transfer energy or power from one side to another side at same frequency. It has two windings, primary, and secondary winding. There is no interconnection between primary and secondary. Its basic principle of operation is based on mutual induction (Figs 11.1 and 11.2).

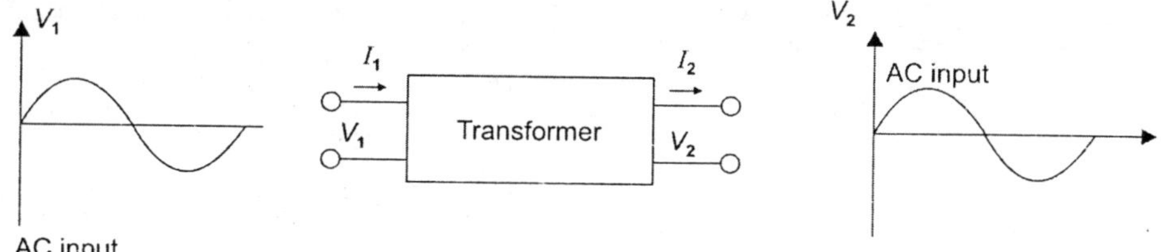

Fig. 11.1

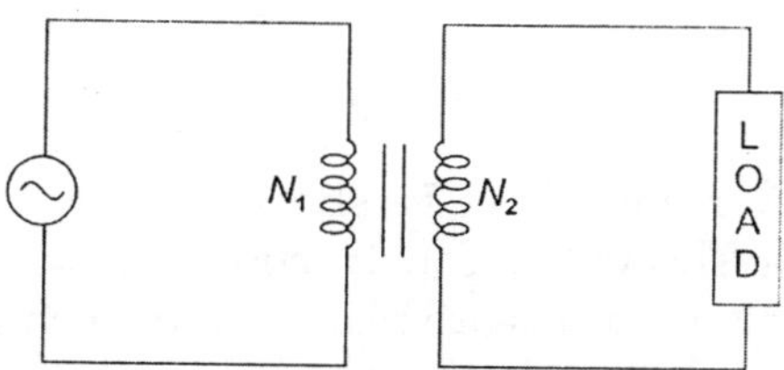

Fig. 11.2: Symbol of transformer

11.3 CLASSIFICATION OF TRANSFORMER

(a) On the basic of phase
   (i) Single phase transformer (ii) Three-phase transformer
(b) On the basic of construction
   (i) Shell type (ii) Core type
   (iii) Berry type
(c) On the basic of application
   (i) Step-up transformer (ii) Step-down transformer

Types of Transformer on the Basic of Construction

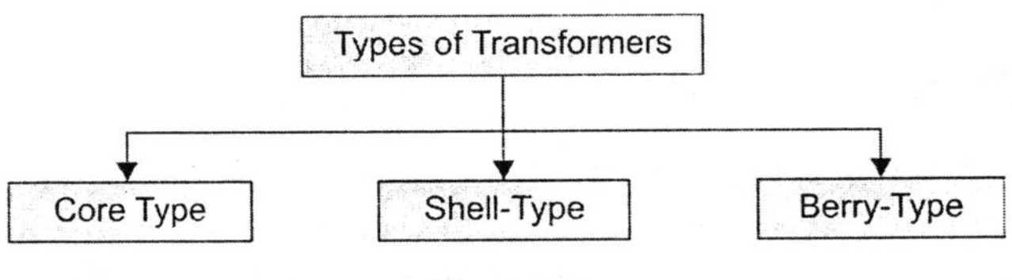

Fig. 11.3

(a) **Core type transformer:** The construction of core type transformer is shown in Fig. 11.3a and 11.4a. The core of this transformer is in the form of a rectangular frame made from laminations. It provides a single magnetic circuit as shown in Fig. 11.4b. The primary and secondary windings are uniformly distributed on two limbs of the core. Both the windings are of cylindrical shape and they are arranged in a concentric manner with the low voltage winding placed near the core. In core type transformer, the windings surround a considerable portion of the core.

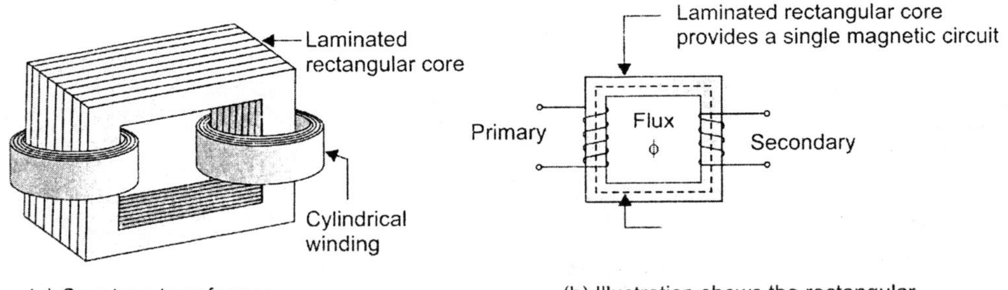

(a) Core type transformer

(b) Illustration shows the rectangular core provides magnetic circuit

Fig. 11.4

(b) **Shell type transformer:** Figure 11.5a shows the construction of a shell type transformer. Fig. 11.5b shows the construction of a shell type transformer. The primary and secondary windings are placed on the central limb of the core. The high voltage and low voltage windings are of sandwich type, which are in the form of interleaved pancakes. This type of core provides double magnetic circuit. This type of core provides a better mechanical support and protection for the windings. In shell-type transformer, the core surround a considerable portion of the windings.

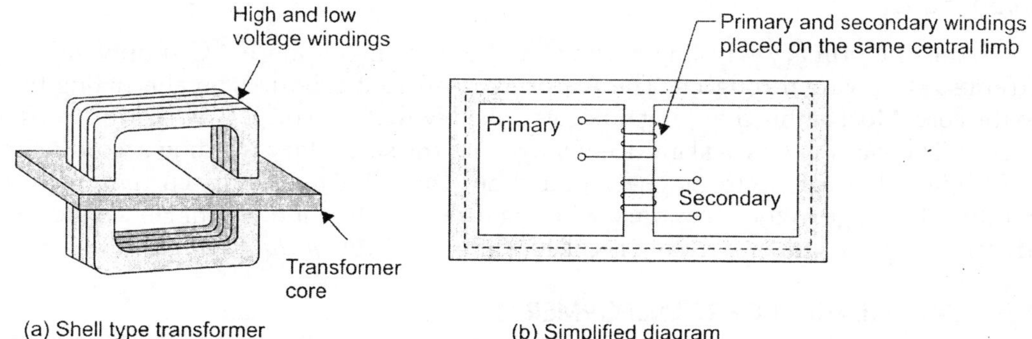

(a) Shell type transformer

(b) Simplified diagram

Fig. 11.5

(c) **Berry type transformers:** The berry type transformer is shown in Fig. 11.6. The construction of the core is such that the yoke radiates out from the centre, similar to the spokes of a wheel. Due to this construction, the berry type transformer has a distributed magnetic circuit. The high voltage and low voltage windings are placed as shown in Fig. 11.6 with the low voltage winding placed inside the high voltage winding placed outside.

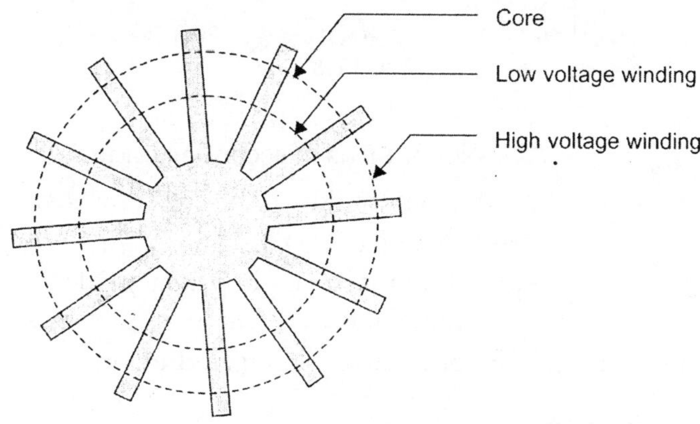

Fig. 11.6: Plane view of berry type transformer

11.4 PRINCIPLE OF OPERATION OF TRANSFORMER

A transformer with primary and secondary windings is shown in Fig. 11.7.

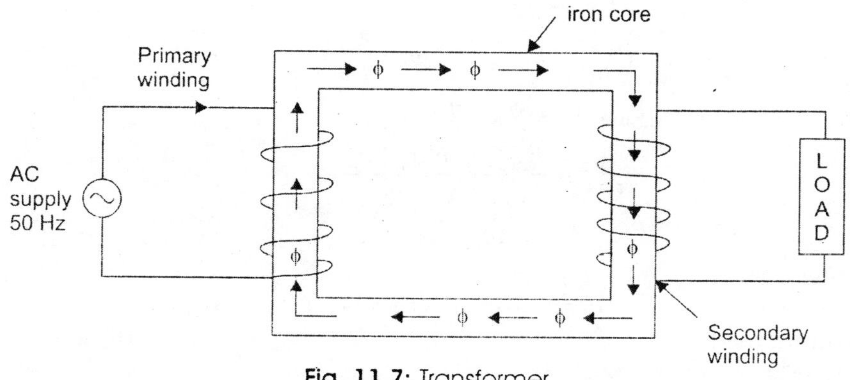

Fig. 11.7: Transformer

Explanations

As soon as the primary winding is connected to the single-phase AC supply, an AC current start flowing through it. The AC primary current produces an alternating flux ϕ in the core. Most of this changing flux gets linked with the secondary winding through the core. The varying flux will induce voltage into the secondary winding according to the Faraday's laws of electromagnetic induction. Thus, due to primary current, there is an induced voltage in the secondary winding due to mutual induction. Hence the emf induced in the secondary winding is called as the *mutually induced emf.*

11.5 EMF EQUATION OF TRANSFORMER

[UPTU 2009-10, 2010-11]

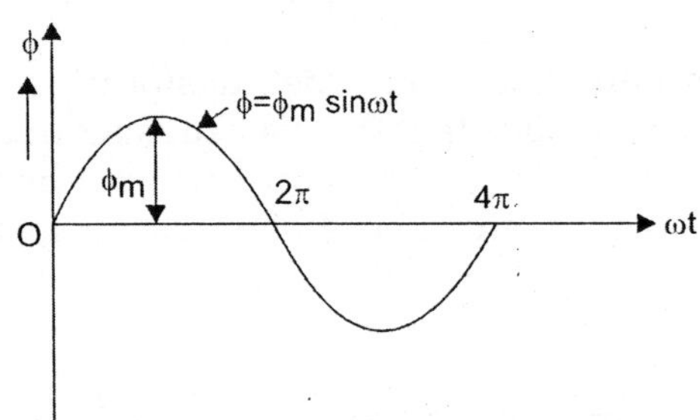

Fig. 11.8

Let

N_1 = No. of turns in primary side

N_2 = No. of turns in secondary side

ϕ_m = maximum flux in the core in weber

f = frequency (Hz)

E_1 = self induced emf in primary side

E_2 = mutual induced emf in secondary side

According to the Faraday's law of electromagnetic induction

$$\therefore \quad \text{Induced emf} = -\frac{Nd\phi}{dt}\,\text{V}$$

$$e = -\frac{Nd(\phi_m \sin\omega t)}{dt}\,\text{V}$$

$$= -N\phi_m\,\omega(\cos\omega t) = N\phi_m\,\omega \sin\left(\omega t - \frac{\pi}{2}\right)$$

$$= E_{max} \sin\left(\omega t - \frac{\pi}{2}\right)$$

where $E_{max} = N\phi_m\, 2\pi f$

$$\therefore \quad E_{rms} = \frac{E_{max}}{\sqrt{2}} = \frac{N\phi_m\, 2\pi f}{\sqrt{2}}$$

$$= 4.44\phi_m f N \text{ volts}$$

For primary side

$$E_1 = 4.44\phi_m f N_1 \text{ volts}$$

For secondary side

$$E_2 = 4.44\phi_m f N_2 \text{ volts}$$

11.6 TRANSFORMATION RATIO (K)

The transformation ratio for voltage is defined as the ratio of secondary voltage to the primary voltage of a transformer. It is denoted by *K*.

$$K = \frac{V_2}{V_1} = \frac{E_2}{E_1} = \frac{N_2}{N_1}$$

For ideal transformer, i.e. no losses

$\therefore$ Input power = output power

$$V_1 I_1 = V_2 I_2$$

$$\frac{V_2}{V_1} = \frac{I_1}{I_2}$$

$$K = \frac{V_2}{V_1} = \frac{I_1}{I_2} = \frac{E_2}{E_1} = \frac{N_2}{N_1}$$

Note: $K > 1$ for step-up transformer. $K < 1$ for step-down transformer.

SOLVED EXAMPLES ON ABOVE THEORY

Example 1: The maximum flux density in the core of a 250/3000 V, 50 Hz single phase transformer is 1.2 Wb/m^2. If the emf per tunrs is 8 volt. Determine (i) primary and secondary turns (ii) area of the core.

Solution: Given data

$$E_1 = 250 \text{ V}$$
$$E_2 = 3000 \text{ V}$$
$$B_m = 1.2 \text{ wb/m}^2$$

(i) $E_1 = N_1 \times$ emf indcued/turns

$$N_1 = \frac{E_1}{\text{emf induced/turns}} = \frac{250}{8} = 32$$ **Ans.**

Similarly, $N_2 = \frac{3000}{8} = 375$ **Ans.**

(ii) $E_2 = 4.44 \text{ N}_2 \text{ B}_m \text{ A}$ [since $\phi_m = B_m A$]

$$A = \frac{3000}{4.44 \times 375 \times 50 \times 1.2} = 0.03 \text{ m}^2$$

Example 2: A single phase transformer has 400 primary and 1000 secondary turns. The net cross-sectional area of the core is 60 cm^2. If the primary winding be connected to a 50 Hz supply at 520 V. Calcualte (i) the peak value of flux density in the core (ii) Voltage induced in the secondary winding.

Solution: Given data

$$N_1 = 400, \; N_2 = 1000$$
$$f = 50 \text{ Hz}, \; E_1 = 520 \text{ V} = \text{V}_1$$

(i) $E_1 = 4.44\phi f N_1$

$$E_1 = 4.44 B_m A f N_1$$
$$520 = 4.44 \times B_m \times 60 \times 10^{-4} \times 50 \times 400$$

$\therefore$ $B_m = 0.976 \text{ wb/m}^2$ **Ans.**

(ii)
$$\frac{E_2}{E_1} = K$$

$$\therefore \quad K = \frac{N_2}{N_1} = \frac{1000}{400} = 2.5$$

$$E_2 = KE_1 = 2.5 \times 520 = 1300 \text{ V}$$ **Ans.**

11.7 IDEAL TRANFORMER

An ideal transformer is an imaginary transformer and possesses the following properties:

(a) Its primary and secondary winding resistance are negligible.

(b) It has no losses thus efficiency is 100%.

(c) Leakage flux is zero, i.e. 100% flux produced by primary links with the secondary.

11.8 PRACTICAL TRANSFORMER

In discussion, we considered the properties of an ideal transformer, certain assumptions were made which are not valid in a practical transformer. For example in a practical transformer the winding have resistance, the core has finite permeability and there is a leakage flux. The efficiency of a practical transformer is not 100% due to the losses. Therefore, in practical transformer, we shall consider all these imperfections (Fig. 11.1).

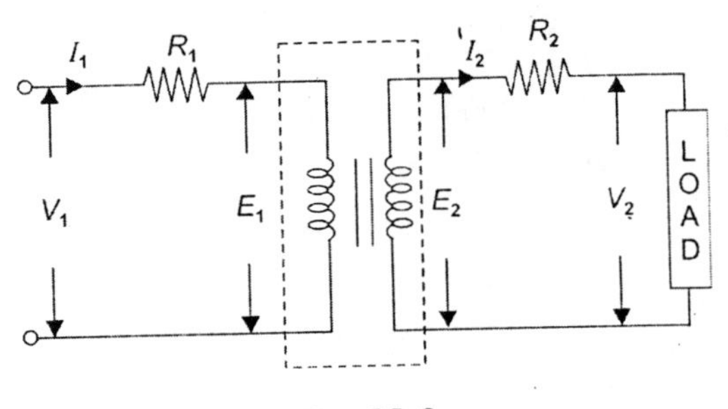

Fig. 11.9

Winding Resistance

An ideal transformer is supposed to posses no resistance, but in actual transformer there is always some resistance of primary and secondary windings as shown in the Fig. 11.9. The primary and secondary windings resistance will causes a copper loss and voltage drop in the windings.

Leakage Reactance

In an ideal transformer it is assumed that all the flux produced by the primary winding links both the primary and secondary winding. However, in an actual transformer not all of the flux remains within the magnetic core. A portion of this flux is diverted to the nonferromagnetic material surrounding the winding (generally air or oil). This is because the surrounding medium also has a definite permeability although it is very much less than that of the core. This small portion of the flux which transverses an external path is known as *primary leakage flux*.

11.9 PRACTICAL TRANSFORMER ON NO-LOAD

A transformer is said to be at no load when the secondary winding is open circuited. The secondary current is thus zero. When an alternating voltage is applied to the primary, a small current I_0 is flows in the primary. The current I_0 is called the no-load current of the transformer. It is made up of two components as shown in the block-diagram (Fig. 11.10).

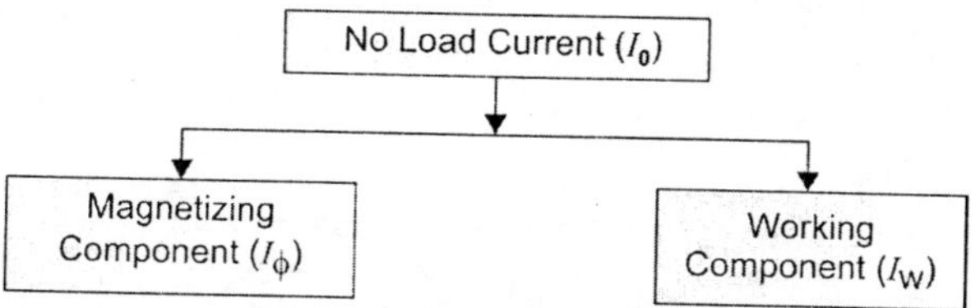

Fig. 11.10: Block diagram

(a) **Magnetizing component:** This is a purely reactive component of no-load current I_0. It magnetizes the core and produces flux in the core therefore I_ϕ in phase with flux ϕ as shown in Fig. 11.11. The current I_ϕ is also called reactive or wattless component of no load current.

(b) **Working component:** The function of working component to supply the total loss under no load condition, i.e. it supplies hysteresis and eddy current losses in the core and the negligible I^2R loss in the primary winding. It is at 90° with respect to the magnetizing component (I_ϕ) as shown in the phasor diagram shown in Fig. 11.11. It is also called watt full component or coreloss component.

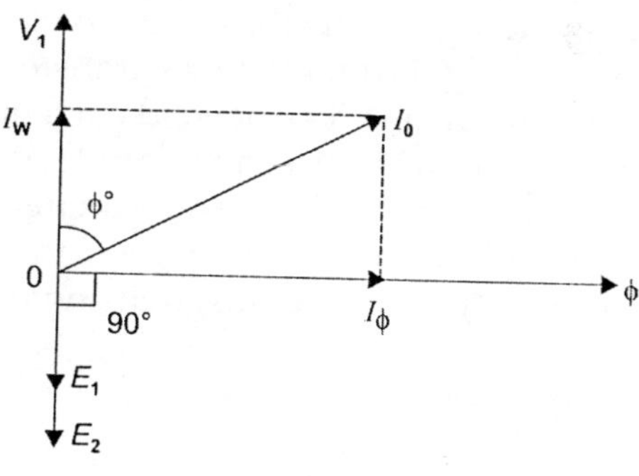

Fig. 11.11: Phasor diagram

The total no load current I_0 is the vector addition of I_f and I_W

$$\therefore \quad I_0 = I_\phi + I_w$$

where

$$I_\phi = I_0 \sin \phi_0$$

$$I_W = I_0 \cos \phi_0$$

The magnitude of the no load current is given by

$$I_0 = \sqrt{I_\phi^2 + I_w^2}$$

while ϕ_0 = no load primary power factor angle

The total power input on no-load is denoted by W_0

$$\therefore \quad W_0 = V_1 I_0 \cos\phi_0$$

11.10 TRANSFORMER ON LOAD

A transformer is said to be on load if its secondary side is connected to the load. When the secondary is loaded, the secondary current I_2 flows through it. The phase angle of secondary current I_2 with respect to V_2 depends upon the nature of load, i.e. whether the load is resistive, inductive or capacitive. If load is resistaive I_2 is in phase with V_2. If load is inductive, I_2 lags V_2 while for capacitive load, I_2 leads V_2.

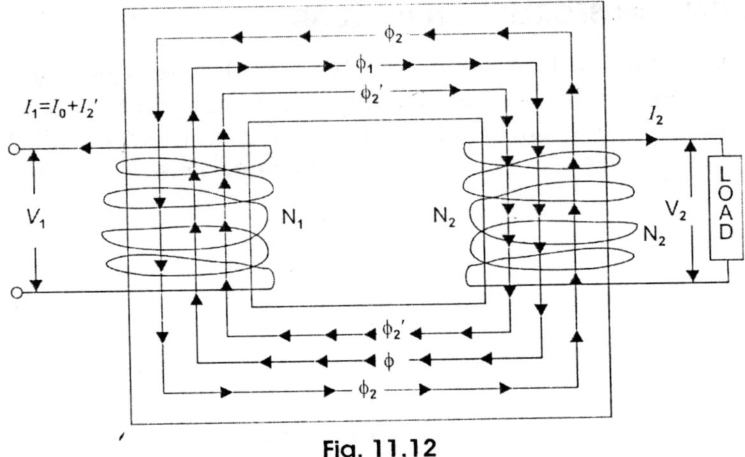

Fig. 11.12

Explanation

The working of transformer on load can easily be explained with the help of diagram shown in Fig. 11.12. When the transformer is at no-load it draws no-load current I_0 from the supply mains. The no load current I_0 produces mmf N_1I_0 which set up flux ϕ in the core. When the transformer is at load, current I_2 flows in the secondary winding. This secondary current I_2 produces an mmf N_2I_2 which is set up flux in the core. According to Lenz's law, this flux ϕ_2 opposes the flux ϕ which is set up by the current I_0. Hence the mmf $N = I_2$ is called demagnetizing ampere turns. This is shown in Fig. 11.13.

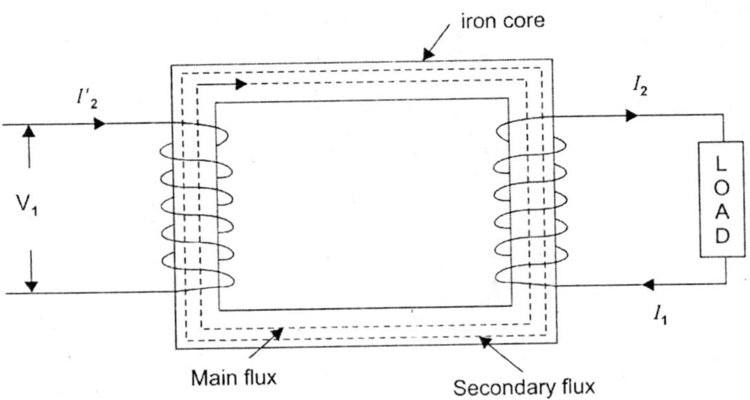

Fig. 11.13: ϕ_2 opposes ϕ

The flux ϕ_2 momentarily reduces the main flux ϕ_2 due to which the primary induced emf E_1 also reduces. Hence the vector difference $\boldsymbol{V_1 - E_1}$ increases due to which primary draws more current from the supply. This additional current drawn by primary is due to the load hence called load component of primary current denoted as I_2' as shown in the Fig. 11.14. This current I_2' is in anti-phase with I_2. The current I_2' sets up its own flux ϕ_2' which opposes the flux ϕ_2 and helps the main flux ϕ. This flux ϕ_2' neutralizes the flux ϕ_2 produced by I_2. The mmf, i.e. ampere turns $N_1 I_2'$, balance the ampere turns N_2I_2, hence the net flux in the core is again maintained at constant level. The load components current I_2' always neutralises the changes in the load. As practically flux in core is constant, the core loss is also constant for all the loads. Hence the transformer is called *constant flux machine*.

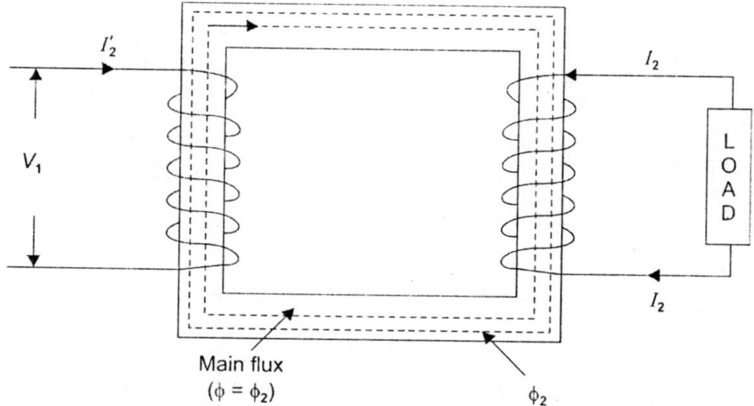

Fig. 11.14: Illustration shows primary draws more current

Phasor Diagram on Load

As the ampere turns are balanced, we can write

$$N_2 I_2 = N_1 I_2'$$

$$I_2' = \frac{N_2}{N_1} I_2 = K I_2$$

Thus when transformer is loaded, the primary current I_1 has two compenents. The no load current I_0 which lags V_1 by angle ϕ_0. It has two components I_m and I_c. The load component I_2' which is in anti-phase with I_2 and phase of I_2 is decided by the load.

Hence primary current $\boldsymbol{I}_1$ is vector sum of I_0 and I_2'.

$$\boldsymbol{I}_1 = \boldsymbol{I}_0 + \boldsymbol{I}_2' = I_0 + I_2'$$

Now, let us discuss the three cases of load and phasor diagram neglecting the voltage drop in winding as shown in Fig. 11.15.

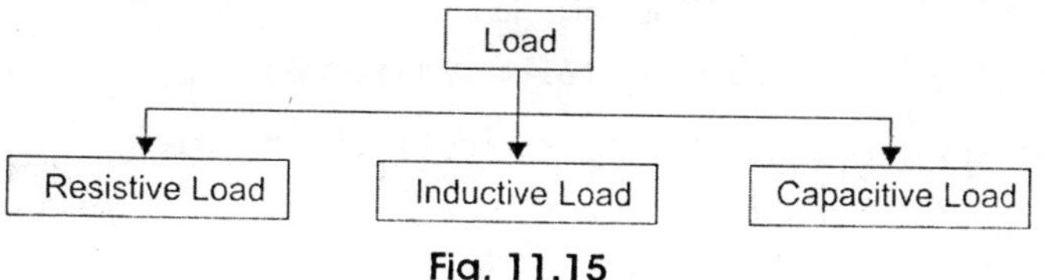

Fig. 11.15

Steps to draw phasor diagram

Voltage drop in winding of transformer is neglected

$$\therefore \quad V_1 = E_1 \text{ and } E_2 = V_2$$

Consider flux ϕ as a reference phasor as it is linked to both primary and secondary sides. Draw I_0 as it is constant for all loads.

E_1 lags ϕ by 90°, reverse E_1 to get $-E_1$ $(V_1 = -E_1)$.

E_1 and E_2 are in phase.

(*a*) For purely resistive load, I_2 in phase with V_2 or E_2.

(*b*) For inductive load, I_2 lags E_2 by ϕ_2.

(*c*) For capacitive load, I_2 leads E_2 by ϕ_2.

Counter balance current $I_2' = KI_2$, let $K = 1$ then $I_2' = I_2$ is 180° out of the phase with I_2. (I_2' is always is anti-phase with I_2).

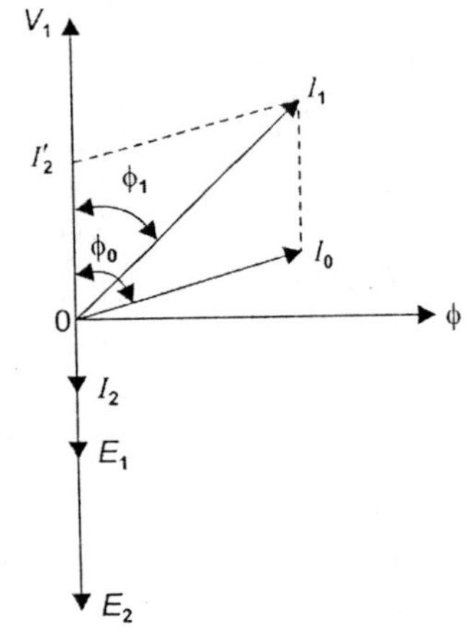

(a) Resistive load

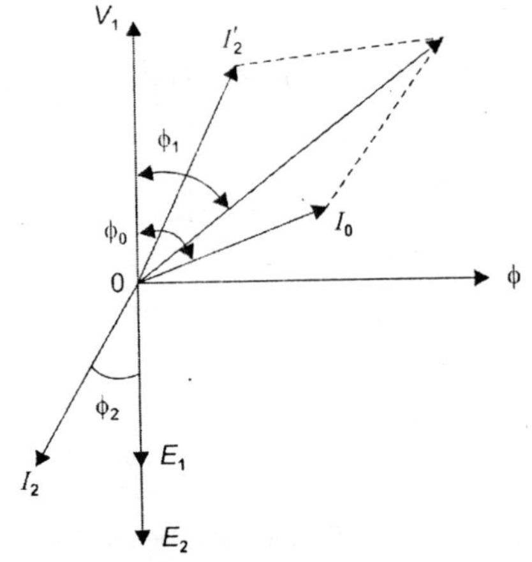

(b) Inductive load

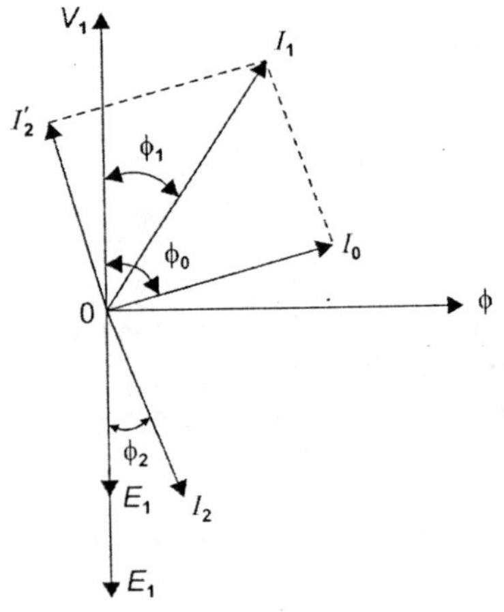

(c) Capacitive load

Fig. 11.16: Phasor diagram

The total primary current I_1 is vector sum of no load current I_0 and counter balance current I_2', i.e.

$$I_1 = I_0 + I_2' = I_0 + I_2'$$

11.11 EQUIVALENT CIRCUIT DIAGRAM

Importance of Equivalent Circuit Diagram

Equivalent circuit diagram makes calculation easy. We can analyse and investigate any electrical device with the help of equivalent circuit. Equivalent circuit can be studied and analysed easily by the electric circuit theory.

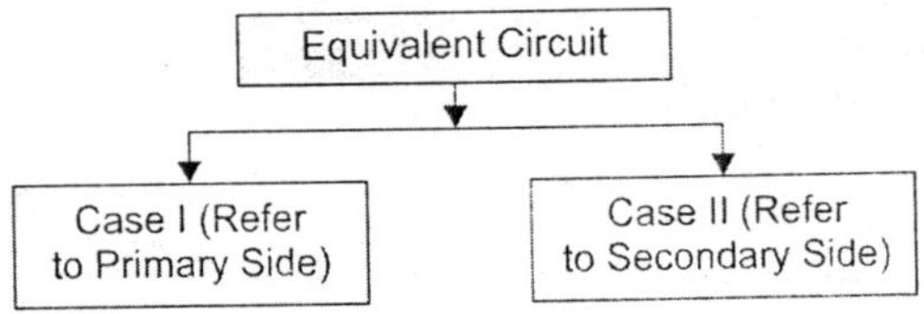

Fig. 11.17

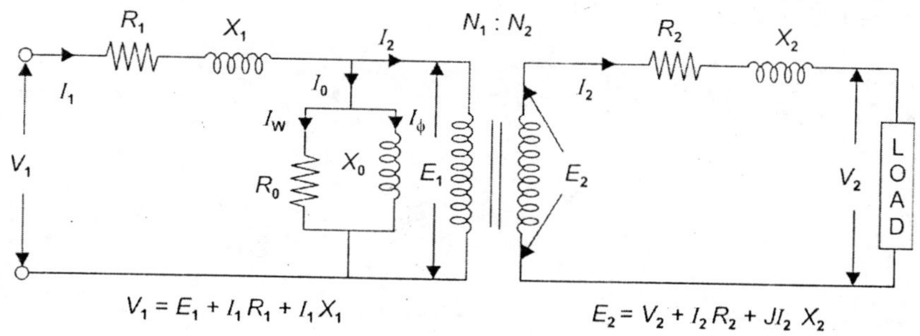

Fig. 11.18

$$I_1 = I_0 + I_2'; \quad I_0 = I_w + I_\phi$$

Case I: Equivalent Circuit Refer to Primary Side

When we are shifting all the secondary side parameters into primary side then it is known as equivalent circuit refer to primary.

We know that, total copper loss

$$P_{cu} = I_1^2 R_1 + I_2^2 R_2$$

$$= I_1^2 \left(R_1 + \left(\frac{I_2}{I_1}\right)^2 R_2 = I_1^2 \left(R_1 + \frac{R_2}{K^2} \right) \right) \qquad \left(\text{since } K = \frac{I_1}{I_2} \right)$$

$$\therefore \quad = I_1^2 R_{01}$$

$$\therefore \quad R_{01} = R_{1eq} = R_1 + R_2' = R_1 + \frac{R_2}{K^2}$$

$$R_2' = \frac{R_2}{K^2}$$

$R_{01} = R_{1eq} =$ Equivalent resistance of transformer transferred to primary side.
Similarly for reactance

$X_{01} = X_1 + X_2' = X_{1eq} =$ Equivalent reactance of transformer transferred to primary sides.

$$X_2' = \frac{X_2}{K^2}$$

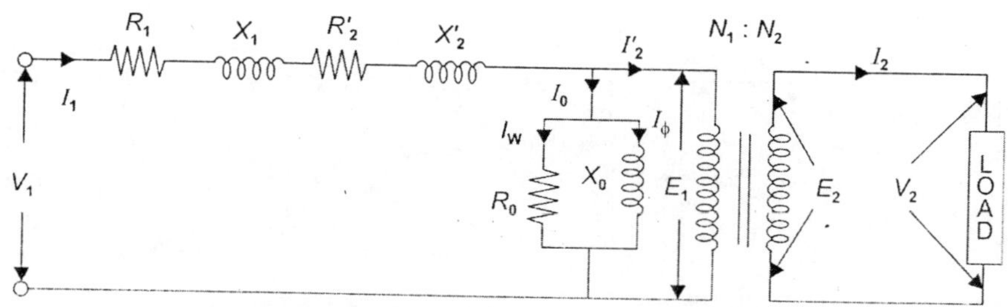

Fig. 11.19: Equivalent circuit

Also redraw the above circuit diagram.

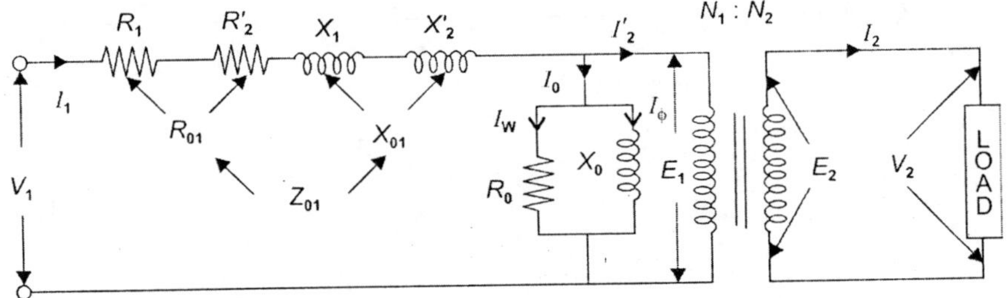

Fig. 11.20: Equivalent circuit diagram referred to primary side

$$Z_{01} = R_{01} + JX_{01}$$

$$= \sqrt{(R_{01})^2 + (X_{01})^2}$$

= equivalent impedance of transformer transferred to primary side.

Case II: Equivalent Circuit Refer to Secondary Side

When we are shifting all the primary side parameters into secondary side then it is known as equivalent circuit refer to secondary side. We know that, total copper loss.

$$P_{cu} = I_1^2 R_1 + I_2^2 R_2$$

$$= I_2^2 \left[\left(\frac{I_1}{I_2} \right)^2 R_1 + R_2 \right] \qquad \left(K = \frac{I_1}{I_2} \right)$$

$$= I_2^2 \left(K^2 R_1 + R_2 \right) = I_2^2 \left(R_{02} \right)$$

where

$$R_{02} = R_{2eq.} = R_2 + R_1'$$

$$R_1' = R_1 \, K^2$$

$R_{02} = R_{2eq}$ = equivalent resistance of transfermer transferred to secondary side.

Similarly for reactance

$$X_{02} = X_{2eq} = X_2 + X_1'$$

$$X_1' = X_1 . K^2$$

$X_{02} = X_{2eq}$ = equivalent reactance of transfermer transferred to secondary side.

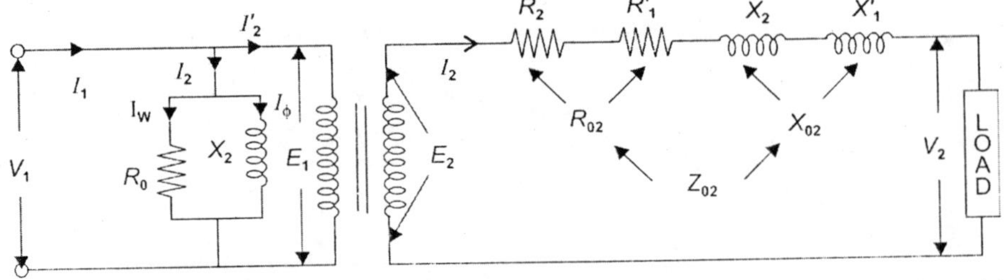

Fig. 11.21: Equivalent circuit diagram of transfermer transferred to secondary side

$$Z_{02} = R_{02} + jX_{02} = \text{equivalent impedance of transformer transferred to secondary site}$$

11.12 LOSSES IN TRANSFORMER

We know that the transformer is a static electromagnetic device which is used to transfer electrical energy from one circuit to another, but whole of energy cannot be transferred into other circuit because certain amount of energy is lost in the core and winding. There are two types of losses occur in transformer as shown in the block diagram (Fig. 11.22).

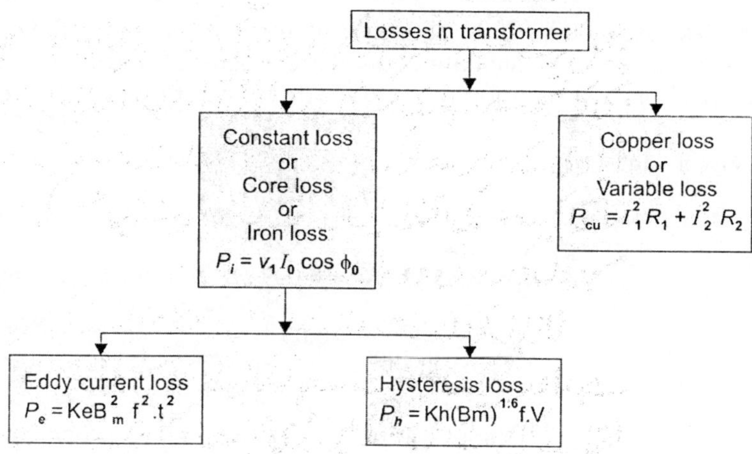

Fig. 11.22: Block diagram of losses

Iron Loss (P_i)

Iron loss P_i is the power loss taking place in the iron core of the transformer.

$$\therefore \quad P_i = \text{Hystersis loss + eddy current loss}$$
$$= P_h + P_e$$

Hysteresis Loss (P_h)

The area inclosed by the hysteresis loop of a material represents the hysteresis loss. The hysteresis loss is frequency dependent. As we increase the frequency of operation, the hysterisis loss will increase proportionally.

$$\therefore \quad P_h = K_h (B_m)^{1.6} fV \text{ W}$$

where
K_h = hysteresis constant depends on the material
B_m = maximum flux density
f = frequency
V = volume of the core

Eddy Current Losses

Due to the time varying flux, there is some induced emf in the transformer core. This induced emf causes some currents to flow through the core body. These currents are known as the eddy currents. The eddy current losses are minimized by using the liminated core.

$$\therefore \quad P_e = K_e (B_m)^2 f^2 t^2 \ \Omega/\text{unit volume}$$

where, K_e = eddy current constant
B_m = maximum flux density
f = frequency
t = thickness of the core

Copper Loss (P_{cu}): The total power loss taking place in the winding resistances of a transformer is known as the copper loss.

$$\therefore \quad P_{cu} = I_1^2 R_1 + I_2^2 R_2$$

SOLVED EXAMPLES ON ABOVE THEORY

Example 1: A 25 kVA, 4000 V/200 V, 50 Hz transformer has $R_1 = 3.45\ \Omega$, $R_2 = 0.009\ \Omega$, $X_1 = 5.2\ \Omega$ and $X_2 = 0.051\ \Omega$, calculate equivalent resistance and equivalent reactance referred to (i) primary (ii) secondary. Also calculate net power loss due to winding resistance. **[UPTU 2004-05, 09-10]**

Solution: Given data

$$S = 25 \text{ kVA}, \frac{E_1}{E_2} = \frac{4000}{200}, f = 50 \text{ Hz}$$

$$R_1 = 3.45\ \Omega,\ R_2 = 0.009\ \Omega,\ X_1 = 5.2\ \Omega,\ X_2 = 0.051\ \Omega$$

$$K = \frac{V_2}{V_1} = \frac{200}{4000} = 0.05$$

(i)
$$R_{01} = R_1 + \frac{R_2}{K^2} = 3.45 + \frac{0.009}{(0.05)^2} = 7.05\ \Omega \quad \textbf{Ans.}$$

$$X_{01} = X_1 + \frac{X_2}{K^2} = 5.2 + \frac{0.051}{(0.05)^2} = 25.6\ \Omega \quad \textbf{Ans.}$$

(ii)
$$R_{02} = R_2 + R_1 K^2 = 0.009 + 3.45 \times (0.05)^2$$
$$= 0.0176\ \Omega \quad \textbf{Ans.}$$

$$X_{01} = X_2 + X_1 K^2 = 0.051 + 5.2 \times (0.05)^2 = 0.064\ \Omega \quad \textbf{Ans.}$$

$$S = V_1 I_1$$

$$I_1 = \frac{25 \times 10^3}{4000} = 6.25 \text{ A} \quad \textbf{Ans.}$$

$$P_{cu} = I_1^2 R_{01} = (6.25)^2 \times 7.05 = 275.04 \text{ watt} \quad \textbf{Ans.}$$

Example 2: A 30 kVA, 2000/200 V, single phase, 50 Hz transformer has a primary resistance of 3.5 Ω and reactance of 4.5 Ω. The secondary resistance and reactance are 0.015 Ω and 0.02 Ω respectively. Find: (i) equivalent resistance, reactance and impedance referred to the primary side (ii) total Culoss in the transformer.

Solution: Given data

$$S = 30 \text{ kVA}, E_1 = 2000,\ E_2 = 200 \text{ V}$$

$$R_1 = 3.45\ \Omega,\ X_1 = 4.5\ \Omega,\ R_2 = 0.015\ \Omega,\ X_2 = 0.02\ \Omega$$

$$K = \frac{V_2}{V_1} = \frac{200}{2000} = 0.1$$

(i)
$$R_{01} = R_1 + \frac{R_2}{K^2} = 3.5 + \frac{0.015}{(0.1)^2} \quad \textbf{Ans.}$$

$$X_{01} = X_1 + \frac{X_2}{K^2} = 4.5 + \frac{0.02}{(0.1)^2}$$

$$R_{02} = \sqrt{(R_{01})^2 + (X_{01})^2}$$

$$S = V_1 I_1$$

$$I_1 = \frac{30 \times 10^3}{2000} = 15 \text{ A}$$

$$I_2 = \frac{30 \times 10^3}{200} = 150 \text{ A}$$

$$P_{cu} = I_1^2 R_1 + I_2^2 R_2$$

$$= (15)^2 \times 3.5 + (150)^2 \times 0.015 = 1125 \text{ W}$$ **Ans.**

11.13 TRANSFORMER EFFICIENCY

It is the ratio of the output power to the input power of a transformer. It is denoted by η.

$$\therefore \quad \eta = \frac{\text{Output power}}{\text{Input power}} = \frac{\text{Output power}}{\text{Output power + losses}}$$

Let

$$\text{power input} = V_1 I_1 \cos\phi_1$$

$$\text{power output} = V_2 I_2 \cos\phi_2$$

So, efficiency of transformer

$$\eta = \frac{V_2 I_2 \cos\phi_2}{V_1 I_1 \cos\phi} \times 100$$

But, we know that

$$\text{Output} = \text{Input} - \text{losses}$$

$$\text{Power input} = \text{Power output} + \text{losses}$$

$$V_1 I_1 \cos\phi_1 = V_2 I_2 \cos\phi_2 + Pi + P_{cu}$$

$$\therefore \quad \eta = \frac{V_2 I_2 \cos\phi_2}{V_2 I_2 \cos\phi_2 + Pi + P_{cu}}$$

Some important formulae used to determine efficiency

(a)

$$\% \eta = \frac{sx \cos\phi_2}{sx \cos\phi_2 + Pi + x^2 P_{cu}} \times 100$$

where S = rating of transformer (VA)

$$x = \frac{\text{Actual load}}{\text{Full load}}$$

Example: $x = 1$ for full load

$$x = \frac{1}{2} \text{ for half load}$$

(b) Load at maximum efficiency

$$= S \times \sqrt{\frac{P_i}{P_{cu}}}$$

11.13.1 Condition for Maximum Power Efficiency

When a transformer works on a constant input voltage and frequency then efficiency varies with the load. As load increases, the efficiency increases. At a certain load current, it achieves a maximum value. If the transformer is loaded further the efficiency starts decreasing. The graph of efficiency against load current I_2 is shown in Fig. 11.23.

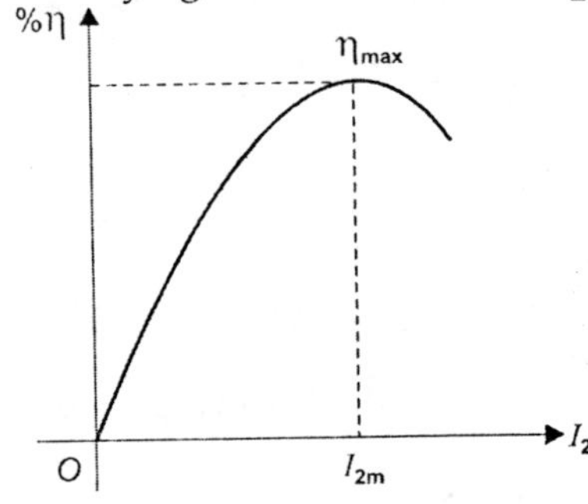

Fig. 11.23: η curve

Proof:

$$\%\eta = \frac{\text{Output power}}{\text{Input power}} \times 100 = \frac{V_2 I_2 \cos\phi_2}{V_1 I_1 \cos\phi_1} \times 100$$

$$\text{Input power} = \text{Output power} + \text{Losses}$$

$$V_1 I_1 \cos\phi_1 = V_2 I_2 \cos\phi_2 + P_i + P_{cu}$$

$$\therefore \quad V_2 I_2 \cos\phi_2 = V_1 I_1 \cos\phi_1 - (P_i + P_{cu})$$

$$\%\eta = \frac{V_1 I_1 \cos\phi_1 - (P_i + I_1^2 R_1)}{V_1 I_1 \cos\phi_1}$$

$$\eta = 1 - \frac{P_i}{V_1 I_1 \cos\phi_1} - \frac{I_1 R_1}{V_1 \cos\phi_1}$$

For maximum

$$\frac{d\eta}{dI_1} = 0$$

$$\frac{d\eta}{dI_1} = 0 + \frac{P_i}{V_1 I_1^2 \cos\phi_1} - \frac{R_1}{V_1 \cos\phi_1}$$

$$\Rightarrow \quad \frac{P_i}{V_1 I_1^2 \cos\phi_1} = \frac{R_1}{V_1 \cos\phi_1}$$

$$P_i = I_1^2 R_1$$

At maximum efficiency

Iron loss = copper loss or

$$P_i = I_1^2 R_1$$

$$= x^2 P_{cu} \text{ at maximum efficiency}$$

11.13.2 Voltage Regulartion of a Transformer

Ideally the secondary terminal voltage V_2 (or load voltage) of a transformer should remain constant independent of the load current as shown in Fig. 11.24. But practically the load voltage decreases with increase in load current I_1 as shown in Fig. 11.24.

(a) **No load voltage:** The no load voltage is the secondary terminal voltage corresponding to zero load current. For a transformer

$$\text{No load voltage} = E_2 \text{ V} \quad ...(11.1)$$

(b) **Full load voltage:** It is the secondary terminal voltage corresponding to the specified load current. Let us denote it by V_2. The percent voltage regulation is given mathematically as:

$$\% \text{ Regulation} = \frac{E_2 - V_2}{E_2} \times 100$$

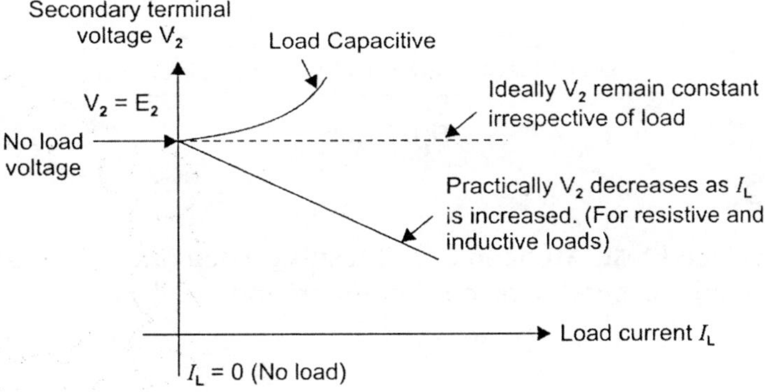

Fig. 11.24: Concept of voltage regulation

Thus with increase in load current, the value of V_2 decreases and the percent regulation increases (becomes poor). Ideal value of voltage regulation is 0%.

Defintion of Voltage Regulation

The voltage regulation of a transformer is defined as the change in secondary terminal voltage (V_2) from no load to full load with the primary source voltage (V_1) and the temperature of the transformer maintained constant.

Reason for Reduction in Voltage

The drop in secondary terminal voltage takes place due to the voltage drop taking place across the primary and secondary impedances. As the load current increases, the voltage drop across these impedances will increase. This will reduce the secondary terminal voltage V_2 with increase in I_L.

Does the Secondary Terminal Voltage Depend only on the Load Current?

The answer is NO. The secondary terminal voltage does not depend only on the magnitude of I_L, but it also depends on the type of the load. As shown in Fig. 11.24, the secondary terminal voltage decreases for resistive or inductive loads whereas it increases with increase in I_L if the load is capacitive.

Note: The regulation is positive for the resistive and inductive loads and it can be negative for the capacitive loads.

11.13.3 Efficiency from Transformer Tests

Transformer tests are performed to determine efficiency, voltage regulation and equivalent circuit parameters without actually loading the transformer. Transformer tests give more accurate result these obtained by taking measurements on fully loaded transformer. Also, the power consumption in these tests is very small compared with the full load output of the transformer. Usually two types of transformer tests are conducted to find the efficiency, regulation and equivalent circuit parameters as shown in Fig. 11.25.

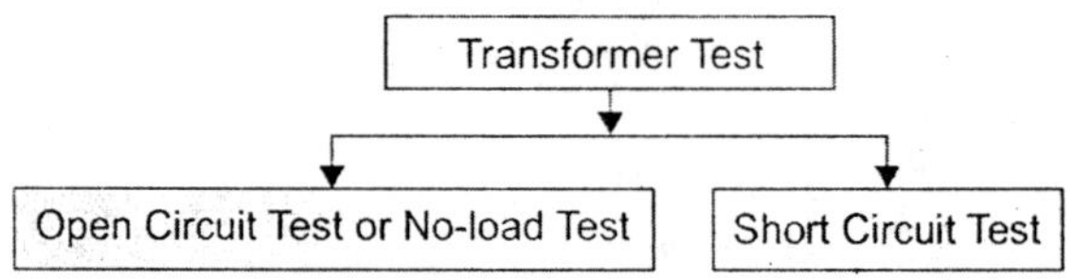

Fig. 11.25

Open Circuit Test

It is also called no load test. An open circuit test is carried out to find core loss or iron loss (p_i) and no load current I_0 which is helpful in finding R_0 and X_0.

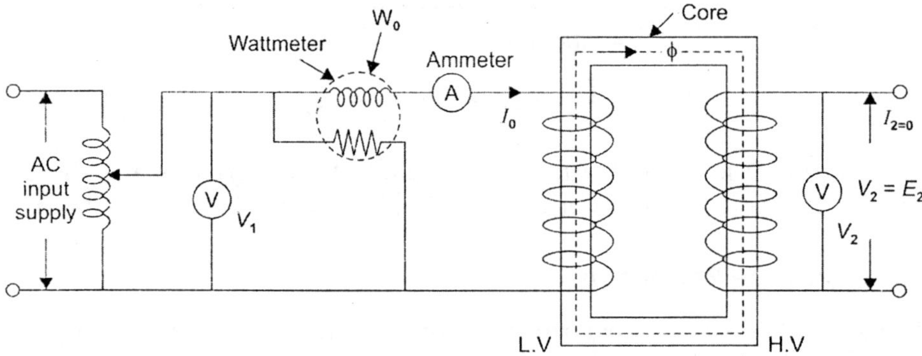

Fig. 11.26: Open circuit test

Figure 11.26 shows the connection diagram for the open circuit test, the high voltage (HV) side is left open. In this test, the rated voltage is applied to the primary (usually low voltage side) while the secondary is left open circuited. The applied primary voltage V_1 is measured by the voltmeter, the no-load current I_0 by ammeter and no-load input power W_0 by wattmeter as shown in Fig. 11.26.

Calculation of Parameters

$$I_W = I_0 \cos\phi_0 \, ; \, I_\phi = I_0 \sin\phi_0 \, ; \, W_0 = V_1 I_0 \cos\phi_0$$

No load power factor $= \cos\phi_0 = \dfrac{W_0}{V_0 I_0}$

Magnetising current $I_\phi = I_0 \sin\phi_0$

Working component $I_w = I_0 \cos\phi_0$

$$\therefore \qquad R_0 = \frac{V_0}{I_W}\ \Omega$$

$$X_0 = \frac{V_0}{I_\phi}\ \Omega$$

Short Circuit Test

An short circuit test is carried out to find copper loss and equivalent resistance, reactance and impedance of the transformer referred to the winding in which the measuring instruments are connected.

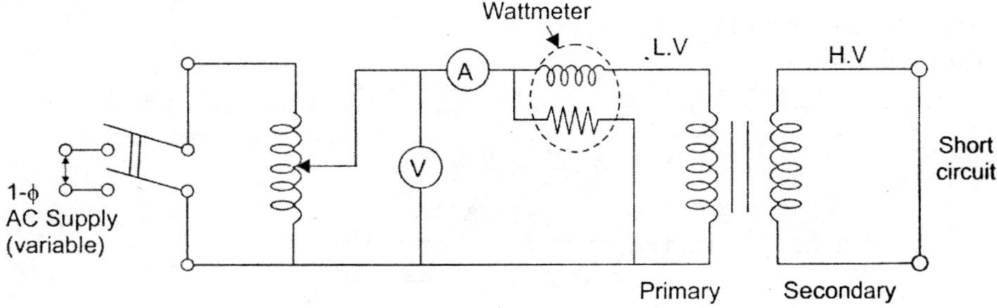

Fig. 11.27: Short circuit test

Explanation

The high voltage winding is supplied at the reduced voltage from a variable voltage supply. The supply voltage is gradually increased until full load primary current flows. When the rated full load current flows in the primary winding rated full load current will flow in the secondary winding by transformer action. Reading of the ammeter, voltmeter and wattmeter are noted. The wattmeter reading is the power loss which is equal to full load copper loss as iron loss is very low.

$$W_{SC} = (P_{cu}) \text{ full load} = \text{full load copper loss}$$

Calculations

$$W_{SC} = V_{SC}\, I_{SC} \cos\phi_{SC}$$

$$\therefore \quad \cos\phi_{SC} = \frac{W_{SC}}{V_{SC} \cdot I_{SC}} = \text{short circuit power factor}$$

$$W_{SC} = I_{SC}^2 . R_{1e} = \text{copper loss}$$

$$R_{1e} = \frac{W_{SC}}{I_{SC}^2}\ \Omega$$

$$Z_{1e} = \frac{V_{SC}}{I_{SC}} = \sqrt{(R_{1e})^2 + (X_{1e})^2}$$

$$\therefore \quad X_{1e} = \sqrt{(Z_{1e})^2 - (R_{1e})^2}$$

11.13.4 Calculation of Efficiency from OC and SC Test

We know that

From OC test $\quad W_O = P_i$

From SC test $\quad W_{SC} = (P_{cu})\ FL$

$$\%\eta \text{ on full load} = \frac{V_2 (I_2)_{FL} \cos\phi_2 \times 100}{V_2 (I_2)_{FL} \cos\phi_2 + W_O + W_{SC}}$$

SOLVED EXAMPLES ON ABOVE THEORY

Example 1: Find the efficiency of a 150 kVA transformer at 25% full load at 0.8 pf lagging. The copper loss at full load is 1600 watts and the iron loss is 1400 watt. Ignore the effect of temperature rise and magnetizing current.

Solution: Given data

$$S = 150 \text{ kVA}, pf = \cos\phi = 0.8; P_{cu} = 1600 \text{ watt}, P_i = 1400 \text{ W}$$

$$x = \frac{1}{4} = .25 = 25\%$$

$$\%\eta \text{ at } 25\% \text{ load} = \frac{x S \cos\phi}{x S \cos + P_i + x^2 P_{cu}} \times 100$$

$$\%\eta = \frac{0.25 \times 150 \times 0.8 \times 10^3}{0.25 \times 150 \times 0.8 + 1400 + (0.25)^2 \times 1600} \times 100 = 95.25\% \textbf{ Ans.}$$

Example 2: In a 25 kVA, 2000/250 V transformer the constant and variable losses are 350 watt and 400 watt respectively. Calculate the efficiency on unity power factor at (a) full load (b) half load.

Solution: Given

$$S = 25 \text{ kVA}; V_1 = 2000 \text{ V}; V_2 = 250 \text{ V}; P_i = 350 \text{ W}; P_{cu} = 400 \text{ W}; pf = \cos\phi = 1$$

(a) At full load $x = 1$

$$\%\eta = \frac{x S \cos\phi}{x S \cos\phi + P_i + x^2 P_{cu}}$$

$$= \frac{1 \times 25 \times 1}{1 \times 25 \times 1 + \frac{350}{1000} + \frac{400}{1000}} \times 100 = 97.08\% \quad \textbf{Ans.}$$

(a) At full load $x = \frac{1}{2}$

$$\%\eta = \frac{\frac{1}{2} \times 25 \times 1}{\frac{1}{2} \times 25 \times 1 + 0.35 + \left(\frac{1}{2}\right)^2 \times 0.4} \times 100 = 96.53\% \quad \textbf{Ans.}$$

11.14 AUTO TRANSFORMER

Auto transformer is a special transformer in which primary and secondary shares same common single winding. So auto-transformer consists of only one winding (AB) on a laminated magnetic core, with rotary movable contact. *Auto transformer used as step-down transformer.*

AB is connected to a single phase AC supply V_1, so AB winding of N_1 turns is acting as a primary winding. CB is connected to load, so CB winding of N_2 turns is acting as secondary winding.

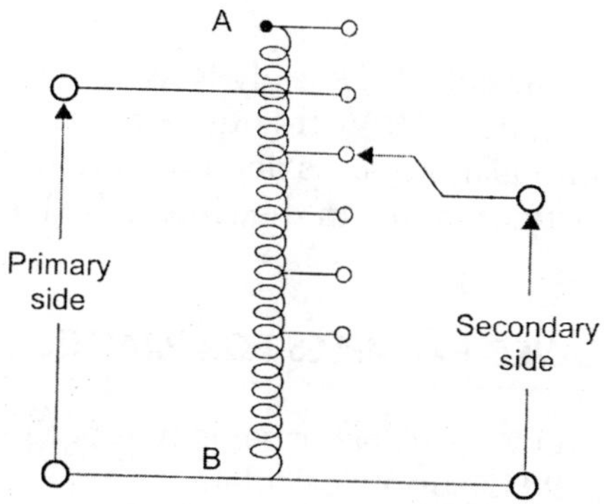

Fig. 11.28: Auto transformer

Now $$V_2 = \frac{N_2}{N_1} \times V_1$$

$$N_2 < N_1 \text{ , } V_2 < V_1$$

Auto transformer used as step-up transformer

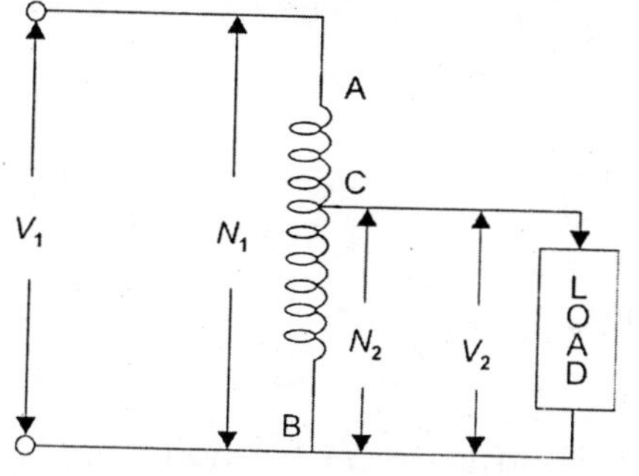

Fig. 11.29: Step-down transformer

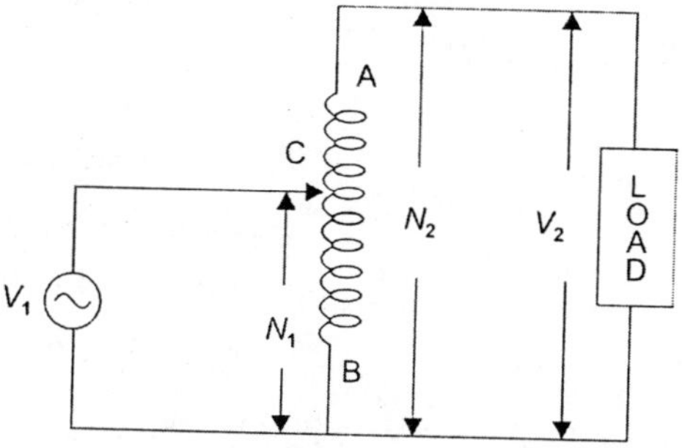

Fig. 11.30: Step-up transformer

Now AB of N_2 turns is connected to load, so acting as secondary winding and CB of N_1 turns is connected to input AC supply voltage V_1 so acting as primary winding.

$$V_2 = \frac{N_2}{N_1} \times V_1$$

Now $$N_2 > N_1, \ V_2 > V_1$$

Thus auto transformer used as step-up transformer.

Advantages

As only one winding is used. Copper required for the transformer is very less. So size and cost is reduced compared to two winding transformer. The losses taking place in the winding are reduced. Hence the efficiency is higher than two winding transformer.

Disadvantages

There is no electrical isolation between the primary and secondary winding. Thus can prove to be dangerous for high voltage applications.

Applications

It can be used as variac, i.e. variable AC supply to vary the AC voltage applied to the load smoothly from 0 V to about 270 V. It is used to start to AC machines such as induction motor or synchronous motors. As demonstrated; when the auto transformer is used to control the intensity of lamps in the cinema hall, etc. It is called as dimmer-state.

SOLVED EXAMPLES FOR PRACTICES

Example 1: The no load current of a transformer is 10 A at a power factor of 0.25 lagging when connected to 400 V, 50 Hz supply calculate:

(a) Magnetizing component of no load current.
(b) Iron loss.
(c) Maximum value of flux in the core.

Assume primary winding turns as 500. **[UPTU 2005-06]**

Solution: Given data

$$I_0 = 10\text{ A}, \cos\phi_0 = 0.25, V_1 = 400\text{ V}, f = 50\text{ Hz}; N_1 = 500$$

(a)
$$I_\phi = I_0 \sin\phi_0$$
$$= 10\sqrt{1-(\cos\phi_0)^2} = 10\sqrt{1-(0.25)^2} = 9.68\text{ A}$$ **Ans.**

(b) Iron loss (P_i)

$$\therefore \quad P_i = W_0 = V_1 I_0 \cos\phi_0 = 400\times 10\times 0.25$$
$$P_i = 1000\text{ watt}$$ **Ans.**

(c)
$$E_1 = 4.44\phi_m f N_1$$
$$400 = 4.44\times 500\times \phi_m \times 500$$
$$\phi_m = 3.61\text{ mWb}$$ **Ans.**

Example 2: A 10 kVA, 2000/400 V, single phase 50 Hz transformer at no load, has resistance and leakage reactance of primary winding of 5.5 Ω and 12 Ω respectively. The corresponding values of secondary winding being 0.2 Ω and 0.45 Ω. Determine the value of secondary voltage at full-load 0.8 power factor lagging when the primary applied voltage is 2000 V. **[UPTU 2006-07]**

Solution: Given data

$$S = 10\text{ kVA}, V_1 = 2000\text{ V}, V_2 = 400\text{ V}, R_1 = 5.5\ \Omega; X_1 = 12\ \Omega, R_2 = 0.2\ \Omega, X_2 = 0.45\ \Omega$$

We know that
$$K = \frac{V_2}{V_1} = \frac{400}{2000} = 0.2$$

$$R_{01} = R_1 + R_2' = R_1 + \frac{R_2}{K^2} = 5.5 + \frac{0.5}{(0.2)^2} = 10.5\ \Omega$$

$$X_{01} = X_1 + X_2' = X_1 + \frac{X_2}{K^2} = 12 + \frac{0.45}{(0.2)^2} = 23.25\ \Omega$$

$$I_2 = \frac{S}{V_2} = \frac{10\times 10^3}{400} = 25\text{ A}$$

$$R_{02} = K^2 R_{01} = 0.42\ \Omega \text{ and } X_{02} = K^2 X_{01}$$

$$X_{02} = 20.93\ \Omega$$

Full load voltage drop

$$= I_2[R_{02}\cos\phi + X_{02}\sin\phi]$$

$$= 25[0.42\times0.8 + 0.93\times0.6] = 22.35 \text{ V}$$

The value of secondary voltage is given by

$$E_2 = V_2 + \text{voltage drop}$$

$$V_2 = 400 - 22.35 = 377.65 \text{ V}$$

Ans.

Example 3: A 10 kVA, single phase, 500/250 volt transformer gave the following test:

OC test: 250 V, 3 A, 200 W

SC test: 15 V, 30 A, 300 W

Calculate the efficiency at full load 0.8 lagging power factor.

Solution: The given rating

$$S = 10 \text{ kVA},\ V_1 = 500 \text{ V},\ V_2 = 250 \text{ V}$$

We know that OC and SC tests give iron and core losses as follows:

from OC test = P_i = 200 watt (given)

SC test gives copper losses P_{cu} = 300 W

$$\frac{P_{cu}}{P_{cu(fl)}} = \frac{I_{SC}^2}{I_{1(fl)}^2}$$

$$= \frac{20^2}{30^2} \times 300 = 133.33 \text{ W}$$

$$P_{cu}(fl) = 133.33 \text{ W}$$

Ans.

The efficiency at full load and 0.8 power factor is given by

$$\%\eta_{(fl)} = \frac{VA \text{ rating} \cos\phi}{VA \text{ rating} \cos\phi + P_i + P_{cu(fl)}} \times 100$$

$$= \frac{10\times10^3\times0.8}{10\times10^3\times0.8 + 200 + 133.33} \times 100 = 96\%$$

$$\eta_{(fl)} = 96\%$$

Ans.

Example 4: A 20 kVA, 2000/200 V, 50 Hz single phase transformer has iron loss of 120 watt and full load copper loss of 300 W, low voltage side of the transformer is loaded at 0.8 lagging power factor. Calculate maximum efficiency of transformer.

Solution: Given rating

$$S = 20 \text{ kVA},\ V_1 = 2000V,\ V_2 = 200 \text{ V}$$

$$P_i = 120 \text{ W},\ P_{cu} = 300 \text{ W},\ \cos\phi = 0.8$$

$$\text{kVA for } \eta_{max} = \text{kVA} \times \sqrt{\frac{P_i}{P_{cu(fl)}}} = 20\times\sqrt{\frac{120}{300}} = 12.649 \text{ kVA}$$

We know that at η_{max}, $P_{cu} = P_i = 120$ W

$$\eta_{max} = \frac{\text{KVA for } \eta_{max} \times \cos\phi}{\text{KVA for } \eta_{max} \times \cos\phi + 2P_i}$$

$$= \frac{12.649\times1000\times0.8}{12.649\times1000\times0.8 + 2 + 120} \times 100 = 97.682\%$$

Ans.

Example 5: The ohmic values of the circuit parameter of a transformer, having a turns ratio of 5 are $R_1 = 0.5\ \Omega$, $R_2 = 0.21\ \Omega$, $X_1 = 3.2\ \Omega$, $X_2 = 0.12\ \Omega$, $R_C = 350\ \Omega$ and $X_m = 98\ \Omega$ referred to primary. Draw the approximately equivalent circuit of the transformer referred to secondary. Show the numerical values of the circuit parameters.

Solution: Given turn ratio = 5, $R_1 = 0.5\ \Omega$, $R_2 = 0.21\ \Omega$, $X_1 = 3.2\ \Omega$, $X_2 = 0.12\ \Omega$, $R_C = 350\ \Omega$ and $X_m = 98\ \Omega$

The turn ratio

$$\frac{N_1}{N_2} = \frac{5}{1}$$

$$K = \frac{N_2}{N_1} = \frac{1}{5} = 0.2$$

The equivalent parameters referred to secondary side is calculated as follows:

$$R_{2e} = R_2 + K^2R_1 = 0.021 + (0.2)^2 \times 0.5 = 0.041\ \Omega$$ **Ans.**

$$X_{2e} = X_2 + K^2X_1 = 0.12 + (0.2)^2 \times 3.2 = 0.248\ \Omega$$ **Ans.**

$$R'_e = K^2R_C = (0.2)^2 \times 350 = 14\ \Omega$$ **Ans.**

$$X'_m = K^2X_m = (0.2)^2 \times 98 = 3.92\ \Omega$$ **Ans.**

Example 6: Following results were obtained on a 100 kVA, 11000/220 V single phase transformer:

OC test (LV side): 220 V, 45 A, 2 KW

SC test (HV side): 500 V, 9.09 A, 3 KW

Determine equivalent circuit parameters of the transformer referred to low voltage side. **[UPTU 2009-2010]**

Solution: Given rating

$$= 100\ \text{kVA},\ V_1 = 11000\ \text{V},\ V_2 = 200\ \text{V}$$

As OC test is performed on LV side, the parameters are also referred to low voltage side.

$$W_0 = 2\ \text{kW},\ V_0 = 220\ \text{V},\ I_0 = 45\ \text{A}$$

$$\cos\phi_0 = \frac{W_0}{V_0I_0} = \frac{2\times10^3}{220\times45} = 0.202$$

$$I'_C = I_0\cos\phi_0 = 9.09\ \text{A and } I'_m = I_0\sin\phi_0 = 44.07\ \text{A}$$

$$R'_0 = \frac{V_2}{I'_C} = 24.20\ \Omega \text{ and } X'_0 = \frac{V_2}{I'_m} = 4.9918\ \Omega$$ **Ans.**

As SC test is performed on HV side, the parameters to be obtained from results are referred to high voltage side, i.e. primary side must be transferred to low voltage side, i.e. secondary

$$W_{SC} = 3\ \text{KW},\ V_{SC} = 500\ \text{V},\ I_{SC} = 9.09\ \text{A (given)}$$

$$R_{1e} = \frac{W_{SC}}{I_{SC}^2} = \frac{3000}{(9.09)^2} = 36.3072\ \Omega$$

$$Z_{1e} = \frac{V_{SC}}{I_{SC}} = \frac{500}{9.09} = 55\ \Omega$$

$$X_{1e} = \sqrt{Z_{1e}^2 - R_{1e}^2} = \sqrt{55^2 - (36.3072)^2} = 41.3132\ \Omega$$

$$K = \frac{220}{11000} = 0.02$$

$$R_{2e} = K^2 R_{1e} = (0.02)^2 \times 36.3072 = 0.0145\ \Omega$$

$$X_{2e} = K^2 X_{1e} = (0.02)^2 \times 41.3132 = 0.01652\ \Omega$$

$$Z_{2e} = K^2 Z_{1e} = (0.02)^2 \times 55 = 0.022\ \Omega$$

$$R_{2e} = 0.0145\ \Omega,\ X_{2e} = 0.01652\ \Omega,\ Z_{2e} = 0.022\ \Omega$$ **Ans.**

Example 7: A 250/500 V single-phase transformer gave the following test results:
SC test: 20 V, 12 A, 100 W (LV short circuited)
OC test: 250 V, 1 A, 80 W (low voltage side)
Determine the efficiency of the transformer when output is 12 ampere, 500 V at 0.85 power factor lagging **[UPTU 2010-11]**

Solution: Given

$$V_1 = 250\text{ V},\ V_2 = 500\text{ V}$$

We know that short circuit test gives copper loss P_{cu}
= 100 W at 12 A
and open circuit test gives iron loss (P_i)
= 80 W

The efficiency $\%\eta$ is

$$= \frac{V_2 I_2 \cos\phi}{V_2 I_2 \cos\phi + P_i + P_{cu(fl)}} \times 100$$

$$= \frac{500 \times 12 \times 0.85}{500 \times 12 \times 0.85 + 80 + 100} \times 100 = 96.59\%$$ **Ans.**

Example 8: The efficiency of a given 400 kVA, singe phase transformer is 98.77% at full load 0.8 power factor and 99.13% at half full load unity power factor.
Find: (a) Iron losses at full and half full loads
(b) Copper losses at full and half full loads. **[UPTU 2010-11]**

Solution: Given rating

$S = 400$ kVA, $\eta_{(fl)} = 98.77\%$, $\cos\phi = 0.8$, $\eta_{nl} = 99.13\%$, $\cos\phi = 1$ (at half load)

For full load $x = 1$

$$\%\eta_{fl} = \frac{xS\cos\phi}{xS\cos\phi + P_i + P_{cu(fl)}} \times 100$$

$$0.9877 = \frac{400 \times 10^3 \times 0.8}{400 \times 10^3 \times 0.8 + P_i + P_{cu(fl)}}$$

$$P_i + P_{cu(fl)} = 3985.015 \qquad \ldots(1)$$

The half load efficiency of transformer is given by, *i.e.* $x = \frac{1}{2}$

$$\%\eta_{hl} = \frac{xs\cos\phi}{xs\cos\phi + P_i + x^2 P_{cu(fl)}} \times 100$$

$$\therefore \quad 0.9913 = \frac{0.5 \times 400 \times 10^3 \times 1}{0.50 \times 400 \times 10^3 \times 1 + P_i + (0.5)^2 P_{cu(fl)}}$$

$\therefore \quad P_i + 0.25P_{cu(fl)} = 1755.2708$ ...(2)

Now subtracting Eq. (2) from Eq. (1)

$$0.75P_{cu(fl)} = 2229.744 \text{ i.e. } P_{cu(fl)} = 2972.993 \text{ W}$$

$$P_i = 1012.0225 \text{ W}$$

Iron losses remain same on full road and half load which are $P_i = 1012.0225$ W **Ans.**

Copper losses on full load $= P_{cu(fl)} = 2972.993$ W **Ans.**

Copper losses on half load $= (0.5)^2 P_{cu(fl)} = 743.248$ W **Ans.**

Example 9: The maximum efficiency of a 100 kVA transformer is 98.40% and operates at 90% full load unity power factor. Calculate the efficiency of a transformer at unity power factor at full load.

Solution: Given rating

$S = 100$ kVA, $\eta_{max} = 98.40\%$, KVA and $\eta_{max} = 90\%$ of full load, $\cos\phi = 1$

For calculating efficiency, first we calculate the loss as follows:

$$\%\eta_{max} = \frac{Sx \text{ for } \eta_{max} \times \cos\phi}{Sx\cos\phi \text{ for } \eta_{max} + 2P_i} \times 100$$

$$0.984 = \frac{0.9 \times 100 \times 10^3 \times 1}{0.9 \times 100 \times 10^3 \times 1 + 2P_i}$$

$$P_i = 731/7073 \text{ W}$$

We know that at maximum efficiency, copper losses = iron losses

$$P_{cu} = 731.7073 \text{ W at 0.9 of full load, i.e. } n = 0.9$$

$$P_{cu} \propto I^2 \propto (VA)^2$$

$$\frac{P_{cu(fl)}}{P_{cu}} = \left[\frac{VA_{fl}}{0.9VA_{fl}}\right]^2$$

$$P_{cu(fl)} = 731.7073 \times \left(\frac{1}{0.9}\right)^2 = 903.3432 \text{ W}$$

$$\%\eta_{fl} = \frac{VA\cos\phi}{VA\cos\phi + P_i + P_{cu(fl)}} \times 100$$

$$= \frac{100 \times 10^3 \times 1}{100 \times 10^3 + 731.7073 + 903.3423} \times 100 = 98.3912\% \text{ **Ans.**}$$

Example 10: The following test results were obtained on a 20 kVA; 2200/220 V transformer.

OC test (LV): 220 V, 1.1 A, 125 W; **SC test (HV):** 52.7 V, 8 A, 287 W

The transformer is loaded at 0.8 power factor on secondary side with a voltage of 220 V. Determine the efficiency at 80% of full load, the maximum efficiency and load at which it occurs.

Solution: Given that

First we calculate the full load primary current as follows:

$$I_{fl} = \frac{20 \times 1000}{2200} = 9.09 \text{ A}$$

Full load copper loss, P_{cu}= power loss with short circuit current of

$$= 8.4 \text{ A} \times \frac{I_{fl}}{I_{SC}}$$

$$= 287 \times \left(\frac{9.09}{8.4}\right)^2 = 336 \text{ W}$$

The input, output and copper loss of full load at 80% is given by
Output at 80% of full load = 0.8 × rated kVA × *pf* = 0.8 × 20 × 0.8 = 12.8 kW
Input at 80% of full load = 12.8 + 0.125 + 0.215 = 13.14 kW
Copper loss at 80% of full load = $(0.8)^2$ × 336 = 215 W
The efficiency is given by

$$\eta = \frac{\text{Output}}{\text{Input}} \times 100 = \frac{12.8}{13.14} \times 100 = 97.41\%$$ **Ans.**

Let us assume that maximum efficiency occur at n times full load then

$$n = \sqrt{\frac{P_i}{\text{full load copper loss}}} = \sqrt{\frac{125}{336}} = 0.372$$

The load at which maximum efficiency occur

$$\eta_{max} \text{ load} = 0.372 \times 20 = 7.44 \text{ kVA}$$

The output at which maximum efficiency occurs = 7.44 × 0.8 = 5.952 kW
The maximum efficiency, η_{max} is given by

$$\frac{5.952}{5.952 + 0.125 + 0.125} \times 100 = 95.97\%$$

$$\eta_{max} = 95.97\%$$ **Ans.**

Example 11: The maximum efficiency of a 100 kVA, 1100/440 V, 50 Hz transformer is 96%. This occurs at 75% of full load at 0.8 pf lagging. Find the efficiency of transformer at 3/4 full load at 0.6 pf leading.

Solution: Given data

$$S = 100 \text{ KVA}, V_1 = 1100, V_2 = 440, F = 50 \text{ Hz}$$

Power output corresponding to maximum efficiency is given by

$$P_{out} = \text{kVA} \cos\phi$$
$$= 100 \times 0.75 \times 0.8 = 60 \text{ kW}$$

Efficiency

$$\eta = \frac{\text{Output}}{\text{Output} + P_i + P_{cu}}$$

or $$0.96 = \frac{60}{60 + P_i + P_{cu}}$$

or $$P_i + P_{cu} = \frac{60}{0.96} - 60 = 2.5 \text{ kW}$$

$$P_i = \frac{2.5}{2} = 1.25 \text{ kW}$$

$$P_i = P_{cu} = 1.25 \text{ kW}$$

At 3/4th full load copper loss = 1.25 kW
iron loss = 1.25 kW

The power output at 3/4 full load and 0.6 power factor leading is given by

$$P_{out} = \frac{3}{4} \times 100 \times 0.6 = 45 \text{ KW}$$

$$\text{Efficiency } \eta = \frac{\text{Output}}{\text{Output} + P_i + P_{cu}} = \frac{45}{45 + 1.25 + 1.25} \times 100$$

$$\eta = 94.7\%$$

Ans.

Example 12: The maximum efficiency of a 100 kVA transformer is 98.40% and operates at 90% full load unity power factor. Calculate the efficiency of a transformer at unity power factor at full load.

Solution: The output of transformer is 100 kVA and load power factor, $\cos\phi = 1$. The output at 90% of full load is given by

$$P_{out} = \text{kVA} \cos\phi$$

$$= 100 \times 0.9 \times 1.0 = 90 \text{ kW}$$

The power input at 90% of full load and total losses is given by

$$P_{in} = \frac{P_{out}}{\eta} = \frac{90}{0.98} = 91.463 \text{ kW}$$

$$\text{Total loss} = P_{in} - P_{out} = 9.146 - 90 = 1.46 \text{ kW}$$

The maximum efficiency occurs when iron loss equal to copper loss so

$$P_i = \frac{P_{in} - P_{out}}{2} = \frac{1.463}{2} = 7315 \text{ kW}$$

So full load copper loss, $P_{cu} = \dfrac{0.7315}{0.9^2} = 0.903 \text{ kW}$

The power output at full load and unity power factor is given by

$$100 \times 1.0 = 100 \text{ kW}$$

The total losses at full load

$$P_i + P_{out} = 0.7315 + 0.903 = 1.6346 \text{ kW}$$

The transformer efficiency at unity power factor and at full load is given by

$$\eta = \frac{\text{Power}}{\text{Power output} + \text{Total losses}} \times 100$$

$$= \frac{100}{100 + 1.6346} \times 100 = 98.39\%$$

Ans.

EXERCISES

1. Explain basic principle of operation of a single-phase transformer. Where are they used? **[UP Technical Univ; Elec. Engineering, Second Semester 2005-06]**
2. Derive emf equation for a single-phase transformer. **[UP Technical Univ; Electrical Engineering, June 2001, January 2003]**
3. Explain the working of an ideal transformer under (i) no-load and (ii) loaded conditions and derive expressions for voltage and current ratio; relating to trans-former turns ratio. **[UP Technical Univ; Elec. Engineering, First Semester 2004-05]**
4. Derive emf equation of a single-phase transformer and obtain relation for secondary to primary winding voltages. **[GB Technical Univ; Electrical Engineering, First Semester 2009-10]**

5. Draw and explain phasor diagram of transformer under loaded condition.
[UP Technical Univ; Electrical Engineering February 2002]
6. Draw and explain phasor diagram of single-phase transformer on load with lagging power factor. **[UP Technical Univ; Elec. Engineering, First Semester 2005-06]**
7. Draw the phasor diagram of a single-phase transformer for leading power factor load. **[UP Technical Univ; Electrical Engineering, Second Semester 2007-08]**
8. Draw and explain the no-load and full-load phasor diagrams for a single-phase transformer. **[GB Technical Univ; Electrical Engineering, Second Semester 2009-10]**
9. Derive an emf expression of power transformer. Also draw an equivalent circuit of it. **[GB Technical Univ; Electrical Engineering, First Semester 2011-12]**
10. Derive an emf / voltage expression of power transformer. Also draw an equivalent circuit of it. **[Mahamaya Technical Univ; Electrical Engineering, Second Semester 2010-11]**
11. Develop the equivalent circuit of a single phase transformer on no load and on load conditions. **[UP Technical Univ; Electrical Engineering, Second Semester 2009-10]**
12. Draw exact equivalent circuit and corresponding phasor diagram of a single-phase transformer on load and explain them. Why no-load current is kept small and how it is reduced? **[UP Technical Univ; Electrical Engineering, First Semester 2006-07]**
13. Explain the following for single phase transformer.
[UP Technical Univ; Electrical Engineering, Second Semester 2007-08]
    (i) Phasor diagram for inductive load
    (ii) Equivalent circuit.
    (iii) Voltage regulation.
14. Develop the equivalent circuit of a single-phase transformer. Mention the physical significance of all its parameters.
[UP Technical Univ; Electrical Engineering, September 2001]
15. (i) What is meant by leakage flux and leakage reactance in reference to a transformer?
    (ii) Define voltage regulation of a transformer and deduce expression for lagging power factor load.
[UP Technical Univ; Electrical Engineering, Second Semester 2003-04]
16. Explain the working of a transformer with the derivation of the emf equation for a transformer. Also discuss the losses in the transformer.
[GB Technical Univ; Electrical Engineering, Second Semester 2010-11]
17. Explain why the hysteresis and eddy current losses occur in the transformer. How does change in frequency affect the operation of given transformer?
[GB Technical Univ; Electrical Engineering, Second Semester 2009-10]
18. Explain the efficiency of transformer.
[GB Technical Univ; Electrical Engineering, First Semester 2010-11]
19. Write down the expression of efficiency for a transformer. How is it affected by change in power factor?
[GB Technical Univ; Electrical Engineering, First Semester 2011-12]

20. List various losses occurring in a transformer and mention the condition for maximum efficiency. **[UP Technical Univ; Electrical Engineering, First Semester 2006-07]**
21. Explain the OC and SC tests performed on a single-phase transformer. Determine the equivalent circuit based on the above tests. Derive the condition for maximum efficiency of a transformer. **[UP Technical Univ; Electrical Engineering, First Semester 2007-08]**
22. Discuss in brief about auto-transformer.
[GB Technical Univ; Electrical Engineering, Second Semester 2011-12]
23. Describe the working of an auto-transformer.
[GB Technical Univ; Electrical Engineering, First Semester 2010-11]
24. Explain single-phase auto-transformer and give its application.
[GB Technical Univ; Electrical Engineering, First Semester 2009-10]
25. What is an auto-transformer? How does it differ from conventional two-winding transformer? State its one applications.
[GGSIP Delhi Univ; Electrical Science, May 2005]
26. Explain working of a single phase auto-transformer and mention its applications. Show that there will be saving of copper in auto-transformer in comparison to same rating of two winding transformer.

PROBLEMS FOR PRACTICE

1. The maximum flux density in the core of 250/3000 V, 50 Hz single-phase transformer is 1.2 Wb/m^2. If the emf per turn is 8 V, determine (i) primary and secondary turns (ii) area of the core.
[Nagpur Univ; Elec. Engineering-I, 1991] [**Ans.** (i) 32384 (ii) 0.03 m^2]
2. A single-phase transformer has 500 turns in the primary and 1200 turns in the secondary. The cross-sectional area of the core is 80 cm^2. If the primary winding is connected to a 50 Hz supply at 500 V, calculate peak flux density, and voltage induced in the secondary. **[Bharathiyar Univ; November 1997]**
[**Ans.** 0.553 T; 1200]
3. A 200 kVA, 6600/400 V, 50 Hz single phase transformer has 80 turns on the secondary. Calculate (i) the approximate values of the primary and secondary currents (ii) the approximate number of primary turns and (iii) the maximum value of flux. **[Punjab Univ; Elec Engineering I, 1994]**
[**Ans.** (i) 30.3 A, 500 A; (ii) 1320 (iii) 22.5 mWb]
4. The no-load current of a transformer is 5 A at 0.25 *pf* when supplied at 235 V, 50 Hz. The number of turns on the primary winding is 200. Calculate (i) the maximum value of flux in the core, (ii) the core loss (iii) the magnetizing component.
[Nagpur Univ; Elec Machines I, 1991]
[**Ans.** (i) 5.293 mWb (ii) 293.75 W (iii) 4:84 A]
5. A single-phase transformer with auto of 449/110 V takes a no-load current of 5 A at 0.2 power factor lagging. If the secondary supplies a current of 120 A at a pf of 0.8 lagging, estimate the current taken by the primary.
[Elec. Machines-I, Bangalore Univ 1992; SCE and TEWB 1996 and Elec. Engg. Punjab Univ 1991]
[**Ans.** (i) 33.9 A, 42.49° (lag)]
6. A 10 kVA, 1-phase transformer with 2,000/400 V at no load, has resistance and leakage reactance of primary winding 5.5 Ω and 12 Ω respectively, the

corresponding values of secondary winding being 0.5 Ω and 0.45 Ω. Determine the value of secondary voltage at full load, 0.8 *pf* lagging, when the primary applied voltage is 2,000 V. **[UP Technical Univ; Electrical Engineering; July 2001]**

[**Ans.** 377.65]

7. 50 kVA, 4400/200 V transformer has $R_1 = 3.45\ \Omega$, $R_2 = 0.009\ \Omega$. The values of reactances are $X_1 = 5.2\ \Omega$ and and $X_2 = 0.015\ \Omega$. Calculate for the transformer (i) equivalent resistance as referred to primary (ii) equivalent resistance referred to secondary (iii) equivalent reactance as referred to both primary and secondary (iv) equivalent impedance as referred to both primary and secondary (v) total copper loss, first using individual resistances of the two windings and secondly using equivalent resistances as referred to each side.

[Nagpur Univ; Elec. Engineering-I, 1993]

8. A 5 kVA, 2,200/220 V single phase transformer has the following parameters.
HV side : $r_1 = 3.4\ \Omega$, $x_1 = 7.2\ \Omega$; LV side : $r_2 = 0.028\ \Omega$, $x_2 = 0.060\ \Omega$
The transformer is made to deliver rated current at 0.8 lagging power factor to a load corrected to LV side. If the load voltage is 220 V, calculate the terminal voltage on the HV side. Also find the voltage regulation at this load.

[RGPV Bhopal, Basic Electrical Engineering, December 2003]

[**Ans.** 2229.28 V; 1.33%]

9. If in a transformer core, the hysteresis and eddy current losses are 80 Ω and 50 Ω at normal voltage and frequency, Calculate the losses when voltage and frequency are increased by 20°. **[UP Technical Univ; Elec. Engineering, First Semester 2004-05]**

[**Ans.** 96 W, 72 W]

10. A transformer is connected to 2200 V, 40 Hz supply. The core loss is 800 watts out of which 600 watts are due to hysteresis and remaining eddy current losses. Determine the core loss if the supply voltage and frequency are 3300 V and 60 Hz respectively. **[Bhrathiyar Univ; Nov. 1997]** [**Ans.** 1350 W]

11. The following data were obtained on a 50 kVA, 2400/120 V transformer.
Open-circuit test, instruments on *LV* side:
Wattmeter reading = 396 W; Ammeter reading = 9.65 A, Voltmeter reading = 120 V
Short-circuit test, instruments on *hv* side:
Wattmeter reading = 810 W; Ameter reading = 20.8 A, Voltmeter reading = 92 V
Find the equivalent circuit parameters referred to high voltage side.

[Punjab Technical Univ; Electrical Engineering, May 2002]

[**Ans.** 14.5 kΩ, 5.3 kΩ, 1872 Ω, 4 Ω]

12. The parameters of the equivalent circuit of a 200 kVA, 2500/250 V single phase transformer are as follows:

Primary resistance = 0.2 Ω
Secondary resistance = 2 mΩ
Primary leakage reactance = 0.45 Ω
Secondary leakage resistance = 4.5 Ω
Core loss resistance = 10 kΩ
Magnetizing reactance = 1.55 kΩ

Using the circuit referred to primary, determine (a) voltage regulation (b) efficiency of the transformer at rated load with 0.8 lagging power factor.

[Punjab Technical Univ; Electrical Engineering, May 2001]

[**Ans.** (a) 2.686% (b) 98.048%]

13. In a 25 kVA, 2000/200 V transformer, the constant and variable losses are 350 W and 400 W respectively. Calculate the efficiency on unity power factor at (*i*) full load and (*ii*) half-full load. **[Punjab Technical Univ; Electrical Engineering, 1999]** [**Ans.** (i) 97.09% (ii) 96.53%]

14. The no load transformation ratio in a 200 kVA, 50 Hz single phase transformer is 4,000/250 V. For a maximum core flux of 0.06 Wb, find
    (i) the efficiency at half the rated kVA and at unity power factor,
    (ii) the efficiency at full load, 0.8 power factor lagging and
    (iii) kVA load for maximum efficiency, given that the full-load copper losses are 1.8 kW and core losses, are 1.5 kW.
    [UP Technical Univ; Electrical Machines, 2001-2002]
    [**Ans.** (i) 98.08% (ii) 97.98% (iii) 482.574 kVA]

15. In a 25 kVA, 2000/200 V transformer, the iron and copper losses are 350 watts and 400 watts respectively. Calculate the efficiency at full load and 0.8 power factor lagging. Determine the maximum efficiency and the corresponding load. **[UP Technical Univ; Elec. Engineering, February 2001]** [**Ans.** 96.39%; 23.38 kVA; 97.1%]

16. The maximum efficiency of a 100 kVA, single phase transformer is 98% and occurs at 80% of full load. If the leakage impedance of the transformer is 5%, find the voltage regulation at rated load of 0.8 *pf* lagging. **[Nagpur Univ; Elec. Machines-I, 1993]** [**Ans.**3.74%]

17. A 600 kVA, single-phase transformer when working at unity power factor, has an efficiency of 92% at full-load and also at half-load. Determine its efficiency when it operates at unity *pf* and 60% of full-load. **[UP Technical Univ; Electrical Machines, 2003-04]** [**Ans.**93.53%]

18. A transformer rated 200 V/50 V, 10 kVA has a core loss of 100 W. What is the maximum efficiency of the transformer at 0.8 lagging power factor ? Assume full-load copper loss as 200 W. At what load this maximum efficiency is obtained? How and why would your answer be different if the power factor were unity? **[RGPV Bhopal; Basic Electrical Engineering, December 2004]** [**Ans.** 7.07 kVA, 96.585%, 97.249%]

19. The efficiency of a 100 kVA single-phase transformer is 98.77% when delivering full-load at 0.8 *pf* and 99.13% at half load and unity power factor. Calculate: (*i*) Iron losses (*ii*) The full-load copper losses. **[RGPV Bhopal; Basic Electrical Engineering, Jan/Feb. 2006]** [**Ans.** 1.012 kW, 2.973 kW]

20. Find all-day efficiency of a transformer having maximum efficiency of 98% at 15 kVA at unity power factor and loaded as follows:
    12 hours — 2 kW at 0.5 pf lag:
    6 hours — 12 kW at 0.8 pf lag
    6 hours— at no load. **[Nagpur Univ; Elec. Machines, 1993]** [**Ans.** 95.31%]

21. A transformer has a primary voltage rating of 11500 V and secondary voltage rating of 2300 V. Two winding are connected in series and the primary is connected to a supply of 11500 V, to act as a step-up auto-transformer. Determine the ouput voltage of the transformer. **[Madras Univ; 1997]** [**Ans.** 13800 *V*]

22. A 11500/2300 V transformer is rated at 100 kVA as a two-winding transformer. If the two windings are connected in series to form an auto-transformer, what will be the possible voltage ratio? **[Manonmanium Sundarnar Univ; April, 1998]** [**Ans.** 13800/2300 V, 13800/11500 V]

VIVA VOCE QUESTIONS ANSWERS

1. **What is the function of transformer?**

Ans. The basic function of a transformer is to transform energy from one voltage level to another (may be from low voltage to high voltage or vice versa).

2. **What do you understand by step-up and step-down transformers?**

Ans. When transformer raises the voltage, i.e. when the ouput voltage is higher than its input voltage, it is called the step-up transformer. When the transformer lowers the voltage, it is called the step-down transformer.

3. **Why does a transformer has iron core? [PTU, December 2000]**

Ans. The use of iron or steel for transformer core ensures a high permeability of the magnetic circuit and because of high permeability the magnitude of exciting current necessary to create the required flux in the core is small. The presence of steel core also causes 100% of magnetic flux created by primary to be linked with secondary.

4. **Why is the efficiency of a transformer maximum among electrical equipments? Explain. [PTU 1999]**

Ans. Owing to lack of rotating parts in a transformer, there are no friction and windage losses. The other losses such as iron losses are also comparatively small because of better magnetic material and less handling of the material. So the efficiency of a transformer is maximum among electrical equipments.

5. **What is normally the efficiency of a transformer?**

Ans. Typical transformer efficiencies at full load lie between 96% and 97% and with extremely large transformers they may be as high as 99%.

6. **What name is given to the coils through which current flows from the source?**

Ans. Primary winding.

7. **What name is given to the coils across which load is connected?**

Ans. Secondary winding.

8. **Why the transformer is also called the static transformer?**

Ans. Since basic construction of transformer does not require any moving part, it is also called the static transformer.

9. **What is one-to-one transformer? What is its application? [RGPV Bhopal; June 2002]**

Ans. The transformer having equal turns in primary and secondary windings is called the one-to-one transformer. Such transformers are used for isolating the load from supply.

10. **Explain with reasons what happens when a power transformer is connected to DC supply of the same voltage rating?**

Ans. If a rated DC voltage is applied to the primary of the transformer, the flux produced in the transformer core will not vary but remain constant in magnitude and, therefore, there will be no self-induced emf in the primary winding (which is only possible with varying flux linkage) to oppose the applied voltage and since the resistance of the primary winding is quite low, a heavy current will flow through the primary winding that may cause burning out of the primary winding.

11. What are the properties of an ideal transformer?

[GGSIP Delhi Univ; May, 2000]

Ans. The properties of an ideal transformer are (i) no winding resistance (ii) no magnetic leakage (iii) no iron loss and (iv) zero-magnetizing current, i.e. an ideal transformer is assumed to consist of two pure inductive coils wound on a loss free core.

12. What is the difference between an ideal and practical transformer?

[PTU; January 2000]

Ans. An ideal transformer is an imaginary transformer that has no winding resistance, no magnetic leakage, no iron loss and zero reluctance while a practical transformer is an actual transformer which operates at a particular frequency and has winding resistance, magnetic leakage, iron loss, copper loss, and magnetic reluctance.

13. The primary of a single-phase transformer having a turn ratio 1:2 is connected to a 10 V DC source while its secondary is connected to a 10 W resistor? What is the value of the steady-state current in the resistor?

Ans. Zero

14. Is there a definite relationship between the number of turns and voltages in transformers?

Ans. The voltage varies in exact proportion to the number of turns connected in series in each winding.

15. What is transformer and transformation ratio? **[M.D. Univ; July, 2001]**

Ans. The transformer is an AC machine that (i) transfers electrical energy from one electric circuit to another (ii) does so without a change of frequency (iii) does so by the principle of electromagnetic induction and (iv) has electric circuits that are linked by a common magnetic circuit. Voltage transformation ratio is defined as the ratio of secondary induced emf to primary induced emf.

16. Does the flux linking both the windings of a transformer remain same?

Ans. Yes; the flux linking the primary and secondary windings is the same.

17. Does the transformer draw any current when its secondary is open?

Ans. Yes; no-load primary current.

18. What is meant by magnetising current?

Ans. Magnetising current is quadrature or watt less component of exciting current of transformer and is used to create alternating flux in the core.

19. What do you know about the no-load current of a transformer?

Ans. The current drawn by primary winding of a transformer on no load is called the no-load or exciting current. It is very small in magnitude in comparison to the full-load primary current (2 to 5 per cent of full-load current). It has two components—energy component (comparatively very small) to meet the iron loss in addition to small amount of copper loss occuring in the primary winding and magnetising component relatively large to create the alternating flux in the core.

20. Does the magnetising current of a transformer lie in phase with the applied voltage?

Ans. No; the magnetising current of a transformer lags behind the applied voltage by 90°.

21. Ordinarily, what is the phase relationship between the primary and secondary voltages of a transformer?

Ans. 180° out of phase.

22. Explain how in a transformer, as the secondary current increases, primary current also increases. **[PTU; May 2002]**

Ans. When the secondary current of a transformer increases, the secondary ampere-turns (N_2I_2) creates more secondary flux. This increased secondary flux opposes the main flux ϕ set up by the exciting current I_0. Thus main flux ϕ is weakened momentarily by the opposing increased secondary flux ϕ_2, and, therefore, difference of applied voltage V_1 and back emf E_1 increases, consequently, more current is drawn from the source of supply flowing through the primary winding until the original value of flux ϕ restores. The extra current drawn from the supply source increases the primary ampere-turns (N_1I_1) and compensates the extra secondary ampere-turns i.e. $N_1I_1 = N_2I_2$.

Thus in a transformer when the secondary current increases, primary current also increases.

23. Why the main flux in a transformer remains practically constant from no-load to full-load?

Ans. When the transformer is on no load, it draws no-load or exciting current I_0 from the supply mains. The no-load current I_0 sets up mmf N_1I_0 which produces flux ϕ in the core. When an impedance is connected across the secondary terminals, current I_2 flows through the secondary. The secondary current I_2 sets up its own mmf and hence creates a secondary flux ϕ_2 opposing the main flux ϕ. In other words, the secondary ampere-turns weaken the main flux in the core. Momentarily, self-induced emf E_1 decreases due to which primary draws extra current from the supply source. This extra current drawn from the supply source increases the primary ampere-turns (N_1I_1) and current sates the secondary ampere-turns N_2I_2.

Since the secondary flux ϕ_2 produced by secondary mmf N_2I_2 is neutralized by the flux ϕ_1 produced the mmf N_1I_1 set up by counterbalancing primary current I_1', the flux in the transformer core remains constant from no-load to full load.

24. How does the leakage flux occur in a transformer? **[PTU; December 2001]**

Ans. In actual practice the total flux created does not link the primary and secondary windings but is divided into three parts namely the main flux ϕ linking both the primary and secondary windings, primary leakages, flux ϕ_{L1}, linking with primary winding only and secondary leakage flux ϕ_{L2}, linking with secondary winding only.

The flux set up by the primary or secondary which is set up in the core linking with its own turns and not linking with the other is known as *leakage flux*.

25. What is leakage reactance of transformers? **[PTU; December 2003]**

Ans. Leakage fluxes of primary and secondary produce self inductances L_1 given as $\frac{N_1\phi_{L1}}{I_1}$ and L_2 given as as $\frac{N_2\phi_{L2}}{I_2}$ in respectively windings, i.e. primary and secondary. These inductances, in turn, produce inductive reactances X_1 given as $2\pi L_1$ and X_2 given as $2\pi L_2$ which cause voltage drop in respective windings lagging behind the currents I_1 and I_2 respectively by 90°. The reactances produced by leakage fluxes are called the leakages reactance.

26. What is the effect of leakage flux in a transformer. What is meant by magnetising current? **[PTU; June 2000]**

Ans. The effect of leakage flux is to develop into their respective windings emfs of self-inductance which are proportional to the current, and are, therefore, equivalent in effect to the addition of an inductive coil in series with each winding. The component of no-load current used to create the flux in the transformer core is known as magnetising current.

27. Explain with reasons what happens when the primary terminals of a single phase transformer are connected to the rated AC supply while secondary terminals are short circuited.

Ans. The transformer with secondary short circuited becomes equivalent to a coil having an impedance equal to impedance of both windings, which is quite small. When the primary terminals of the transformer are connected to the rated AC supply, heavy current will flow through primary and secondary winding, that may cause burning out of these windings.

28. Define voltage regulation of a transformer.

[UP Technical Univ. Second Semester 2003-04; GGSIP Univ. Delhi; May 2005]

Ans. Voltage regulation of a transformer is defined as the change in magnitude of terminal or secondary voltage, when full load (rated load) of specified power factor supplied at rated voltage is thrown off (reduced to no load) with primary voltage and frequency held constant, as percentage of the rated terminal voltage.

29. Is voltage regulation better or worse at 0.6 pf lagging than 0.8 pf lagging for the same kVA output explain. [UTU May 2001]

Ans. The voltage regulation will be the maximum and worst when power factor becomes equal to $\cos \tan^{-1} \frac{X_{02}}{R_{02}}$ (lagging).

Since equivalent reactance of transformer is usually more than double its equivalent resistance, the voltage regulation will increase, (i.e. become more and more worse) till power factor falls even below $\cos \tan^{-1} 2$, i.e. 0.45 (lagging), the voltage regulation will worsen of 0.6 *pf* lagging than at 0.6 *pf* lagging.

30. Is the regulation at rated load of a transformer same at 0.8 pf lag and 0.8 pf lead?

Ans. No, the regulation obtained is different at leading and lagging power factors.

31. On what factors does the hysteresis loss depend? Why can this loss be assumed to be constant?

Ans. Hysteresis loss depends upon the type of material, volume of the material, frequency of reversal of magnetic field and

$P_h = \eta (B_{max})^{1.6} fv$ watts

Since from no load to full load the flux linking with the core and supply frequency remains constant, hysteresis load is assumed to remain constant.

32. On what factors does the eddy current loss depend? Why this loss can be assumed to be constant? [PTU; June 2000]

Ans. The eddy current loss depends on the maximum value of flux density in the core and supply frequency for a given core (i.e nature of magnetic material, volume of the core, and thickness of laminations remaining unchanged). Since from no load to full load the flux linking with the core and supply frequency remain constant, the eddy current loss remains constant.

33. Classify the losses in power transformer. [GBTU; First Semester 2011-12]

Ans. Transformer losses may be classified into two categories namely constant losses and variable losses. Iron losses are independent of load, and therefore, are called the constant losses. These losses consist of hysteresis and eddy current losses and occur in the core and yoke of the transformer due to alternating flux.

Copper losses vary as the square of load current or kVA, and therefore, they are called variable losses. These losses occur in primary and secondary windings of the transformer due to their resistances when the transformer is loaded.

34. Name the constant losses taking place in a transformer.

[GBTU; Second Semester 2011-12]

Ans. Iron losses are constant losses that take place in a transformer. Eddy current loss and hysteresis loss constitute the iron losses.

35. Does eddy current loss of a transformer depends on the applied voltage?

Ans. Yes, eddy current loss depends upon the applied voltage. If the transformer is operated with increased voltage but at the same frequency the eddy current loss increases due to increase in value of peak value of flux density and if applied voltage is increased with increase in frequency, the proportion of increase being the same in both, the eddy current loss increases due to increase in supply frequency.

36. If the supply frequency is doubled, which loss component in transformer will double?

Ans. Due to doubling of supply frequency, the hysteresis loss component will be double.

37. What is the purpose of the markings on transformer leads?

Ans. They are there for standardization, so that the transformer polarities may be recognizable for any type of use.

38. How can eddy current loss be minimised?

Ans. By using laminated iron core.

39. What is meant by equivalent circuit of a transformer?

Ans. An electrical circuit that can represent behaviour of the transformer to an approximation is called its equivalent circuit.

40. How may the iron loss be reduced to a minimum in a transformer?

Ans. The iron loss may be minimised by using steel of high silicon content for the transformer core and by using very thin laminations (0.35 to 0.5 mm thick) insulated from each other by insulating varnish or by layers of papers.

41. Why are iron or core losses assumed to remain constant from no load to full load in a power transformer?

Ans. Since iron or core losses depend on the flux density and supply frequency for a given transformer core and flux density and supply frequency remain the same from no load to full load, iron or core losses are assumed to remain constant from no load to full load.

42. Why is the iron loss in a transformer substantially independent of the load current? Explain.

Ans. Iron or core loss is caused by the alternating flux in the core and consists of hysteresis and eddy current losses which depend upon the maximum flux density in the core and supply frequency. Since it has been determined that the mutual flux varies some what with the load (its variation being 1 to 3 per cent from no load to full load), the core loss will vary some what with the load and its power factor. It may be emphasized here that core loss is assumed to remain constant from no load to full load, the variations in losses from no load to full load being very small and negligible.

43. Write the condition for efficiency in transformer to be maximum.
[MTU; First Semester 2011-12]

Ans. Efficiency of transformer will be maximum when variable loss (copper loss) is equal to constant loss (iron loss)

$$\text{i.e. } x^2 P_{cu} = P_i$$

where P_i is the iron loss, P_{cu} is the copper loss on full load and x is the fraction of full-load kVA at which efficiency is maximum.

44. Is the efficiency of a transformer same at the same load at 0.8 pf lag and 0.8 pf lead?

Ans. Yes, the efficiency of a transformer remains the same for a given load at a given power factor irrespective of the fact whether the *pf* is lagging or leading.

45. What is meant by all-day efficiency of a power transformer and why is it lower than commercial efficiency?

Ans. The all-day efficiency, also known as energy efficiency or operational efficiency, is defined as the ratio of energy (kWh) output over 24 hours to the energy input, over-the same period,

$$\text{i.e. all-day efficiency} = \frac{\text{Output in kWh}}{\text{Input in kWh}}$$

There are certain types of transformers, such as distribution transformers, which remain energized for 24 hours but they supply very light loads for major part of the day. Thus iron or core loss occurs for the whole day but the copper loss occurs only when the transformer is loaded and so the all-day efficiency of transformer is lower than its commercial efficiency.

46. Why is laminated core used in the transformer? [MD Univ., May 2003]

Ans. Laminated core is used in the transformer to reduce the eddy current loss.

47. Why is an iron-silicon alloy core used in a transformer?
[PTU, December, 2005]

Ans. Iron-silicon alloy core is used in a transformer to ensure a high permeability of the magnetic circuit and keep the iron loss the minimum possible.

48. Why silicon content in electrical sheet steel is limited to 4.5 to 5%?

Ans. Silicon content exceeding 5% makes the sheet steel brittle and so causes problem in punchings.

49. Where may auto-transformer be used?

Ans. Auto-transformers are used when transformation ratio is nearly equal to unity and where there is no objection to direct electrical connection between primary and secondary.

50. A 2-winding transformer is used to step-down the voltage from 220 V to 110 V. If an auto-transformer is used for the same purpose, what would be the ratio of copper weight in them?

Ans. 0.5.

Chapter

12 DC Machines

12.1 INTRODUCTION

Rotating electrical machines can be broadly classified into two categories: DC machines and AC machines. All those machines which either generate or use DC supply falls under the category of DC machines. These machines are further divided into two categories, i.e. DC generators and DC motors. The major advantages of DC machines are their easy speed and torque regulation. These machine works on the concept of electro-mechanical energy conversion.

12.2 CONCEPT OF ELECTRO-MECHANICAL ENERGY CONVERSION

The term electro-mechanical energy conversion refers to conversion of electrical energy into mechanical energy or vice versa. This energy conversion is achieved through a magnetic medium as the intermediary stage between electrical and mechanical forms of energy.

The device used to convert mechanical energy to electrical energy is known as *generator*, while the device which converts electrical energy to mechanical energy is called as *motor*. In generator, mechanical energy is provided by a prime-mover, such as in a diesel engine, this mechanical energy rotates the armature of generator in magnetic field to get electrical output. While in motor, electrical energy is provided to armature conductors placed in a magnetic field to produce a mechanical torque. The block diagram representation is shown in Fig. 12.1.

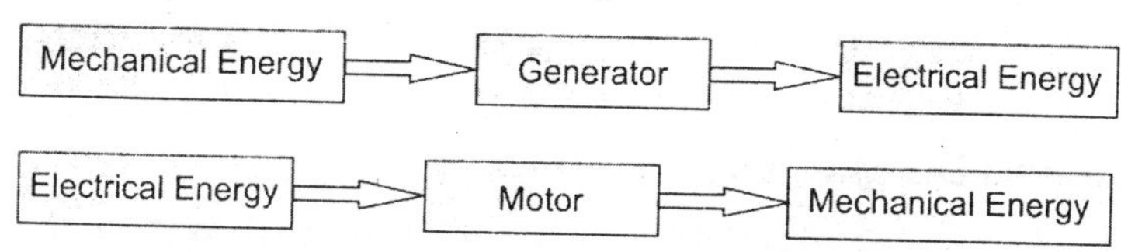

Fig. 12.1: Block diagram representation of concept of elector–mechanical energy conversion

12.3 TYPES OF DC MACHINES

Based on type of excitation used in field winding to set up magnetic field, DC machines can be classified as given in Fig. 12.2.

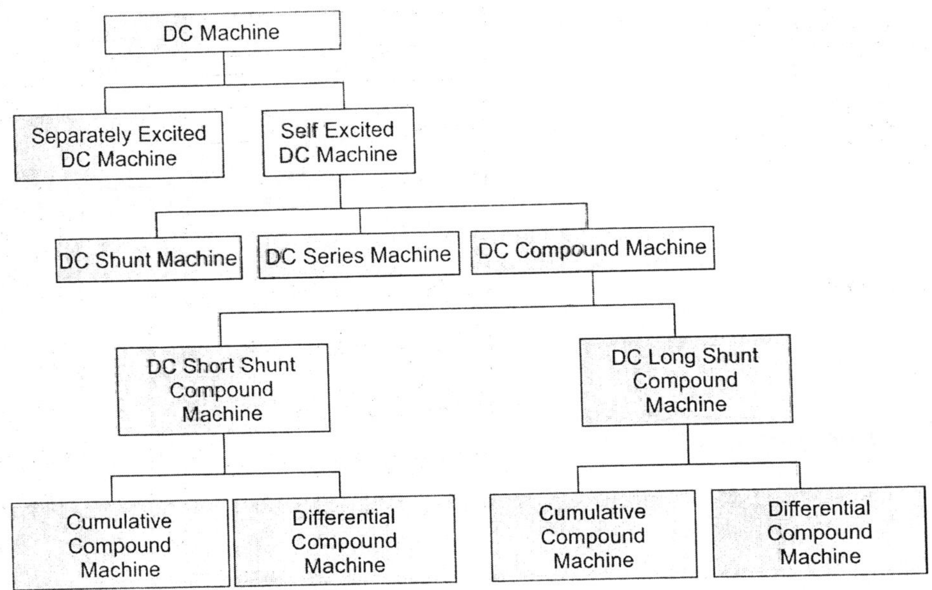

Fig. 12.2

12.3.1 Separately Excited DC Machine

When the field coils of a DC machine are excited or energised from an external DC source, the machine is known as separately excited machine.

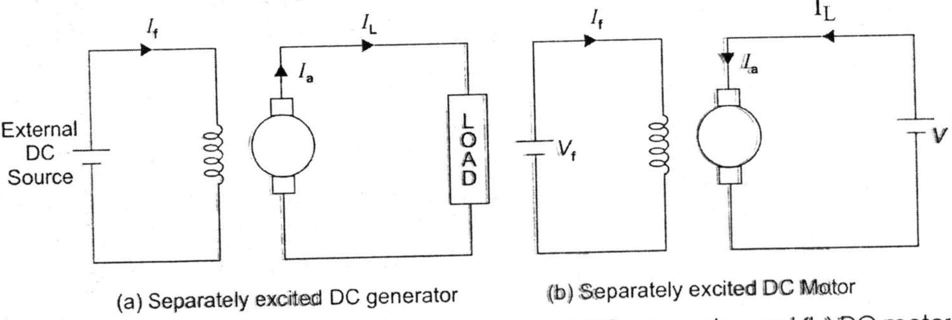

Fig. 12.3: Circuit diagram of separately excited (a) DC generator and (b) DC motor

12.3.2 Self Excited DC Machine

In self excited DC machine, the field coils are energised from the current supplied by the generator itself (in case of DC generator) or the current supplied by DC source connected with armature (in case of DC motor). Therefore, no external source is required to excite field winding. These machines are further classified based on the way field winding is connected with armature winding.

DC Shunt Machine

In DC shunt machine field winding is connected in parallel with the armature winding. Therefore, the voltage across armature and field windings remain same.

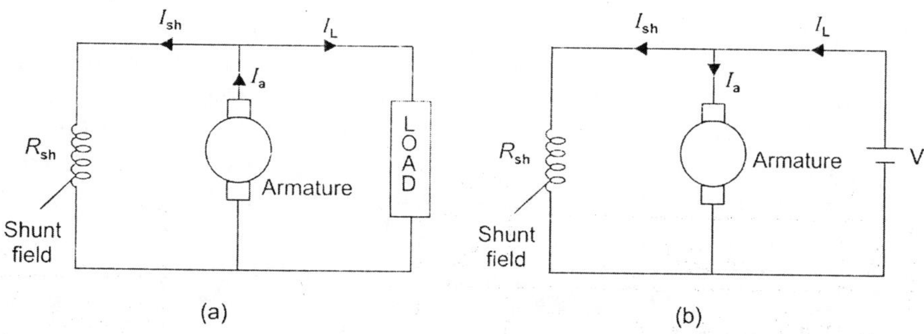

Fig. 12.4: Circuit diagram of DC shunt (a) Generator (b) Motor

DC Series Machine

In DC series machine, field winding is connected in series with armature circuit. Therefore, current flowing through armature and field windings remain same. As the series field winding has to carry large armature current, it is made of thick conductors with less number of turns.

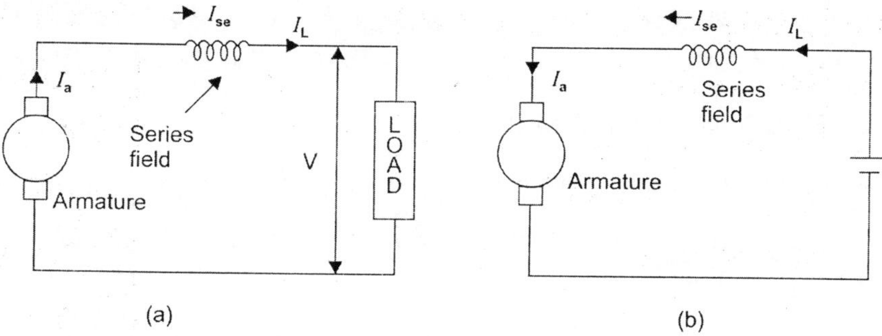

Fig. 12.5: Circuit diagram of DC series (a) Generator (b) Motor

DC Compound Machine

In DC compound machines, two field coils are used. One of these coils is connected in parallel with the armature, while other is connected in series with the armature. Based on the connection of shunt winding with armature these machines are classified as short shunt or long shunt.

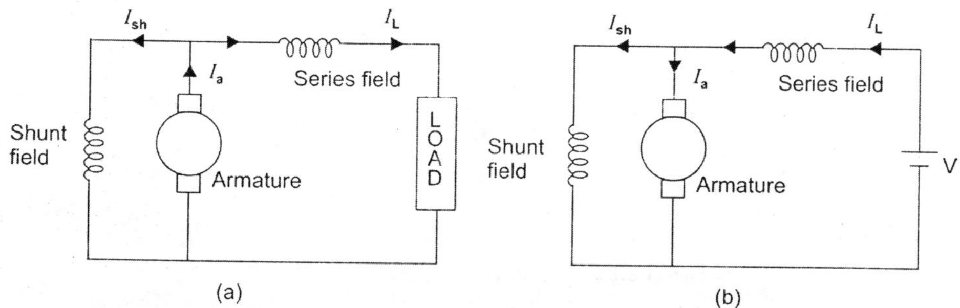

Fig. 12.6: Circuit diagram of short shunt (a) DC generator (b) DC motor

In short shunt machines, shunt winding is connected in parallel with armature winding, as shown in Fig. 12.5. In long shunt machines, shunt winding is connected in parallel with armature and series field winding as represented in Fig. 12.6.

Compound motors can further be classified as cumulative compound and differential compound. In cumulative compound machines, two field windings are arranged in such a way that direction of field current through them is same, then flux due to series field strengthen the flux due to shunt field winding. In differential compound machines, the direction of field currents in shunt and series field opposes each other, therefore, flux due to series field weakens the flux due to shunt field winding.

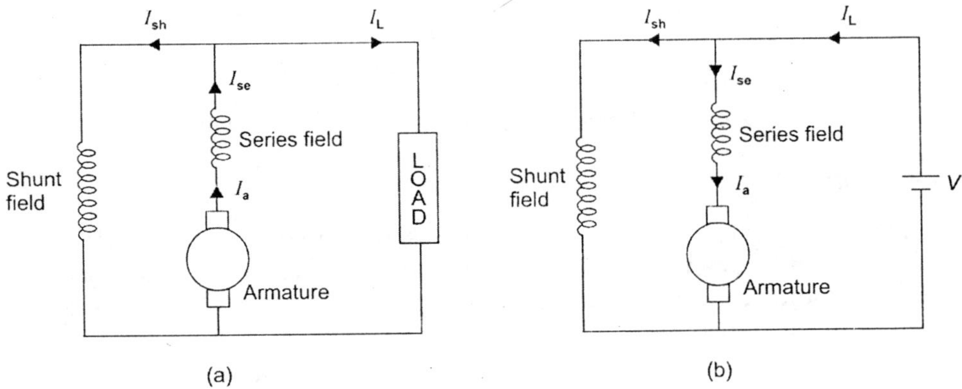

Fig. 12.7: Circuit diagram of long shunt (a) DC generator (b) DC motor

12.4 CONSTRUCTION OF DC MACHINE

The construction of a DC machine is shown in Fig. 12.8.

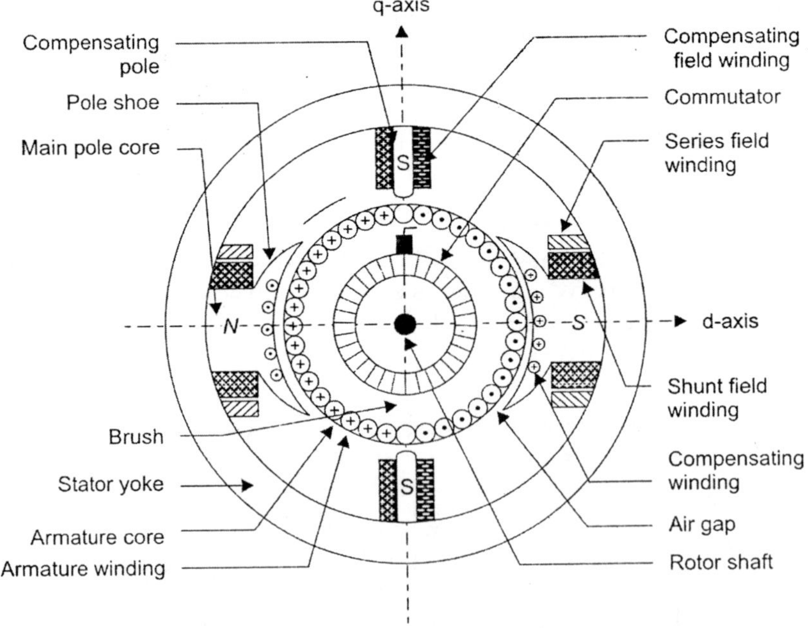

Fig. 12.8: Construction of a DC machine

A DC machine has following essential parts:

(i) Yoke or outer enclosure/frame
(ii) Pole core and pole shoes
(iii) Field coils
(iv) Armature core
(v) Armature winding
(vi) Commutator
(vii) Brush assembly and brush gear
(viii) Bearings

12.4.1 Yoke

The outer enclosure of a DC machine is known as yoke. It serves the following purposes:

(i) It provides protection to the machine from dust, moisture etc.

(ii) It provides low reluctance path to magnetic flux produced by the pole.

(iii) It provides mechanical support to poles.

As yoke is an essential part of magnetic circuit, it is made up of low reluctance material such as cast iron, cast steel or rolled steel etc.

12.4.2 Pole Core and Pole Shoes

A pole consists of pole core and pole shoe. Pole core can be a solid iron piece or laminated one. It houses the field winding. Pole shoes are made up of thin laminations. It is an extended part of pole core and due to its typical shape serves following purposes:

(i) It acts as a support to the field coil.

(ii) It reduces the reluctance of magnetic circuit (due to large cross-sectional area).

(iii) It spread out the flux in the air gap

Based on the pole construction, the pole core and pole shoe are shown in Fig. 12.9. Pole core and pole shoes are made of low reluctance material such as cast iron or cost steel.

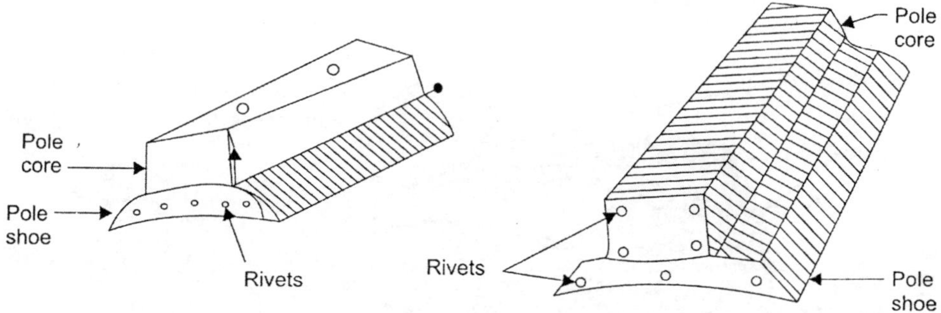

Fig. 12.9: Constructional view of (a) Solid pole core with laminated pole shoe (b) Laminated pole core and pole shoe

12.4.3 Field Coils

Field coils are used to setup flux in the pole core. When field coils are energised they electromagnetise the poles and sets up flux in the magnetic circuit. Field coils are made up of copper wire or strip. Wound coil is placed over the pole core as shown in Fig. 12.10.

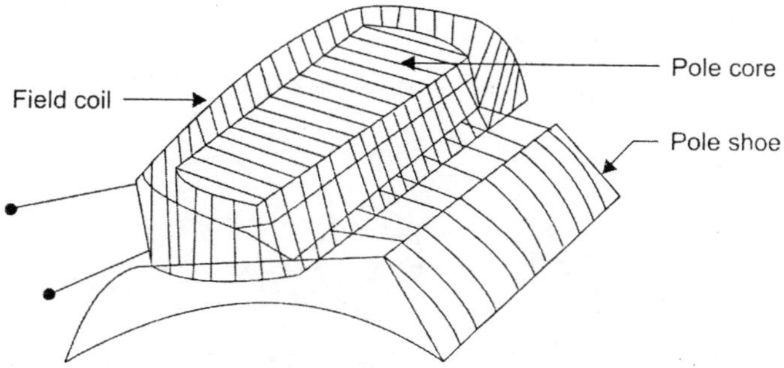

Fig.12.10: Field coil wound over pole

12.4.4 Armature Core

Armature core provides low reluctance path to magnetic lines of flux linking from north pole to south pole. It also houses the armature winding and secure them firmly in armature slots. It is cylindrical in shape and made up of thin laminations to reduce eddy current losses. In DC machines armature is the rotating part of machine. Armature core is made up of high permeability silicon steel laminations. Fig. 12.11a shows a single armature core lamination, while 12.11b represents armature core housing armature winding.

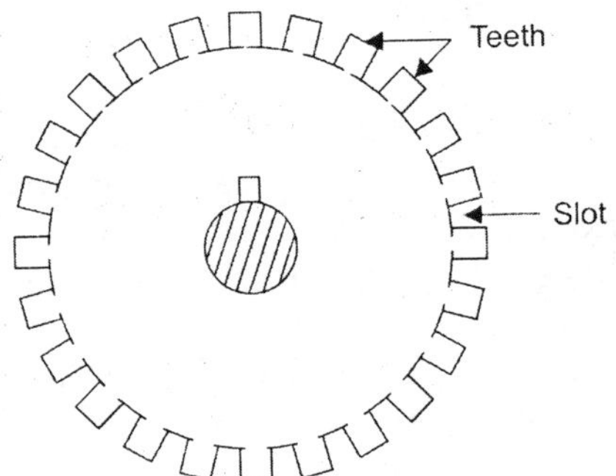

Fig. 12.11a: Armature core lamination

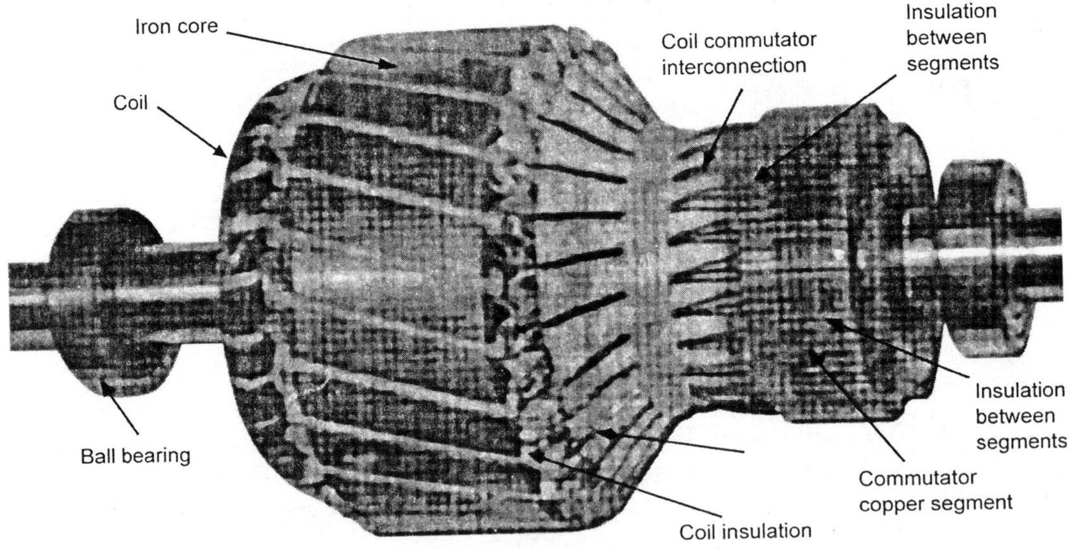

Fig. 12.11b: Armature core housing armature winding

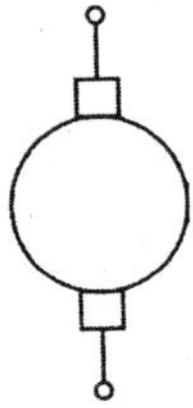

Fig. 12.11c: Symbol of DC machine

12.4.5 Armature Winding

Copper wires housed in armature slots are suitably connected to form armature winding. As per the number of parallel path provided for armature current, armature windings are classified into two categories, i.e. lap winding and wave winding.

In lap winding, conductors are connected such that number of parallel paths are equal to number of poles. In wave winding, the armature conductors provide two parallel path to armature currents.

12.4.6 Commutator

Commutator serves the purpose of collecting the alternating current from armature circuit (in case of generator) and supply it to external circuit by making it unidirectional, while its function is vice versa in case of motor. It is made up of multiple segments of copper which are insulated by mica as shown in Fig. 12.12.

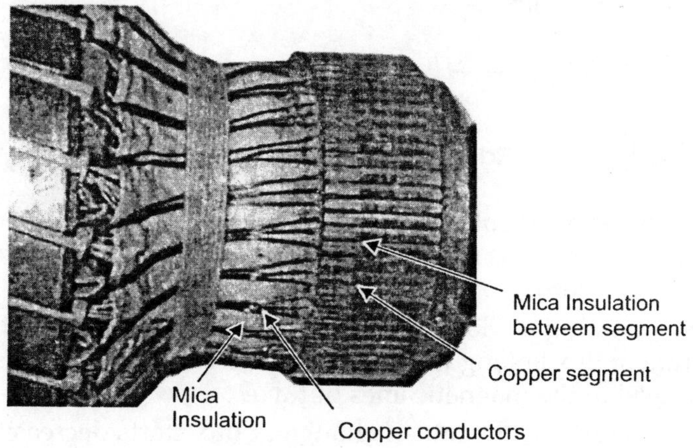

Fig. 12.12: Commutator

12.4.7 Brush Assembly and Brush Gear

Brushes are used to collect current from commutator and supply it to external circuit (in case of generator) and vice-versa in case of a motor. Brushes are made up of carbon or graphite. These brushes are housed in brush holders and are kept pressed on commutator by a spring. Entire arrangement of brush holder, spring and its tension adjusting mechanism is referred to as brush gear.

12.4.8 Bearings

Rotor of DC machines is supported on both ends by bearings to provide almost friction less rotation. For low and medium rating machines ball bearings are used while for heavy duty machines roller bearings are preferred.

12.5 WORKING OF DC GENERATOR

The DC generator works on the principle of Faraday's law of electromagnetic induction, i.e. whenever a conductor cuts magnetic flux, dynamically induced emf is produced in it. The magnitude of this induced emf is directly proportional to rate of change of flux and its direction is given by Fleming's right hand rule.

Working: To understand the working of DC generator, let us consider a single turn rectangular copper coil ABCD as shown in Fig. 12.13. Let this coil rotates in magnetic field, two ends of this coil are joined to two slip rings *a* and *b*. The current is collected from slip rings with the help of brushes 1 and 2.

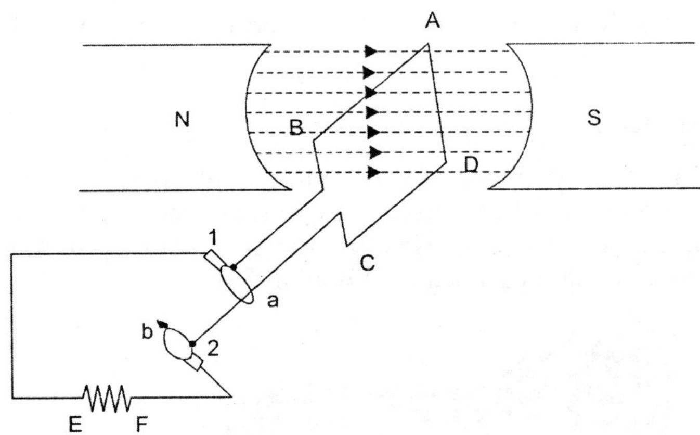

Fig. 12.13: Single turn generator

When the coil is perpendicular to the magnetic line of fluxes as shown in Fig. 12.13, the flux linking with the coil is maximum but its rate of change is zero. Hence induced emf in this position is zero.

Let the coil is rotating in clockwise direction, as the coil starts taking successive positions, the rate of flux linking with coil sides increases and reaches maximum value when coil is parallel to the magnetic lines of fluxes.

As the coil turns further, the rate of change of flux starts decreasing and reaches to zero as the coil rotates by 180°.

When coil rotates further rate of change of flux starts increasing in negative direction up to negative maximum at 270°. On further rotation, the rate of change of flux decreases towards zero as the coil complete one turn at 360°. Therefore, the induce emf has alternating nature as shown in Fig. 12.14.

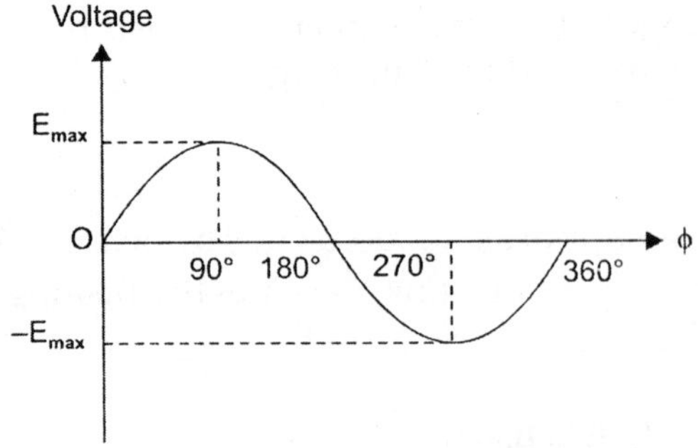

Fig. 12.14: Waveform of induced emf of single turn generator

To make this emf unidirectional, split rings are used in place of slip rings, as shown in Fig. 12.15.

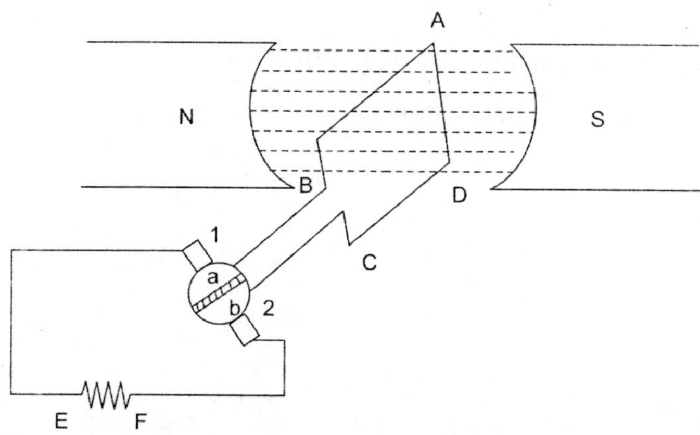

Fig. 12.15: Single turn DC generator

The corresponding wave form of emf is shown in Fig. 12.16.

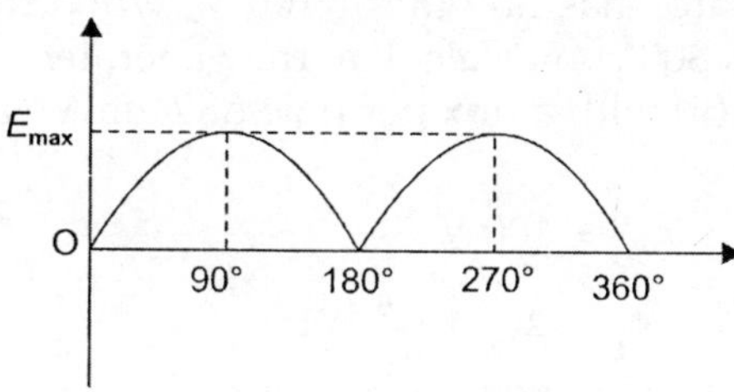

Fig. 12.16: Waveform of induced emf with split ring and no. of coil turns

As number of segments of split rings are increased, the pulsating undirection emf becomes constant DC. A multiple segment split ring arrangement is called *commutator*, which makes alternating emf of armature as a constant DC for external circuit.

12.6 EMF EQUATION OF DC GENERATOR

Let

ϕ = flux/pole, weber
P = no. of poles
N = number of revolution/minute made by armature
Z = total No. of armature conductors
= no. of slots × no. of conductors/slot
A = no. of parallel paths in armature
E_g = generated emf

$$\text{Average emf generated/conductor} = \frac{d\phi}{dt}\text{ volt}$$

$$\text{Flux cut/conductor in one revolution } d\phi = P\phi \text{ Wb}$$

$$\text{Time taken to complete one revolution } dt = \frac{60}{N}\text{ sec}$$

(as N revolutions are completed in 60 sec)

$$\text{Average emf generated/conductor} = \frac{d\phi}{dt} = \frac{p\phi}{60/N}$$

$$= \frac{\phi PN}{60}$$

$$\text{No. of armature conductors/parallel path} = \frac{Z}{A}$$

$$\text{Generator emf, } E_g = \text{Avg. emf generator/parallel path}$$

$$E_g = \frac{\phi PN}{60}\frac{Z}{A}$$

or $$E_g = \frac{\phi ZPN}{60\ A}\text{ volt}$$

For lap winding $A = P$

For wave winding $A = 2$

$$E_g \propto \phi N$$

SOLVED EXAMPLES ON ABOVE THEORY

Example 1: A DC generator has an emf of 100 V, when the useful flux per pole is 20 mWb and the speed is 800 rpm. Calculate the generated emf (i) with the same flux and a speed of 1000 rpm (ii) with a flux per pole of 24 mWb and a speed of 900 rpm. **[UPTU, 2003]**

$$E_{g1} = 100\text{ V}$$

$$\phi_1 = 20 \times 10^{-3}\text{ Wb}$$

$$N_1 = 800\text{ rpm}$$

As $$E \propto \phi N$$

So, $$\frac{E_{g2}}{E_{g1}} = \frac{\phi_2}{\phi_1} \times \frac{N_2}{N_1}$$

(i) $$\phi_2 = \phi_1,\ N_2 = 1000\text{ rpm}$$

$$\frac{E_{g2}}{E_{g1}} = \frac{\phi_1}{\phi_1} \times \frac{1000}{800}$$

or $$E_{g2} = E_{g,1} \times \frac{1000}{800} = 100 \times \frac{1000}{800} = 125\text{ V}$$

(*ii*) $$\phi_2 = 24 \times 10^{-3}\text{ Wb},\ N_2 = 900\text{ rpm}$$

or $$E_{g2} = E_{g,1} \times \frac{\phi_2}{\phi_1} \times \frac{N_2}{N_1} = 100 \times \frac{24 \times 10^{-3}}{20 \times 10^{-3}} \times \frac{900}{800} = 135\text{ V}$$ **Ans.**

Example 2: A four-pole, wave wound generator has 51 slots, each slot containing 20 conductors. Calculate generated voltage, when it is running at 1500 rpm. Assume flux per pole as 7 mWb. **[Allahabad University, 1993]**

Solution:

$$E_g = \frac{\phi ZN}{60}\left(\frac{P}{A}\right)$$

$$\phi = 7\text{ mWb} = 7 \times 10^{-3}\text{ Wb}$$

$$Z = 51 \times 20 = 1020\text{ conductors}$$

$$N = 1500 \text{ rpm}$$
$$P = 4$$
$$A = 2$$

$$E_g = \frac{7 \times 10^{-3} \times 1020 \times 1500}{60}\left(\frac{4}{2}\right) = 357 \text{ V}$$ **Ans.**

Example 3: In a DC generator, what will be the change in induced emf, if flux is reduced by 20% and speed is increased by 20%? **[UPTU 2005-06]**

Solution:

$$\frac{E_{g2}}{E_{g1}} = \frac{\phi_2}{\phi_1} \times \frac{N_2}{N_1}$$

$$\phi_2 = 0.8\ \phi_1$$

$$N_2 = 1.2\ N_1$$

$$E_{g2} = E_{g1} \times \frac{0.8\phi_1}{\phi_1} \times \frac{1.2N_1}{N_1}$$

$$E_{g1} = 0.96 \cdot E_{g1}$$

$\therefore$ Change in induced emf $= E_{g1} - 0.96\ E_{g1} = 0.04\ E_{g1}$

or induced emf is reduced by 4% **Ans.**

12.7 IMPORTANT RELATIONS FOR VARIOUS TYPES OF DC GENERATORS

12.7.1 Separately Excited DC Generator

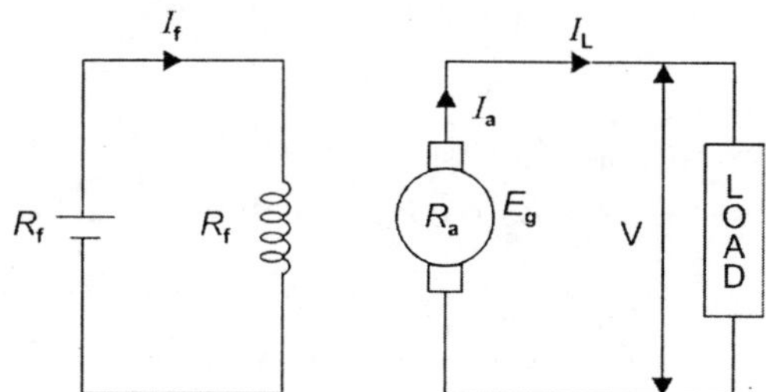

Fig. 12.17: Separately excited DC generator

For separately excited DC generator, shown in Fig. 12.17.

Let V_f = field voltage provided by external source

I_f = field current

R_f = field resistance

I_a = armature current

I_L = load current

R_L = armature resistance

E_g = generated emf

V = output voltage

$$I_a = I_L$$

$$I_f = \frac{V_f}{R_f}$$

$$V = E_g - I_a R_a - \text{brush contact drop (if any)}$$

Power developed $P_g = Eg\, I_a$

Power delivered $P_L = VI_L$

12.7.2 Shunt Wound DC Generator

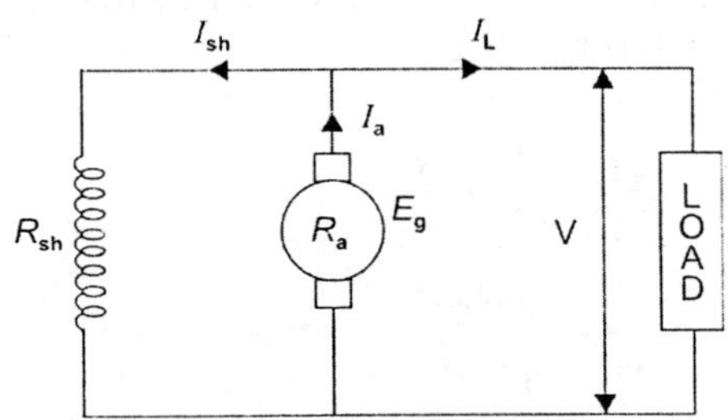

Fig. 12.18: DC shunt generator

For shunt wound DC generator as shown in Fig. 12.18.

Let I_{sh} = shunt field current

R_{sh} = shunt field resistance

V = output voltage

E_g = generated voltage

I_a = armature current

I_L = load current

R_a = armature resistance

$$I_{sh} = \frac{V}{R_{sh}}$$

$$I_a = I_L + I_{sh}$$

$$V = E_g - I_a R_a - \text{Brush contact drop (if any)}$$

Power developed $P_g = E_g I_a$

Power delivered $P_L = V I_L$

12.7.3 Series Wound DC Generator

For DC series generator shown in Fig. 12.19.

Let I_{se} = series field current

R_{se} = series field resistance

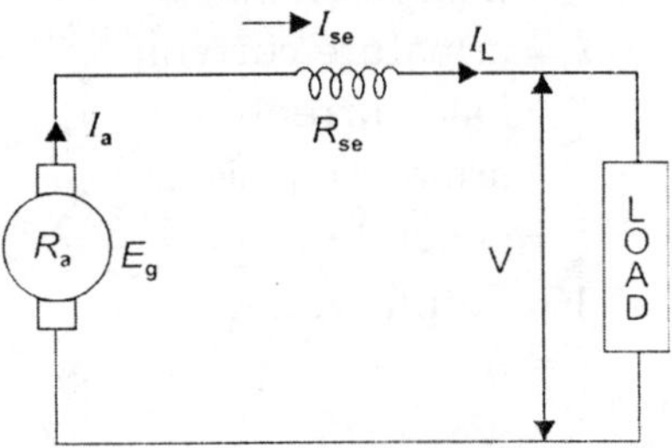

Fig. 12.19: DC series generator

$V =$ Output voltage
$E_g =$ Generated voltage
$I_a =$ Armature current
$I_L =$ Load current
$R_a =$ Armature resistance
$I_{se} = I_a = I_L$

$V = E_g - I_a(R_a + R_{se})$ – Brush contact drop (if any)

Power developed $P_g = Eg\, I_a$

Power delivered $P_L = V I_L$

12.7.4 Compound Wound DC Generator

Case 1: Short shunt DC compound generator

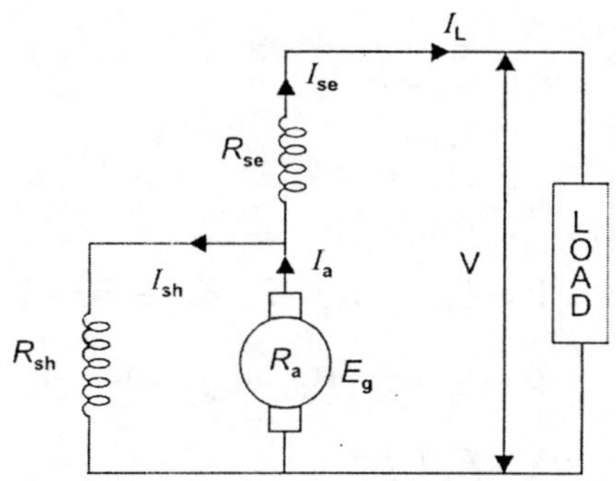

Fig. 12.20: Short shunt DC compound generator

For short shunt DC compound generator shown in Fig. 12.20.

Let $I_{sh} =$ shunt field current
$I_{se} =$ series field current
$R_{sh} =$ shunt field resistance
$R_{se} =$ series field resistance
$V =$ output voltage
$I_L =$ load current
$E_g =$ generated voltage
$I_a =$ armature current

$$I_a = I_{sh} + I_{se}$$

$$I_{se} = I_L$$

$$I_{sh} = \frac{V + I_{se} R_{se}}{R_{sh}}$$

$V = E_g - I_a R_a - I_{se} R_{se} -$ brush contact drop (if any)

Power developed $P_g = E_g I_a$

Power delivered $P_L = VI_L$

Case 2: Long Shunt DC Compound Generator

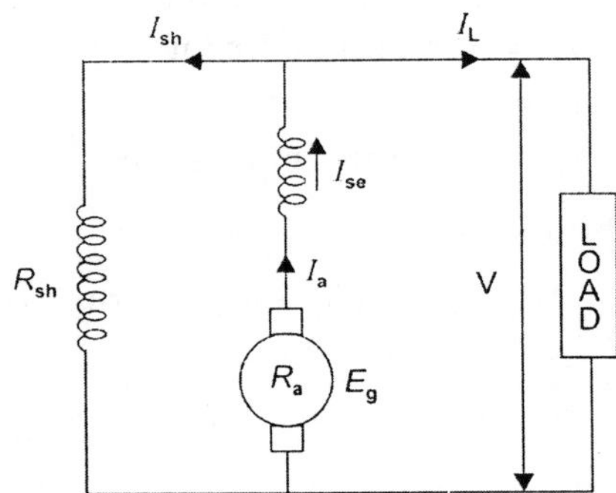

Fig. 12.21: Long shunt DC compound generator

For long shunt DC compound generator shown in Fig. 12.21, we have

$$I_a = I_{se}$$

$$I_a = I_{sh} + I_L$$

$$I_{sh} = \frac{V}{R_{sh}}$$

$$V = E_g - I_a R_a - I_{se} R_{se} - \text{brush contact drop (if any)}$$

or $$V = E_g - I_a (R_a + R_{se}) - \text{brush contact drop (if any)}$$

Power developed $\quad P_g = E_g I_a$

Power delivered $\quad P_L = VI_L$

SOLVED EXAMPLES ON ABOVE THEORY

Example 1: A 20 kW, 200 V shunt generator has an armature resistance of 0.05 Ω, and a shunt field resistance of 200 Ω. Calculate power developed in armature, when it delivers rated output. **[UPTU 2006-07]**

Solution: Given data

$$P_L = 20 \text{ kW};\ V = 200 \text{ V};\ R_{sh} = 200\ \Omega;\ R_a = 0.05\ \Omega$$

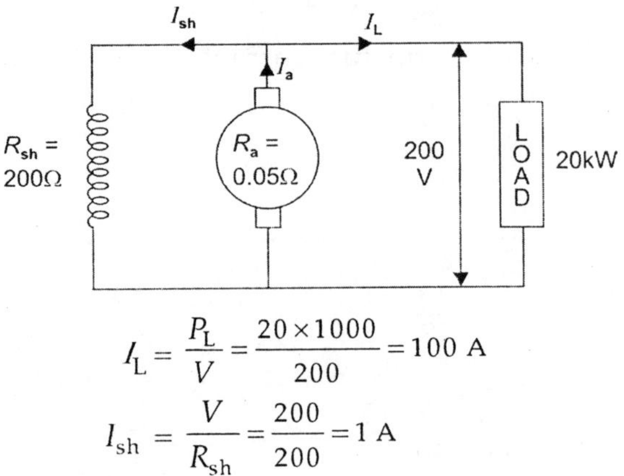

$$I_L = \frac{P_L}{V} = \frac{20 \times 1000}{200} = 100 \text{ A}$$

$$I_{sh} = \frac{V}{R_{sh}} = \frac{200}{200} = 1 \text{ A}$$

$$I_a = I_L + I_{sh} = 100 + 1 = 101 \text{ A}$$
$$E_g = V + I_a R_a = 200 + 101 \times 0.05 = 205.05 \text{ V}$$
$$P_g = Eg\, I_a = 205.05 \times 101 = 20710 \text{ W} = 20.71 \text{ kW}$$ **Ans.**

Example 2: In a 120 V compound generator, the resistances of armature, shunt and series field windings are 0.06 Ω, 25 Ω and 0.04 Ω, respectively. Load current is 100 A. Find the induced emf and armature current, when the machine is connected as (i) short shunt, (ii) long shunt.

Solution: Given data

$$V = 120 \text{ V};\ R_a = 0.06\ \Omega;\ R_{sh} = 25\ \Omega;\ R_{se} = 0.04\ \Omega;\ I_L = 100 \text{ A}$$

(i) When working as short shunt

$$I_{se} = I_L = 100 \text{ A}$$
$$I_{sh} = \frac{V + I_{se} R_{se}}{R_{sh}} = \frac{120 + 100 \times 0.04}{25} = 4.96 \text{ A}$$

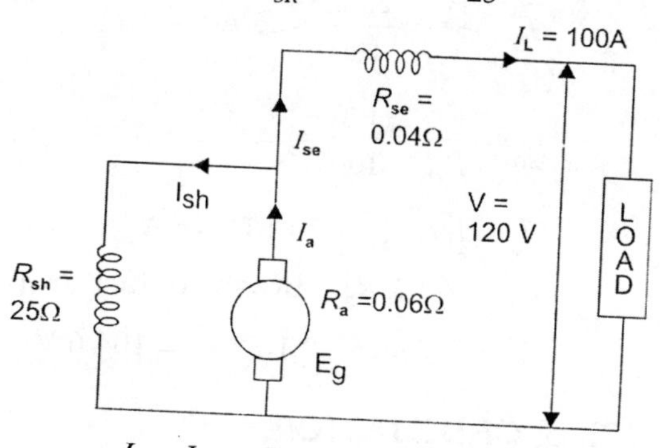

$$I_a = I_{sh} + I_{se} = 104.96 \text{ A}$$
$$E_g = V + I_a R_a + I_{se} R_{se}$$
$$= 120 + 104.96 \times 0.06 + 100 \times 0.04 = 130.30 \text{ V}$$ **Ans.**

(ii) When working as long short

$$I_{sh} = \frac{V}{R_{sh}} = \frac{120}{25} = 4.8 \text{ A}$$
$$I_a = I_{se} = I_L + I_{sh}$$
$$I_a = 100 + 4.8 = 104.8 \text{ A}$$
$$E_g = V + I_a (R_a + R_{se})$$
$$= 120 + 104.96(0.06 + 0.04) = 130.48 \text{ V}$$

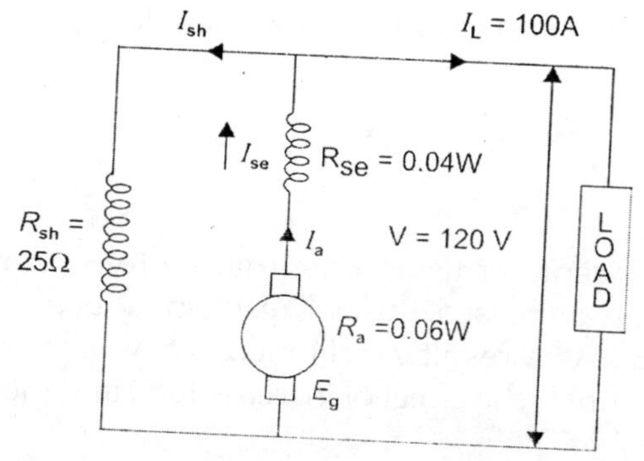

Example 3: A dc shunt generator having armature and field resistance of 0.1 Ω and 0.1 Ω, respectively. It supplies power to fifty 100 V, 50 W bulbs. Calculate armature current and generated emf. Consider brush contact drop of 1 V/brush.

Solution:

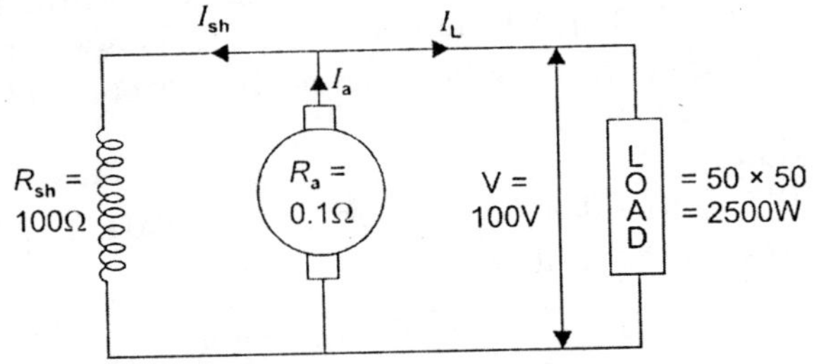

$$P_L = 50 \times 50 \text{ W} = 2500 \text{ W}$$

$$I_L = \frac{P_L}{V} = \frac{2500}{100} = 25 \text{ A}$$

$$I_{sh} = \frac{V}{R_{sh}} = \frac{100}{100} = 1 \text{ A}$$

$$I_a = I_L + I_{sh} = 25 + 1 = 26 \text{ A}$$

$$E_g = V + I_a R_a + \text{brush contact drop}$$

$$= 100 + 26 \times 0.1 + 2 \times 1 = 104.6 \text{ V}$$ **Ans.**

12.8 WORKING PRINCIPLE OF DC MOTOR

The working of a DC motor is based on the principle that when a current carrying conductor is placed in a magnetic field it experiences a force, whose direction is governed by Fleming's left hand rule. The magnitude of this mechanical force is given by:

$$f = BIl \text{ newton}$$

When this force acts on conductors armature starts rotating. As armature conductor rotates in magnetic field, an emf called as back emf induces in them. This back emf (E_b) apposes the applied voltage and its magnitude is same as that was for generated emf in DC generator, i.e.

$$E_b = \frac{\phi Z N}{60}\left(\frac{P}{N}\right)$$

12.8.1 Significance of Back EMF in DC Motor

The presence of back emf makes a DC motor a self regulating machine. The expression for back emf is given as

$$E_b = V - I_a R_a$$

or

$$I_a = \frac{V - E_b}{R_a}$$

To understand the concept, let us assume that motor is running in steady state. Suppose its load is suddenly increased, this will result in reduction of speed which means reduction in back emf E_b. As a result I_a will increase, which will make the motor to develop more torque to counter the effect of increase load and motor will regain its rated speed.

Similarly, if load from a motor is suddenly removed. It will try to accelerate, thereby increasing back emf and reducing armature current. This reduction in current will reduce the developed torque of armature. This reduced torque will oppose the acceleration of motor and motor will regain its rated speed.

Therefore, presence of back emf maintains a DC motor in stable zone of operation.

12.8.2 Important Relations for Different Types of DC Motors

Separately excited DC motor

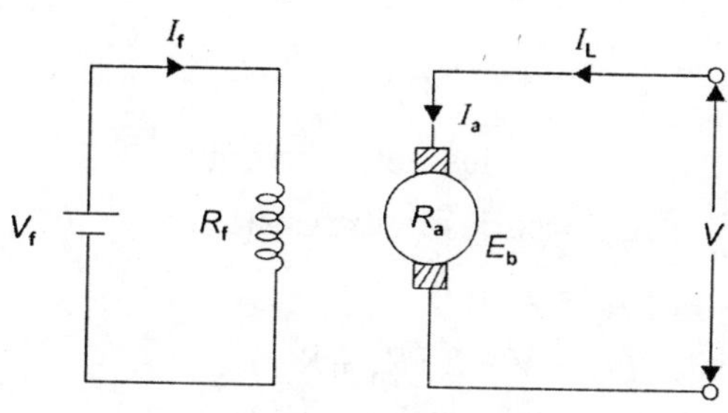

Fig. 12.22

Let

I_a = Armature current

R_a = Armature resistance

I_L = Line current

V = Input voltage

R_f = Field resistance

V_f = Field voltage

I_f = Field current

$$I_f = \frac{V_f}{R_f}$$

$$I_a = I_L$$

$$E_b = V - I_a R_a$$

Input power $P_{in} = VI_L$

Output power $P_{out} = E_b I_a$

DC Shunt Motor

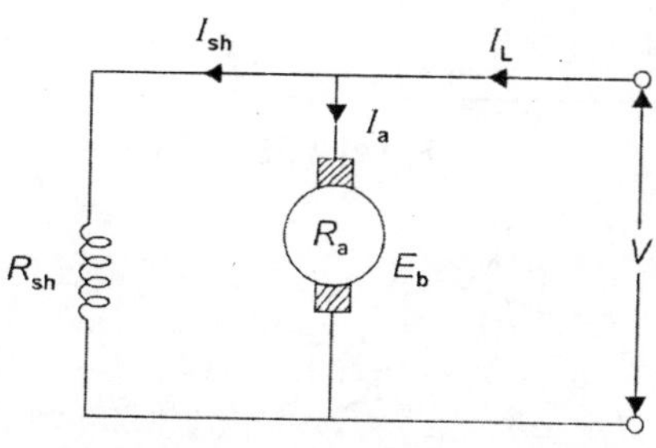

Fig. 12.23

Let, I_{sh} = shunt field current

R_{sh} = shunt field resistance

then
$$I_{sh} = \frac{V}{R_{sh}}$$

$$I_L = I_a + I_{sh}$$

$$E_b = V - I_a R_a$$

Input power $P_{in} = V I_L$

Output power $P_{out} = E_b I_a$

DC Series Motor

Let, I_{se} = series field current

R_{se} = series field resistance

$$I_a = I_L = I_{se}$$

$$E_b = V - I_a (R_a + R_{se})$$

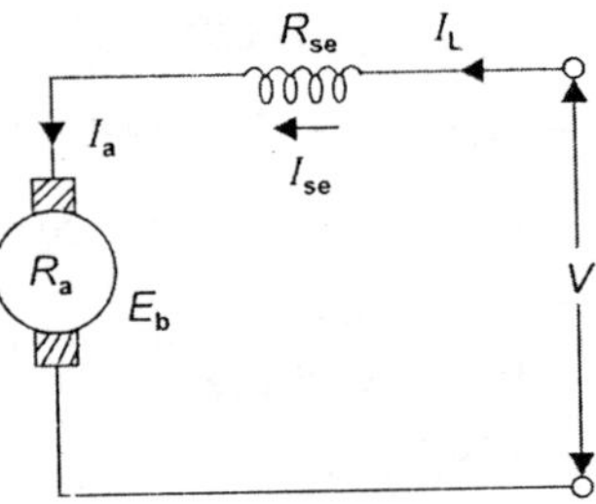

Fig. 12.24

Input power $P_{in} = V I_L$

Output power $P_{out} = E_b I_a$

Short Shunt DC Compound Motor

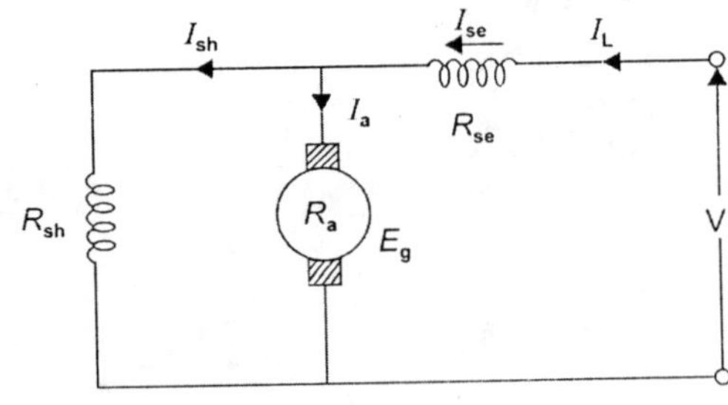

Fig. 12.25

$$I_L = I_a + I_{sh}$$

$$I_L = I_{se}$$

$$I_{sh} = \frac{V - I_{se} R_{se}}{R_{sh}}$$

or $$I_{sh} = \frac{E_b + I_a R_a}{R_{sh}}$$

$$E_b = V - I_a R_a - I_{se} R_{se}$$

Input power $P_{in} = VI_L$

Output power $P_{out} = E_b I_a$

Long Shunt DC Compound Motor

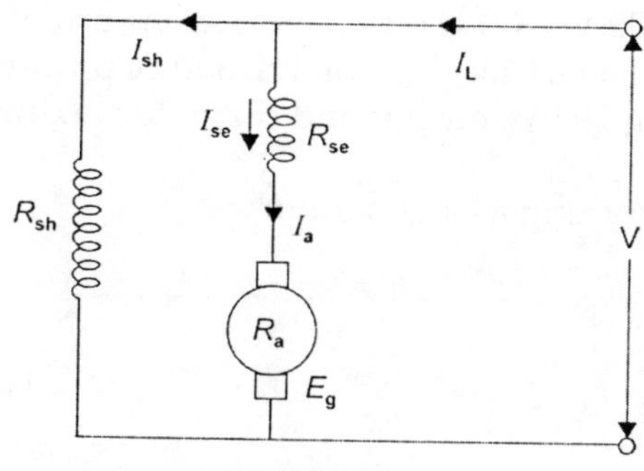

Fig. 11.26

$$I_L = I_{se} + I_{sh}$$

$$I_L = I_a + I_{sh}$$

$$I_a = I_{se}$$

or $$I_{sh} = \frac{V}{R_{sh}}$$

$$E_b = V - I_a (R_a + R_{se})$$

Input power $P_{in} = VI_L$

Output power $P_{out} = E_b I_a$

SOLVED EXAMPLES ON ABOVE THEORY

Example 1: A 500 V, DC shunt motor has an armature resistance of 0.5 Ω and field resistance of 250 Ω. Calculate the value of back emf, when motor is taking a power of 10 kW from supply.

Solution:

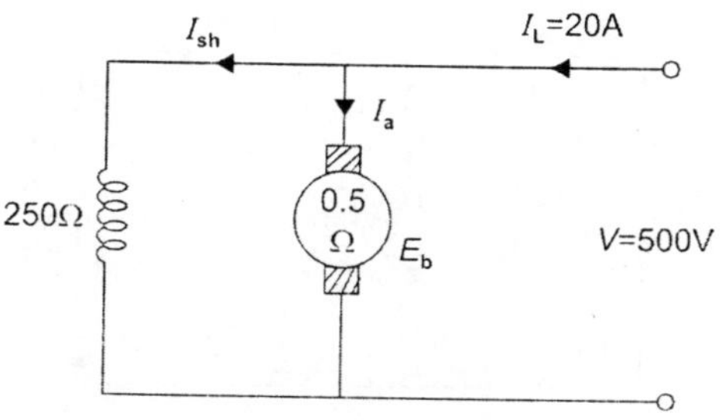

$$\text{Input power} = VI_L = 10 \times 1000\ W$$

$$\text{Line current} = \frac{10 \times 1000}{V} = \frac{10 \times 1000}{500} = 20\ \text{A}$$

$$I_{sh} = \frac{V}{R_{sh}} = \frac{500}{250} = 2 \text{ A}$$

$$I_L = I_a + I_{sh}$$

or $$I_a = I_L I_{sh} = 200 - 2 = 18 \text{ A}$$

$$E_b = V - I_a R_a$$

$$= 500 - 18 \times 0.5 = 491 \text{ V}$$ **Ans.**

Example 2: A 10 kW, 200 V DC shunt generator has armature and field resistance of 0.05 Ω and 200 Ω respectively. Calculate total armature power developed when (i) works as a generator supplying 10 kW output and (ii) motor taking 10 kW input power from supply.

Solution: (i) When working as a generator

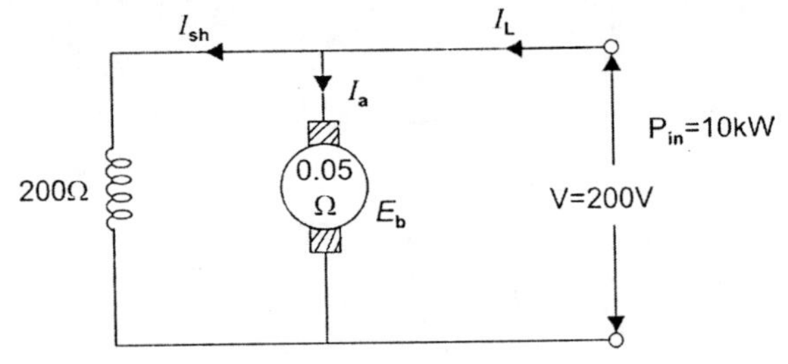

$$I_{sh} = \frac{V}{R_{sh}} = \frac{200}{200} = 1 \text{ A}$$

$$\text{Output power} = V I_L = 10 \times 1000 \text{ W}$$

or $$I_L = \frac{10 \times 1000}{200} = 50 \text{ A}$$

$$I_a = I_L + I_{sh} = 50 + 1 = 51 \text{ A}$$

$$E_g = V + I_a R_a = 200 + 51 \times 0.05 = 202.55 \text{ V}$$

Total power developed in armature

$$= E_g I_a = 202.55 \times 51$$

$$= 10330.05 \text{ W} = 10.33 \text{ kW}$$ **Ans.**

(ii) When working as a motor

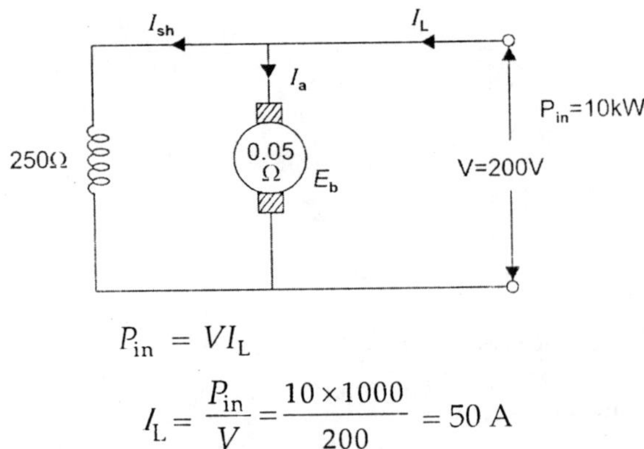

$$P_{in} = V I_L$$

$$I_L = \frac{P_{in}}{V} = \frac{10 \times 1000}{200} = 50 \text{ A}$$

$$I_{sh} = \frac{200}{200} = 1\text{ A}$$

$$I_a = I_L - I_{sh} = 50 - 1 = 49\text{ A}$$

$$E_b = V - I_a R_a$$

$$= 200 - 49 \times 0.05 = 197.55\text{ V}$$

Power developed by armature $= E_b I_a$

$$= 197.55 \times 49 = 9679.95\text{ W} = 9.68\text{ kW}$$ **Ans.**

Example 3: A 250 V, shunt motor runs at 1200 rpm with a line current of 50 A. Its armature and field resistance are 0.2 Ω and 250 Ω respectively. Find the speed at which motor runs with a line current of 25 A.

Solution:

$$\frac{N_2}{N_1} = \frac{E_{b,2}}{E_{b,1}} \times \frac{\phi_1}{\phi_2}$$

For shunt motor flux remains constant

So, $$\frac{N_2}{N_1} = \frac{E_{b,2}}{E_{b,1}}$$

$$E_{b,1} = V - I_{a,1} R_a$$

$$I_{sh} = \frac{V}{R_{sh}} = \frac{250}{250} = 1\text{ A}$$

$$I_{a,1} = I_{L,1} - I_{sh} = 50 - 1 = 49\text{ A}$$

$$E_{b,1} = 250 - 49 \times 0.2 = 240.2\text{ V}$$

$$I_{a,2} = I_{L,2} - I_{sh} = 25 - 1 = 24\text{ A}$$

$$E_{b,2} = 250 - 24 \times 0.2 = 245.2\text{ V}$$

$$N_2 = N_1 \times \frac{E_{b,2}}{E_{b,1}}$$

$$= 1200 \times \frac{245.2}{240.2}$$

$$= 1224.97 = 1225\text{ rpm}$$

12.9 TORQUE DEVELOPED IN A MOTOR

Let T_a be the torque developed by the armature of a DC motor, running at N rpm.

Mechanical power developed by this torque

$$P_m = T_a \omega = T_a \times \frac{2\pi N}{60}\text{ W}$$

where ω = angular velocity of armature in radian/sec

Electrical power developed at armature

$$P_e = E_b I_a$$

This electrical power should be equal to mechanical power developed at armature.

$$T_a \times \frac{2\pi N}{60} = E_b I_a$$

or $$T_a \times \frac{2\pi N}{60} = \frac{\phi Z N}{60}\left(\frac{P}{A}\right) I_a$$

or $$T_a = \frac{1}{2\pi}\phi Z\left(\frac{P}{A}\right) I_a$$

$$= 0.159\ \phi Z\ I_a\left(\frac{P}{A}\right) N-m$$

So, $T_a \propto \phi I_a$

For shunt motor ϕ is constant $T_a \propto I_a$

For series motor $\phi \propto I_a$, Hence $T_a \propto I_a^2$

Note: The direction of torque is dependent on direction of flux and armature current. If either of the two is reversed, the direction of torque will reverse and this will load to reversal of direction of rotation.

Shaft torque $$(T_{sh}) = \frac{E_b I_a - \text{Iron and friction losses}}{2\pi N/60}$$

or $$T_{sh} = T_a - T_f \text{ Nm}$$

where T_f= Friction torque

$$= \frac{\text{Iron and friction losses}}{2\pi N/60}$$

Also $$T_{sh} = \frac{\text{Output of motor in watts}}{2\pi N/60} \text{Nm}$$

SOLVED EXAMPLES ON ABOVE THEORY

Example 1: A 300 V, 4 pole DC series motor has 800 wave wound conductors. The motor has total armature and series field resistance of 0.5 Ω and motor takes 50 A from supply. If flux per pole is 70 mWb, find speed and gross torque (armature torque) produced by the motor.

Solution:

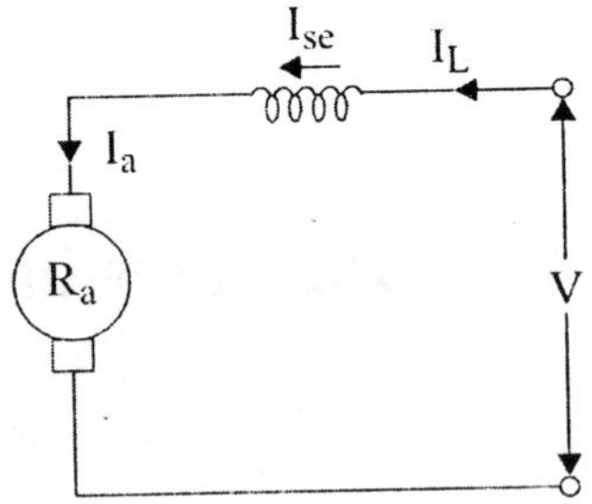

$$I_a = I_L = I_{se} = 50 \text{ A}$$

$$E_b = V - I_a (R_a + R_{se})$$

$$= 300 - 50 \times 0.5$$

$$= 275 \text{ V} = \frac{\phi Z N}{60}\left(\frac{P}{A}\right)$$

$$275 = \frac{70 \times 10^{-3} \times 800 \times N}{60}\left(\frac{4}{2}\right)$$

$$N = 147.32 \text{ rpm}$$

$$T_a = 0.159\phi Z\ I_a\left(\frac{P}{A}\right)$$

$$= 0.159 \times 70 \times 10^{-3} \times 800 \times 50 \times \left(\frac{4}{2}\right) = 890.4 \text{ Nm}$$ **Ans.**

12.10 CHARACTERISTICS OF DC MOTORS

The application of a DC motor is determined by its characteristics which shows relationships between the following:

1. Torque vs Armature current (T/I_a)
2. Speed vs Armature current (N/I_a)
3. Speed vs Torque (N/T)

12.10.1 Characteristics of DC Shunt Motor

1. Torque vs Armature Current (T/I_a)

$$T_a \propto \phi I_a$$

For shunt motors, flux is assumed to be constant (although at heavy loads it reduces slightly due to armature reaction).

So $T_a \propto I_a$

This relation represents a straight line passing through the origin.

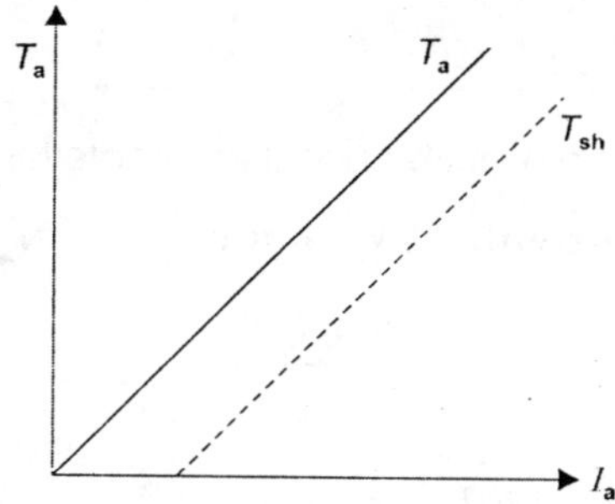

Fig. 12.27: Torque vs armature current (characteristics of a DC shunt motor)

$T_{sh} < T_a$ for same armature current.

2. Speed vs Armature current (N/I_a)

$$N \propto \frac{E_b}{\phi}$$

or

$$\propto \frac{V - I_a R_a}{\phi}$$

as ϕ is almost constant

$$N \propto V - I_a R_a$$

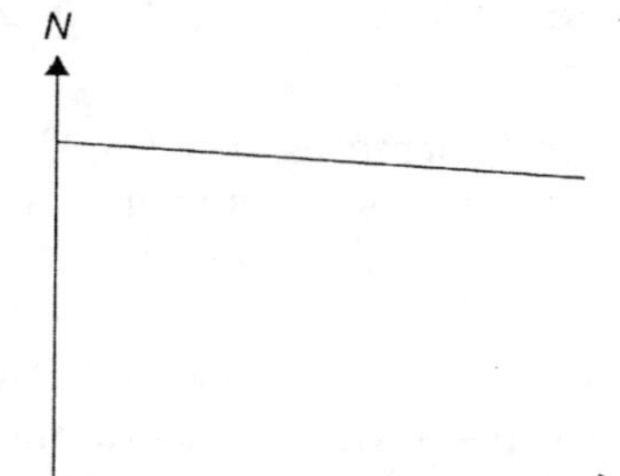

Fig. 12.28: Speed vs armature current (characteristics of a DC shunt motor)

With increase in armature current, speed will drop slightly. These motors are suitable for constant speed applications.

3. Speed vs Torque (N/T_a): In case of DC shunt motors torque is proportional to I_a. So torque follows the profile of armature current. Hence speed torque characteristic follows the similar trend as a speed-armature current characteristics as shown in Fig. 12.29.

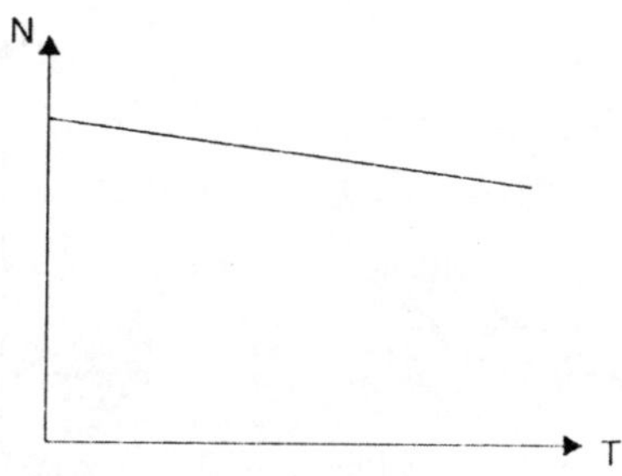

Fig. 12.29: Speed vs torque characteristics of a DC shunt motor

12.10.2 Characteristics of DC Series Motor

1. Torque vs Armature Current

For series motors $\phi \propto I_a$

and $T_a \propto \phi I_a$ so $T_a \propto I_a^2$

As I_a increases, T_a also increases as the square of the armature current. After saturation flux becomes almost constant and the characteristics curve becomes a straight line after magnetic saturation.

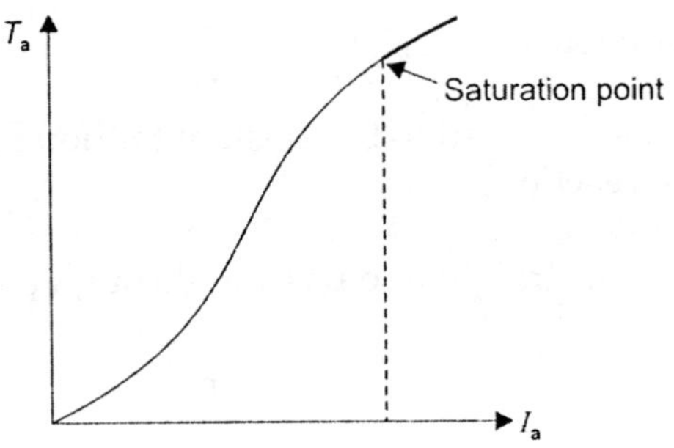

Fig. 12.30: Torque vs armature current (characteristics of DC series motor)

2. Speed vs Armature Current: As we know

$$N \propto \frac{E_b}{\phi} \propto \frac{V - I_a R_a}{\phi}$$

and in case of series motor $\phi \propto I_a$

So $$N \propto \frac{V - I_a R_a}{I_a}$$

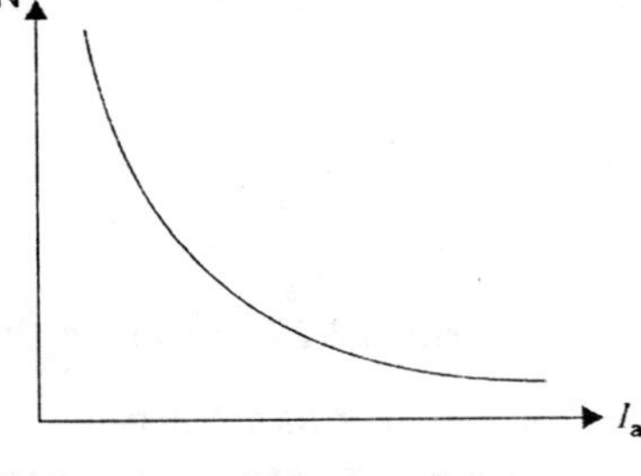

Fig. 12.31: Speed vs armature current (characteristics of DC series motor)

As I_a increases, $V - I_a R_a$ decreases slightly but more increase in denominator, (i.e. I_a), speed decreases with a much higher rate. When $I_a = 0$, speed tends towards infinity as shown in Fig. 12.31.

DC series motor should never be run on no load otherwise it will gain tremendous high speed, which may damage the motor.

3. Speed vs Torque Characteristics: This characteristic curve is drawn on the conclusions of above two characteristics conditions (1) and (2) as shown in Fig. 12.32.

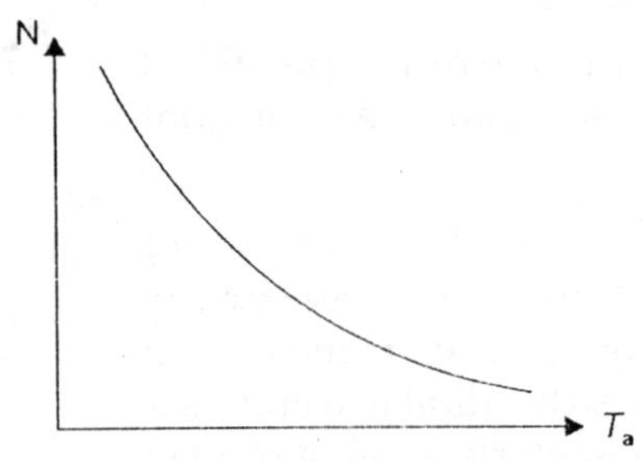

Fig. 12.32: Speed vs torque (characteristics of DC series motor)

12.10.3 Characteristics of DC Compound Motors

1. Torque vs Armature Current: $T \propto \phi I_a$ In cumulative: compound, series field supports shunt field. As I_a increases, net flux increases. So torque will initially follow the characteristics similar to shunt motor and as I_a increases it starts showing the characteristics of series field as represented in Fig. 12.33.

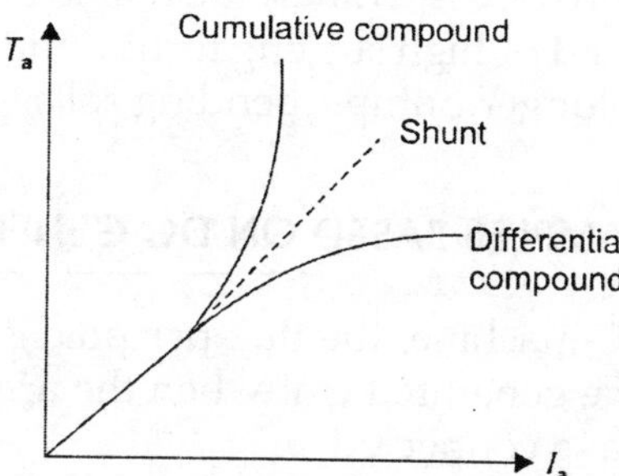

Fig. 12.33: Torque vs armature current characteristics

In case of differential compound flux will decrease as armature current increases. Therefore, characteristics curve will move downwards after following straight line.

2. Speed vs Armature Current:

$$N \propto \frac{V - I_a R_a}{\phi}$$

Initially motor will follow the shunt characteristics as flux increases with increase in armature current, in case of cumulative compound, motor speed will reduce with large rate. In case of differential compound, speed will increase due to reduced flux as shown in Fig. 12.34.

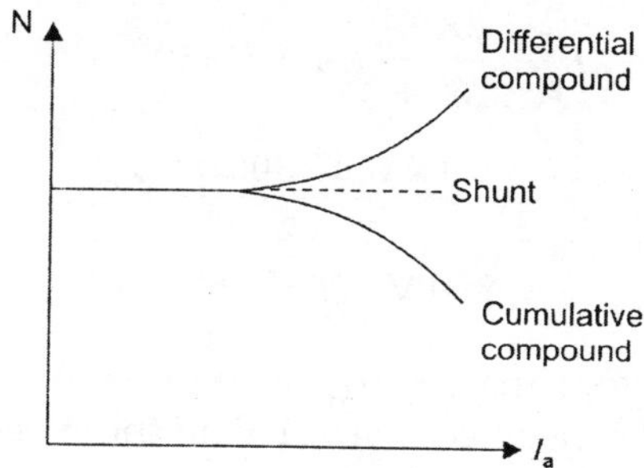

Fig. 12.34: Speed vs armature current characteristics

3. Speed vs Torque Characteristics: From above two characteristics, this curve can be drawn as shown in Fig. 12.35.

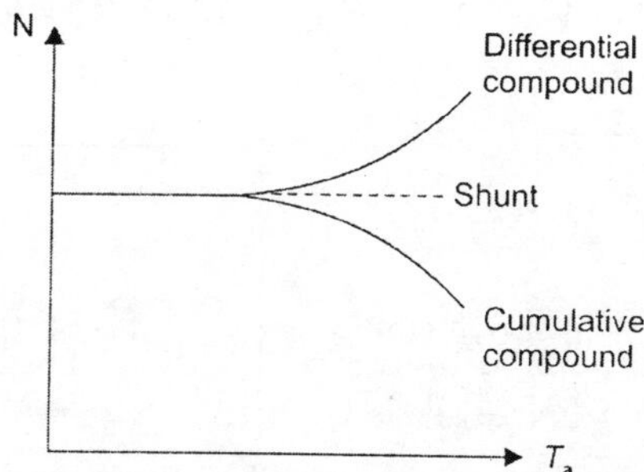

Fig. 12.35: Speed vs torque characteristics

Applications of DC Motors: Based on performance characteristics, the applications of various motors are given below.

1. **DC Shunt Motor:** For constant speed loads, such as centrifugal pumps, fan, blowers, conveyers, machine tools etc.
2. **DC Series Motor:** For very high starting torque and variable speed applications such as electric traction, hoists, cranes, moveable bridges.
3. **DC Compound Motor:** For high starting torque and constant speed applications as shears, crushers, plunger pumps, bending rolls, press etc.

UNIVERSITY SOLVED EXAMPLES BASED ON DC GENERATOR AND DC MOTOR

Example 1: In an 8-pole DC machine, the flux per pole is 0.1 Wb, 400 conductor and speed 300 rpm. Calculate the generated emf when the armature is:

(a) Lap connected (b) Wave connected. **[UPTU 2005-06]**

Solution: Given data

$$P = 8;\ \phi = 0.1 \text{ Wb};\ Z = 400;\ N = 300 \text{ rpm}$$

(a) For lap connected armature

$$E_g = \frac{\phi ZNP}{60\ A} \quad A = P = 8$$

$$\therefore \quad = \frac{0.1 \times 400 \times 300 \times 8}{60 \times 8} = 200$$

$$= 200 \text{ V}$$

(b) For wave connected

$$E_g = \frac{\phi ZNP}{60 A} \quad A = P = 2$$

$$\therefore \quad = \frac{0.1 \times 400 \times 300 \times 8}{60 \times 2} = 800$$

$$= 800 \text{ V}$$

Ans.

Example 2: A DC shunt motor runs at 600 rpm taking 60 A from a 230 V supply armature resistance is 0.2 Ω and field resistance is 115 Ω. Find the speed when the current through the armature is 30 A. **[UPTU 2006-07, 2008]**

Solution: Given data

$$N_1 = 600 \text{ rpm},\ I_{L_1} = 60 \text{ A}$$

$$V = 230 \text{ V},\ R_{sh} = 115\ \Omega,\ R_a = 0.2\ \Omega,\ I_a = 30 \text{ A}$$

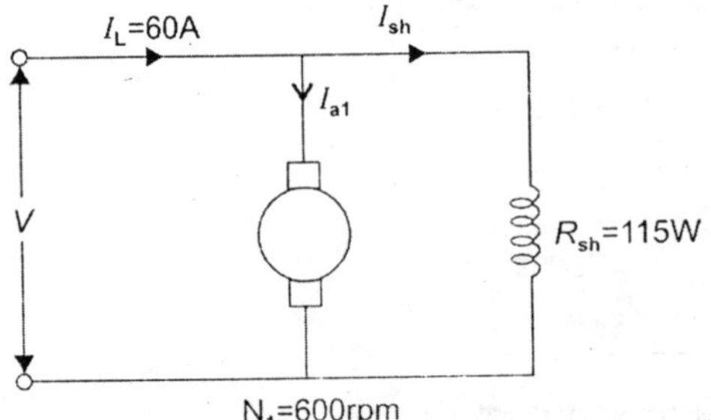

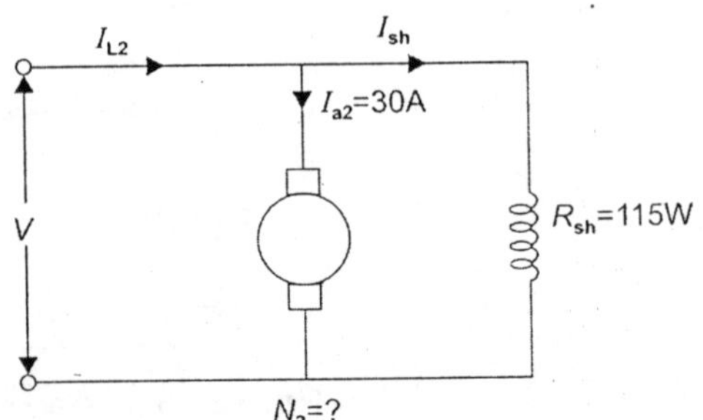

$$I_{sh} = \frac{V}{R_{sh}} = \frac{230}{115} = 2\text{ A}$$

$$I_{a1} = I_{L1} - I_{sh} = 60 - 2 = 58\text{ A}$$
$$E_{b1} = V - I_{a1}R_a = 230 - 58 \times 0.2 = 21814\text{ V}$$
$$E_{b2} = V - I_{a2}R_a = 230 - 30 \times 0.2 = 224\text{ V (Since } \phi = \text{Constant)}$$

We know that

$$\frac{N_2}{N_1} = \frac{E_{b2}}{E_{b1}}$$

$$= \frac{E_{b2}}{E_{b1}} \times N_1 = \frac{224}{218.4} \times 600 = 615.38\text{ rpm}$$ **Ans.**

Example 3: A 6 pole lap wound shunt motor has 500 conductor in the armature. The resistance of armature path is 0.05 Ω. The resistance of shunt field is 25 Ω. Find the speed of the motor when it takes 120 A from DC mains of 100 V supply. Flux per pole is 2×10^{-2} Wb. **[UPTU 2007-08]**

Solution: Given data

$$P = A = 6,\ Z = 500;\ R_a = 0.05\ \Omega,\ R_{sh} = 25\ \Omega$$
$$V = 100\text{ V}, I_L = 120\text{ A}, \phi = 2 \times 10^{-2}\text{ Wb}$$

We know that

$$I_{sh} = \frac{V}{R_{sh}} = \frac{100}{25} = 4\text{ A}$$

$$I_a = I_L - I_{sh} = 120 - 4 = 116\text{ A}$$

$$E_b = V - I_aR_a = 100 - 116 \times 0.05 = 94.2\text{ V}$$

$$N = \frac{E_b}{\phi} \times \left(\frac{60\text{ A}}{2P}\right) = \frac{94.2 \times 60 \times 6}{2 \times 10^{-2} \times 6 \times 500} = 565\text{ rpm}$$ **Ans.**

Example 4: A 25 kW, 250 V DC shunt generator has armature and field resistance of 0.06 Ω and 100 Ω respectively. Determine the total armature power developed when working: (i) as a generator delivering 25 kW output and (ii) as a motor taking 25 kW input. **[UPTU 2009-10]**

Solution: Given data

(i)

$$P_L = 25 \times 10^3\text{ W}$$

$$I_L = \frac{25 \times 10^3}{250} = 100\text{ A}$$

$$I_{sh} = \frac{V}{R_{sh}} = \frac{250}{100} = 2.5\text{ A}$$

∴

$$I_a = I_L + I_{sh} = 100 + 2.5 = 102.5\text{ A}$$
$$E_g = 250 + 102.5 \times 0.56 = 256.15\text{ V}$$
$$P_g = E_g \times I_a = 256.15 \times 102.5 = 26.255\text{ kW}$$ **Ans.**

(ii) As motor

$$P_{in} = 25 \times 10^3$$

$$I_L = \frac{25 \times 10^3}{250} = 100\text{ A}$$

$$I_{sh} = \frac{V}{R_{sh}} = \frac{250}{100} = 2.5$$

$$I_a = I_L - I_{sh} = 100 - 2.5 = 97.5 \text{ A}$$

$\therefore$ $$E_b = V - I_a R_a = 250 - 97.5 \times 0.06\ 244.15 \text{ V}$$

$\therefore$ $$P_m = \text{Power developed} = E_b \times I_a = 244.15 \times 97.5$$

$$= 23.846 \text{ kW}$$ **Ans.**

Example 5: The armature of a 4-pole DC machine has 100 turns and runs at 600 rpm. The emf generated in open circuit is 220 V. Find the useful flux per pole. When armature is (a) Lap connected (b) Wave connected. **[UPTU 2010-11]**

Solution: Given data

$$P = 4, \text{ turns} = 100, N = 600 \text{ rpm}; E_g = 220 \text{ V}$$

Now, as we know that two conductors constitute one turn

$$Z = \text{Total conductors} = 2 \times 100 = 200$$

(a) Lap connected $A = P = 4$

$$E_g = \frac{\phi ZNP}{60\ A}$$

$$\phi = \frac{220 \times 60 \times 4}{600 \times 4 \times 200} = 0.11 \text{ Wb}$$ **Ans.**

(b) for wave connected winding

$$A = 2$$

$$\phi = \frac{220 \times 60 \times 2}{600 \times 4 \times 200} = 0.055 \text{ Wb}$$ **Ans.**

Example 6: A 6 pole lap wound DC generator has 720 conductor, a flux of 80 mWb/pole is driven at 1000 rpm. Find the generated emf. **[GBTU 2010-11]**

Solution: Given data

$$P = 6, A = P = 6 \text{ for lap}$$

$$Z = 720$$

$$\phi = 80 \times 10^{-3} \text{ Wb}$$

$$N = 1000 \text{ rpm}$$

$$E_g = \frac{\phi ZNP}{60\ A} = \frac{80 \times 10^{-3} \times 720 \times 1000 \times 6}{60 \times 6} = 960 \text{ V}$$ **Ans.**

Example 7: The armature of a four pole DC machine has 1000 turns and runs at 500 rpm. The emf generated in open circuit is 220 V. Find the useful flux per pole when armature is (*a*) lap connected (*b*) wave connected. **[UPTU 2011-12]**

Solution: Given data

$$P = 4, N = 500 \text{ rpm}$$

$$E_g = 220 \text{ V, turns} = 1000$$

$\therefore$ $$Z = 2 \times \text{turns} = 2 \times 1000 = 2000$$

(a) Lap connected

$$A = P = 4$$

$$\phi = \frac{220 \times 60 \times 4}{500 \times 4 \times 2000} = 0.012 \text{ Wb}$$ **Ans.**

(b) Wave connected

$$A = 2$$

$$\phi = \frac{220 \times 60 \times 2}{500 \times 4 \times 2000} = 0.006 \text{ Wb}$$ **Ans.**

Example 8: A DC shunt generator delivers 50 kW at 250 V, and 400 rpm. The armature and field resistances are 0.02 Ω and 50 Ω respectively. Calculate the speed of the machine running as shunt-motor and taking 50 kW input at 250 V, allow brush drop of 1 V per brush. **[MTU 2012-13]**

Solution: Given that

$P_L = 50$ kW; $V = 250$ V; $N_g = 400$ rpm; $R_a = 0.02\ \Omega$; $R_{sh} = 50\ \Omega$

For generator

$$I_{sh} = \frac{V}{R_{sh}} = \frac{250}{50} = 5 \text{ A}$$

$$I_L = \frac{P_L}{V} = \frac{50 \times 10^3}{250} = 200 \text{ A}$$

$$I_a = I_L + I_{sh} = 200 + 5 = 205 \text{ A}$$

$$E_g = V + I_a R_a + BDV$$

$$= 250 + 205 \times 0.02 + 2 \times 1 = 256.1 \text{ V}$$ **Ans.**

For motor $I_L = 200$ A, V = 250; $I_{sh} = 5$ A

$$I_a = I_L - I_{sh} = 200 - 5 = 195 \text{ A}$$

$$E_b = V - I_a R_a - BDV$$

$$= 250 - 195 \times 0.02 - 2 \times 1 = 244.1 \text{ V}$$

$$\frac{N_m}{N_g} = \frac{E_b}{E_g} \Rightarrow N_m = \frac{E_b}{E_g} \times N_g$$

$$N_m = \frac{244.1}{256.1} \times 400 = 381.3 \text{ rpm}$$ **Ans.**

Example 9: A DC shunt motor develops an open circuit emf of 250 V, at 1500 rpm. Find the developed torque for an armature current of 20 Amp. **[GBTU 2012-13]**

Solution: Given data

$E_b = 250$ V, $N = 1500$ rpm; $I_a = 20$ A

$$T_e = \frac{9.55 \times E_b I_a}{N} = \frac{9.55 \times 250 \times 20}{1500} = 31.822 \text{ Nm}$$ **Ans.**

Example 10: The armature resistance of a 200 V DC shunt motor is 0.12 Ω. It runs at 600 rpm at constant torque load and draws a current of 21 A. Calculate its new speed if the field current is reduced to 10%. **[GBTU 2012-13]**

Solution: Given data

$V = 200$ V; $I_{L_1} = 21$ A

Assuming $I_{a_1} = I_{L_1} = 21$ A

$$N_1 = 600 \text{ rpm}$$

For motor $E_{b_1} = V - I_{a1} R_a$

$$= 200 - 21 \times 0.12 = 197.48 \text{ V}$$

The given $T_2 = T_1$

$$I_{a2}\phi_2 = I_{a1}\phi_1$$

$$I_{a2} = I_{a1} \times \frac{\phi_1}{\phi_2} = I_{a1} \times \frac{I_{sh1}}{I_{sh2}}$$

$$= 21 \times \frac{1}{0.9} = 23.33 \text{ A} \qquad \begin{bmatrix} \phi \propto I \\ I_{sh2} = 0.9 I_{sh1} \end{bmatrix}$$

$$E_{b_2} = V - I_{a2}R_a = 200 - 23.33 \times 0.12 = 197.2 \text{ V}$$

$$N_2 = \frac{E_{b2}}{E_{b1}} \times \frac{\phi_1}{\phi_2} \times N_1 = \frac{197.2}{197.4} \times \frac{1}{0.9} \times 600 = 665.7 \text{ rpm}$$ **Ans.**

EXERCISES

1. What is the principle of electro-mechanical energy conversion?
2. What is the principle of DC Generator. Write down the emf equation of DC generator. **[UPTU 2009-10]**
3. What is back emf and its significance in DC motor? Write down the equation of back emf. **[UPTU 2008-09]**
4. What are the application of DC motor?
5. Explain the constructional features of the DC machine with neat sketch. **[UPTU 2003-04-05]**

Short Answer Questions

1. Derive the emf equations for the DC generator. Explain with the help of neat diagram the different types of DC machine. **[UPTU 2004-05-06-08]**
2. Derive the expression for the electromagnetic torque developed in a DC motor. **[UPTU 2008-09]**
3. Sketch and explain the speed-current, speed-torque and torque-current characteristics of a shunt motor, series motor and compound motor. **[UPTU 2009-10, 2011-12]**
4. A 10-pole DC machine having lap winding with 400 armature conductor. Calculate the emf generated when the machine is driven by a 1000 rpm and the flux per pole is 0.065 Wb. [**Ans.** 4.33.34 V]
5. A 4-pole DC shunt generator with LAP-connected armature has field and armature resistance of 80 W and 0.1 Ω respectively. It supplied power to 50 lamps rated for 100 volts, 60 W each. Calculate the total armature current and the generated emf by allowing a contact drop of 1 V per brush. **[UPTU 2009-10]** [**Ans.** 31.25 A, 105.125 V]

Descriptive Questions

1. Derive the emf equation of a DC generator. What will be change in emf induced if the flux is reduced by 20% and the speed is increased by 20%? **[UPTU 2005-06]**
2. Derive the expression for torque in a DC motor. Draw the torque armature current, speed-armature current and torque speed characteristics of following DC motor.
   (a) DC shunt motor (b) DC series motor
   (c) DC compound motor

Chapter

13

Induction Motors

13.1 THREE PHASE INDUCTION MOTOR

The induction motors are basically AC motors, i.e. they need an alternating voltage for their operation. They can operate on single phase or three phase AC supply, however the single phase induction motors find very limited area of applications. In almost 85% applications, the three phase induction motors are preferred. Depending on the type of rotor, the induction motor are classified into two types.

(a) Squarrel cage induction motor
(b) Slip ring induction motor.

Advantages

(i) Low maintenance
(ii) Ruggedness, smaller size, weight.
(iii) Low cost.
(iv) They can operate in dusty and explosive environments, because the brushes are not used.
(v) They can operate at a higher speed of the order of 12000 rpm
(vi) It can produce sufficient torque.

Disadvantages

(i) Low starting torque
(ii) Lagging and low pf.
(iii) Speed control by electrical methods is not easy.

Applications

(i) Fans
(ii) Pumps
(iii) Extruders
(iv) Conveyors
(v) Chemical industries
(vi) Paper and sugar industries, etc.

13.2 CONSTRUCTION OF 3-ϕ INDUCTION MOTOR

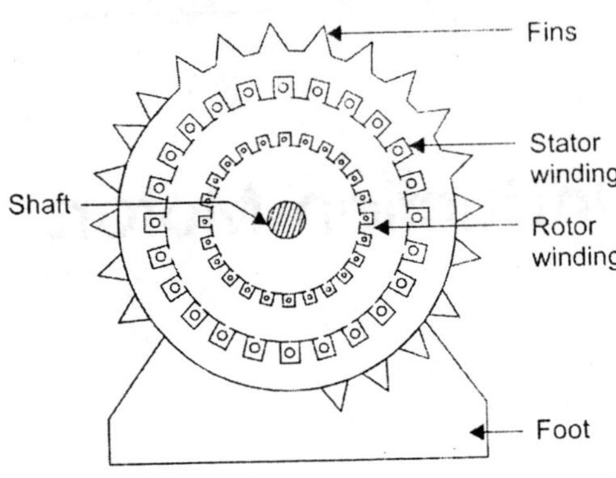

Parts:

- Outer frame: (Stationary)—Mechanical protation.
- Stator: (Stationary)—Stationary part is known as stator.
- Rotor: (Rotating)—Rotating part is known as rotor.

Fig. 13.1

Types of 3-ϕ Induction Motor

1. Single squarrel cage.
2. Double squarrel cage.
3. Slip ring IM or wound rotor.

13.3 OPERATION OF 3-ϕ INDUCTION MOTOR

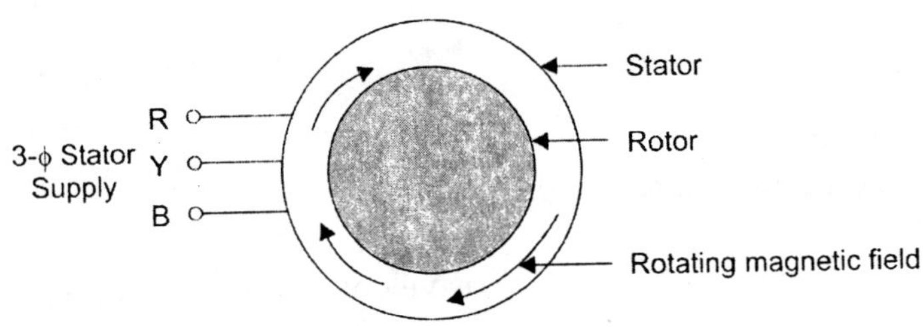

Fig. 13.2

The three phase stator winding of induction motor is connected to the three phase AC supply as shown in Fig. 13.2. Due to AC voltage applied, current starts flowing in the stator conductors. Due to three phase stator current a rotating magnetic field of constant amplitude is rotating at a constant speed is set up in the air gap between stator and rotor. The rotating magnetic field rotates at a speed called as *synchronous speed* (N_S).

$N_S = \frac{120 f}{P}$, f = stator supply frequency, P = No. of poles of the motor. The rotor winding is still stationary so the rotating magnetic field cuts the stationary rotor conductor and induces an emf in the rotor winding. The rotor induced voltage gives rise to rotor currents. The direction of the rotor current is such that it will oppose very cause that produces the current. And the cause behind producing the rotor current is the relative velocity between the rotating field and the rotor.

So the rotor current will flow in a such a direction that the rotor will experience a force that accelerates it in the same direction as that of the rotating magnetic field as shown in Fig. 13.2. At no load ideally speaking the rotor should rotate at the same speed as that of the rotating magnetic field, i.e. N_S. But practically it rotates at slightly less speed than N_S due to friction and winding.

Motor on load: When the induction motor is loaded mechanically, its speed (N_r) decreases to produce the required amount of torque. The reduction in the motor speed (N_r) will stop as soon as the torque produced by the rotor (T) is exactly equal to the load torque (T_L). The percentage difference between the synchronous speed (N_S) and actual speed (N_r) is known as slip (S).

$$S = \frac{N_S - N_r}{N_r}$$

13.4 SLIP SPEED, SLIP, SYNCHRONOUS SPEED

Synchronous speed: It is constant speed.

$$N_S = \frac{120f}{P}$$

P= No. of poles

f= Supply frequency

Slip speed: It is the speed difference between stator (N_S) and rotor or motor (N_r). It is also known as relative speed.

$$\text{Slip speed} = (N_S - N_r)\ \text{rpm}$$

$$= (\omega_s - \omega_r)\ \text{rad/sec} \qquad \left[\omega_s = \frac{2\pi N_S}{60}\right]$$

% (percentage) of slip =

$$s\% = \frac{N_S - N_r}{N_S} \times 100$$

$$N_r = (1 - s)N_s \text{ or } \omega_r = (1 - s)\,\omega_s$$

13.4.1 Rotor Frequency (f_r)

$$f_r = sf$$

Proof: We know that $\quad N_S = \dfrac{120f}{P}$ ...(13.1)

$$N_S - N_r = \frac{120F_r}{P} \qquad \text{...(13.2)}$$

Dividing Eq. (13.2) by Eq. (13.1) we get

$$\frac{N_S - N_r}{N_S} = \frac{F_r}{f} \Rightarrow S = \frac{F_r}{f}$$

$\therefore$ $$F_r = Sf$$

F_r = rotor frequency

13.4.2 Rotor Current, Rotor Power Factor

Rotor current, $I_2 = \dfrac{E_2}{\sqrt{\left(r^2/s\right)^2 + (x_2)^2}}$ or $I_2 = \dfrac{sE_2}{\sqrt{r_2^2 + (sx_2)^2}}$

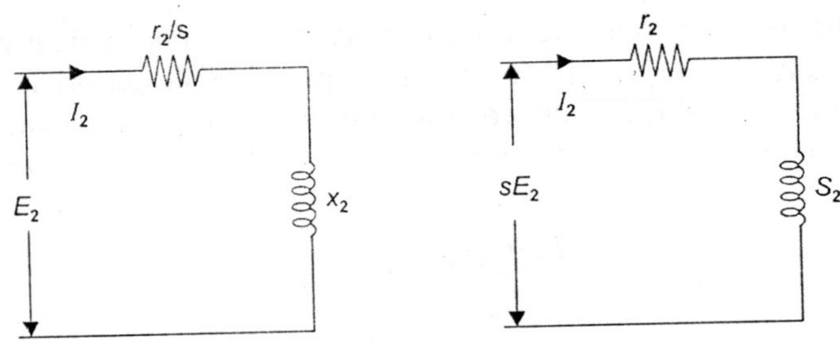

Fig.13.3: Equivalent circuit

$$\text{Power factor, } \cos\phi_2 = \frac{r_2/s}{\sqrt{\left(r^2/s\right)^2 + (x_2)^2}} \quad \cos\phi_2 = \frac{r_2}{\sqrt{r_2^2 + (sx_2)^2}}$$

13.5 POWER STAGES IN 3-ϕ INDUCTION MOTOR

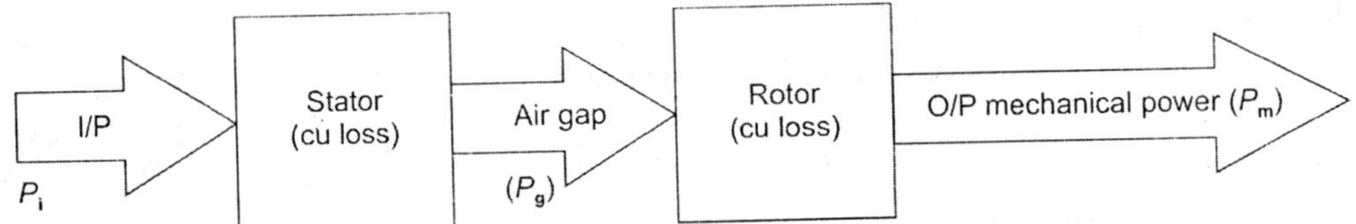

Fig. 13.4

$$P_g = \text{Air gap power} = E_2 I_2 \cos\phi_2$$

$$= I_2 \times \sqrt{(r_2/s)^2 + x_2^2} \times \frac{I_2 \times r_2/s}{\sqrt{(r_2/s)^2 + x_2^2}}$$

$$E_2 = I_2 \times \sqrt{(r_2/s)^2 + x_2^2}$$

$$\cos\phi_2 = \frac{r^2/s}{\sqrt{\left(r^2/s\right)^2 + x_2^2}}$$

Putting all values, we get

$$P_g = I_2^2 \frac{r_2}{s}$$

$$sP_g = I_2^2 r_2 \text{ (rotor copper loss)}$$

We can write the above expression

$$P_g = I_2^2 r_2 + \frac{(1-s)}{s} I_2^2 r_2$$

$$= sP_g + (1-s)P_g$$

$$1 : s : 1 - s$$

$$P_g = \text{Rotor copper loss} + \text{mechanical power } (P_m)$$

$$\therefore \quad P_m = (1 - s)P_g$$

13.6 ELECTROMAGNETIC TORQUE EXPRESSION FOR 3-ϕ INDUCTION MOTOR

$$\omega_r (T_e) = P_m$$

$$\omega_r T_e = (1-s) P_g$$

$$T_e = \frac{(1-s)P_g}{(1-s)\omega_s} \qquad [\omega_r = (1-s)P_g]$$

$$= \frac{P_g}{\omega_s}$$

$$= \frac{I_2^2 \times r_2/s}{\omega_s} \qquad I_2 = \frac{E_2}{\sqrt{\left(\frac{r_2}{s}\right)^2 + x_2^2}}$$

$$= \frac{1}{\omega_S}\frac{E_2^2 \times r_2/s}{\left[\left(\frac{r_2^2}{s}\right) + x_2^2\right]} \qquad \omega_S = \frac{2\pi N_S}{60}$$

$$= \frac{60}{2\pi N_S}\frac{E_2^2 \times r_2/s}{\left[\left(\frac{r_2^2}{s}\right) + x_2^2\right]} \qquad N_S = \frac{120f}{P}$$

for 3-ϕ

$$= \frac{3\times 60}{2\pi N_S} = \frac{E_2^2 r_2/S}{\left[\left(\frac{r_2^2}{S}\right) + x_2^2\right]}$$

For maximum torque, $\frac{\partial T_e}{\partial s} = 0$

After solving, we get $s = \frac{r^2}{x^2}$

$$\therefore \quad T_{max} = \frac{3\times 60}{2\pi N_s}\frac{E_2^2}{2x_2}$$

13.7 TORQUE SLIP AND TORQUE-SPEED CHARACTERISTICS OF 3-ϕ INDUCTION MOTOR

For motoring: The forward motoring region corresponds to the values of slip between 0 and 1.

At starting $s = 1, \left[s = \frac{N_s - N_r}{N_s}\right], N_r = 0$

The torque increases as the slip increases while the air gap flux remains constant. Once the torque reaches its maximum value T_{max}, at $s = s_m$ (max slip), the torque decreases, with increases in slip due to reduction in air gap flux.

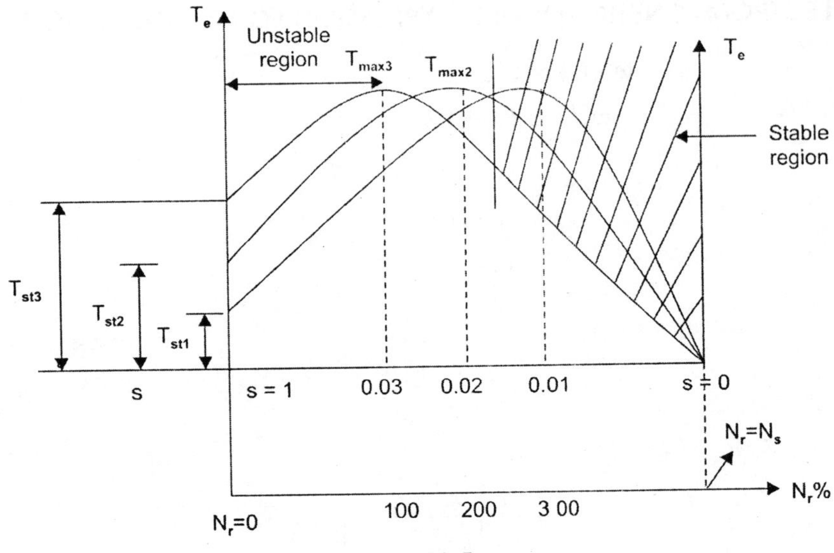

Fig. 13.5

Stable Region of Operation

Region ($0 \leq s \leq 1$) of the torque speed characteristics. The region $s_m \leq s \leq 1$ is unstable region.

$$T_{max} = K\left(\frac{E_2^2}{2x_2}\right)$$

$$T \propto S$$

13.8 NEED OF A STARTER FOR 3-ϕ INDUCTION MOTOR AND STARTING METHOD OF 3-ϕ INDUCTION MOTOR

$$I_2 = \frac{sE_2}{\sqrt{r_2^2 + (sx_2)^2}}$$

at standstill $\qquad s = 1$

$\therefore$

$$I_2 = \frac{E_2}{\sqrt{r_2^2 + x_2^2}}$$

$$E_2 = \frac{N_2}{N_1} \times E_1 \text{ at standstill}$$

$\therefore$

$$I_2 = \frac{KV_1}{\sqrt{r_2^2 + (x_2)^2}}$$

It a rated voltage is applied to the motor at the time of starting, then the motor will draw heavy starting current. So due to $I_2^2 R$ will over heat the motor. The heavy starting current may damage the motor windings.

$\therefore$ Starter is needed.

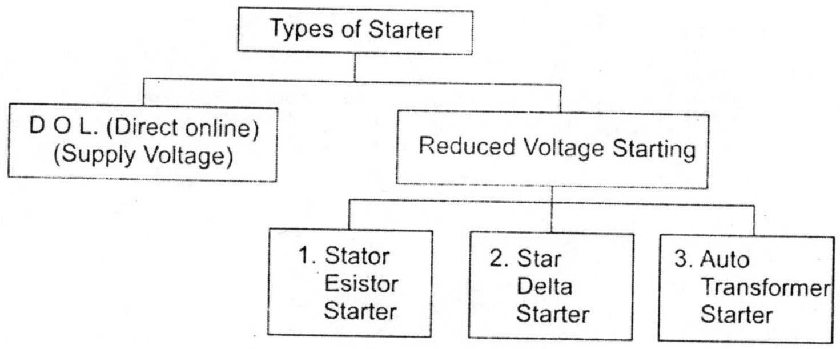

Fig. 13.6

13.8.1 DOL (Direct Online Starter)

It consist of fuse links connected in each line, relay contacts in series with each line, conductor, contacts and start stop logic. Contactor operates.

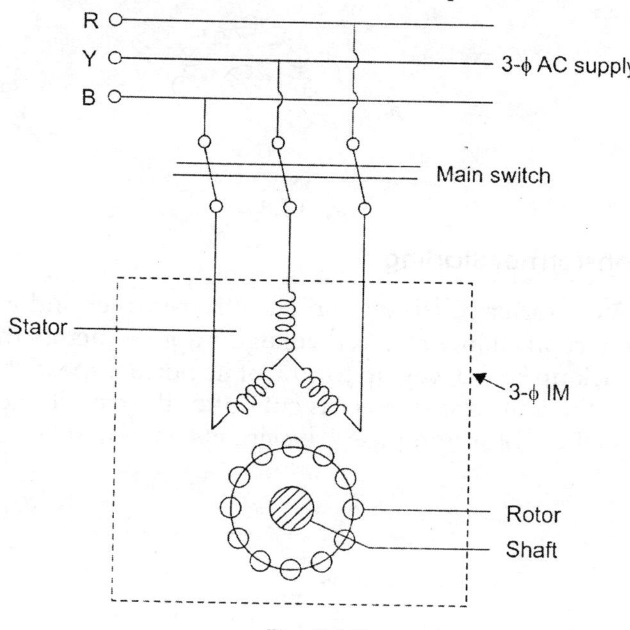

Fig. 13.7

Operations

The motor is started by connecting it directly to 3-ϕ supply. The impedance of the motor at standstill is relatively low and when it is directly connecting to the supply system, the starting current will be high at a low power factor, consequently this method of starting is relatively small (up to 7.5 kW) motor or 3 HP only.

13.8.2 Reduced Voltage Starting

In this method of starting a 3-ϕ squarrel cage, IM reduced voltage is obtained by means of resistors (or reactor) that are connected in series with each stator during the starting period. The voltage drop in resistors causes a reduced voltage across the motor terminals. As the motor picks up the speed, the resistor are cut out in steps and finally short circuited when the motor attains the operating speed (Fig. 13.7).

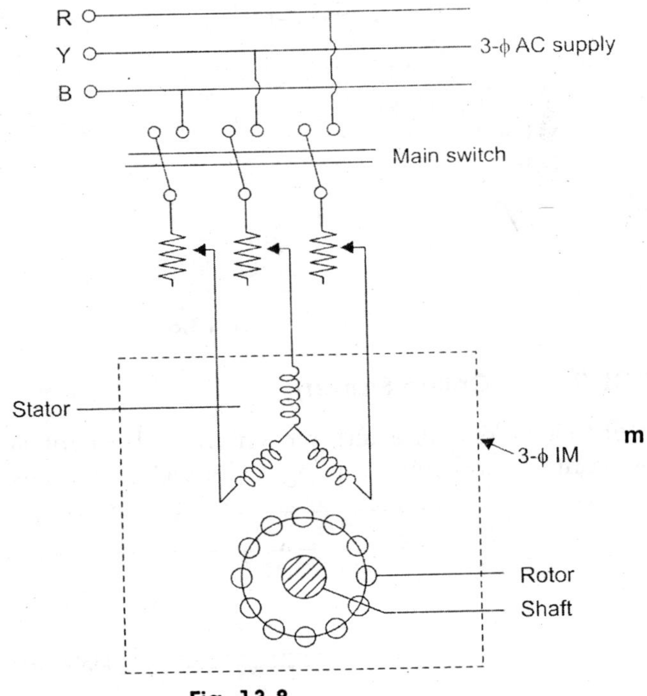

Fig. 13.8

13.8.2 Auto-Transformer Starting

An auto transformer starter consists of an auto-transformer and a switch. When the switch *S* is put on start position, a reduced voltage is applied across the motor terminals. When the motor pick up speed, say up to 80% of its normal speed, the switch is put on run position. Then the auto-transformer is cut out of the circuit and full rated voltage gets applied across the motor terminals. The circuits shown in Fig. 13.9.

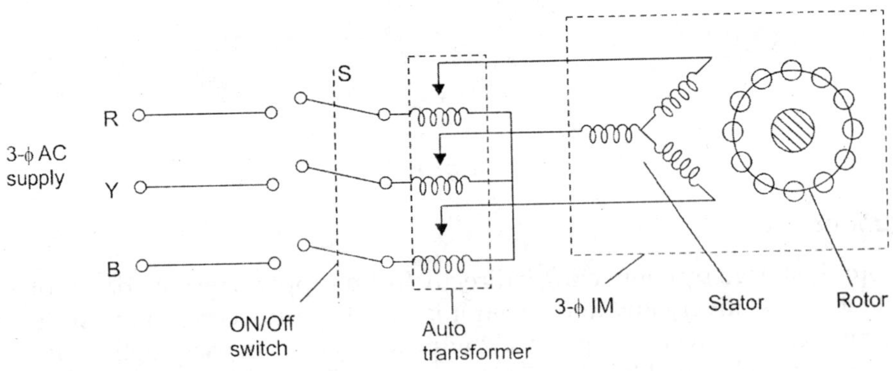

Fig. 13.9

13.8.3 Star-Delta Method of Starting

The stator phase winding first connected in star and full voltage is connected across its three terminals. As the motor picks up speed, the windings are disconnected through a switch and they are reconnected in delta across the supply terminals. The current drawn by the motor from the lines is reduced to 1/3 as compared to the current it would have drawn if connected in delta.

$$I_P = I_{LY} = \frac{V}{\sqrt{3}Z_P}$$

Z_P = impedance per phase

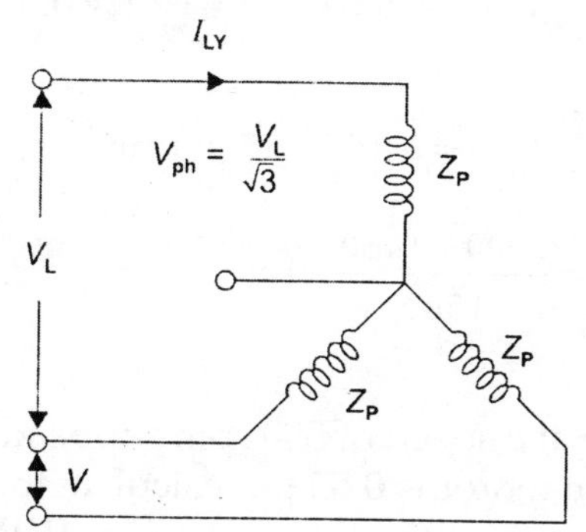

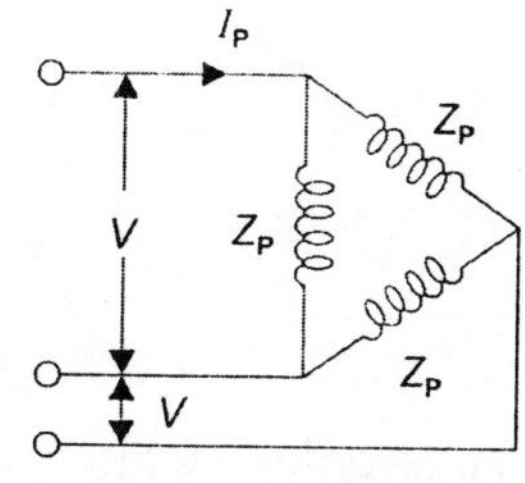

Fig. 13.10

13.9 SOME IMPORTANT FORMULAE

1. Synchronous speed

$$N_S = \frac{120f}{P}; \; f = \text{supply frequency}; \; P = \text{no. of pole}$$

2. Rotor frequency $= f_r = sf$

3. Slip speed $= (N_S - N_r)$ rpm

$= \omega_s - \omega_r$ radian/sec

4. % Slip $s = \frac{N_S - N_r}{N_S} \times 100$

5. Rotor speed (N_r) $N_r = (1-s)N_S$ $\left(\omega_s = \frac{2\pi N_S}{60}\right)$

or $\omega_r = (1-s)\omega_s$ $\left(\omega_r = \frac{2\pi N_r}{60}\right)$

6. Rotor current $I_2 = \frac{E_2^2 \, r_2/s}{\sqrt{(r_2/s)^2 + x_2^2}}$

7. Power factor $\cos\phi_2 = \frac{r_2/s}{\sqrt{(r_2/s)^2 + x_2^2}}$

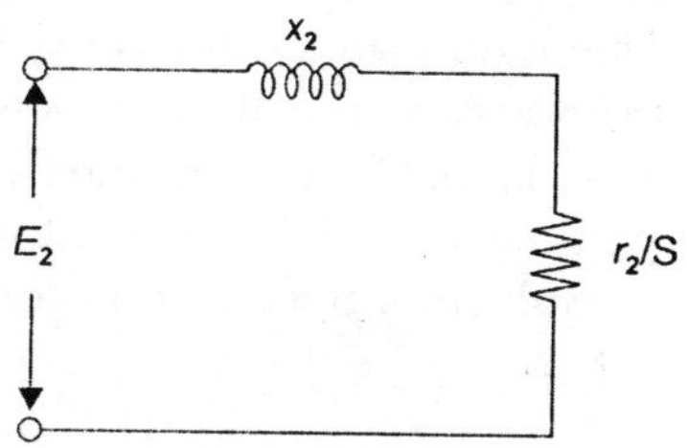

Fig. 13.11

8. Air gap power $P_g = E_2 I_2 \cos\phi_2 = I_2^2 r_2/s$

9. Rotor copper loss $sP_g = I_2^2 r_2$

10. Torque $T_e = 3 \times \frac{60}{2\pi N_S}\left[\frac{E_2^2 \, r_2/s}{(r_2/s)^2 + x_2^2}\right]$

12. Mechanical power $P_m = (1-s)P_g$

SOLVED EXAMPLES FOR PRACTICE

Example 1: A 3-ϕ, 4 pole, 50 Hz induction motor runs at 1460 rpm. Determine the slip. **[UPTU 2003-04]**

Solution:

$$N_S = \frac{120f}{P} = \frac{120 \times 50}{1500} = 3 \times 50 = 1500 \text{ rpm}$$

$$s = \frac{N_S - N_r}{N_S} = \frac{1500 - 1460}{1500} \times 100$$

$$s\% = 2.667\%$$ **Ans.**

Example 2: A 12-pole, 3-ϕ alternator driven at a speed of 500 rpm supplied power to an 8-pole 3-ϕ induction motor. If the slip of the motor is 0.03 pu, calculate the speed. **[UPTU 2002-03]**

Solution:

$$N_S = \frac{120f}{P} = f = \frac{500 \times 12}{120} = 50 \text{ Hz}$$

$$= \frac{120f}{P} = \frac{120 \times 50}{8} = 750 \text{ rpm}$$

$$N_r = N_S(1-s) = 750(1-0.03) = 727.5 \text{ rpm}$$ **Ans.**

Example 3: A 3-ϕ, 4 pole IM is supplied from diesel-generator set running at 600 rpm. The generator has 10 poles, find the synchronous speed of the IM and also the actual speed for a slip of 4%.

Solution:

$$f = \frac{P \times N}{120} = \frac{10 \times 600}{120} = 50 \text{ Hz}$$

$$N_S = \frac{120f}{P} = \frac{120 \times 50}{4} = 1500 \text{ rpm}$$

$$N_r = N_S(1-s) = 1500(1-0.04) = 1440 \text{ rpm}$$ **Ans.**

Example 4: A motor generator set used for providing variable frequency AC supply consists of a 3-ϕ 10 pole synchronous motor and a 24-pole, 3-ϕ synchronous generator. The motor-generator set is fed from a 25 Hz, 3-ϕ AC supply. A 6-pole, 3-ϕ induction motor is electrically connected to the terminals of the synchronous generator and runs at a slip of 5%. Determine (i) the frequency of the generator voltage of the synchronous generator (ii) The speed at which the induction motor is running.

Solution: Speed of motor generator set

$$N_S = \frac{120 \times \text{Supply frequency } f_1}{\text{No. of poles on synchornous motor}}$$

$$= \frac{120 \times 2.5}{10} = 300 \text{ rpm}$$

(i) Frequency of generated value voltages

$$f_2 = \frac{\text{Speed of motor gen set} \times \text{No. of pole of syn gen.}}{120}$$

$$f_2 = \frac{300 \times 24}{120} = 60 \text{ Hz}$$

(ii) Speed of induction motor

$$N_r = (1-s)N_S = \frac{120 \times 60}{6}(1-0.05) = 1140 \text{ rpm}$$ **Ans.**

Example 5: A 3-ϕ, 4 pole induction motor is supplied from 3-ϕ, 50 Hz AC supply. Calculate (i) synchronous speed (ii) rotor speed when slip is 4% and (iii) rotor frequency when rotor runs at 600 rpm. **[UPTU 2005-06]**

Solution: The synchronous speed

(i) $$N_S = \frac{120 \times f}{P} = \frac{120 \times 50}{4} = 1500 \text{ rpm}$$

(ii) $$N_r = N_S(1-s) = 1500(1-0.04) = 1440 \text{ rpm}$$

(iii) Slip at 600 rpm $$= \frac{1500-600}{1500} = 0.06$$

Rotor frequency $$f_r = s \times f = 0.06 \times 50 = 3 \text{ Hz}$$

Example 6: A 12-pole, 3-ϕ alternator is coupled to an engine running at 500 rpm it is supplied with a 3-ϕ IM having a full-load speed of 1440 rpm. Find the percentage slip, frequency of rotor current and no. of poles of the motor. **[UPTU 2006-07]**

Solution: Frequency of supply from alternator

$$f = \frac{P_a \times N_a}{120} = \frac{12 \times 500}{120} = 50 \text{ Hz}$$

Full-load speed $$N_F = 1440 \text{ rpm}$$

(Motor must have 4 pole) $$P = \frac{120 f}{N} = \frac{120 \times 50}{1440} \approx 4$$

$$N_S = \frac{120 \times 50}{4} = 1500 \text{ rpm}$$

$$s = \frac{N_S - N_r}{N_S} = \frac{1500-1440}{1500} \times 100 = 4\%$$

$$f_r = sf = 0.04 \times 50 = 2 \text{ Hz}$$ **Ans.**

$$P = 4$$ **Ans.**

Example 7: In a 3-ϕ slip ring, four pole induction motor, the rotor frequency is found to be 2 Hz while connected to a 400 V, 3-ϕ, 50 Hz supply. Determine the motor speed in rpm. **[UPTU 2003-04]**

Solution:

$$N_S = \frac{120 \times f}{P} = \frac{120 \times 50}{4} = 1500 \text{ rpm}$$

$$s = \frac{f_r}{f} = \frac{2}{50} = 0.04$$

$$N_r = 1500(1-0.04) = 1440 \text{ rpm}$$ **Ans.**

Example 8: A 3-ϕ, 50 Hz induction motor has 6 poles and operates with a slip of 5% at a certain load. Determine **[UPTU 2002-03]**

(i) The speed of the rotor with respect to the stator
(ii) The frequency of rotor current
(iii) The speed of the rotor magnetic field with respect to rotor
(iv) The speed of the rotor magnetic field with respect to stator and
(v) The speed of the stator magnetic field.

Solution: Given data

$$f = 50,\ P = 6,\ s = 0.05$$

$$N_S = \frac{120 \times 50}{6} = 1000 \text{ rpm}$$

(i) $$N_r = N_S(1-s) = 1000(1-0.05) = 950 \text{ rpm}$$ **Ans.**

(ii) $$f_r = sf = 0.05 \times 50 = 2.5 \text{ Hz}$$ **Ans.**

(iii) $$N_r = \frac{120 \times f_r}{P} = \frac{120 \times 2.5}{6} = 50 \text{ rpm}$$ **Ans.**

(iv) $$N_S = 1000 \text{ rpm}$$ **Ans.**

(v) Rotor and stator fields are revolving at the same speed of 1000 rpm.

∴ Speed between stator at rotor is zero.

Example 9: A 3-ϕ, 440 V, 50 hp, 50 Hz induction motor runs at 1450 rpm, when it delivers rated output power. Determine

(i) No of poles in the machines.
(ii) Speed of rotating air gap.
(iii) Rotor induced voltage if stator to rotor turns ratio is 1:0.8. Assume the winding factors are the same.
(iv) Frequency of rotor current. **[UPTU 2007-08]**

Solution:

(i) $$P = \frac{120 \times f}{N} = \frac{120 \times 50}{1450} \approx 4$$ **Ans.**

(ii) Speed of rotating air gap field

$$N_S = \frac{120 \times 50}{4} = 1500 \text{ rpm}$$ **Ans.**

(iii) Induced emf in rotor at stand still = kE_1

$$= kV_1 = 0.8 \times 440 = 352 \text{ V}$$

$$s = \frac{N_S - N_r}{N_S} = \frac{1500 - 1450}{1500} = 0.033$$

Rotor induced voltage = $sk\,V_1 = 0.033 \times 352 = 11.733$ V **Ans.**

(iv) $$f_r = sf = 0.033 \times 50 = 1.66 \text{ Hz}$$ **Ans.**

Example 10: A 3-ϕ delta connected to 440 volts, 50 Hz, 4-pole induction motor has a rotor stand still emf per phase of 130 V. If the motor is running at 1440 rpm, Calculate for this speed:

(i) The slip
(ii) The frequency of rotor induced emf
(iii) The value of the rotor induced emf per phase
(iv) Stator to rotor turn ratio. **[UPTU 2009-10]**

Solution:

$$N_S = \frac{120 \times 50}{4} = 1500 \text{ rpm}$$

(i) $$s = \frac{1500 - 1400}{1500} = 0.04 = 4\%$$ **Ans.**

(ii) $$f_r = sf = 0.04 \times 50 = 2 \text{ Hz}$$ **Ans.**

(iii) Rotor induced emf per phase

$$= sE_2$$

$$= 0.04 \times 130 = 5.2 \text{ volts}$$ **Ans.**

(iv) Stator for rotor turn ratio

$$= \frac{E_{P1}}{E_{P2}} = \frac{440}{130} = \frac{44}{13}$$ **Ans.**

Example 11: A 4-pole, 50 Hz, 3-ϕ IM running at full load, develops a torque of 160 N-m. When the rotor makes 120 cycle per minute. Calculate the shaft output power. **[MTU 2008-09]**

Solution:

$$f = 50$$

$$f_r = \frac{120}{60} = 2 \text{ Hz}$$

$$s = \frac{f_r}{f} = \frac{2}{50} = 0.04$$

$$N_S = \frac{120 \times 50}{4} = 1500 \text{ rpm}$$

$$N_r = N_S(1 - s) = 1500(1 - 0.04) = 1440 \text{ rpm}$$ **Ans.**

$$P_{out} = \omega T_{sh} = \frac{2\pi \times N_r}{60} \times T_{sh}$$

$$= \frac{2\pi \times 1440}{60} \times 160$$

$$= 24.127 \text{ kW}$$ **Ans.**

SOLVED EXAMPLES

Example 1: A 3-pole, 440 V, 50 Hz, induction motor runs at 1450 rpm when it delivers rated output power. Determine: **[UPTU 2006-07]**

(a) No. of poles in the machine.
(b) Speed of rotating air gap field.
(c) Rotor induced emf of stator to rotor turn ratio is 1 : 0.8. Assume the winding factors are the same.
(d) Frequency of rotor current.

Solution: Given data

$$V = 440 \text{ V}; f = 50 \text{ Hz}$$

$N_r = 1450$ rpm (as N_r and N_S are nearly equal)

(a) No. of poles is given by

$$P = \frac{120f}{N_S} = \frac{120f}{1450} = \frac{120 \times 50}{1450} = 4.13 \approx 4$$

$\therefore$ No. of poles will be 4. **Ans.**

(b) Speed of rotating air gap field.

$$N_S = \frac{120f}{P} = \frac{120 \times 50}{4} = 1500 \text{ rpm}$$

(c) We know $k = \frac{0.8}{1} = 0.8$

Induced emf in rotor at stand still

$$= kE_1 = kV_1 = 0.8 \times 440 = 352 \text{ V}$$

slip $s = \frac{N_S - N_r}{N_S} = \frac{1500 - 1400}{1500} \times 100 = 3.33\%$ **Ans.**

$\therefore$ Rotor induced voltage $= ksV_1 = 0.0333 \times 0.8 \times 440 = 11.733$ V **Ans.**

(d) Frequency of rotor current (f_r)

$\therefore$ $f_r = sf = 0.0333 \times 50 = 1.66$ Hz **Ans.**

Example 2: A 8 pole, three phase induction motor is supplied from 50 Hz, AC supply. On full load, the frequency of induced emf in rotor is 2 Hz. Find the full-load slip and the corresponding speed. **[UPTU 2006-07] [MTU 2009-10]**

Solution: Given data

$$P = 8,\ f = 50 \text{ Hz},\ f_r = 2 \text{ Hz}$$

The full load slip is calculated with the help of rotor frequency as

$$f_r = sf$$

$\therefore$ $2 = s50$

$$s = \frac{2}{50} = 0.04$$

$\therefore$ $\%s = 0.04 \times 100 = 4\%$ **Ans.**

The corresponding speed is given by

$$N_r = (1 - s)N_S$$

where $N_S = \frac{120f}{P} = \frac{120 \times 50}{8} = 750$ rpm

$\therefore$ $N_r = (1 - 0.04)750 = 720$ rpm **Ans.**

Example 3: A 4-pole, 50 Hz, 3-ϕ induction motor has a rotor resistance of 0.024 Ω per phase and stand still reactance of 0.06 Ω per phase. Determine the speed at which maximum torque is developed. **[UPTU 2007-08] [MTU 2009-10]**

Solution: The given data

$$r_2 = 0.024\Omega/\text{phase}$$

$$x_2 = 0.6\ \Omega/\text{phase}$$

We know that the slip corresponding to maximum torque can be calculated as below.

$$S = \frac{r_2}{x_2} = \frac{0.024}{0.6} = 0.04$$

∴ Speed corresponding to maximum torque

$$N_r = (1-s)N_S = (1-0.04)\frac{120 \times f}{P}$$

$$= (1-0.04) \times \frac{120 \times 50}{4} = 1440 \text{ rpm} \qquad \textbf{Ans.}$$

Example 4: A 4-pole, 3-ϕ induction motor is energized from a 60 Hz supply and is running at a load condition for which the slip is 0.03. Determine

(i) Rotor speed in rpm.

(ii) Rotor current frequency in Hz.

(iii) Speed of the rotors rotating magnetic fields with respect to the stator frame in rpm. **[UPTU 2008-09, MTU 2008-09]**

Solution: Given data $P = 4, f = 60 \text{ Hz}, s = 0.3$

(i) $$N_S = \frac{120f}{P} = \frac{120 \times 60}{4} = 1800 \text{ rpm}$$

∴ $$N_r = (1-S)N_S = (1-0.03)1800 = 1740 \text{ rpm} \qquad \textbf{Ans.}$$

(ii) The speed of rotor magnetic field with respect to stator frame is calculate as

$$f_r = sf = 0.03 \times 60 = 1.8 \text{ Hz}$$

(iii) Rotor magnetic field rotates at speed

$$= \frac{120 f_r}{P} = \frac{120 \times 1.8}{4} = 54 \text{ rpm} \qquad \textbf{Ans.}$$

Example 5: A three phase, 50 Hz induction motor has a full load speed of 960 rpm calculate: **[UPTU 2009-10] [MTU 2011-12]**

(i) Slip

(ii) Frequency of rotor induced emf.

(iii) No. of poles.

(iv) Speed of rotor field with respect to rotor structure.

(v) Speed of rotor field with respect to stator field.

Solution: Given data

$$N_r = 960 \text{ rpm}; f = 50 \text{ Hz}$$

(i) If $N_r = 960$ rpm, then we assume

$$N_S = 1000 \text{ rpm}$$

$$\%s = \frac{N_S - N_r}{N_S} \times 100 = \frac{1000 - 960}{1000} \times 100 = 4\% \qquad \textbf{Ans.}$$

(ii) The frequency of rotor induced emf

$$f_r = sf = 0.04 \times 50 = 2 \text{ Hz} \qquad \textbf{Ans.}$$

(iii) The no. of poles is given by

$$N_S = \frac{120f}{P}, \text{ i.e. } 1000 = \frac{120 \times 50}{P}$$

∴ $$P = 6$$

(iv) The speed of field rotor structure is given by with the help of rotor frequency

$$\therefore \qquad \frac{120.f_r}{P} = \frac{120 \times 2}{6} = 40 \text{ rpm} \qquad \textbf{Ans.}$$

(v) Both stator and rotor fields are rotating at N_S with respect to stator structure hence speed of rotor field with respect to stator field is zero.

Example 6: A 3-ϕ, 4-pole induction motor is running with 4% slip. The supply frequency is 50 Hz. Find out the speed of induction motor. **[GBTU 2010-11]**

Solution: Given data

$$P = 4; s = 0.04; f = 50 \text{ Hz}$$

$$N_S = \frac{120 f}{P} = \frac{120 \times 50}{4} = 1500 \text{ rpm}$$

$$N_r = (1 - s)N_S = (1 - 0.04)1500 = 1440 \text{ rpm} \qquad \textbf{Ans.}$$

13.10 SINGLE PHASE INDUCTION MOTOR

As the name suggests, these motor's are used on single phase supply. These are the most familiar of all electric motors because they are extensively used in domestics, commercial and industrial applications. These are used in ceiling fans, hair drier, food mixers, washing machines, vacuum cleaners, food processors and refrigerators. These are small size motors of fractional killowatt rating and similar to three phase induction motors except for the fact that the stator has a single-phase winding instead of three phase winding. These are not self-starting. Hence certain extra circuit or auxillary devices are used to make them self-starting.

13.11 CONSTRUCTION OF A SINGLE PHASE INDUCTION MOTOR

The construction of a single phase induction motor is very similar to that of a three phase induction motor.

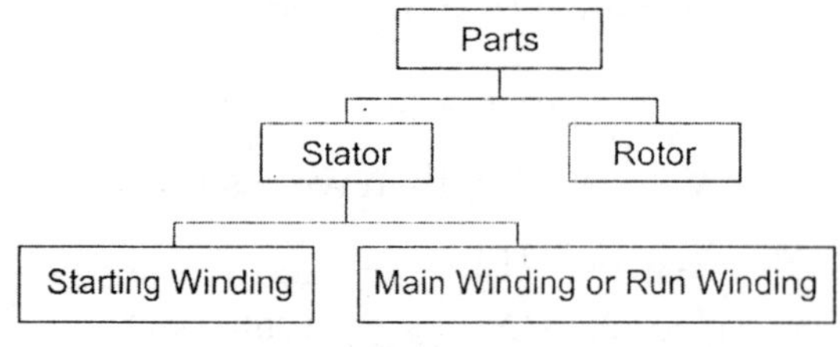

Fig. 13.12

13.12 WORKING PRINCIPLE OF SINGLE PHASE INDUCTION MOTOR

A single-phase induction motor consist of a single-phase winding mounted on the stator and a cage winding on the rotor. When a single-phase supply is connected to the stator winding a **pulsating** magnetic field is produced. By **pulsating** field we mean that the field build up in one direction, falls to zero, and then builds up in the opposite direction. Under the condition, the rotor does not rotate due to inertia. Therefore, a single phase induction motor is in generally not self-starting and requires some special starting means. If, however, the single-phase stator winding is excited and the rotor of the motor is started by an auxiliary means, and the starting devices is then removed, the motor continuous to rotate in the direction in which it is started.

13.13 WHY SINGLE PHASE INDUCTION MOTOR IS NOT SELF-STARTING

When a single phase supply is connected to the stator winding, a pulsating or alternating magnetic field is produced. This pulsating field build up in one direction, fall to zero and then build up in the opposite direction. Under this condition, the resultant torque is zero and pulsating magnetic field can not produce rotation in rotor. Therefore, a single phase induction motor is not a self starting motor. Now let us see why single phase induction motor are not self starting with the help of a theory called **double revolving field theory**.

13.13.1 Double Revolving Field Theory

According to this theory, any alternating quantity can be resolved into two rotating components which rotates in opposite directions and each having magnitude as half of the maximum magnitude of the alternating quantity.

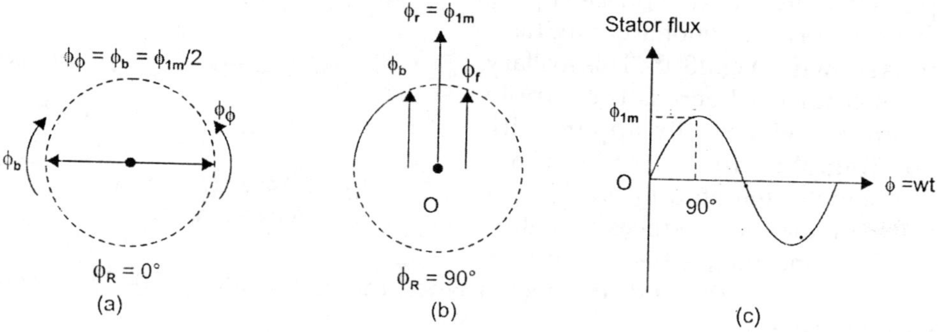

Fig. 13.13: Stator flux and its two components

In case of single phase induction motors, the stator winding produces an alternating magnetic field having maximum magnitude of $\phi_1 m$. According to double revolving field theory consider the two components of the stator flux, each having magnitude half of maximum magnitude of stator flux, i.e. $\left(\frac{\phi_1 m}{2}\right)$. Both these components are rotating in opposite directions at the synchronous speed N_S which is dependant on frequency and stator poles. Let ϕ_f is the forward component rotating in anticlockwise direction while ϕ_b is the backward component rotating in clockwise direction. The resultant to these two components at any instant gives the instantaneous value of the stator flux at that instant. So resultant of these two is the original stator flux.

Figure 13.13 shows the stator flux and its two components ϕ_f and ϕ_b. Both the components are shown opposite to each other in Fig. 13.13a. Thus the resultant $\phi_R = 0$. This is flux at start. After 90° as shown in Fig. 13.13b. The two components are rotates in such away that both are pointing in the same direction. Hence the resultant ϕ_R is the algebraic sum of the magnitudes of the two components.

So $\phi_R = \left(\frac{\phi_{1m}}{2}\right) + \left(\frac{\phi_{1m}}{2}\right) = \phi_{1m}$. This is nothing but the instantaneous value of the stator flux at $\phi_R = 90°$ as shown in Fig. 13.13c. Thus continuous rotation of the two components gives the original alternating stator flux.

Both the components are rotating and hence get cut by the rotor conductors. Due to cutting of flux, emf gets induced in rotor which circulates rotor current. The rotor current produces rotor flux. This flux interacts with forward components ϕ_f to produce a torque in one particular direction say anticlockwise direction. While rotor flux interacts with backward comparent ϕ_b to produce a torque in the clockwise direction. So if anti-clockwise torque is positive then clockwise torque is negative.

At the start these two torques are equal in magnitude but opposite in direction. Each torque tries to rotate the rotor in its direction. Thus net torque experienced by rotor is zero at start hence the single phase induction motor are not self starting.

13.13.2 Single Phase Induction Motor is Self-starting

As we know that, the single phase induction motor is not self starting. To make a single phase induction motor self-starting, we should produce a **rotating magnetic field** in stator. This may achieved by converting a single phase supply into two phase supply through the use of an additional or **auxiliary** winding as shown in Fig. 13.14. This axillary winding is connected across the supply voltage and 90° electrically appart with **main winding.** With the help of auxiliary winding the motor temporarily working as a two phase motor and produces a rotating magnetic field and makes the motor self-start. A centrifugal switch is disconnected when the motor attains 70–80 percent of normal running speed.

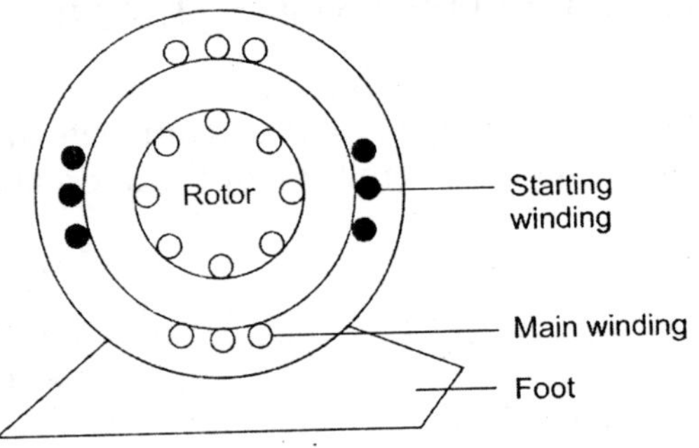

Fig. 13.14: Single phase induction motor

13.14 TYPES OF SINGLE PHASE INDUCTION MOTOR OR PHASE SPLITING METHOD OF STARTING

Single phase induction motors are usually classified according to the auxiliary means used to start the motor. They are classified as follows.

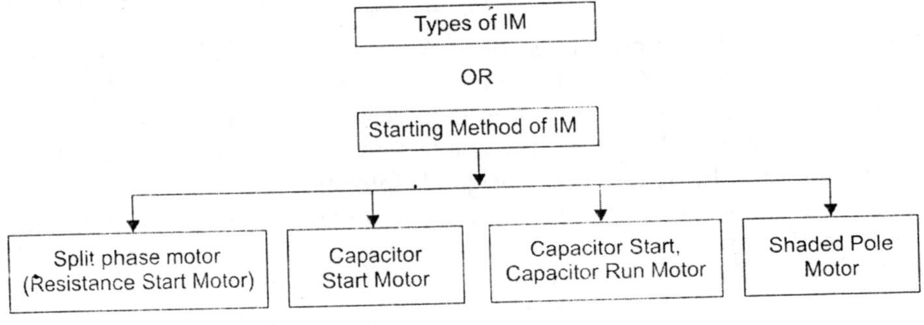

Fig. 13.15

13.14.1 Split Phase Induction Motor

Split phase induction motor is also called as resistance start motor Fig. 13.16 shows a split phase induction motor. It has a single cage type rotor and its stator has two windings a main winding and a starting (auxiliary) winding. The main field winding and the starting winding are displaced 90° like the winding in a two phase induction motor. The main winding has very low resistance and high inductive reactance.

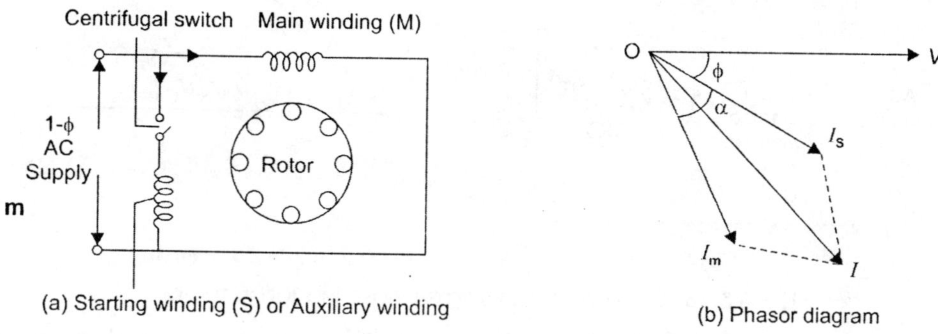

Fig. 13.16: Split phase induction motor

Operation

When the two stator windings are energised from a single phase supply, the main winding carries current I_m, while the starting winding carries current I_S. Since main winding is made highly inductive while the starting winding highly resistive, the current I_m and I_S have a reasonable phase difference angle a (25° to 35°) between them as shown in Fig. 13.17. Consequently, a weak rotating magnetic field approximating to that of a two phase machine is produced which start the motor. When the motor reaches about 75% of synchronous speed, the centrifugal switch open the circuit of the starting winding. The motor then operates as a single phase induction motor and contirtue to accelerate till it reaches the normal speed.

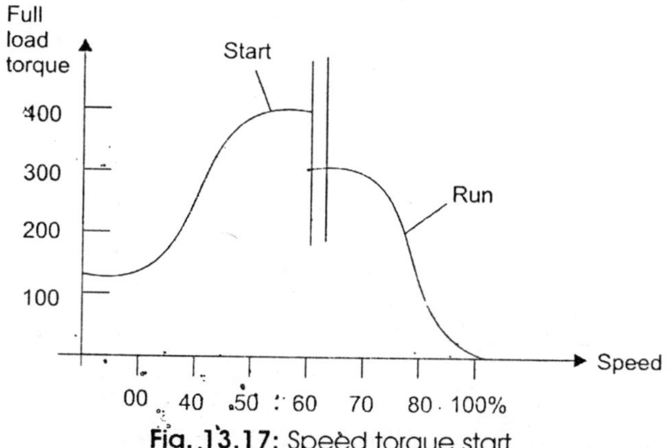

Fig. 13.17: Speed torque start

Applications

(a) Fans and blowers
(b) Washing machines and refrigerators
(c) Food processing machine, grinders and wood working tools

13.14.2 Capacitor Start Induction Motor

These are single phase induction motors that employ a *electrolyte type capacitor* in the auxiliary winding as shown in Fig. 13.18.

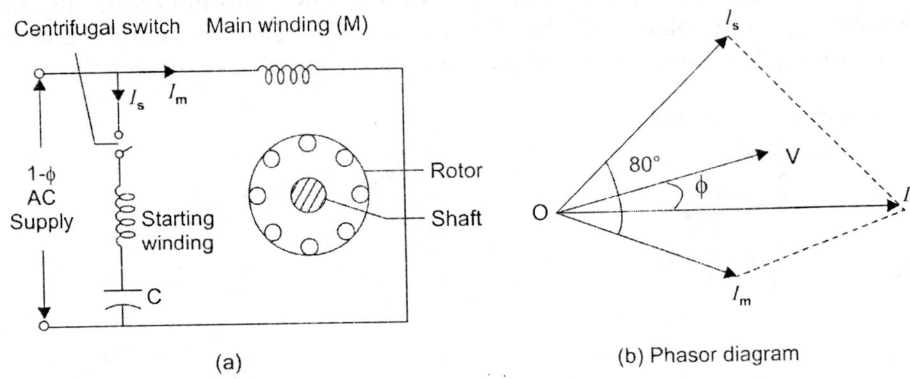

Fig. 13.18: Capacitor start single phase induction motor

It has a cage rotor and its stator has two winding. The main winding and the auxiliary winding. The two winding are displaced 90° in space. A capacitor C is connected in series with the starting winding to produce a greater phase difference the current in the main and auxiliary windings, as shown in Fig. 13.18. The value of capacitor is so chosen that I_s leads I_m by about 80° which is considerably greater than 25° found in split phase motor. Consequently, starting torques much more than that of a split-phase motor. Again, the starting winding is opened by the centrifugal switch when the motor attains about 75% of synchronous speed. The motor then operates as a single phase induction motor and continue to accelerate till it reaches the normal speed.

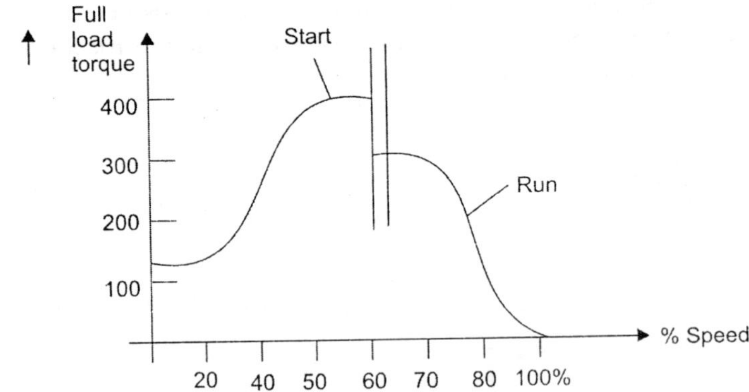

Fig. 13.19: Torque-speed characteristics

Applications

(a) Pumps (b) compressor (c) air conditioners (d) conveyors.

13.14.3 Capacitor Start Capacitor Run Motor

There are two types

(a) Single value capacitor run motor
(b) Two value capacitor run motor

(a) **Single value capacitor run motor:** Capacitor starts and run motor similarly to capacitor start motor except that starting winding and capacitor are connected in the circuit at all times. It has one main winding and one starting winding in series with a capacitor since capacitor remains in the circuit permanently. This motor is often referred to as permanently split capacitor run motor.

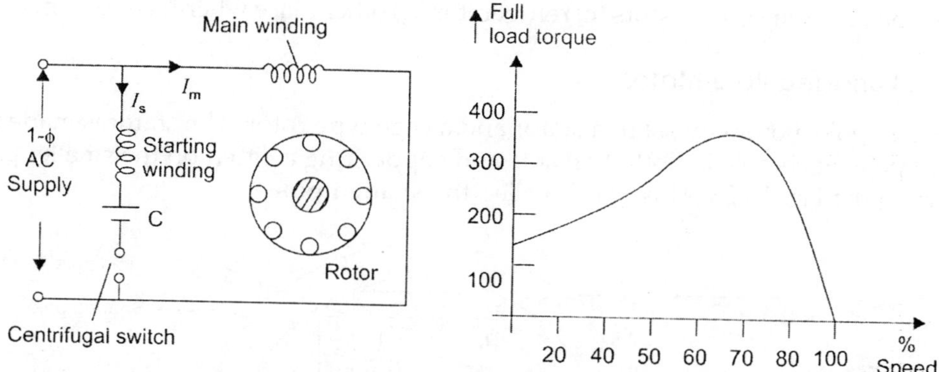

Fig. 13.20: Single value capacitor run motor

(b) **Two-value capacitor run motor:** This motor starts with a high capacitor in series with the starting winding so that the starting torque is high.

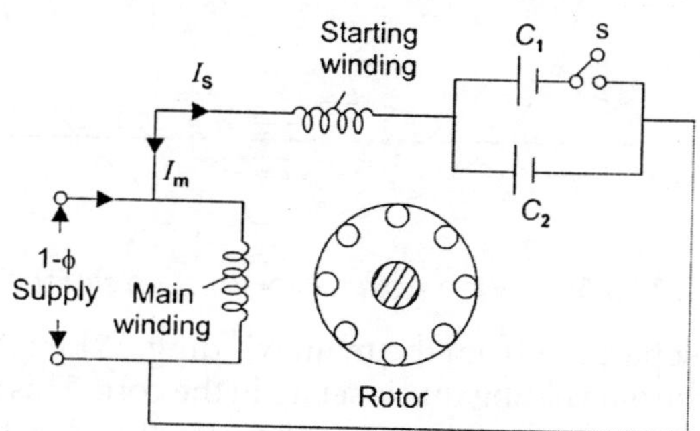

Fig. 13.21: Two value capacitor run motor

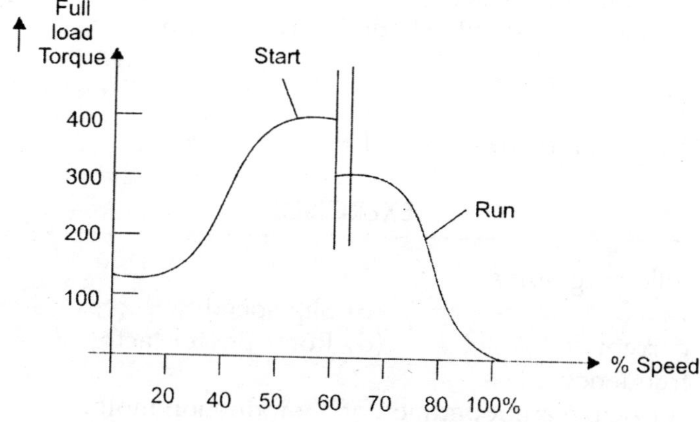

Fig. 13.22: T-H characteristics

For running, a low capacitor is substituted by switch both starting and running winding remains in the circuit. By using two capacitors in parallel at the start and the switching out one for low value run.

Applications

(a) Hospitals (b) air compressors (c) refrigerator (d) other place where silence is important

13.14.4 Shaded Pole Motor

A shaded pole motor consist of a stator and a cage type rotor. The stator is made up of salient pole. Each pole is slotted on side and copper ring is fitted on the smaller part as shown in the Fig. 13.23. This part is called the **shaded pole**.

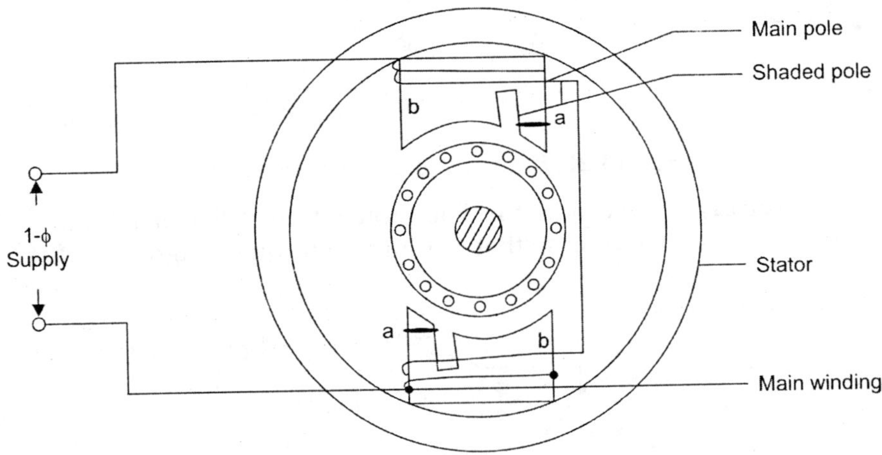

Fig. 13.23: Shaded pole motor with two stator poles

The shaded coil is separated from the main winding. When AC supply is connected to the main winding, the alternating flux is set up in the core. This alternating flux induces the current in a shading coil which opposes the core flux due to long low. The flux in the shaded portion of the pole lags the flux in the unshaped portion of it. This result the rotating field moving in the direction from unshaped portion to shaded portion of pole and the starting torque is produced. The shaped pole motor is always rotates in the direction from unshaded portion to shaded portion of pole.

Applications

(a) Small fans (b) toys (c) hairdrayers and electric chocks.

EXERCISES

1. Define the following terms:
   (a) Slip (b) Slip speed
   (c) Rotor current (d) Rotor power factor
   (e) Rotor frequency
2. Explain the principle and operation of 3-ϕ induction motor.
3. Draw slip/speed torque characteristics of 3-ϕ induction motor.
4. What are the application of squirrel cage induction motors?

5. The rotor speed of a 6-pole, 50 Hz induction motor is 960 rpm. Find the percentage slip. [UPTU 2008-09]
6. Why single phase induction motor is not self starting?
7. Explain the types of single-phase induction motor and its applications.

Short Answer Questions

1. Explain the working principle of 3-phase induction motor. [UPTU 2003-04]
2. Draw and explain the torque–slip characteristics of 3-phase induction motor. [UPTU 2004-05, 06]
3. Draw the torque–slop characteristics of a 3-ϕ induction motor and explain its various region of operations.
4. Give the application of the following: (a) 3–ϕ induction motor (b) 1–ϕ induction motor.
5. Explain why a single phase induction motor is not self starting and discuss briefly and two method used to produces starting torque is such motor? [UPTU 2005-06,07] [MTU 2009-10]
6. Using double-revolving field theory explain the principle of operation of a 1-ϕ induction motor.
7. Explain the starting method of 1-ϕ induction motor. [UPTU 2010-11-12-13] [MTU 2009-10-11-12]

Descriptive Type Questions

1. Discuss why single-phase induction motors do not have self starting. Explain its principle of operation and explain various methods of staring. [UPTU 2005, 06-07]
2. Explain principle of operation of a single phase induction motor using revolving field theory. Explain various method of starting. [MTU 2008-09-10] [UPTU 2008-09-10]
3. What are the different types of induction motor? Explain the principle of operation of 3-ϕ induction motor.
   A 12 pole, 3-ϕ induction alternator is coupled to an engine running at 1500 rpm. It supplied a 3-ϕ induction motor having a full load speed of 1440 rpm. Find the percentage slip, frequency of rotor current and number of poles of motor. [**Ans.** %5 = 4%, f_r = 2 Hz, P = 4]
4. Derive the torque equation of a 3-ϕ induction motor. Draw the torque-slip characteristics of 3-ϕ induction motor. [UPTU 2003-04, 05, 06, 07, 08] [MTU 2009-10, 2011-12]

Chapter

14

Three Phase Synchronous Machines

14.1 INTRODUCTION

AC system has a number of advantages over DC system. Now-a-days electric supply used for commercial as well as domestic purpose is of alternating type. A synchronous machine is a doubly excited machine, i.e. excitation is needed for both stator as well as rotor. Generally the stator is connected to AC supply and rotor is connected by DC supply. The mechanical power is converted into electrical power with the help of AC machine called synchronous generator. Same machines can be used to convert electrical power into mechanical power is known as *synchronous motor*.

14.2 CONSTRUCTION OF AN ALTERNATOR

Similar to other rotating machine, an alternator consists of two main parts namely.

Stator: It is the stationary part of the machine. It carries the armature winding in which the voltage is generated. The output of the machine is taken from the stator. It is the rotating part of the machine.

Rotor: It carries a field winding, which is supplied with direct current through two slip rings by a separate DC source. The DC source (called exciter) is generally a small DC shunt or compound generator mounted on the shaft of the alternator.

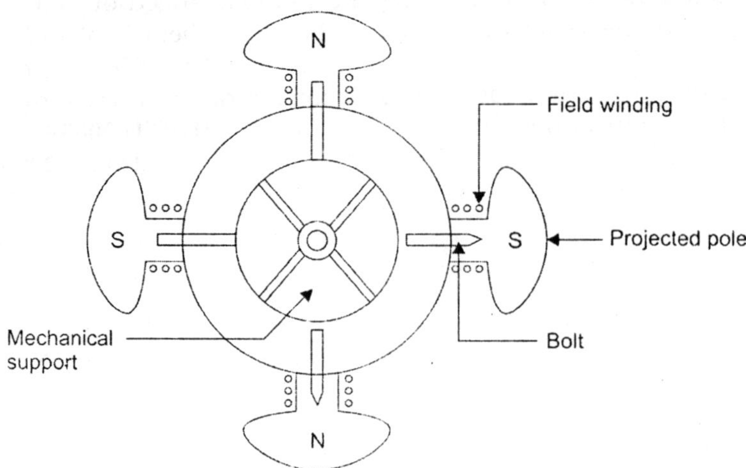

Fig. 14.1: Salient pole type rotor

They are two types of rotor. (1) salient pole type (2) nonsalient (cylindrical) pole type

1. Salient pole type: The salient pole rotor consists of poles projecting outside from the surface of the rotor core as shown in Fig. 14.1.

Salient features:

(i) It is used in low and medium speed (125–750 rpm) alternators.
(ii) These rotors having large diameters and small axial length.
(iii) The prime movers used to drive such rotor are generally water turbine.
(iv) Salient pole alternator driven by water turbine are called hydro-alternators.

2. Nonsalient pole rotor: This is also called smooth in cylindrical type rotor. The rotor consists of smooth solid steel cylinder, having a number of slots to accommodate the field coils.

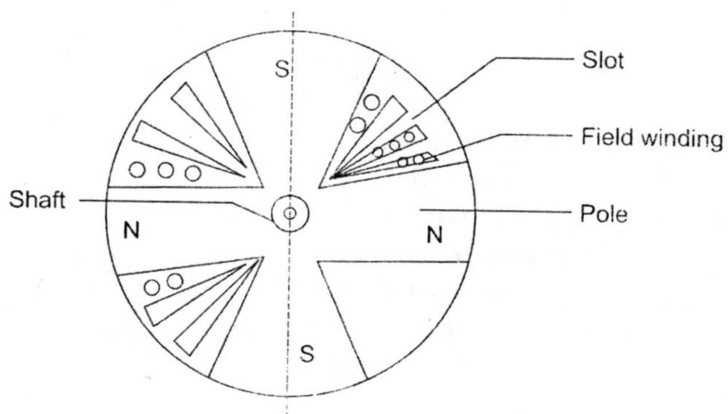

Fig. 14.2: Nonsalient pole type rotor

Salient features:

(i) It is used in high speed (750–3000 rpm) alternators.
(ii) These rotors having small diameter and large axial length.
(iii) Prime movers used to drive such type of rotors are generally steam turbine.
(iv) Such high speed alternators are called *turbo alternator.*

14.3 PRINCIPLE OF OPERATION OF AN ALTERNATOR

The alternator works on the principle of electromagnetic induction. According to this when a rotor is rotated by means of prime mover, the armature conductors cut the magnetic flux, therefore an emf is induced in the armature conductors, due to electromagnetic induction. The direction of induced emf can be found by Fleming's right hand rule and frequency is given by

$$f = \frac{NP}{120}$$

where N = speed of rotor in rpm

P = no. of poles

We know that when there is a relative motion between the conductors and the flux emf gets induced in the conductors. Consider a relative motion of a single conductor under the magnetic field produced by two stationary poles.

Let the conductor starts rotating from position 1. At this instant, the entire velocity component is parallel to the flux lines by the conductor, so $\frac{d\phi}{dt}$ at this instant is zero and hence emf induced in the conductor is zero.

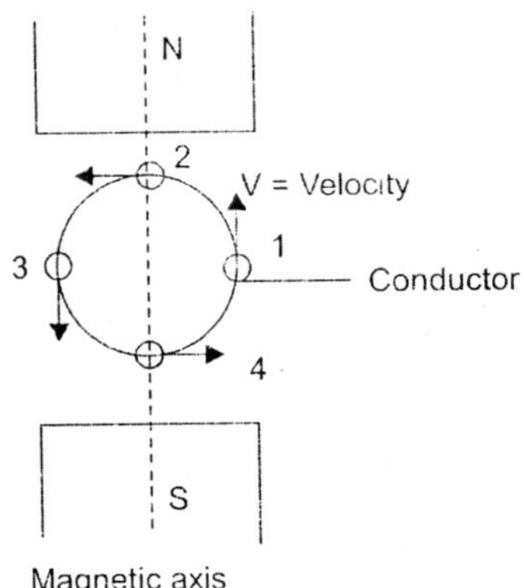

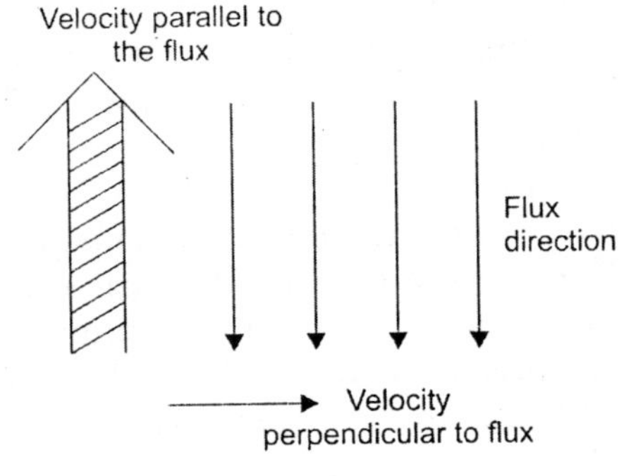

Fig. 13.3

As the conductor moves from position 1 towards position 2, the part of the velocity component becomes perpendicular to the flux lines and emf gets induced inside the conductor. The induced emf increases slowly as it moves from position 1 to position 2.

At position 2, the entire velocity component is perpendicular to the flux lines and at this instant, the induced emf in the conductor is at its maximum.

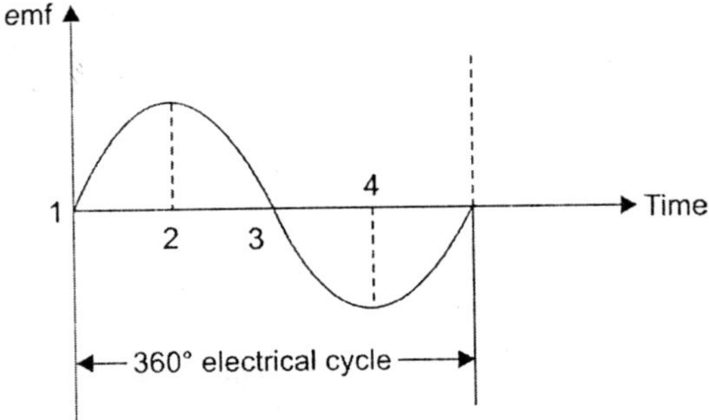

Fig. 14.4: Alternating nature of the induced emf

At position 3, again the entire velocity component is parallel to the flux lines and hence at this instant induced emf in the conductor is zero.

As the conductor moves from position 3 towards 4, the velocity component perpendicular to the flux component but in opposite direction. At position 4, it achieves maximum in the opposite direction.

Again from position 4 to 1, induced emf decreases and finally at position 1, again becomes zero. This cycle continues as conductor rotates at a certain speed.

14.4 FREQUENCY OF INDUCED EMF

The frequency of induced emf in the armature conductors depend upon speed and no. of the poles

Let P = no. of poles

N = speed of the rotor (rpm); f = frequency of the induced emf

One mechanical revolution of rotor = $\frac{P}{2}$ cycles of emf electrically

Thus, there are $\frac{P}{2}$ cycles per revolution.

At speed N rpm, in one second, rotor will complete $\left(\frac{N}{60}\right)$ revolution

But cycles/sec = frequency (f)

Frequency = (no. of cycles per revolution) × number of revolutions per second

$$f = \frac{P}{2} \times \frac{N}{60} = \frac{PN}{120} \text{ Hz (cycle per second)}$$

14.5 SYNCHRONOUS MOTOR

A synchronous motor is a machine which converts electric power into mechanical power at a constant speed called synchronous speed. Synchronous motor works only at synchronous speed and can not work other than synchronous speed. Its speed is constant.

Construction

A synchronous motor has the following two parts:

1. **Stator:** It is the stationary part of the machine. The three phase armature winding is placed in the slots of stator core and is wound for the same number of poles as the rotor as shown in Fig. 14.5.

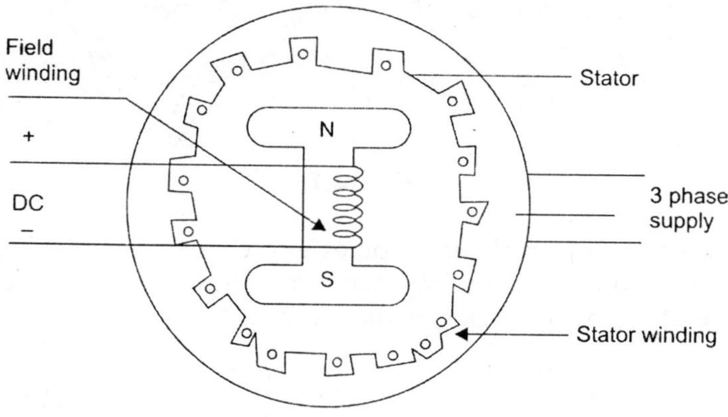

Fig. 14.5

2. **Rotor:** The rotor of synchronous motor can be of the salient pole or cylindrical pole (nonsalient) type construction. The practically most of the synchronous motor use salient, i.e. projected type construction, except for exceedingly high speed machines.

14.6 OPERATING PRINCIPLE

Synchronous motor works on the principle of magnetic locking.

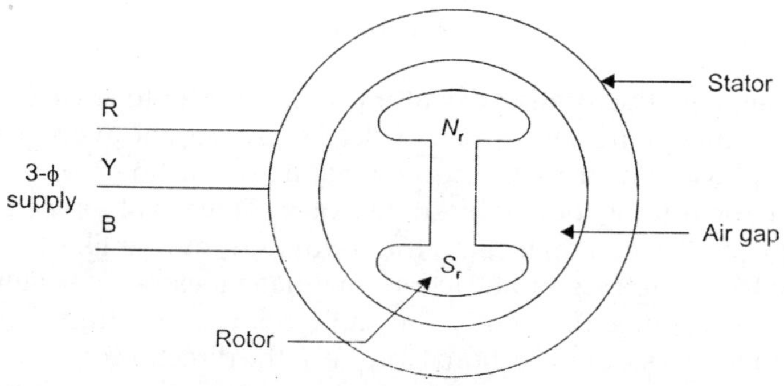

Fig. 14.6

N_S, S_S → Stator north and south poles

N_r, S_r → Rotor north and south poles

When a three phase supply is given to the stator winding, a rotating magnetic field is produced in stator. Due to rotating magnetic field, let the stator poles $N_S < S_S$ rotate with synchronous speed. At a particular time stator pole N_S coincides with N_r and S_S concides with S_r, i.e. like poles of stator and experiences and repulsive force, so rotor poles experiences a repulsive force F_r. Assume that the rotor tends to rotate in anticlockwise direction as shown in Fig. 14.7

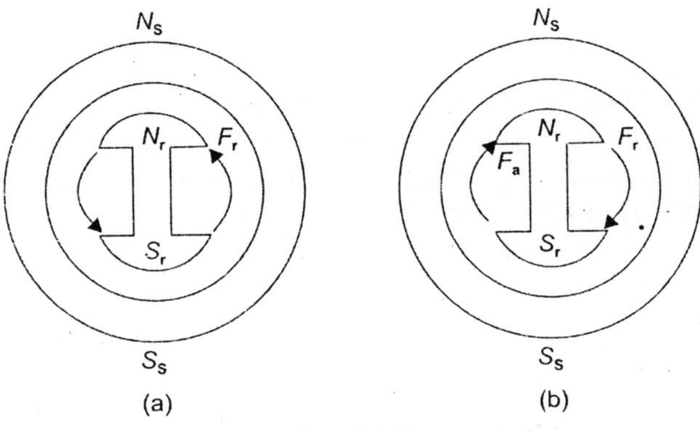

Fig. 14.7

After half cycle or half period, stator poles into change their position as shown in Fig. 14.8. Now unlike poles concluding each other and rotor experience the attractive force ϕ_a and tends to rotate is clockwise direction.

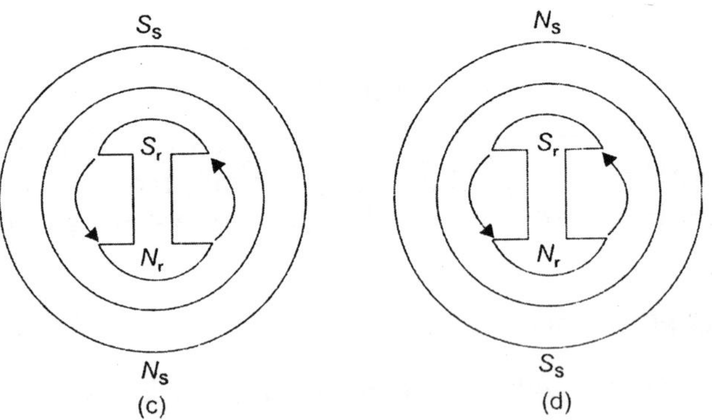

Fig. 14.8

We can say that, with the rotation of stator poles, the rotor tends to drive in clockwise and anticlockwise direction in every half cycle. As a result, the average torque on rotor is zero. Hence 3 phase synchronous motor is not a self starting motor.

Now suppose the rotor is rotated by some external means at a speed almost equal to synchronous speed. At a certain instant, the stator and rotor unlike poles will face each other, then due to strong face of attraction, magnetic locking is established, the rotor and stator poles continues to occupy the same relative position. Due to this, rotor continuously experiences a unidirectional torque in the direction of the rotating magnetic field. Hence, 3 phase synchronous motor must run at synchronous speed.

14.7 METHOD OF STARTING A SYNCHRONOUS MOTOR

Synchronous motor is not self starting. They are various methods of starting of synchronous motor.

1. Using small induction motor.
2. Using small DC machine.
3. Using damper winding.

14.8 V-CURVES

The curve plotted between field current (I_f) and armature current (I_a) is called *V* curves. Figure 14.8 shows a typical V curve at no load, half load and full load. When the level of excitation of a synchronous motor is changed gradually from underexcitation to overexcitation for different load, the following effects are observed.

1. When the motor is underexcited, the armature current and power factor is lagging. In this case the motor behaves like an inductive load.

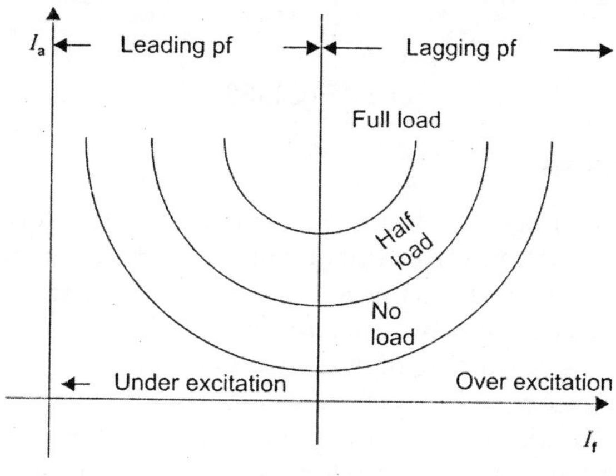

Fig. 14.9

2. When the motor is normally excited, the power factor is a unity. In this case, the armature current is minimum and is in phase with the terminal voltage.
3. When the motor is over excited, the power factor is leading. In this case, the motor behaves like a capacitive load.

14.9 APPLICATION OF THREE PHASE SYNCHRONOUS MOTOR

1. Synchronous motors were mainly used in constant speed applications.
2. Overexcited synchronous motors can be used in improve the power factor.
3. Synchronous motors are used to improve the voltage regulation of transmission lines.
4. Synchronous motors only runs at synchronous speed, therefore it is used in textile, paper mill, etc.
5. Synchronous motors are particularly attractive for low speed ($<$ 300 rpm) because the power can always be adjusted to unity and efficiency is high.

14.10 DISADVANTAGES OF SYNCHRONOUS MOTORS

1. It is not self starting.
2. Its cost is higher in companion to other motors.

3. It needs frequent maintenance.
4. The construction of a synchronous motor is more complicated then 3-f induction motor.
5. External DC source is necessary for providing excitations.

Example: A 4-pole AC generator is running and producing the frequency of 50 Hz. Calculate the rpm of the generator. If the frequency is reduced to 15 Hz, how many number of poles will be required if the generator is to be run at the same speed.

Solution: Frequency generated, $f = 50$ Hz

Number of poles $P = 4$

$$\text{Speed, N} = \frac{120f}{P} = \frac{120 \times 50}{4} = 1500 \text{ rpm } \textbf{Ans.}$$

When frequency $f = 15$ Hz

$$\text{Number of poles required } P' = \frac{120f}{N} = \frac{120 \times 15}{1500} = 1.2 \cong 2 \textbf{ Ans.}$$

EXERCISES

Short Answer Questions

1. What are the advantages of stationary armature in an alternator?
2. Write down the equation for frequency of emf induced in an alternator?
3. Name the types of alternators based on their rotor construction.
4. What are V curves of a synchronous motor.
5. Name the methods of starting of synchronous motor.
6. How the synchronous motor is made self starting?
7. State the characteristics features of synchronous motor.
8. Which type of synchronous generator are used in hydroelectric plants and why.

Descriptive Type Questions

1. Explain the principle of operation of a three phase synchronous motor.
2. Explain the following
   (a) Synchronous motor always run at synchronous speed.
   (b) Field winding of synchronous generators is placed on rotor.
3. Three phase induction motor is self starting but three phase synchronous motor is not self starting? Explain why? Give applications of 3-phase synchronous motor.
4. State the advantages of having rotating field system rather than a rotating armature system in a synchronous machine. What is the effect of charge of excitation of a synchronous motor on its power factor for different loads.
5. Give the constructional details of salient pole of synchronous machine. Explain *V* curve and give the applications of synchronous motor.

Index